Chemistry and Molecular Biology of the Intercellular Matrix

Volume 1

EDITORIAL BOARD

Chemistry and Molecular Biology of the Intercellular Matrix

Edited by ENDRE A. BALAZS
Boston, Mass., U.S.A.

Volume I

Collagen, Basal Laminae

Elastin

1970

ACADEMIC PRESS · LONDON and NEW YORK

ACADEMIC PRESS INC. (LONDON) LTD
Berkeley Square House
Berkeley Square
London, W1X 6BA

U.S. Edition published by
ACADEMIC PRESS INC.
111 Fifth Avenue
New York, New York 10003

Library of Congress Catalog Card Number: 75–114219
SBN: 12–077001–6

Printed in Great Britain by
Spottiswoode, Ballantyne and Co. Ltd
London and Colchester

LIST OF CONTRIBUTORS

ABBOTT, J.	Department of Biological Sciences, Columbia University, New York, New York
ACCINNI, L.	II Clinica Medica della Università di Roma, Rome, Italy
ANDERSEN, S.O.	Department of Zoology, Cambridge University, Cambridge, England
ANDRES, G.	II Clinica Medica della Università di Roma, Rome, Italy
ASCENZI, A.	Istituto di Anatomia e Istologia Patologica, Rome, Italy
BAILEY, A.J.	Agricultural Research Council, Meat Research Institute, Langford, Bristol, England
BALAZS, E.A.	Department of Connective Tissue Research, Boston Biomedical Research Institute and Harvard Medical School, Boston, Massachusetts
BALDUINI, C.	Institute of Biological Chemistry, Faculty of Science, University of Pavia, Pavia, Italy
BAZIN, S.	Service de Pathologie Experimentale, Institut Pasteur, Garches, France
BENJAMINI, E.	Laboratory of Medical Entomology, Kaiser Foundation Research Institute, Oakland, California
BENSUSAN, H.B.	The Bejamin Rose Hospital of the Bejamin Rose Institute, Cleveland, Ohio
BENTLEY, J.P.	Department of Biochemistry, University of Oregon Medical School, Portland, Oregon
BERMAN, E.R.	Department of Ophthalmology, Biochemistry Research Laboratory, Hebrew University School, Hadassah Medical School, Jerusalem, Israel

BHATNAGER, R.S. — University of California Medical Center, Department of Periodontology, San Francisco, California

BLUMENFELD, O.O. — Department of Biochemistry and The Unit for Research in Aging, Albert Einstein College of Medicine, Yeshiva University, New York, New York

BONUCCI, E. — Istituto di Anatomia e Istologia Patologica, Rome, Italy

BORNSTEIN, P. — Departments of Biochemistry and Medicine, University of Washington, Seattle, Washington

BOWNESS, J.M. — Department of Biochemistry, University of Manitoba, Bannatyne and Emily, Winnipeg, Manitoba

BRÄUMER, K. — Max-Planck-Institut für Eiweiss-und Lederforschung, Munich, Germany

BROVELLI, A. — Institute of Biological Chemistry, Faculty of Science, University of Pavia, Pavia, Italy

BRUNS, R.R. — The Developmental Biology Laboratory, Department of Medicine, Harvard Medical School and the Massachusetts General Hospital, Boston, Massachusetts

BUTLER, W.T. — Institute of Dental Research and Department of Biochemistry, University of Alabama in Birmingham, Birmingham, Alabama

BRANDT, K. — Boston University School of Medicine, Arthritis and Connective Tissue Diseases Section, Boston, Massachusetts

CASTELLANI, A.A. — Institute of Biological Chemistry, Faculty of Science, University of Pavia, Pavia, Italy

CERIMELE, D. — Instituto di Clinica Dermatologica Policlinico, S. Matteo, Pavia, Italy

CHACKO, S. — Department of Pathology, School of Veterinary Medicine, University of Pennsylvania, Philadelphia, Pennsylvania

CIFERRI, A. Laboratorio di Tecnologia dei polimeri e reologia, Napoli, Italy

CIFONELLI, J.A. Department of Pediatrics and Biochemistry, Joseph P. Kennedy, Jr. Mental Retardation Research Center and the La Rabida-University of Chicago Institute, University of Chicago, Chicago, Illinois

CLELAND, R.L. Department of Chemistry, Dartmouth College, Hanover, New Hampshire

COHEN, A.S. Boston University School of Medicine, Arthritis and Connective Tissue Diseases Section, University Hospital, Boston, Massachusetts

CROMBIE, G. Boston University School of Medicine, Department of Biochemistry, Boston, Massachusetts

DAMON, H. Department of Medicine, Albert Einstein College of Medicine, Departments of Pediatrics and Biochemistry, University of Chicago, Chicago, Illinois

DARRELL, R.W. Corneal Center, Institute of Ophthalmology, College of Physicians and Surgeons, Columbia University, New York, New York

DAVIDSON, E.A. Department of Biological Chemistry, The Milton Hershey Medical Center, Pennsylvania State University, Hershey, Pennsylvania

DEAN, M.F. Department of Biochemistry, The Mathilda and Terence Kennedy Institute of Rheumatology, Bute Gardens, London, England

DE BERNARD, B. Institute of Biological Chemistry, University of Trieste, Trieste, Italy

DELAUNAY, A. Service de Pathologie Experimentale, Institut Pasteur, Garches, France

DELLOVO, M.C. — University of Alabama Medical Center, Birmingham, Alabama
The Regina Elena Institute for Cancer Research, Rome, Italy

DE LUCA, S. — Oral Disease Research Laboratory, Boston Veterans Administration Hospital, Boston, Massachusetts

DESHMUKH, A. — Department of Medicine, Rheumatic Disease Laboratory, University of Southern California, School of Medicine, Los Angeles, California

DESHMUKH, K. — Department of Medicine, Rheumatic Disease Laboratory, University of Southern California, School of Medicine, Los Angeles, California

DI FERRANTE, N. — Laboratories of Connective Tissue Research of The Department of Biochemistry, Baylor College of Medicine, Houston, Texas

DISCHE, Z. — College of Physicians and Surgeons, Department of Ophthalmology, Columbia University, New York, New York

DORFMAN, A. — Departments of Pediatrics and Biochemistry, Joseph P. Kennedy, Jr. Mental Retardation Research Center and the La Rabida-University of Chicago Institute, University of Chicago, Chicago, Illinois

DURWARD, J.J. — Department of Biochemistry, St. Salvator's College, University of St. Andrews, St. Andrews, Fife, Scotland

DZIEWIATKOWSKI, D.D. — Department of Oral Biology, School of Dentistry, University of Michigan Ann Arbor, Michigan

ENGEL, J. — Max-Planck-Institut für Eiwess-und Lederforschung, Munich, Germany

ESPINOSA, E. — Department of Medicine, Case-Western Reserve University School of Medicine and Metropolitan General Hospital, Cleveland, Ohio

EVANSON, J.M. Division of Metabolism, Department of Medicine, Royal Infirmary, Manchester, England

FARIS, B. Department of Biochemistry, Boston University School of Medicine, Boston, Massachusetts

FAVILLI, G. Istituto di Patologia Generale, Università di Bologna, Bologna, Italy

FESSLER, J.H. Molecular Biology Institute and Department of Zoology, University of California, Los Angeles, California

FERNANDEZ-MADRID, F. Rheumatology Section, Wayne State University School of Medicine, Detroit, Michigan

FITTON JACKSON, S. Nuffield Biophysics Laboratories, Strangeways Research Laboratory, Cambridge, England

FLOREANI, L. Department of Biochemistry, St. Salvator's College, University of St. Andrews, St. Andrews, Fife, Scotland

FOWLER, L.J. Agricultural Research Council, Meat Research Institute, Langford, Bristol, England

FRANSSON, L.-Å. Department of Physiological Chemistry, Chemical Center, University of Lund, Lund, Sweden

FRANZBLAU, C. Department of Biochemistry, Boston University School of Medicine, Boston, Massachusetts

GALLOP, P.M. Department of Biochemistry and The Unit for Research in Aging, Albert Einstein College of Medicine, Yeshiva University, New York, New York

GEE, D.R. Department of Chemistry and Applied Chemistry, University of Salford, Salford, England

GIANNETTI, A. Istituto di Clinica Dermatologica Policlinico, S. Matteo, Pavia, Italy

GIBBS, D.A. Department of Connective Tissue Research, Boston Biomedical Research Institute, Boston, Massachusetts
Dewey and Almy Chemical Division W.R. Grace and Company, Cambridge, Massachusetts

GLIOZZI, A. Istituto di Fisica dell Università, Genova, Italy

GOLDSTEIN, E.R. National Institute of Dental Research, National Institutes of Health, Bethesda, Maryland

GOTTE, L. Institute of Histology of the University of Padua, Padua, Italy

GONZÁLEZ, E. Departmento de Bioquimica, Instituto Nacional de la Nutrición, Mexico City, Mexico

GOULD, B.S. Department of Biology, Massachusetts Institute of Technology, Cambridge, Massachusetts

GREGORY, J.D. The Rockefeller University, New York, New York

GREILING, H. Rheumaforschungsinstitut, Aachen, Germany

GROSS, J. The Developmental Biology Laboratory, Department of Medicine, Harvard Medical School and the Massachusetts General Hospital, Boston, Massachusetts

HALLÉN, A.A. Department of Medical Chemistry, University of Uppsala, Uppsala, Sweden

HALME, J. Children's Hospital and Department of Medical Chemistry, University of Helsinki, Helsinki, Finland

HAMABATA, A. Departmento de Bioquimica, Instituto Nacional de la Nutrición, Mexico City, Mexico

HAMERMAN, D. Medical Service, Montefiore Hospital and Department of Medicine, Albert Einstein College of Medicine, Yeshiva University, New York, New York

HARKNESS, R.D. — Department of Physiology, University College London, London, England

HARPER, E. — The Developmental Biology Laboratory, Department of Medicine, Harvard Medical School and the Massachusetts General Hospital, Boston, Massachusetts

HASCALL, V.C. — Department of Oral Biology, School of Dentistry University of Michigan, Ann Arbor, Michigan

HAYDUK, U. — Max-Planck-Institut für Eiweiss-und Lederforschung, Munich, Germany

HELLSING, K. — Institute of Clinical Chemistry, University Hospital, Uppsala, Sweden

HERINGTON, A.C. — Department of Biochemistry, Monash University, Clayton, Victoria, Australia

HILZ, H. — Institut für Physiologische Chemie der Universität, Hamburg, Germany

HOFFMAN, P. — Research Institute for Skeletomuscular Diseases, Hospital for Joint Disease and Medical Center, New York, New York

HOLTZER, H. — Department of Anatomy, School of Medicine, University of Pennsylvania, Philadelphia, Pennsylvania

HOLTZER, S. — Department of Anatomy, School of Medicine, University of Pennsylvania, Philadelphia, Pennsylvania

HÖRMANN, H. — Max-Planck-Institut für Eiweiss-und Lederforschung, Munich, Germany

HORNER, A.A. — Charles H. Best Institute, University of Toronto, Toronto, Canada

HSU, K.C. — Department of Microbiology, Columbia University, New York, New York

IVERIUS, P.-H. Institute of Medical Chemistry, University of Uppsala, Uppsala, Sweden

JACKSON, D.S. Department of Medical Chemistry, Lapworth Laboratories, University of Manchester, Manchester, England

JACOBSON, B. Department of Connective Tissue Research, Boston Biomedical Research Institute, Boston, Massachusetts

JAFFE, R. Department of Biochemistry, Boston University School of Medicine, Boston, Massachusetts

JEANLOZ, R.W. Laboratory for Carbohydrate Research, Departments of Biological Chemistry and Medicine, Harvard Medical School and Massachusetts General Hospital, Boston, Massachusetts

KANG, A.H. The Developmental Biology Laboratory, Department of Medicine, Harvard Medical School and Massachusetts General Hospital, Boston, Massachusetts

KAPLAN, M.H. Department of Medicine, Case-Western Reserve University School of Medicine and Metropolitan General Hospital, Cleveland, Ohio

KATZMAN, R.L. Laboratory for Carbohydrate Research, Departments of Biological Chemistry and Medicine, Harvard Medical School and Massachusetts General Hospital, Boston, Massachusetts

KEFALIDES, N.A. La Rabida-University of Chicago Institute and Department of Medicine, University of Chicago, Chicago, Illinois

KEIDITSCH, E. Institut für Pathologie, Munich, Germany

KELLER, S. Columbia University, College of Physicians and Surgeons, New York, New York

KISTERS, R. Rheumaforschungsinstitut, Aachen, Germany

KIVIRIKKO, K.I. Children's Hospital and Department of Medical Chemistry, University of Helsinki,
Helsinki, Finland

KLEINE, T.O. Institut für Physiologische Chemie der Universität,
Hamburg, Germany

KONIGSBERG, I.R. Department of Biology, University of Virginia,

KÜHN, K. Max-Planck-Institut für Eiweiss-und Lederforschung,
Munich, Germany

KULONEN, E. Department of Medical Chemistry, University of Turku,
Turku, Finland

LANE, D.A. Department of Biochemistry, Monash University,
Clayton, Victoria, Australia

LAPIERE, Ch.M. Laboratoire de Dermatologie expérimentale, Hopital de Bavière, Université de Liège,
Liège, Belgium

LAURENT, T.C. Institute of Medical Chemistry, University of Uppsala,
Uppsala, Sweden

LENT, R.W. Department of Biochemistry, Boston University School of Medicine,
Boston, Massachusetts

LEVI, M. Columbia University, College of Physicians and Surgeons,
New York, New York

LIEFLÄNDER, M. Max-Planck-Institute for Experimental Medicine, Department of Biochemical Pharmacology,
Gottingen, Germany

LINDAHL, U. Institute of Medical Chemistry, University of Uppsala,
Uppsala, Sweden

LOWTHER, D.A. Department of Biochemistry, Monash University,
Clayton, Victoria, Australia

MAC GREGOR, E.A. Department of Biochemistry, University of Manitoba,
Bannatyne and Emily, Winnipeg

MAMMI, M. — Institute of Organic Chemistry, University of Padua, Padua, Italy

MANDL, I. — Columbia University, College of Physicians and Surgeons, New York, New York

MAROUDAS, A. — Biomechanics Unit, Mechanical Engineering Department, Imperial College of Science and Technology, London, England

MARTIN, G.R. — Laboratory of Biochemistry, National Institute of Dental Research, Bethesda, Maryland

MASHBURN, JR.,T.A. — Research Institute for Skeletomuscular Diseases, Hospital for Joint Diseases and Medical Center, New York, New York

MATALON, R. — Department of Pediatrics, Joseph P. Kennedy, Jr. Mental Retardation Research Center and the LaRabida-University of Chicago Institute, University of Chicago, Chicago, Illinois

MATHESON, D.W. — Department of Anatomy, The Milton S. Hershey Medical Center, Pennsylvania State University, Hershey, Pennsylvania

MATHEWS, M.B. — Departments of Pediatrics and Biochemistry The University of Chicago, Chicago, Illinois

MATUKAS, V.J. — Laboratory of Biochemistry, National Institute of Dental Research, National Institutes of Health, Bethesda, Maryland

MECHANIC, G. — Dental Research Center, University of North Carolina, Chapel Hill, North Carolina

MELIA, T.P. — Department of Chemistry and Applied Chemistry, University of Salford, Salford, England

MEYER, K. — Department of Chemistry, Yeshiva University, Belfer Graduate School of Science, New York, New York

MICHAELI, D. Laboratory of Medical Entomology, Kaiser Foundation Research Institute, Oakland, California

MILLER, E.J. Laboratory of Biochemistry, National Institute of Dental Research, National Institutes of Health, Bethesda, Maryland

MOCZAR, E. Laboratoire de Biochimie du Tissue Conjonctif, Equipe de Recherche du CNRS No. 53, Paris, France

MOCZAR, M. Laboratoire de Biochimie du Tissu Conjonctif, Equipe de Recherche du CNRS No. 53, Paris, France

MORCHIO, R. Istituto di Fisica dell Università, Genova, Italy

MORGAN, R.E. University of Alabama Medical Center, Birmingham, Alabama

MORRISON, R.I.G. Strangeways Research Laboratory, Cambridge, England

MUIR, H. The Mathilda and Terence Kennedy Institute of Rheumatology, Bute Gardens, London, England

NIMNI, M.E. Department of Medicine, Rheumatic Disease Laboratory, University of Southern California, School of Medicine, Los Angeles, California

NORDWIG, A. Max-Planck-Institut für Eiweiss-und Lederforschung, Munich, Germany

NUSGENS, B.V. Laboratoire de Dermatologie expérimentale, Hopital de Bavière, Université de Liege, Liege, Belgique

ÖBRINK, B. Institute of Medical Chemistry, University of Uppsala, Uppsala, Sweden

OGSTON, A.G. Department of Physical Biochemistry, John Curtin School of Medical Research, Canberra City, Australia

PADDAY, J.F. Research Laboratories, Kodak Limited, Harrow, England

PAGE-THOMAS, D.P. Medical Research Council,
Rheumatism Research Unit, Canadian Red Cross Memorial Hospital,
Taplow, England

PARTRIDGE, S.M. Meat Research Institute,
Langford, Bristol, England

PAZ, M.A. Department of Biochemistry and the Unit for Research in Aging, Albert Einstein College of Medicine, Yeshiva University,
New York, New York

PEACH, C.M. Agricultural Research Council, Meat Research Institute,
Langford, Bristol, England

PEZZIN, G. Institute of Physical Chemistry of the University of Padua
Padua, Italy

PHILLIPS, G.O. Department of Chemistry and Applied Chemistry, University of Salford,
Salford, England

PIERCE, G.B. Department of Pathology, University of Colorado Medical Center,
Denver, Colorado

PIEZ, K.A. Laboratory of Biochemistry, National Institute of Dental Research, National Institutes of Health,
Bethesda, Maryland

PIKKARAINEN, J. Department of Medical Chemistry, University of Turku,
Turku, Finland

PINNELL, S.R. The Arthritis Unit, Massachusetts General Hospital,
Boston, Massachusetts

PITA, JR., J. Department of Medicine and Biochemistry, University of Miami School of Medicine,
Miami, Florida

PUGLIARELLO, M.C. Istituto di Chimica Biologica, Università di Trieste,
Trieste, Italy

PROCKOP, D.J. General Clinic Research Center, Philadelphia General Hospital,
Philadelphia, Pennsylvania,
Departments of Medicine and Biochemistry, University of Pennsylvania,
Philadelphia, Pennsylvania

QUINTARELLI, G. University of Alabama Medical Center, Birmingham, Alabama, The Regina Elena Institute for Cancer Research, Rome, Italy

RAUTERBERG, J. Max-Planck-Institut für Eiweiss-und Lederforschung, Munich, Germany

RENDÒN, G. Departmento de Bioquimica, Instituto Nacional de la Nutrición, Mexico City, Mexico

REVEL, J-P. Department of Anatomy, Harvard Medical School, Boston, Massachusetts

REXRODT, F. Max-Planck-Institut für Eiweiss-und Lederforschung, Munich, Germany

ROBERT, A.M. Laboratoire de Biochimie du Tissu Conjonctif, Equipe de Recherche du CNRS No. 53, Paris, France

ROBERT, B. Laboratoire de Biochimie du Tissu Conjonctif, Equipe de Recherche du CNRS No. 53, Paris, France

ROBERT, L. Laboratoiré de Biochimie du Tissu Conjonctif, Equipe de Recherche du CNRS No. 53, Paris, France

RODÉN, L. Department of Pediatrics, University of Chicago Medical School, Chicago, Illinois

ROGALL, E. Max-Planck-Institut für Eiweiss-und Lederforschung, Munich, Germany

ROJKIND, M. Departmento de Bioquimica, Instituto Nacional de la Nutrición, Mexico City, Mexico

ROKOSOVA, B. Department of Biochemistry, Univeristy of Biochemistry, University of Oregon Medical School, Portland, Oregon

ROSS, R. Department of Pathology, University of Washington, Seattle, Washington

SAJDERA, S.W. The Rockefeller University,
New York, New York

SALCEDO, L.L. Department of Biochemistry, Boston
University School of Medicine,
Boston, Massachusetts

SANDSON, J. Department of Medicine, Albert Einstein
College of Medicine, Yeshiva University,
New York, New York

SCOTT, J.E. M.R.C. Rheumatism Unit, Canadian Red Cross
Hospital,
Taplow, England

SEEGAL, B.C. Department of Microbiology, Columbia
University,
New York, New York

SERAFINI-FRACASSINI, A. Department of Biochemistry, St. Salvator's
College, University of St. Andrews,
St. Andrews, Fife, Scotland

SHULMAN, H.J. Department of Medicine, Columbia University
College of Physicians and Surgeons, and
The Edward Daniels Faulkner Arthritis
Clinic of the Presbyterian Hospital,
New York, New York

SIEGEL, R.C. National Institute of Dental Research,
National Institutes of Health,
Bethesda, Maryland

SILBERT, J.E. Oral Disease Research Laboratory, Boston
Veterans Administration Hospital and the
Departments of Medicine and Biochemistry
Tufts University School of Medicine,
Boston, Massachusetts

SIMONS, K. Department of Serology and Bacteriology,
University of Helsinki,
Helsinki, Finland

SMITH, B. Department of Biochemstry, Boston University
School of Medicine,
Boston, Massachusetts

SMITH, C. Medical Service, Montefiore Hospital and
Department of Medicine, Albert Einstein
College of Medicine,
New York, New York

SMITH, J.W. Department of Anatomy, St. Salvator's College, University of St. Andrews, St. Andrews, Fife, Scotland

SMITH, L.A. Molecular Biology Unit and Department of Zoology, University of California, California

SPENCER, A.F. Oral Disease Research Laboratory, Boston Veterans Administration Hospital, Boston, Massachusetts

SPIRO, R.G. Departments of Biological Chemistry and Medicine, Harvard Medical School, The Elliott P. Joslin Research Laboratory, and the Peter Bent Brigham Hospital, Boston, Massachusetts

STEVEN, F. Department of Medical Biochemistry, Lapworth Laboratories, University of Manchester, Manchester, England

STIMSON, W.H. Department of Biochemistry, St. Salvator's College, University of St. Andrews, St. Andrews, Fife, Scotland

STONE, A.L. Laboratory of Neurochemistry, National Institute of Mental Health, Bethesda, Maryland

STOOLMILLER, A.C. Departments of Pediatrics and Biochemistry, Joseph P. Kennedy, Jr. Mental Retardation Research Center and the La Rabida-University of Chicago Institute, University of Chicago, Chicago, Illinois

STRAUCH, L. Max-Planck-Institut für Eiweiss-und Lederforschung, Munich, Germany

STUHLSATZ, H.W. Rheumaforschungsinstitut, Aachen, Germany

SWANN, D.A. Department of Connective Tissue Research, Boston Biomedical Research Institute and Harvard Medical School, Boston, Massachusetts

SZIRMAI, J.A. Institute for Rheumatism Research, University Hospital, Leiden, The Netherlands

TANZER, M.L. Department of Biochemistry, University of Connecticut Medical School, Farmington, Connecticut

TOOLE, B.P. The Developmental Biology Laboratory, Department of Medicine, Harvard Medical School and Massachusetts General Hospital, Boston, Massachusetts

TRISTRAM, G.R. Department of Biochemistry, University of St. Andrews, Bute Medical Buildings, St. Andrews, Fife, Scotland

TSIGANOS, C.P. The Mathilda and Terence Kennedy Institute of Rheumatology, Bute Gar Bute Gardens, London, England

UDENFRIEND, S. Roche Institute of Molecular Biology Nutley, New Jersey

VEIS, A. Department of Biochemistry, The Medical School, Northwestern University, Chicago, Illinois

VITTUR, F. Institute of Biological Chemistry, University of Trieste, Trieste, Italy

VOLPIN, D. Institute of Histology, University of Padua, Padua, Italy

VON DER MARK, K. Max-Planck-Institut für Eiweiss-und Lederforschung, Munich, Germany

WASTESON, Å. Institute of Medical Chemistry, University of Uppsala, Uppsala, Sweden

WEIS-FOGH, T. Department of Zoology, Cambridge University, Cambridge, England

WELLS, P.J. Department of Biochemistry, St. Salvator's College, University of St. Andrews, St. Andrews, Fife, Scotland

WESSLER, E. Institute of Medical Chemistry, University of Uppsala, Uppsala, Sweden

WOESSNER, J.F. Laboratories for Cardiovascular Research
Howard Hughes Medical Institute and
Department of Biochemistry, University
of Miami,
Miami, Florida

ZIMMERMANN, B. Max-Planck-Institut für Eiweiss-und Leder-
forschung,
Munich, Germany

PREFACE

It is now generally realized that the output of biomedical, biophysical and biological knowledge has become so great that new subspecialities have to be developed. The danger is that new subspecialities may lead to excessive fragmentation in our attempts to understand integrated biological systems. A new subspeciality, however, need not represent only a new methodological approach or a concentration on a minute aspect of a rather narrow existing field. Rather it could bring together scientists of various methodological backgrounds in a joint effort to focus their attention on a newly emerging biological problem. The life processes occurring in the multicellular organism outside the cell membrane seem to represent such a new problem area. Thus a new branch of biology appears on the scene, matrix biology, which concerns itself with the structure and function of the organized extracellular environment of the cell. It addresses itself to such fundamental questions as how is the life of the individual cell influenced and controlled by its microenvironment, and what is the role of the matrix in assembling cells into organized populations, and how does the matrix maintain the specific functions of cell systems.

Extracellular matrix, or, briefly, matrix, is defined as organized solid or semi-solid extracellular matter on the surface of individual cells and on the surface or in between cells of multicellular organisms. The basal lamina contained substance in which the cells of the connective tissue are embedded, the cell coats, the "sweet husks" of cells (glycocalyx), the capsule of bacteria and eggs, the chitinous exoskeletons of insects, the mucus covering endothelial cells, and the substance between closely packed cells of the epithelial, endothelial, neural and some muscle tissues are all part of the extra- and intercellular matrix.

Most molecular biologists today focus their attention on those intracellular molecules which are involved in the storage of information and the control of cell processes. The assembly, organization, and specialization of cells in multicellular systems, however, occurs only when the intercellular matrix develops -- protecting, connecting, binding and organizing the cells into one functional system of tissue, organ or organism. The intercellular matrix produced by the cells forms their external environment. This environment may play a primary role in the control of cell processes. Thus, the cellular function of the multicellular organism cannot be understood fully without complete knowledge of the structure and function of the matrix.

The primary objective of this book is to review the established aspects of matrix biology and, secondly, to explore the forefront of research in this field. The field is too large, however, to be reviewed in three volumes, hence the subject is limited to the matrix of connective tissue. In order to remind the reader that, in Revel's words "the same type of molecules which are characteristic of the reaches of the connective tissue are also found in close association with cell surfaces" the matrix and cell coats of epithelial cells are also briefly discussed.

The topics of this book include the chemical and physical structure and metabolism of the structural and macromolecular components of the connective tissue matrix as well as the biological role of matrix in health and disease.

The first volume is devoted to the isolation, characterization, and metabolism of collagen; to the chemistry, fine structure, development, and function of the basal laminae in healthy and diseased tissues. It also discusses the characterization, fine structure, mechanical properties and biosynthesis of elastin.

The second volume presents the chemistry, structure and metabolism of glycosaminoglycans and proteoglycans. It also deals with the interaction between cationic dyes, organic and inorganic cations and glycosaminoglycans, as well as the interaction between collagen and glycosaminoglycans.

The third volume deals with such functional aspects of matrix as the control of transport of molecules, ion binding, lubrication, shock absorption, and with the role of matrix in structural organization of such tissues as skin, bone, cartilage, synovial tissue and fluid, and intervertebral disc. Furthermore, it presents the immunological, and some pathological aspects of the matrix; the chemical expression of the differential function of connective tissue cells; the degradation of the matrix by tissue enzymes during regeneration, granulation, embryogenesis, tumor growth and experimental and rheumatoid arthritis; and the role of matrix in wound healing and development.

No book can ever be completely up to date. The authors, editors and publisher, however, can make a special effort to produce a book in the shortest time that modern technology and economy will allow. The publication of these three volumes represents such an effort. The desire for speedy publication created a considerable logistic problem in the editing, retyping and printing of 134 manuscripts written by 202 authors. It is my hope that the readers will agree that some unavoidable compromise with uniformity and stylistic perfection was justified.

The authors and members of the editorial board, however, have in no way compromised the quality of their contributions. Without their unstinting cooperation and patience a task of this magnitude, within the given limitations, could never have been completed. For this, I wish to express my sincere thanks.

Endre A. Balazs

Boston, Massachusetts
December 1969

ACKNOWLEDGEMENTS

The publication of this book would not have been possible without the meeting of nearly 150 scientists at the Imperial Palace Hotel in Santa Margherita Italy between the 16th and 28th of May, 1969. The meeting, under the co-directorship of E.A. Balazs and G.R. Tristram was an Advanced Study Institute on the Chemistry and Molecular Biology of the Intercellular Matrix, sponsored by the Scientific Affairs Division of the North Atlantic Treaty Organization (NATO).

The Directors and the members of the Organization and Program Committees (C. Cessi, A.A. Castellani, J.T. Dingle, A. Dorfman, L. Gotte, J. Gross, D.S. Jackson, T.C. Laurent, H. Muir, G.B. Pierce, G. Quintarelli, J.E. Scott and J.A. Szirmai) wish to thank the Scientific Affairs Division of NATO for financial support and Dr. H. Arnth-Jensen, Head, Pure Science Bureau of NATO for his kind cooperation in the organization of this meeting.

We also wish to extend our thanks to the following organizations for their generous financial support of the many participants of the meeting: Ethicon Inc., Somerville, New Jersey; Ethicon Limited, Edinburgh, United Kingdom; Hoffman La Roche, Nutley, New Jersey; Imperial Chemical Industries Limited, London, England; National Research Council, Italy; National Institutes of Health, Bethesda, Maryland; Roche Pharmaceutical Company, Italy; Smith, Kline and French Laboratories, Philadelphia, Pa.; Surel Inc., Philadelphia, Pa.; Uniliver Limited, London, England; and the Selco Electronic Company, Italy for providing and installing a closed-circuit television system.

The Editor of this book wishes to thank Miss Elizabeth Walsh and Mrs. Carol Stockwood for their competent, tireless and devoted work in the preparation of the manuscript for publication, and to express appreciation to Dr. Bernard Jacobson and Miss Sylvia Landers for copy editing, Miss Margareta Svänsson for preparing the author index, Dr. Donald Scheufele for assisting in the preparation of the subject index and Miss Gunnel Jutheden for general assistance.

GUIDE TO NOMENCLATURE

The usage of nomenclature in these three volumes does not represent any major innovation in the field. nor does it present the reader with cumbersome technicalities. The trivial names of chemical compounds are used almost exclusively. Nomencature is a necessary evil which undergoes constant revision to make communication in science clear and efficient. Thus, the expressions and their application as suggested in these volumes should be used only until a more detailed definition of the chemical and physical structure of these macromolecules permits the use of better specific names.

The major points in nomenclature as they apply to the material presented in these three volumes are summarized as follows:

<u>Mucopolysaccharides</u>: this term was suggested by Karl Meyer, and it was used for the first time in the title of a paper on The Chemistry and Biology of Mucopolysaccharides and Glycoproteins by him (Cold Spring Harbor Symposia on Quantitative Biology, Vol. 6, 91, 1938). At that time it meant "hexosamine-containing compounds" ....which "occur in nature either as free polysaccharides or as protein salts" and was intended to be the general term for such heteropolysaccharides as heparin, chondroitin sulfate, hyaluronic acid, some bacterial polysaccharides, and chitin. During the following two decades this colorful expression served the field extremely well. By the late nineteen-fifties, however, the indiscriminate use of the term mucopolysaccharide resulted in several re-definitions. One of these suggested that the word "mucopolysaccharide" or "mucoprotein" should be used "for firm complexes of protein or peptide with the type of carbohydrate containing hexosamine and neutral sugar but not uronic acid or sulfate" (F.R. Bettelheim-Javons, Advances in Protein Chemistry, Vol. 13, 39, Academic Press, N.Y., 1958). This definition, in obvious contradiction to the original, excluded most of the molecules for which the term was originally coined. In the ensuing confusion, pathologists, histologists, histochemists and cytologists used this term to designate proteins that contain "some"

carbohydrates or polysaccharides that contain "some" amino acids. To suggest that this term should be eliminated from our scientific vocabulary at this time would be impractical. Therefore, we recommend that it may be used as a very broad, collective term when histochemical evidence suggests the presence of a carbohydrate moiety and the available evidence does not settle conclusively the chemical nature of the macromolecule or structure. Such moiety may be part of a glycoprotein, glycosaminoglycan, glycolipid or glycolipoprotein molecule. It is hoped that the continued broad use of mucopolysaccharide will encourage and, in a sense, protect the proper use of more specific trivial names of chemically well-characterized compounds.

Glycosaminoglycans (GAG): this semisystematic name gained considerable popularity in the past decade and is used in this book. It designates polysaccharides which contain one or several types of amino sugar moieties (R.W. Jeanloz, Arthritis and Rheumatism, Vol. 3, 233, 1960). The individual names of glycosaminoglycans of animal cells and matrices are used as suggested in The Amino Sugars, Vol. IIA, page XIII (Editors E.A. Balazs and R.W. Jeanloz, Academic Press, New York, London):

chondroitin 4-sulfate (Ch4-S) for chondroitin sulfate A,
chondroitin 6-sulfate (Ch6-S) for chondroitin sulfate C,
dermatan sulfate (DS) for chondroitin sulfate B,
keratan sulfate, (KS) for kerato sulfate,
heparan sulfate (HS) for heparitin sulfate, as well as
hyaluronic acid (HA), chondroitin (Ch) and heparin (H).

Proteoglycans (PG): This name was suggested in 1967 by the Editor of this book in order to simplify some of the cumbersome expressions in the designation of "protein-polysaccharide complexes". This expression refers to macromolecules in which one or more polysaccharide chains are covalently bound to one or more protein chains. In proteoglycans the carbohydrate moiety is the dominant feature of the macromolecule.

In glycoproteins (GP) where monosaccharides or oligosaccharides are covalently bound to one or more protein chains, the protein moiety is the dominant feature of the macromolecule. The name proteoglycan should be used for a macromolecule in which the glycan moiety or moieties are well defined polysaccharide entities. The prefix proteo will be attached to the trivial name of the polysaccharide, e.g. proteoheparin (PH), proteoheparan sulfate (PHS), proteokeratan sulfate (PKS), proteochondroitin 6-sulfate (PCh6-S), proteochondroitin 4-sulfate (PCh4-S) etc. In case more than one type of glycosaminoglycan is covalently bound to a protein, the name will be, for example, proteokeratan chondroitin 4-sulfate (PKS-Ch4-S).

Peptidoglycan (PepG): this expression refers to macromolecules in which one or more peptides are covalently bound to one or more polysaccharide chains. The peptide(s) may branch off or be attached to the end of a polysaccharide chain or form a bridge between two chains or two points of the same chain.

Proteoglycan complex refers to macromolecular complexes in which one or more proteoglycans alone or with one or more protein, lipid, or polysaccharide molecules are linked together with non-covalent bonds.

Protein-glycosaminoglycan complex or protein-polysaccharide complex is used when proteins and glycosaminoglycans or other polysaccharides are linked by non-covalent bonds.

The Chain Components of Collagen: Based on a mutual agreement between the principal scientists actively working on the structural chemistry of collagen, in this book, the chain components of the tropocollagen molecule are designated as: α1, α2, β11, β12. This convention eliminates the use of subscripts one and two in the symbols designating these components.

ABBREVIATIONS

ACP	aldol condensation product
Ag-Ab	antigen-antibody complex
AO	acridine orange
ASC	acid-soluble collagen
ATP	adenosine triphosphate
BAPN or βAPN	3-aminopropionitrile (β-aminopropionitrile)
BL	basal lamina(e)
BUDR or BUdR	2'-deoxy-5-bromouridine
CB	cyanogen bromide
CD	circular dichroism
CEC	critical electrolyte concentration (see p. 1106)
Ch	chondroitin
ChS	chondroitin sulfate(s)
Ch4-S	chondroitin 4-sulfate
Ch6-S	chondroitin 6-sulfate
CM	carboxymethyl
CPC	cetylpyridinium chloride
C-PG	collagen-proteoglycan complex (see p. 1126)
CPH	cetylpyridinium hyaluronate
CTAB	cetyltrimethyl ammonium bromide
CTC	Ca-Tris-citrate buffer (see p. 1594)
DNA	deoxyribonucleic acid
DNP	dinitrophenyl
2,4-DNPH	2,4-dinitrophenylhydrazine
DS	dermatan sulfate
EBM	epithelial (specific) basement membrane
EDTA	ethylenediaminetetraacetate
EPR	electron paramagnetic resonance

e^{-}_{aq}	hydrated electron
ER	endoplasmic reticulum
ESR	electron spin resonance
FLS	fibrous long-spacing forms of collagen
FUdR or FUDR	2'-deoxy-5-fluorouridine
GAG	glycosaminoglycan
GalN	galactosamine
GalNAc	N-acetylgalactosamine
GBL	glomerular basal lamina
GBM	glomerular basement membrane
GlcN	glucosamine
GlcNAc	N-acetylglucosamine
GlcUA	glucuronic acid
GP	glycoprotein
GPep	glycopeptide
H	heparin
HA	hyaluronic acid
HA-P	hyaluronic acid-protein complex
Hex	hexose
HexA	hexuronic acid
HexN	hexosamine
HexNAc	N-acetylhexosamine
HS	heparan sulfate
IdUA	iduronic acid
IgG	immunoglobulin G
IUDR	2'-deoxy-5-iodouridine
KS	keratan sulfate
KSI	keratan sulfate from cornea (see p. 14)
KSII	keratan sulfate from human rib cartilage (see p. 14)
MEM	minimal essential medium
MeOH	methyl alcohol
MB	methylene blue

MG	methyl green
MPD	most probable distribution (see p. 737)
m-RNA	messenger ribonucleic acid
NBM	neoplastic basement membrane
NIH	National Institutes of Health (Bethesda, Maryland)
NMR	nuclear magnetic resonance
ORD	optical rotary dispersion
PC	polymeric collagen (see p. 45)
PCA	perchloric acid
PChS	proteochondroitin sulfate
PCh4-S	proteochondroitin 4-sulfate
PCh6-S	proteochondroitin 6-sulfate
PDS	proteodermatan sulfate
PepH	peptidoheparin
PGS	proteoglycan subunit
PH	proteoheparin
PHA	proteohyaluronic acid
PHS	proteoheparan sulfate
PKS	proteokeratan sulfate
RNA	ribonucleic acid
RNAse	ribonuclease
SGP	structural glycoprotein (see p. 237)
SGPA	structural glycoprotein of the aorta (see p. 237)
SGPC	structural glycoprotein of the cornea (see p. 237)
SKS	sulfated keratan sulfate
SLS	segment-long spacing form of collagen
TFE	trifluoroethanol
TNBS	2,4,6-trinitrobenzene-1-sulfuric acid
TNP	trinitrophenyl

UA	uronic acid
UDP	uridine diphosphate
UDP-Ar	UDP-arabinose
UDP-Gal	UDP-galactose
UDP-GalNAc	UDP-N-acetylgalactosamine
UDP-Glc	UDP-glucose
UDP-GlcN	UDP-glucosamine
UDP-GlcNAc	UDP-N-acetylglucosamine
UDP-GlcUA	UDP-glucuronic acid
UDP-IdUA	UDP-iduronic acid
UDP-Xyl	UDP-xylose
UMP	uridine monophosphate
UTP	uridine triphosphate

CONTENTS

VOLUME 1

CHAPTER I

VOLUME 2

CHAPTER V

CHEMISTRY, STRUCTURE AND METABOLISM OF HYALURONIC ACID 701

CHAPTER VI

CHEMISTRY, STRUCTURE AND METABOLISM OF SULFATED GLYCOSAMINOGLYCANS AND THEIR PROTEOGLYCANS 795

CHAPTER VIII

INTERACTION BETWEEN PROTEOGLYCAN AND COLLAGEN 1133

VOLUME 3

CHAPTER IX

CHAPTER X

THE PRODUCTION OF PROTEOGLYCANS IN NORMAL AND PATHOLOGICAL CONDITIONS 1419

CHAPTER XI

IMMUNOLOGICAL AND PATHOLOGICAL ASPECTS OF THE MATRIX 1515

INTRODUCTION

G. Favilli

First, I wish to thank the members of the organizing committee of the NATO Advanced Study Institute on the Chemistry and Molecular Biology of the Intercellular Matrix for the distinction they conferred by asking me to preside at this inaugural session.

The Institute, which begins today, brings together for 18 lecture sessions over the next 10 days, distinguished investigators who are well known for their contributions to the knowledge of the biochemistry, biophysics, physiology and pathology of connective tissues. It is very appropriate that the inaugural lecture be given today by Karl Meyer, who described hyaluronic acid for the first time as a chemically well defined component of the "ground substance" of connective tissue, thus becoming the pioneer who opened an ever widening road to the study of connective tissues. Following his work the "ground substance" was no longer regarded as an inert mechanical element in the organization of various systems and structures of the multicellular organism, but as the site of essential vital processes.

I do not think it superfluous to remind you of some dates--dates that mark outstanding events in the field of connective tissue research. I call your attention to the year 1934, when Dr. Meyer, in collaboration with J.W. Palmer, published in the Journal of Biological Chemistry a paper that described the isolation and characterization of a polysaccharide of high molecular weight, and proposed that ".... for convenience, the name of hyaluronic acid, from hyaloid (vitreous) and uronic acid" should be adopted. Thus hyaluronic acid was born, and its birth was an extremely important even in the history of connective tissue. This substance represented a chemically well-identified macromolecule, which soon afterward proved to be the specific substrate of an enzyme that, for this reason, was called "hyaluronidase" by Meyer and his coworkers in 1940.

The identification of the hyaluronic acid-hyaluronidase system was an historic event in the history of connective tissue research because it marks the first time when this tissue was investigated with methods which lead to the understanding of metabolic events in normal and pathological conditions.

It is stated in the Introduction of this program of the Institute "... the cellular functions of multicellular organism cannot be understood fully without total knowledge of the structure and function of the intercellular matrix". This is quite true. I would like to add that when we look upon our present knowledge of hyaluronic acid we realize the enormity of the task accomplished by molecular biologists, physiologist and pathologists in little more than three decades. This is most encouraging.

I am sure that there are many more distinguished and more deserving persons than I who could preside over the inaugural assembly of this important meeting. Why was this honour given to me? Looking back over my long career in the laboratory I cannot find any other justification for this than a youthful love of the structure of capillaries in granulation tissue and of experimental amyloidosis and one event, the memory of which has always been very dear to me. That event was my witnessing of the first investigations on "spreading factors" and having participated in this work--though taking a very modest part--from the beginning and for the many years that followed.

In 1928 Francisco Duran Reynals described the enhancing effect of testicle extracts on lesions induced by vaccinia virus on rabbit skin. This finding was the starting point in our knowledge of the diffusion phenomenon and of spreading factors. From that moment Duran Reynals' brilliant intelligence and indefatigable activity were entirely devoted to the development of those first observations. He worked at the Rockefeller Institute in New York in 1931, a time when I too, was there and was fascinated by the new adventure begun by Duran Reynals when he discovered the diffusion phenomenon. Close to Duran Reynals, then in Florence, and later with Douglas McClean at the Lister Institute in London, I continued to devote myself to research on spreading factors. My own work represents only a small fragment of the structure that an increasing number of investigators had begun in order to discover the nature of diffusion phenomena and of their, at that time, mysterious agents. The building of this structure was to take us very far afield--to knowledge of the intercellular matrix, namely, the discovery of the enzymatic nature of the diffusion phenomenon by Chain and Duthie in 1939. Thanks to Karl Meyer's work this later proved to be the effect of the action of hyaluronidase on the hyaluronic acid of the ground substance in vivo in the dermis connective tissue and in every organ ...?

I beg your pardon, dear colleagues, for these diversions, which you will recognize as personal recollections that will, therefore, have little significance to you. I just wanted to remind you of an episode in the history of the science of connective tissue in which I played a small part. I did this in order to pay homage to one of the greatest contributors--Karl Meyer--and to point out that we must derive a more important lesson, not confined to the study of the intercellular matrix. Such teaching suggests that progress in science has always been the result of man's ability to satisfy his curiosity of natural phenomena, and from the observation of them to derive a stimulus to his imagination to investigate them with perseverance. "Nature gives us the seed of science, not science": this is a saying left to us by the Roman philosopher Lucio Anneo Seneca, which we, in full scientific era, could thus make up to date: nature is made up of mysteries, but man has the means to reveal them.

REFLECTIONS ON "MUCOPOLYSACCHARIDES" AND THEIR PROTEIN COMPLEXES

Karl Meyer

I RETROSPECTION

When the organizers of this meeting, Drs. Bálazs and Tristram, asked me a few months ago to give an Inaugural Lecture of a general nature in an area of connective tissue, I felt greatly honored. When I started to think about the problem I became increasingly alarmed about the magnitude and difficulty of the assignment. I remember a story about another inaugural speaker who asked the chairman what he expected him to talk about; whereupon the chairman, who had of course to be German, answered, "Über Alles, nur nicht über 20 Minuten". It is quite obvious that I cannot speak "Über Alles" not even in the area of my main interest, and according to my instructions by Dr. Tristram, I am supposed to speak for one hour.

I chose as my title, "Reflections on Mucopolysaccharides and Their Protein Complexes", in order to indicate that this will be a subjective essay in a complex multi-faceted field, a field to which many laboratories have contributed and which still has rather hazy outlines.

I am sure you do not expect me to take as my model a recent well known personal account in a far more fashionable and dramatic field. I do not consider my subject nor my literary and other gifts, adequate to compete with the "Double Helix". Thus I decided to begin this lecture with a short description of the circumstances which led me into this field over 35 years ago when I was the chemist in the Institute of Ophthalmology at Columbia University and Assistant Professor of Biochemistry. With one assistant or technician, we had to carry out the clinical analyses for the hospital and were expected to conduct scientific investigations in our spare time.

My colleague, Dr. Richard Thompson, the microbiologist of the Institute, and I were supposed to work on ophthalmological problems. We decided to cooperate in a study of lysozyme, at that time a mysterious agent of unknown chemical composition and unknown mechanism of action. Early in 1934, our two laboratories reported in Science that lysozyme was a basic polypeptide which acted on a substrate of "mucoid" nature located in the outer layers of susceptible micro-organisms (Meyer, Thompson, Palmer, and Khorazo, 1934). My colleague John Palmer and I then began searching for defined substrates of lysozyme. At that time the available information on substances of "mucoid" nature was contained in a monograph by P.A. Levene entitled: Hexosamines and Mucoproteins (Levene, 1925). Levene had to his credit some very important contributions such as the structure of chondrosamine as 2-deoxy-2-amino-D-galactose and the nature of the sugar in DNA as 2-deoxy-D-ribose. Substances of mucoid nature, according to Levene, fell into two groups, both sulfate esters, one of which was the already known chondroitin sulfate, the other mucoitin sulfate. Mucoitin sulfate was supposed to be present in all connective tissues, in serum, in egg white, in umbilical cord and in vitreous humor. Levene had proposed that mucoitin sulfate was an isomer of chondroitin sulfate. Both were considered non-reducing tetrasaccharides composed of two moles each of N-acetylhexosamine O-sulfate and glucuronic acid, with D-glucosamine in mucoitin and D-galactosamine in chondroitin sulfate. Levene heated the tissues of fluids with $Ba(OH)_2$ then concentrated the solution on a steam bath and removed Ba with dilute H_2SO_4. With this background we decided to isolate mucoitin sulfuric acid from vitreous humor. However, we avoided the use of hot alkali and extracted the acetone precipitates of bovine vitreous humor with water or salt solutions at room temperature, removed the protein by mild methods such as precipitation with Zn (OH_2) and fractionation from acetate buffer with alcohol. We obtained ropy precipitates which in water gave sulfate-free, non-dialysable solutions of high viscosity which could be spun into threads. On analysis, the substance was composed of equimolar quantities of a hexuronic acid, hexosamine and acetyl. The hexosamine was isolated, crystalized and characterized as D-glucosamine; the uronic acid as D-glucuronic acid by oxidation to gluco-saccharic acid. Next we turned to umbilical cord which, according to Levene, also contained "mucoitin sulfuric acid". By extraction with water and neutral salt we isolated again a sulfate-free fraction very similar in composition and physical properties to that isolated from vitreous humor. From the insoluble residue, we isolated by mild alkaline extraction a second hexosamine-containing fraction which contained sulfate and on hydrolysis yielded D-galactosamine. This second fraction we considered chondroitin sulfate. We proposed the term hyaluronic acid for the first component. Neither hyaluronic acid nor the chondroitin sulfate fractions were hydrolysed by lysozyme. We immediately searched for other enzymes which would hydrolyse these polysaccharides. A very lucky coincidence early in 1936 finally led to such enzymes, the hyaluronidases. Dr. René Dubos was working at that time on the autolytic system of pneumococci. Lyophilized solutions obtained from a strain of pneumococcus which Dubos supplied for testing for lysozyme activity were negative for lysozyme but had a remarkable effect on the viscosity of hyaluronate solutions and on longer incubation gave increasing quantities of reducing sugar. In short succession we reported on the isolation of hyaluronic acid from a number of different sources; on hyaluronidases of micro-organisms and of mammalian tissues, on the isolation and properties of chondroitin sulfate of hyaline cartilage, and on the isolation of a neutral mucopolysaccharide of pig gastric mucosa which possessed high blood group A activity. I thus had become immersed for better or for worse in what is now called glycosaminoglycans.

The shifting attitudes toward various fields of science, the ground substances in general and the glycosaminoglycans in particular, offer an interesting subject. As the term "Grund-Substanz", or still better, the French synonym "substance fondamantale" implies, the histologists a hundred years ago considered these extra-cellular components to be the matrix of all formed extracellular elements. By the time we started our work the ground substances were at best a nuisance and of no interest biologically, at least as far as biochemists were concerned. For example, not so many years ago, Francis O. Schmitt referred to the ground substances as "crud" which Webster's Dictionary defines as an "imaginary disease, used as a general term for any vague disorder or ailment". On the other hand, in a symposium on Frontiers in Molecular Neurobiology with the same F.O. Schmitt as chairman and contributor (Schmitt, 1968), we read about the importance of peptidoglycans in the coats of neuronal cells and of "acid mucopolysaccharides" in the synapses, to quote: "The negatively charged groups in the outer surface or coat of the greater neuronal membranes, as well as the occurrence of negatively charged acid mucopolysaccharides in the inter-synaptic space, may be fundamental to exchanges of Na^+ and Ca^{++} ions occurring during excitation and recovery and possibly in learning and memory". Apparently my good friend Frank Schmitt at last has succumbed to the imagined ailment. The recognition of the potential information content of this group of substances is to me very pleasing indeed, since I have attempted to stress this potential for quite a few years. At present, it is admittedly impossible to give form and substance to such a hypothesis, but it seems important to stress the heterogeneity and variability of the glycosaminoglycans and thus to have a good potential of information, even though we do not understand its biological meaning.

II THE HETEROGENEITY AND VARIABILITY OF GLYCOSAMINOGLYCANS

The problem of heterogeneity, of course, is not limited to glycosaminoglycans, but also occurs normally in proteins where it is usually described as polymorphism; for example, in serum albumin, a α1 glycoproteins, in haptoglobins, in isoenzymes, and to an extreme degree, in γ-globulins. Polymorphism of proteins, in general, involves inherited substitutions of one or more amino acids by another, leading to differences in physical properties and in isoenzymes to differences in activity profiles. In polysaccharides, and especially in heteropolysaccharides, we can a priori expect to find a greater degree of errors, and of some degree of randomness, in the biosynthesis since the direct transcription of carbohydrate sequences from a code is absent. For this reason, the substitution in a heteropolysaccharide of one activated glycosyl group by another of similar structure or conformation appears to have a higher degree of probability than the substitution of one amino acid by another in a protein. This of course does not mean that a strictly coded biosynthesis of heteroglycans does not occur. The inheritance of blood group substances or the presence of different types of glycosaminoglycans in different tissues are only explainable by a coded biosynthesis. But even in these substances, heterogeneity of the carbohydrate chains has to be expected, and actually can be demonstrated. The term heterogeneity appears to me preferable to the term polymorphism, which in protein chemistry has been used in a more restrictive sense.

I will limit this discussion for obvious reasons to glycosaminoglycans of connective tissues in which we distinguish heterogeneity from variability. Heterogeneity will denote hybrid molecules, i.e. the replacement of one glycosyl group in the carbohydrate chains by another as well as differences in the linkage region. Variability will be used for differences in the number and sequence of exo groups such as sialyl, fucosyl and sulfate. I firmly believe that heterogeneity in glycosaminoglycans exists to a far higher extent than we can demonstrate by our still very limited methods of separation and of analytical procedures.

Heterogeneity and variability have been demonstrated in all glycosaminoglycans with perhaps hyaluronate as the only exception. The latter aside from polydispersity which will not be considered here, may in some tissues be covalently linked to protein, while in general it is free or at least not covalently linked.

A. DERMATAN SULFATE

The first example of heterogeneity or hybridization in a glycosaminoglycan was found in dermatan sulfate. Hoffman et al. in 1956, (Hoffman, Linker and Meyer, 1956, 1957) reported the presence of both iduronic and glucuronic acid in fractions isolated from pigskin and bull-hide. The two uronosyl groups varied in their proportions from 4:1 in the main dermatan sulfate fraction to 1:1 in the fraction of greatest alcohol solubility. All fractions were resistant to testicular hyaluronidase even after catalytic desulfation. In the original publication the fractions were considered to be mixtures of two glycosaminoglycans--one "chondroitin sulfate B" containing only iduronosyl groups, the other an unknown compound similar to "chondroitin sulfate B" and equally resistant to testicular hyaluronidase, although we debated in the laboratory quite vehemently whether or not we ought to regard these compounds as hybrids. Soon afterwards the latter view won out (Meyer, Hoffman and Linker, 1959). Fransson and Rodén recently confirmed in very elegant experiments the hybrid nature of dermatan sulfate (Fransson and Rodén, 1967, 1968). According to these authors, a minor portion of the glucuronosyl moieties are located near the linkage region. The location and sequence of the rest of the glucuronosyl in the polysaccharide chains remains unknown. In fact, even if a method were available to degrade the polysaccharide sequentially from one end of the molecule, the results, as in all other glycosaminoglycans, could only be considered as statistically valid since no method is available for proving the presence of only a single molecular species in a given preparation.

The proteoglycans of dermatan sulfate are discussed in chapter VI. Only recently such complexes have been described by Toole and Lowther (1968). However, heterogeneity of the linkage region or polymorphism of the protein chains in this group is highly probable. Thus on alkaline elimination, the destruction of serine is only about 30% of that of its analog Ch4-S. Likewise, the number of xyloxyl-groups per chain liberated appears to be very much smaller than in comparable Ch4-S fractions. We thus suspect a considerable number of N-glycosyl or other alkali stable linkages to the protein backbones.

The proteoglycan of dermatan sulfate leads to another important aspect of the ground substances--the interaction of the proteoglycans with the fibrous proteins of the connective tissues, a subject which probably will be of special interest at this meeting. Toole and Lowther described the specific interaction of the isolated proteoglycan of dermatan sulfate with some fractions of tropocollagen (1968). From 1956 on we repeatedly called attention to the association of dermatan sulfate in tissues with coarse collagen fibers. On the basis of this association, we postulated that the occurrence of dermatan fate in cartilage of Hurler's syndrome, in contrast to its absence in the normal, was the cause of the skeletal deformation in this inherited disease (Meyer and Hoffman, 1961).

B. CHONDROITIN 4-S AND CHONDROITIN 6-S AND THEIR PROTEOGLYCANS

Information on occurrence of heterogeneity of Ch4-S and Ch6-S is scanty. The main linkage region of both glycosaminoglycans apparently contains the Ser-xylosyl-digalactosyl grouping (Lindahl and Rodén, 1966; Helting and Rodén, 1968). Katsura and Davidson (1966) reported 1 out of 5 chains of Ch4-S of pig costal cartilage linked via an N-glycosylamine bond to the γ-carboxyl of Glu. Prior to this report we had postulated the presence in ChS of alkali stable bonds since ChS extracted directly from cartilage with alkali was free of amino acids while the same procedure applied to peptidoglycans (after proteolysis) still showed the presence of peptides. This was explained by the presumed loss during the isolation of alkali-stable protein polysaccharide when cartilage itself was extracted instead of peptidoglycans. On the basis of the data of Katsura and Davidson, the presence of heterogeneity in the protein polysaccharide seems indicated at least in the linkage region. The presence of both O- and N-glycosyl linkages in the same protein polysaccharide is known in a number of glycopeptides, as for example, in a glycopeptide isolated from yeast cell wall (Sentandreu and Northcote, 1968) and in γ-globulin of human milk (Descamps, Monsigny and Montreuil, 1968). Information about heterogeneity in the protein moiety of Ch4-S and Ch6-S is very scarce. In fact, it is not known whether or not the protein moiety of Ch4-S and Ch6-S are identical. On the basis of the differences of the peptide-doublets of Ch6-S and KSII (see later) we proposed that the protein backbones of the two isomeric chondroitin sulfates were not identical. Another form of heterogeneity of the proteoglycan concerns the variable number of ChS side chains (Hoffman, Linker and Meyer, 1967). Variations of the SO_4 groups are definitely known, especially in fishes (Mathews, 1967). Although in some types of cartilage the SO_4 to GalN ratio has been reported as remarkably constant, this does not appear to hold true for cartilage in rapid turnover such as epiphyseal cartilage. This also is indicated in recent report on ChS produced in tissue culture, where chondroitin free of or very low in S was demonstrated (Nemeroff and Holtzer, 1967; Shulman and Meyer, 1968; Silbert and DeLucca, 1969).

The problem of sulfation *in vivo* and *in vitro* of the chondroitin sulfates still remains unresolved. We have to assume specific 4- and 6-sulfotransferases. The chondroitin sulfates isolated from the tissues are mixtures of varying proportions of the two isomers depending on the source and age of the species. It is possible, although improbable, that one and the same protein backbone can carry both Ch4-S and Ch6-S sidechains, and even that one carbohydrate chain may contain both primary and secondary sulfate ester groups. What then is the pattern of sulfation *in vitro* with a mixed population of cartilage cells and without the activating and deactivating influences which may be operative *in vivo*?

These considerations and the recent report of the isolation of a 4-6 disulfated *N*-acetyl chondrosine from squid cartilage (Suzuki, Saito, Yamagata, Anno and Kawa, 1968) ought to caution against a too facile interpretation of *in vitro* biosynthetic data.

C. HEPARAN SULFATE (HEPARITIN SULFATE)

Heparan sulfates were the second group of glycosaminoglycans recognized as hybrids (Meyer, Hoffman and Linker, 1957). The chemical structure of heparan sulfates, their origin and biological relation to heparin and in fact their histological location are still largely unknown. Heparan sulfate has been reported to contain variable amounts of iduronic acid substituting for *D*-glucuronic acid. However, the degree of this substitution has been controversial, and is still unknown. In the latest study on the structure of heparan sulfate by Cifonelli (Cifonelli, 1968) iduronic acid was reported present only in minor proportion in all fractions. The oligosaccharide and disaccharide fractions were obtained by degradation with nitrous acid at -20°. This reaction attacks only at the *N*-sulfated glucosaminyl bond while the *N*-acetylated bond is stable. The presence of both *N*-acetyl and *N*-sulfated glucosamine in the same molecule had previously been reported (Linker, Hoffman, Sampson and Meyer, 1958; Cifonelli and Dorfman, 1960). The ratio of *N*-acetyl to *N*-sulfate is variable in different fractions from the same source, and with it the number of O-sulfate which appears to be located mainly in the 6 positions of the hexosaminyl group. This variation in the number and types of the sulfate groups probably indicates a high metabolic activity of heparan sulfates in which this group of compounds may participate as an intermediate in some biosynthetic reaction. However, the differences in distribution of heparan sulfates versus heparin make it improbable that heparan sulfates are precursors or degradation products of heparin. The basic structure of heparan sulfate appears to be that of a branched chain with N-acetylated disaccharide units in the outer branches and the N-sulfated units in an inner core (Linker and Sampson, 1960).

D. KERATAN SULFATES

In these sulfated glycosaminoglycans a high degree of heterogeneity and variation has been demonstrated. This became already evident when we demonstrated the profound chemical differences in alkali stability and composition between keratan sulfate of cornea (KSI) and that of cartilate (KSII) (Seno, Meyer, Anderson and Hoffman, 1965). The latter appears to be identical with that of intervertebral disc. The composition of KSI and KSII is summarized in Table I and the differences in amino acid composition of the peptidoglycans in Table II.

The main repeating unit has been demonstrated as N-acetyl-lactosamine-6-S polymerized via β1→3 bonds in KSI and KSII. The position and structure of the mannosyl group is unknown, as well as the distribution and linkages of the fucosyl and sialyl groups. Aside from variations of fucosyl and sialyl groups, keratan sulfate fractions vary considerably in their sulfate ester content. KSII fractions, especially from cartilage of older persons, are considerably oversulfated. However, both KSI and KSII contain besides glcN-6S, Gal6S at least some of them in disulfated (Bhavanandan and Meyer, 1967, 1968) disaccharide units. In consequence, some of the N-acetyllactosamine units are not sulfated. It seems doubtful to me that the distribution of the SO_4 ester groups explains the anomalous be-

TABLE I

Analysis of KSI (Cornea) and KSII (Human Rib Cartilage)

Analysis	KSI	KSII
Anthrone %	35.3	28.7
Hexosamine %	26.2	24.1
GlcN/Gal N	22:1	8:1
SO_4 %	17.7	18.9
Sialic acid %	trace	3.4
Fucose %	trace	2.7
Mannose %	1-2	2.4
Protein (Lowry) %	2.5	6.6
Protein (A A) %	2.6	6.0
Carbazole %	3.4	2.4
$[\alpha]_D$ (water)	+0.5	-7.2
Alkaline Destruction		
Ser %	13	51
Thr	7	70

TABLE II

Amino Acids of KSI and KSII

(% of total amino acid)

Amino Acids	KSI	KSII
Asp	39.93	13.34
Thr	6.55	13.00
Ser	8.21	10.72
Glu	13.86	23.35
Pro	0.00	14.11
Gly	9.64	8.80
Ala	5.65	5.73
Val	12.05	4.14
Met	0.00	0.28
Ileu	2.18	2.07
Leu	1.13	1.37
Tyr	0.00	0.86
Phen	0.75	1.88

haviour of KS towards quaternary salts, especially their solubility at low salt concentration in excess of CPC together with the high critical salt concentration of the complexes. Some of the properties of keratan sulfate, such as the unexpectedly high solubility of their salts in ethanol, may indicate hydrophobic properties; a behaviour exhibited especially with the desulfated derivatives which are water insoluble, but soluble in formamide, dimethyl formamide and dimethylsulfoxide (Bhavanandan and Meyer, 1967).

The main differences between KSI and KSII are: KSI is alkali stable and apparently linked via N-glucosaminyl bonds, KSII is alkali labile and linked via O-glycosyl bonds between N-acetylgalactosamine and Ser and Thr (Bray, Lieberman and Meyer, 1967) similar to the linkage region in blood group substances (Kabat, Bassett, Pryzwansky and Lloyd, 1965). A few of the galactosamine groups even in hyaluronidase digested samples of KSII, may actually belong to remaining Ch6-S chains, since by gas chromatography Choi, in our laboratory found 0.2% of xylose in KSII even in the best samples exhaustively digested with testicular hyaluronidase, KSII compared to KSI has considerably more side chains of sialic acid and fucose, and has a larger proportion of Gal.-6S. KSII, furthermore, contains a pronase resistant peptide chain. After alkaline elimination, the peptide chain remains attached to the carbohydrate chain, despite the conversion of the N-acetylgalactosaminyl group into a chromogen giving the direct Ehrlich reaction. On this basis we had postulated that the peptide chain is linked to the polysaccharide by a second alkali-stable bond. The peptide chain after alkaline elimination becomes susceptible to digestion by pronase. On the basis of these data, we proposed that the N-acetylgalactosaminyl group was linked by an O-glycosyl bond to Ser and Thr, that it was substituted in carbon 3 to an unknown substituent, and that it was

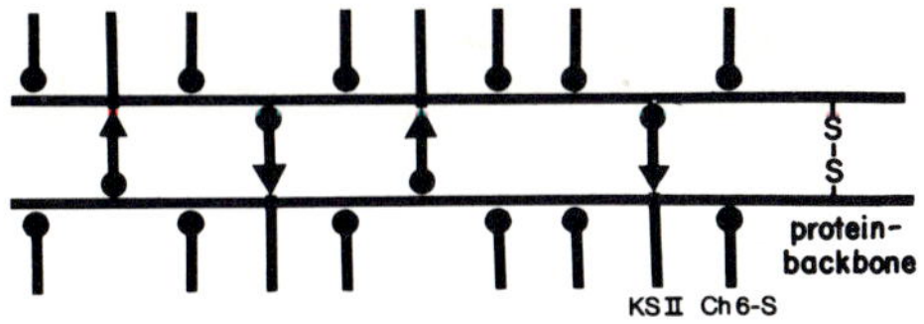

Fig. 1.

linked through carbon 6 to the rest of the carbohydrate chain (Bray, et al., 1967).

The structure summarized information on the proteoglycan of keratan sulfate. The sugar unit following galactosamine is unknown. It may be mannose followed by the repeating units of N-acetyllactosamine. Assuming one mannosyl group per chain, we obtain an average molecular weight of 10,800. A similar figure is obtained from the galactosamine content. We find an excess of about 25% of galactose over glucosamine in KSII. The true excess is somewhat lower if we deduct 2 galactose equivalents calculated from xylose values. This excess of galactose in addition to the considerable loss of galactose together with all the sialyl and fucosyl residues by methanolysis on catalytic desulfation (Bhavanandan and Meyer, 1968) indicates a fair number of substituted galactosyl units in multiple sidechains. The variability of the fucosyl and especially the sialyl groups in KSII is very pronounced in different fractions. The sialic acid content varies between 2 and 7.5%. We do not know whether this variation is based on variation in biosynthesis, or secondarily, by in vivo hydrolysis of these labile groups. In any case, it is obvious that at present the structure of keratan sulfate in many details is still unknown.

The degree of heterogeneity of KSII is difficult to assess at present, while the variability is quite apparent.

We now have to discuss the protein backbone to which KSII is attached. The following facts have been well established: 1) KSII and ChS are covalently linked to one protein chain. This has been demonstrated with the peptidoglycan KSII by Seno, Meyer, Anderson and Hoffman (1965) who further showed that the ChS was exclusively Ch6-S. In the experiments of Hoffman, et al. (1967) it was also demonstrated with the proteoglycan of nasal septum and of articular cartilage, where the main ChS fraction is Ch4-S that the KS on alkaline treatment remained with the protein, while single chains of ChS were obtained. Whether in all cartilagenous tissues KSII is only partly linked to peptides carrying Ch6-S is not known at present but seems to us highly probably. In favor of an obligatory association of KSII with Ch6-S is the simultaneous increase of KSII with Ch6-S in aging cartilage, in nucleus pulposus, and in Marfan's syndrome (Meyer, 1963). Furthermore, we are postulating that the protein backbone of Ch4-S is different and distinct from that of Ch6-S.

The nature of the alkali-stable and pronase-resistant bond between the backbone and the KSII chains is not known. We have considered previously that this bond is an amide formed by the γ-carboxy group of Glu and the amino group of a glucosaminyl moiety. A more appealing type of stable crosslinking is represented by an N-alkylsubstitution of one glycosaminyl group by α-amino caproic acid formed by the reduction of a Schiff base, an analogy with the crosslinkages of elastin and collagen known from the work of Partridge, Paul Gallop and others. Such a stable bond would be more in keeping with crosslinking in fibrous proteins, and might explain the accumulation of KSII in Marfan's syndrome, in which we assume a failure in crosslinking common to collagen and KSII.

Other possible types of crosslinking as an explanation of the properties of the hydrid glycopeptides or peptidoglycans of cartilage are of course possible.

I have summarized the structure of the proteoglycan which contain Ch6-S and KSII in the following speculative drawing.

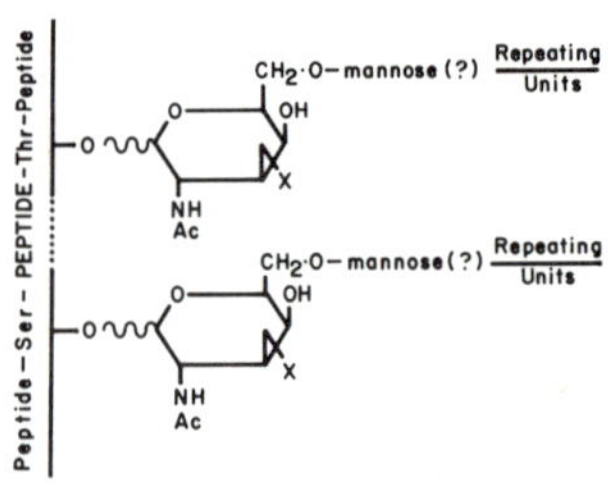

Fig. 2. Scheme of the Proteoglycan of Cartilage

The backbone is a double strand of protein with Ch6-S chains and KSII chains starting from either strand. The two strands are crosslinked by KSII by the second alkali stable bond discussed above. I ought to mention here the very interesting recent paper of Serafini-Fracassini (1968) which came to my attention after I had finished my manuscript. The author proposed a model of PPL after shaking for one hour at room temperature with acetone containing 0.1 M HCl. The author proposes a basic molecular unit of the proteoglycan chains in lateral alignment. The protein-backbones with Val and Asp acid as N-terminal amino acid would have multiple ChS side chains, while the third chain differs in having terminal Ile and KS as side chains. In my opinion a single and separate protein-backbone with only KS side chains is not in accordance with our data on the side by side presence of KS and Ch6-S in the same peptide.

I have attempted in this review to focus on the heterogeneity and variability of the glycosaminoglycans and their proteoglycans. The observed complexity of the substances need to be explained by the cellular biosynthetic mechanisms. A priori, as I mentioned earlier, one ought to expect in the biosynthesis of heteropolysaccharides a greater possibility for "errors" than in proteins. Even in each of the different blood group substances heterogeneity of a minor degree seems possible, although the major part of the structures are inherited and, therefore, their biosynthesis coded. In fact the so-called incompleted chains of Morgan (1960) may be examples of the heterogeneity in blood group substances. In the variability of the exogroups, i.e. fucose, sialic acid and sulfate, the probability of random synthesis is still more obvious. It seems important to be constantly aware of the possibility and probability of heterogeneity when working with glycoproteins or glycosaminoglycans.

III THE BIOLOGICAL FUNCTION OF PROTEOGLYCANS

The last problem which I will now discuss briefly concerns the most puzzling and speculative aspect of the proteoglycans of connective tissues, namely, what are the general functions of these polymers, and why did the organisms develop such an array of similar but distinct anionic polymers? This question of course pre-supposes the tacit assumption that these substances and their multiple variants have distinct and differing functions in the economy of the organism and are not just remnants or fossils of an evolutionary nature like the coccyx in man. The assumption of a purposive and utilitarian nature of these substances is metaphysical, an aspect in general considered beyond the ken and scope of a biologist and certainly of a biochemist. It is known that the glycosaminoglycans are phylogenetically very ancient, and as far as we know, have undergone very little if any evolutionary changes. It is regrettable that there have been very few studies of this kind, the most systematic being the investigations of Martin Mathews (1967), and the demonstration by Anno, Kawai and Seno (1964) of chondroitin in the skin of the squid and a novel variation of some of chondroitin sulfate in squid cartilage (Suzuki et al., 1968) and some rather sketchy and unsystematic studies from our own laboratory. I also find it regrettable that we know so little about the nature and structure of the proteoglycans at early stages of embryo-genesis which might lead to new insights into the phylogeny and functions of the developing organism, namely that they may well be the vanishing organizers of the developing organism.

Any analysis of the function of the proteoglycans has to start with the fact that these compounds are polyanions differing at least formally mainly in the geometry, distances and ionization of the negatively charged group. What are the counterions in situ? If we extrapolate from the _in vitro_ data of Woodward and Davidson (1968) we would expect that Ca in non-ionized form would be the predominant counterion since these authors reported that the proteoglycan of cartilage, i.e. predominantly Ch4-S, bound Ca^{++} in nonionized form in contrast to the peptidoglycan which did not distinguish between Na^{+} and divalent ion. If I interpret the data correctly the Ca^{++} in the protein-complex zippers two or more adjacent polysaccharide chains. On the other hand, how can we reconcile these data with in situ metachromasia or the elegant work of John Scott and his associates? I am not aware of any quantitative data as to how many equivalents of the total anionic group at physiological pH in situ are actually ionized or available to the monovalent dyes or to the quaternary salts of Scott.

In a paper published in 1960, I proposed the hypothesis that the anionic groups of the various glycosaminoglycans are a code of extracellular information for the arrangement or organization of the fibrillar proteins, chiefly collagen fibrils (Meyer, 1960). This hypothesis postulated that cationic groups of collagen fibrils were in register with at least part of the anionic group of the polyanions and thus leading to the arrangement and stabilization of the collagen fibrils or fibres. As a consequence of this hypothesis the proteoglycans would have a rigid and ordered conformation with the protein backbone wound around and parallel to the collagen bundles and the polysaccharide side chains across the bundles. Further the number and sequence of the basic group of collagens from different tissues would differ. I do not know of any experimental evidence of the in situ structure of the proteoglycan or for the differences in the sequence of the basic groups in collagens from various sources. A comparison both chemically and histologically of collagen bundles of cornea in which chondroitin 4-sulfate and keratan sulfate are the polyanions with the deep layers of skin in which dermatan sulfate is the predominant polyanion would best be suitable for comparison. The hypothesis I have outlined here is not meant to exclude other functions of the variations of the polysaccharide. I specifically would mention here their regulatory function in intercellular spaces and their role in differentiation which I have also alluded to above.

I started this lecture on a personal note and would like to close on a similar basis. I consider myself very fortunate to have entered this complex field of glycosaminoglycans and glycoproteins at an early stage of its development. This still is a young field infinitely more complex and difficult operationally than protein or nucleic acid biochemistry. Compared to these two fields, the glycosaminoglycans and related compounds are still very much the poor relatives. I firmly believe this attitude will change when the biological functions of the various members of this group are understood. The increasing interest in the structure and function of cell membranes and their glycoprotein components, the so-called glycochalix of some authors, will inevitably lead to comparison with glycosaminoglycans. There is, after all, only an arbitrary division between the two classes; whether the compounds are sulfated or not, or whether they are derived from mesodermal or epithelial tissues. Undoubtedly what is needed above all, is our ability to attract the young to devote their energy and enthusiasm to these problems.

ACKNOWLEDGEMENT

The studies have been supported by grants from the National Institute of Arthritis and Metabolic Diseases and the National Institute of Child Health and Human Development.

REFERENCES

Anno, K., Kawai, Y. and Seno, N. (1964). Biochem. Biophys. Acta 83, 348.

Bhavanandan, V.P. and Meyer, K. (1967). J. Biol. Chem. 242, 4352.

Bhavanandan, V.P. and Meyer, K. (1968). J. Biol. Chem. 243, 1052.

Bray, B.A., Lieberman, R. and Meyer, K. (1967). J. Biol. Chem. 242, 3373.

Cifonelli, J.A. (1968). Carbohyd. Res. 8, 233

Cifonelli, J.A. and Dorfman, A. (1960). J. Biol. Chem. 235, 3283.

Descamps, J., Monsigny, M. and Montreuil, J. (1968). C.R. Acad. Sc. (Paris) 266, 1775.

Fransson, L. and Rodén, L. (1967). J. Biol. Chem. 242, 4161, 4170.

Fransson, L. and Rodén, L. (1968). J. Biol. Chem. 243, 1504.

Helting, T. and Rodén, L. (1968). Biochem. Biophys. Acta 170, 301.

Hoffman, P., Linker, A. and Meyer, K. (1956). Science 124, 1252.

Hoffman, P., Linker, A. and Meyer, K. (1957). Arch. Biochem. Biophys. 69, 435.

Hoffman, P., Mashburn, T.A. and Meyer, K. (1967). J. Biol. Chem. 242, 3805.

Hoffman, P., Mashburn, T.A., Meyer, K. and Bray, B.A. (1967). J. Biol. Chem. 242, 3799.

Kabat, E., Bassett, E.W., Pryzwansky, K. and Lloyd, K.O. (1965). Biochem. 4, 1632.

Katsura, N. and Davidson, E.A. (1966). Biochem. Biophys. Acta 121, 128.

Levene, P.A. (1925). Hexosamines and Mucoproteins. Longmans, Green and Co., New York.

Lindahl, U. and Rodén, L. (1966). J. Biol. Chem. 241, 2113.

Linker, A., Hoffman, P., Sampson, P. and Meyer, K. (1958). Biochem. Biophys. Acta 29, 443.

Linker, A. and Sampson, P. (1960). Biochem. Biophys. Acta 43, 366.

Mathews, M.B. (1967). Biol. Rev. 42, 499.

Meyer, K. (1960). In Molecular Biology, p. 69. Ed. by Nachmansohn, D., Academic Press.

Meyer, K. (1963). Expos. Ann. Biochim. Masson (Paris), p. 2.

Meyer, K. and Hoffman, P. (1961). Arthr. and Rheumatism 4, 582.

Meyer, K., Hoffman, P. and Linker, A. (1957). In Connective Tissue, a Symposium, p. 86. Blackwell, Oxford.

Meyer, K., Hoffman, P. and Linker, A. (1959). In Connective Tissue, Thrombosis and Atherosclerosis, p. 181. Academic Press.

Meyer, K., Thompson, R., Palmer, J.W. and Khorazo, D. (1934). Science 79, 61.

Morgan, W.T.J. (1960). Proc. Roy. Soc. B. 151, 308.

Nemeroff, M. and Holtzer, H. (1967). Devel. Biol. 16, 250.

Schmitt, F.O. (1968). Proc. Natl. Acad. Sci. 60, 1055.

Seno, N., Meyer, K., Anderson, B. and Hoffman, P. (1965). J. Biol. Chem. 240, 1005.

Sentandreu, R. and Northcote, D.H. (1968). Biochem. J. 109, 419.

Seafini-Fracassini, A. (1968). Biochem. Biophys. Acta 170, 289.

Shulman, H.J. and Meyer, K. (1968). J. Exp. Med. 128, 1353.

Silbert, J.E. (1964). J. Biol. Chem. 239, 1310.

Silbert, J.E. and DeLuca, S. (1969). J. Biol. Chem. 244, 876.

Suzuki, S., Saito, H., Yamagata, T., Anno, K. and Kawa,T.Y. (1968). J. Biol. Chem. 243, 1543.

Toole, B.P. and Lowther, D.A. (1968). Arch. Biochem. Biophys. 128, 567.

Woodward, C. and Davidson, E.A. (1968). Proc. Natl. Acad. Sci. 60, 201.

Chapter I

Chemistry and Structure of Collagen

THE ISOLATION AND CHARACTERISATION OF COLLAGEN FROM THREE INVERTEBRATE TISSUES

A. Nordwig, Erdmute Rogall and Ursula Hayduk

Numerous investigations have been performed on the occurence of collagen in invertebrate tissues (for review see Gross, 1963). However, "most studies have been limited to amino acid analysis of either insoluble collagen or gelatin preparations of uncertain purity" (Piez, 1967). Collagens from earthworm and Ascaris are exceptions relevant here (Maser and Rice, 1962; Josse and Harrington, 1964).

The aim of our investigations is to gain some insight into the phylogeny of collagen at the molecular level. This clearly implies that we have to deal with pure soluble collagen from low developed species. The invertebrate animals we thought useful for this comparative work were Actinia equina, a kind of sea anemone from the group of coelenterates, the liver fluke (Fasciola hepatica), a parasitic flat worm living in the bile ducts of sheep and cattle, and the snail (Helix pomatia).

I ISOLATION AND PURIFICATION

We had to face, as we still must, some difficulties in this field due to poor yields of soluble collagen from the materials selected. The isolation procedure we first used was the well-known extraction of homogenates with acidic media. The amounts obtained were rather disappointing, however (Table I). Using citrate buffer, pH 3.7, the yield was actually zero with Helix pomatia, below 0.1% with Actinia, and satisfactory only with Fasciola, i.e. about 10%. This figure is raised to

TABLE I

Yields of Soluble Collagen from Invertebrate Tissues
(expressed as % of total collagen present)

Preparative method	*Actinia equina* (%)	*Fasciola hepatica* (%)	*Helix pomatia* (%)	calf skin (%)
Citrate buffer (pH 3.7; 0.15 M)	< 0.1	10%(60-80)	0	(15-20)
Acetic acid (1%)	1		6	
Pronase treatment*	5	3	3	50
Acetic acid extraction after pronase treatment	90	45	15	
Pepsin treatment†	80	60-80	8	(90)

*Enzyme:substrate = 1:25; 24 hr at 12°C in 0.05 M Tris + 0.1 M $CaCl_2$, pH 7.8.
†Enzyme:substrate = 1:100; 40 hr at 10°C in 1% acetic acid.

60-80% when young animals collected in late spring or summer are extracted.

Acetic acid in a concentration of 1% proved to be a slightly better, though not really satisfactory, solvent for the two tissues investigated (Table I).

Treatment with the mold enzyme, pronase (Fujii, 1965) gave surprising results. At least 50% of insoluble calf skin collagen readily dissolved during incubation with pronase for 24 hr at neutral pH, but only a small percentage of the invertebrate tissues dissolved under identical conditions (Table I). Unlike calf skin collagen the invertebrate collagens remain insoluble in the neutral pH range after incubation with pronase. Appreciable amounts are obtained, however, when the pronase-treated materials are subsequently extracted with acetic acid (Table I) or citrate buffer. The amounts thus isolated are different from tissue to tissue and are smallest in the case of Helix pomatia collagen.

This situation resembles the results obtained with the pepsin solubilization procedure (Kühn, Fietzek and Kühn, 1966): Under comparable conditions large amounts of calf skin collagen, actinocol (collagen from Actinia) and fasciocol (collagen from Fasciola) became soluble, but only 8% of the collagen present in snail tissue dissolved (Table I). In other words, the cross-linkages of snail collagen appear to be rather stable against proteolytic degradation.

This view was verified for the so-called head-to-tail cross-linkage. When snail collagen dissolved by pepsin treatment was precipitated by ATP, we observed aggregates of the so-called long spacing segment (SLS) fibril type (Fig. 1). The very same result, i.e. segment fibrils, was obtained when collagen from Helix pomatia was dissolved by a new procedure using amines as reagents for the cleavage of cross-linkages in the presence of alkali, and of sodium sulfate which prevents swelling. This method was developed by Fujii (1969) and was successfully applied to the solubilization of steer hide collagen.

Table II summarizes the optimal conditions we have elaborated for the individual tissues. So far, in a variety of experiments we have been unable to find experimental conditions under which collagen from the sea anemone may be solubilized without being degraded by the alkali used in this procedure. The poor yield in the case of Fasciola also is apparently due to degradation, and we cannot completely purify the remaining 11% of our degradation products. (The disc-electrophoretic pattern of this material is shown in Fig. 3). For snail collagen, the conditions presented in Table II are by far the best for the isolation of soluble Helix collagen and are the basis for obtaining pure material. As mentioned before, this collagen is precipitated as segment fibers, not as segments by ATP.

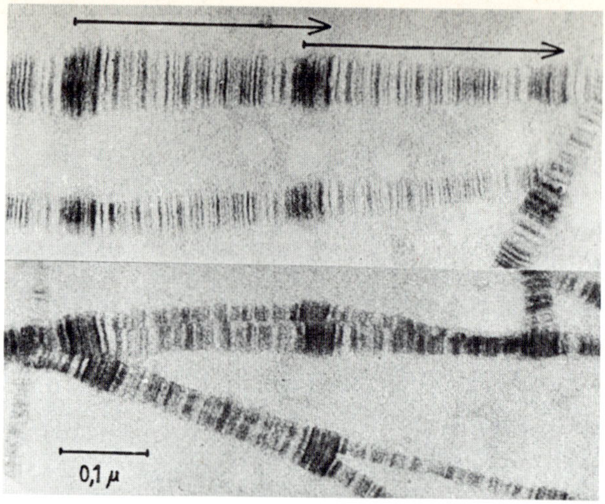

Fig. 1. Long-spacing segment fibrils from calf and snail tissues. Upper part: Long-spacing segment fibril from calf skin (taken from Kühn, et al., 1966). The arrows indicate the orientation of the collagen molecules and the overlap zone in which the "head-to-tail" bonding is located. Lower part: Long spacing segment fibril from snail homogenate treated with pepsin for 17 hr at 25°C in 1% acetic acid (pepsin:collagen = 1:10). Precipitated with ATP at pH 2.5, stained with phosphotungstic acid and uranylacetate. (Picture taken by S. Drews.)

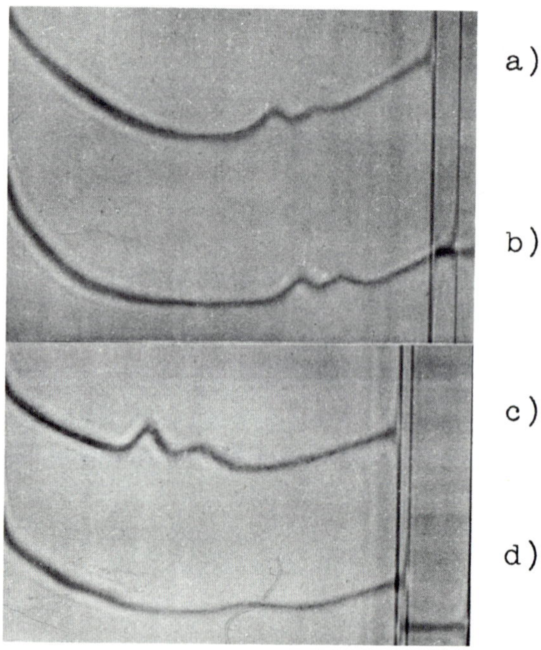

Fig. 2. Sedimentation velocity patterns of denatured collagen solutions. Spinco Model E centrifuge, wedge window cell. Sedimentation from right to left. Medium: 0.25 M citrate buffer, pH 3.7, at 20°C. Phase angle = 10°. Denaturation was performed either by heating or by dialysis of the various preparations against 2 M KSCN. Upper picture taken 88 min, lower picture taken 128 min after reaching 59,780 rev./min. (a) and (b): Collagen from *Actinia equina*, (c): calf skin collagen, (d): collagen from *Fasciola hepatica*.

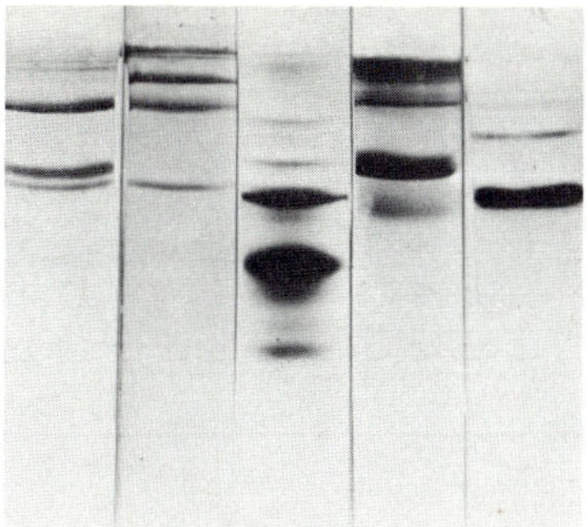

Fig. 3. Disc-electrophoretic patterns of various collagens. (a) calf skin collagen, (b) collagen from Actinia equina, (c) citrate-soluble collagen from Fasciola hepatica, (d) collagen from Fasciola hepatica, dissolved according to Fujii (1965) (cf. text and Table II), (e) collagen from Helix pomatia, dissolved according to Fujii (1965) (cf. text and Table II).

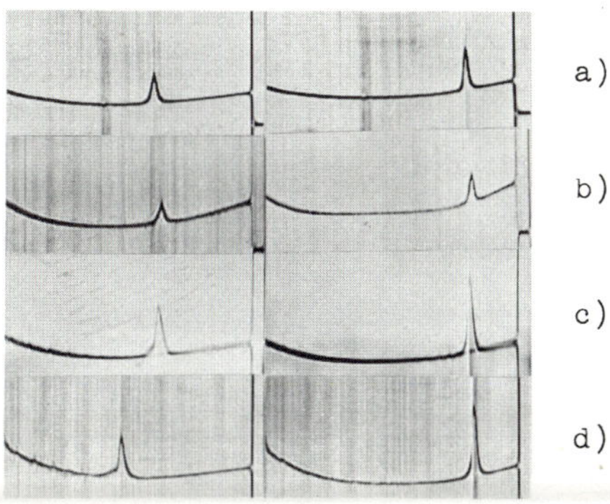

Fig. 4. Sedimentation velocity patterns of native collagen solutions. Sedimentation from right to left. Medium: 0.25 M citrate buffer, pH 3.7. (a) calf skin collagen, c = 1.6 mg/ml. Escher-Wyss centrifuge, phase angle = 12°. Temperature 20°C. Pictures taken 90 min and 165 min after reaching 59,000 rev./min (Fietzek, 1965). (b) collagen from Actinia equina, c = 1 mg/ml. Spinco Model E centrifuge, phase angle = 12°. Temperature 10°C. Pictures taken 96 min and 176 min after reaching 59,780 rev./min. (c) collagen from Fasciola hepatica, stored for 3 weeks at 5°C after preparation, c = 3 mg/ml. Temperature 18°C. For further technical details see b). (d) collagen from Fasciola hepatica, freshly prepared, c = 2.7 mg/ml. Temperature 18°C. For further technical details see a).

TABLE II

Solubilization Experiments with Invertebrate Tissues Using the Amine Procedure

Exptl. conditions	*Actinia equina*	*Fasciola hepatica*	*Helix pomatia*	Steer hide
0.2 M Monomethyl-amine 0.5 N or 0.75 N NaOH 15% Na_2SO_4 14 Days at 20°C	---	---	---	Yield: 89-97% (Fujii, 1969
0.2 M Hydroxyl-amine 0.5 N NaOH 15% Na_2SO_4 14 Days at 10°C	Dissolved: 95-100% After purif: 82%	---	---	---
0.2 M Hydroxyl-amine 0.5 N NaOH 15% Na_2SO_4 14 Days at 15°C	---	Dissolved: 95-100% After purif: 11%	---	---
0.1 M Monomethyl-amine 0.5 N NaOH 15% Na_2SO_4 8 Days at 10°C	---	---	Dissolved: 95-100% After purif: 60%	---

As for purification of our materials, we have precipitated the invertebrate collagens either by dialysis against running tap water or using the KCl-phosphate buffer procedure (Rubin et al., 1965). In each step, the nitrogen and 4-hydroxyproline contents were determined, and we regarded a preparation as pure, when the factor N/Hyp thus measured was constant. Amino acids analysis of the purified collagen was carried out to ensure that the final purification factor determined and the theoretical factor were identical.

The results of these sets of experiments may be summarized as follows:

a. We were able to isolate pure collagens from *Actinia equina* and *Fasciola hepatica*, both by extraction with acidic media or by solubilization using pepsin. A serious limitation to the latter preparations is, however, breakdown in the denatured state due to traces of proteolytic enzymes that cannot be removed.

b. Pure collagen from Helix pomatia has also been obtained by using Fujii's (1969) amine/NaOH/Na_2SO_4-procedure. A prominent feature of snail collagen seems to be the fact that it is insoluble in citrate buffer, pH 3.7.

c. Fujii's (1969) procedure proved useful for solubilizing highly cross-linked collagen, at least in the case of snail tissue. α-Chains from invertebrates appear to be much more labile to alkaline treatment than calf skin collagen subunits. The same is true for the stability of α-chains against proteolytic attack by pronase.

d. The solubilization behaviour of invertebrate collagens is in some cases quantitatively rather different from that of calf skin material. One may speculate whether this might be due to the nature and/or to the quantities of cross-linkages. Certain findings for the head-to-tail bonding have been already mentioned, and it is also of interest that the β-components of invertebrate collagens are converted more slowly to α-chains than are β-chains from vertebrate collagens.

II PROPERTIES

When investigating the properties of the pure collagen from Actinia and Fasciola (Nordwig and Hayduk, 1969), we used calf skin collagen and ichthyocol (the collagen isolated from carp swim bladder) for comparison.

One of the first criteria we applied was amino acid analysis (Table III). The main features of vertebrate collagen are also observed in our invertebrate proteins: one-third of the residues is glycine; high amounts of imino acids are present as well as both Hyp and Hyl. On the other hand, there are significant differences: the amounts of Hyl, for example, are greatly increased compared to those of calf skin collagen and ichthyocol. We further find 15 residues

TABLE III

Amino Acid Composition of Four Collagens from Vertebrate and Invertebrate Tissues*

Amino acid	Calf skin	Carp swim bladder	*Fasciola hepatica*	*Actinia equina*
Gly	335	325	305	309
Ala	107	126	57	66
Val	22	18	35	31
Leu	27	21	31	34
Ile	12	10	26	23
Phe	13	14	7	8
Met	5	13	18	5
Pro	124	116	111	75
4-Hyp	91	81	95	77
3-Hyp	traces	traces	0	15
Tyr	4	2	5	4
Ser	34	37	32	38
Thr	15	29	25	38
Asp	48	47	64	79
Glu	74	71	91	88
His	5	4	5	3
Lys	25	27	17	19
Hyl	7	7	26	28
Arg	50	47	48	62

*Values presented as residues per thousand total residues.

per thousand of 3-Hyp in actinocol, whereas this imino acid occurs in other collagens in only small amounts, if at all (except in earthworm collagen; Fujimoto and Adams, 1964). The contents of Pro and 4-Hyp also vary both as the single imino acids and as their sum. Alanine and methionine also show variations.

Further properties are summarized in Table IV. All of the materials were readily digested by clostridial collagenase. The specific optical rotation decreases to -150° and only 10-15% of the digestion mixture prove undialysable during a period of 48 hr. These results are in full accordance with those obtained by Franzblau, Seifter and Gallop (1964) and Nordwig (1962) for vertebrate collagens. The hexose contents of actinocol and fasciocol are even higher than those reported for other invertebrate collagens. The molecular weight of actinocol, both of acid-soluble and of pepsin-solubilized material, is the same as determined for vertebrate collagens. However, when fasciocol was examined immediately after isolation, it exhibited a higher molecular weight of roughly 500,000; the value was independent of the solubilization procedure. Fasciocol is also exceptional with regard to its specific optical rotation. The value found is about 10% lower than the values measured for the other collagens. On the other hand, the ratio of -[α] as measured at 40°C and 4°C, respectively, is also very close to 3 for this type of collagen. The T_M-values as presented here have been corrected for pure water solutions and will be referred to later.

Determinations of T_M were performed by following the optical rotation at 405 mμ. The range of melting is less narrow in the case of acid-soluble fasciocol, and this is interpreted in terms of breakdown by adhering proteases. There are more results in accord with such a view. As shown in Fig. 2, the sedimentation pattern of denatured actinocol is quite similar to that of calf skin collagen whereas no distinct peaks were found for fasciocol. The disc-electrophoretic pattern of collagen subunit (Fig. 3) exhibited one sharp band in the α-region with actinocol (b), and bands indicative of breakdown products with fasciocol (c). We hope to overcome these difficulties by means of the amine solubilization procedure (see above). The disc pattern obtained with such a material looks more similar to that of calf skin collagen (a), though not completely free of by-products (d). To judge from the comparison of disc-electrophoretic patterns as shown in Fig. 2 there seems to be little doubt that actinocol and most likely also snail collagen (e) consist of only one α-chain type.

TABLE IV

Some Properties of Vertebrate and Invertebrate Collagens

Source of collagen	Digestible by collagenase	Hexose content (weight %)	Molecular weight	$-[\alpha]_{405}$ (at 40°C and 4°C, resp.)	T_M (°C) (at pH 7 and $\mu=0$)
Calf skin	+	0.5	300 000	360°C 1040°C	39°C
Carp swim bladder	+	0.4	300 000	350°C 1080°C	32°C
Fasciola hepatica, liver fluke (whole animal)	+	12.8	500 000	310°C 980°C	36.6°C
Actinia equina, sea anemone (mesogloea)	+	14.1	310 000	345°C 1080°C	26.6°C

Another somewhat unusual result obtained with acid-soluble fasciol in the native state is shown in Fig. 4. The sedimentation behaviour corresponds to a higher molecular weight than normal, if freshly prepared material is used for investigation (d). If fasciocol solutions are stored for some weeks at 4°C, the molecular weight decreases to approximately 300,000 and the sedimentation behaviour becomes normal (c). The electron microscope reveals that the molecule is degraded to fragments of about 1500 Å; the same finding occasionally was made with pepsin solubilized material. These findings seem to indicate a labile bond somewhere in the middle of the fasciocol molecule. Again, the behaviour of actinocol (b) is in full accord with that of calf skin collagen (a). The characteristic sharp boundary was found in any case.

Both invertebrate collagens were able to form SLS when dialysed against ATP-solutions (see below). Our characterization experiments thus show: 1) collagen from Actinia equina appears to be very similar to vertebrate collagens apart from differences in the amino acid composition and from the number of α-chain types; 2) the same conclusions were drawn for the collagen from Fasciola hepatica. However, only preliminary data is available for the denatured protein. An additional point of interest in this material is the molecular weight of 500,000, which requires further investigation.

III PHYLOGENETIC ASPECTS

An important feature of actinocol must be considered. As mentioned before, disc-electrophoretic analysis revealed only one α-chain type, whereas vertebrate collagens contain two or three. The sea anemone is the most primitive animal from which pure collagen was ever prepared and therefore our findings strongly support the view of Pikkarainen and Kulonen (1967), who suggested that collagen was originally composed on only one α-chain type. They assumed that the primordial α-chain gene duplicated at a later stage, perhaps on the level of bony fish, and that independent mutations would have given rise to different α-chains. We intend to check our analytical results by preparative scale work.

Another aspect in which we were interested was the stability of collagen in solution. Our results confirmed that the melting temperature, T_M of collagen is not at all a function of the evolutionary level of the animal from which collagen was derived. Actinocol, like collagens from other aquatic animals (Josse and Harrington, 1964), exhibits rather a low T_M-value, i.e. 26.6°C (Table IV). The liver fluke is at a very low level of development; however, its collagen is much more stable and the T_M-value of 36.6°C (Table IV) approaches the melting temperature of the collagen of its host. This clearly indicates an adaptive effect; in other words, the stability of a collagen is related to the habitat of the animal from which the collagen was prepared. Strong evidence for this view is also provided by Rigby's (1968) results on collagens from ice-fish.

When comparing the cross-striation pattern of the segments of the four species (Fig. 5) we found that the length of 2800 Å was constant. Moreover, the electronmicrographs show the same number of light and dark bands in identical relative positions. The intensity of striations also appears to be very similar. These results suggest that very little change of the quaternary and, therefore, of the tertiary structure of the collagen molecule has taken place during evolution (Nordwig and Hayduk, 1967). This idea was confirmed by electronmicrographs of fibrils (Fig. 6): the band patterns of collagen fibrils from calf, snail or liver fluke are essentially the same. Obviously, all the information necessary for the collagen configuration and for fibril formation is contained, not in the collagen primary structure as a whole, but in certain features of the amino acid sequence, and it is these features that are not subject to variation by mutation processes. These features are undoubtedly the content of one third of glycine and a regular alternation of polar and apolar sequence regions giving rise to the correct charge pattern along the polypeptide chains.

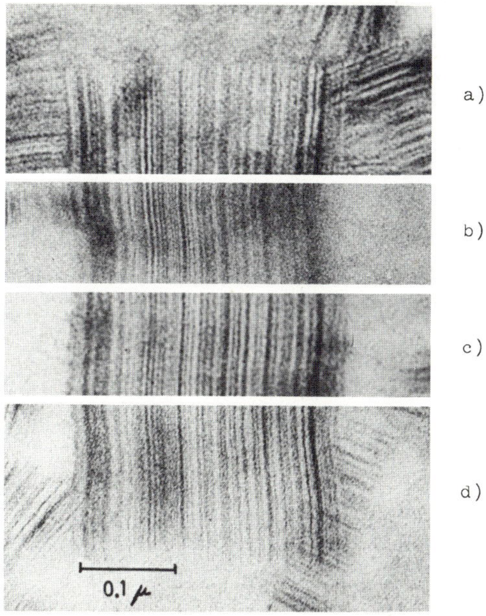

Fig. 5. Electronmicrographs of segments-long-spacing of various collagens. (a) collagen from the mesogloea of Actinia equina, (b) collagen from Fasciola hepatica, (c) collagen from carp swim bladder, (d) collagen from calf skin (courtesy of Prof. K. Kühn). Positive staining with phosphotungstic acid and uranylacetate.

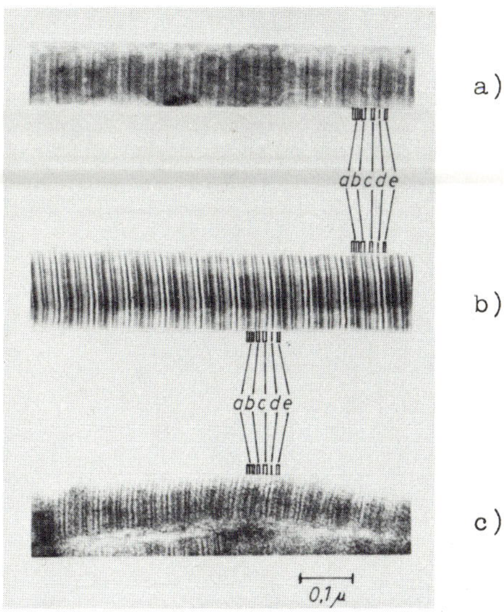

Fig. 6. Electronmicrographs of fibrils of various collagens. (a) fibril of Helix pomatia collagen, (b) calf skin collagen fibril (courtesy of Prof. K. Kühn), (c) fibril of Fasciola hepatica collagen. Positive staining as in Plate V.

To summarize, two main points of the evolution of globular proteins have been verified for collagen as a model of structural proteins: 1) the subunit chains are of homologous sequence [as already shown by Kühn, Tkocz, Zimmerman and Beier (1965), and Tkocz and Kühn (1969), for the α_1- and α_2-chains of calf skin collagen]; 2) the constancy of a certain configuration was the limiting factor for evolutionary processes.

ACKNOWLEDGEMENTS

We gratefully acknowledge the assistance of Dr. Beier and Mrs. Strauch in the ultracentrifugal experiments and the help and advice of Dr. Kühn, Mrs. Wiedemann and Mrs. Scholz with regard to electronmicroscopy.

REFERENCES

Fietzek, P. (1965). Thesis, University of Heidelberg.

Franzblau, C., Seifter, S. and Gallop, P.M. (1964). Biopolymers 2, 185

Fujii, T. (1965). In Biochimie et Physiologie du Tissu Conjonctif, p. 461. Ed. by Comte, P. Lyon.

Fujii, T. (1969). Z. Physiol. Chem. 350, 1257.

Fujimoto, D. and Adams, E. (1964). Biochem. Biophys. Res. Comm. 17, 437.

Gross, J. (1963). In Comparative Biochemistry, vol. 5, p. 307. Ed. by Florkin, M. and Mason, H.S. Academic Press, New York.

Josse, J. and Harrington, W.F. (1964). J. Mol. Biol. 9, 269.

Kühn, K., Fietzek, P. and Kühn, J. (1966). Biochem. Z. 344, 418.

Kühn, K., Tkocz, Ch., Zimmermann, B. and Beier, G. (1965). Nature 208, 685.

Maser, M.D. and Rice, R.V. (1962). Biochim. Biophys. Acta 63, 255.

Nordwig, A. (1962). Das Leder 13, 10.

Nordwig, A. and Hayduk, U. (1967). J. Mol. Biol. 26, 351.

Nordwig, A. and Hayduk, U. (1969). J. Mol. Biol. 44, 161.

Piez, K.A. (1967). In Treatise on Collagen, Vol. 1: Chemistry of Collagen, p. 207. Ed. by Ramachandran, G.N. Academic Press, New York.

Pikkarainen, J. and Kulonen, E. (1967). Scand. J. Clin. Lab. Invest., Suppl. 95, p. 40.

Rigby, B.J. (1968). Nature 219, 166.

Rubin, A.L., Drake, M.P., Davison, P.F., Pfahl, D., Speakman, P.T. and Schmitt, F.O. (1965). Biochemistry 4, 181.

Tkocz, Ch. and Kühn, K. (1969). Europ. J. Biochem. 7, 454.

ISOLATION AND CHARACTERIZATION OF POLYMERIC COLLAGEN FROM COMPLEX CONNECTIVE TISSUES

F.S. Steven

Extraction of young animal skins with dilute solutions of neutral salts of acetic acid led to the purification and isolation of tropocollagen. Tropocollagen has now been studied in great detail by both physical and chemical techniques, with the result that we have a fairly clear picture of its molecular structure. Physicochemical studies on neutral salt soluble tropocollagen indicate that a single molecular species exists in solution, whereas in acetic acid soluble tropocollagen a small percentage of dimers and trimers of the basic tropocollagen monomer molecule are also present.

In mature tendon and skin, the quantity of acetic acid soluble tropocollagen is greatly reduced, in fact for human tissue only 2-5% of the total tissue collagen is soluble as tropocollagen. The remaining 95-98% of the tissue collagen is often referred to as "insoluble collagen". As this is the bulk of the mature tissue collagen, it seems essential that this insoluble collagen be purified and studied in as much detail as tropocollagen. The purpose of the present review is to describe the techniques which have been employed to purify these insoluble collagens from a variety of complex human and bovine connective tissues.

One of the most unusual approaches to the isolation of native insoluble collagen fibrils has recently been reported by McClain (1969). In this procedure, insoluble collagen fibrils from muscle were obtained after disintegrating the muscle at -20°C and passing the muscle powder through a series of sieves. No chemical data have so far been presented to substantiate the claim that this process produces pure collagen. It seems that this sieving process would provide the basic raw material for further purification of muscle collagen by some of the procedures to be described later in this paper.

Veis (1969) and his colleagues have isolated very fine micro-fibrils of collagen from bovine skin by homogenising the tissue in dilute acetic acid and collecting these micro-fibrils in the supernatant fraction after centrifuging. Rubin et al. (1963) and Drake, Davison, Bump and Schmitt (1965) employed an exhaustive neutral salt extraction followed by acetic acid extraction procedure to remove tropocollagen and noncollagenous proteins from mature skin. The swollen residue was centrifuged and the upper layer of swollen collagen fibrils was collected and described by these and later workers as "insoluble collagen". In our experience this insoluble collagen contains rather too much hexosamine to be classed as pure collagen (see Table I).

Nishihara (1962) began two studies on the solubilisation of collagen; the first procedure employed crude bacterial α-amylase in a pretreatment of skin wastes followed by swelling of the treated skin in hydrochloric acid and thermal denaturation to yield a commercially valuable gelatin. The second procedure (Nishihara and Miyata, 1962) involved the thermal denaturation of hide collagen followed by trypsin digestion and extraction of the degraded collagen in 0.1 M acetic acid at 25°C. The extract was further treated with pepsin and the solubilised collagen warmed at neutral pH to form reconstituted collagen fibrils. Although both of these procedures yielded nearly 100% recovery of the original insoluble collagen, as a gelatin in the first procedure, or as reconstituted fibrils in the second procedure, the initial native type fibrils had been denatured and degraded either by HCl treatment or by the proteolytic enzymes.

My objective has been to isolate native type fibrils of pure collagen in high yields by procedures which did not involve chemical or thermal degradation. It seemed that the crude bacterial α-amylase procedure initiated

TABLE I

Carbohydrates Associated with Collagen Preparations
(Grant and Jackson 1968)

	Hexosamine*	Hexose*
Crude tropocollagen	4.26	19.89
Alcohol purified tropocollagen	0.33	9.84
"Insoluble collagen" prepared by the Drake et al. (1966) procedure	6.64	22.78
EDTA treated polymeric collagen	3.87	11.75
Crude α-amylase treated polymeric collagen	0.85	6.37

*Expressed as units per 3000 amino acid residues.

by Nishihara (1962) offered a great opportunity to achieve this aim, provided that the collagen fibrils could be swollen and extracted without the use of HCl.

Adult human tendons were treated with crude bacterial α-amylase (Steven, 1962; Steven and Jackson, 1967) followed by dispersion of the collagen fibrils in dilute acetic acid and isolation of the collagen in 80-100% yield after centrifugation at 300g followed by raising the pH to 7.0 with NaOH or by raising the ionic strength with saturated NaCl solution. Collagen fibrils prepared in this manner can be further purified by repeated dispersion in acetic acid followed by precipitation with NaCl at pH 3.5.

At this point it is essential to realise that the collagen fibrils isolated by the crude bacterial α-amylase procedure are <u>not</u> "reconstituted collagen fibrils" in the sense that the latter are formed by the physical association of tropocollagen monomers under certain conditions of pH, temperature and ionic strength. The α-amylase prepared collagen fibrils are highly cross-linked polymers of tropocollagen (Steven, 1966). A few properties of these fibrils may serve to indicate the main differences between these fibrils which I have termed "polymeric collagen" (PC) and reconstituted collagen fibrils:

1) A dispersion of PC fibrils in dilute acetic acid can be drawn out in the form of a visible fibre.

2) PC fibrils in dilute acetic acid, when placed on an electron microscope grid and shadow cast with gold-palladium have the typical appearance of clean native collagen fibrils of varying diameters (Fig. 1). Under these conditions reconstituted collagen fibrils redissolve as monomeric tropocollagen.

3) PC fibrils stained at pH 4.0 with PTA have the typical appearance of native type fibrils (Fig. 2).

4) PC fibrils from mature human tendon, when boiled for 1 hr at pH 7, yield only 2-8% soluble gelatin, although thermal shrinkage takes place. Reconstituted collagen fibrils yield 100% soluble gelatin under these conditions of denaturation.

5) After extensive degradation with enzymes, NaOH and hydroxylamine, followed by thermal denaturation, mature tendon PC still retains enough cross-linkages to resist complete solubilisation as a gelatin (Steven, 1966).

6) Treatment of PC fibrils with N HCl results in the unwinding of a mass of "protofibrils" (Fig. 3) (Chapman and Steven, 1966; Steven and Jackson, 1967). These protofibrils (Fig. 3) appear to be 4-5 collagen molecules thick and may correspond to the "limiting microfibrils" described by Veis (1969) in his studies on bovine skin.

The mechanism by which crude bacterial α-amylase enables PC to be isolated remains unknown. Pure α-amylase has no action. The enzyme content of the crude α-amylase is difficult to determine because a large percentage by weight of the preparation is carbohydrate and not easily

Legends for Figures 1-3.

All samples of polymeric collagen were obtained from adult human Achilles tendon by the crude bacterial α-amylase procedure. The polymeric collagen fibrils were dispersed in 0.2 M acetic acid and placed on the electron microscope grids before staining as follows: Plate 1. gold-palladium shadow; Plate 2. positive staining with 1% phosphotungstic acid pH 4.0; Plate 3. the grids containing fibrils were momentarily dipped in 1 N HCl, washed exhaustively with water and then stained with 1% phosphotungstic acid.

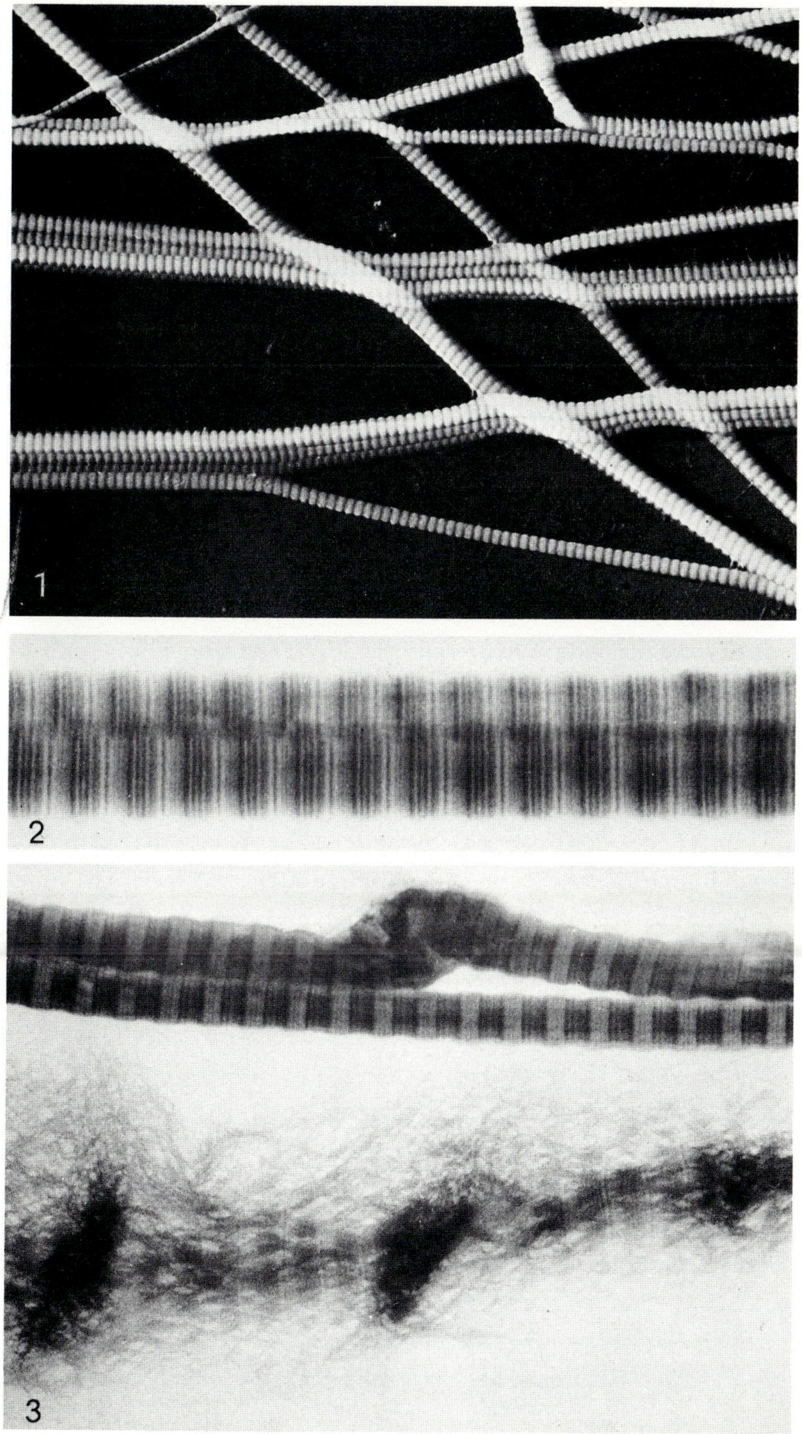

4

removed from the enzymes. So far nine carbohydrases have been identified (Muzaffar, 1968). These carbohydrases were identified as follows:

α - glucosidase (EC 3,2,1,20)
β - glucosidase (EC 3,2,1,21)
α - galactosidase (EC 3,2,1,22)
β - galactosidase (EC 3,2,1,23)
α - mannosidase (EC 3,2,1,24)
β-D-N - acetylaminodeoxyglucosidase (EC 3,2,1,30)
β - xylosidase (EC 3,2,1,37)
α - L - fucosidase
β - L - fucosidase

Hyaluronidase (EC 3,2,1,34,35) was not present. There appears to be very little (if any) protease present as judged by attack on gelatin, denatured ovalbumin and haemoglobin.

Analysis of the carbohydrate content of α-amylase prepared PC fibrils (Table 1) indicated only traces of amino sugars and the expected quantity of hexoses (Grant and Jackson, 1968). A low amino sugar content is perhaps the best criterion of a highly purified collagen; a similar amino sugar content for tropocollagen was obtained after an alcohol fractionation procedure. Since this highly purified tropocollagen contained amino sugar content similar to that of α-amylase prepared PC, it is clear that the enzymes have not selectively removed amino sugars from the collagen fibrils, but have removed amino sugar-containing impurities which were associated with the PC in the original tissue. It is also possible that crude α-amylase treatment may have split off a small quantity of hexose from collagen fibrilles.

It has often been suggested that the effective enzyme in the crude α-amylase preparation is a proteolytic enzyme. Two observations suggest that any proteolytic attack during the crude α-amylase digestion has no effect on the collagen fibrils. The telopeptides released by pepsin digestion of tropocollagen and polymeric collagen are identical (Steven, 1965); it would therefore seem unlikely that the PC had been subjected to prior proteolytic attack since the telopeptide regions are most susceptible to attack and would be cleaved off. Secondly, the amount of soluble gelatin obtained by denaturing PC is greatly increased by prior treatment with proteolytic enzymes, whereas untreated PC from aged tendon yields only 2-6% gelatin.

A second procedure has been developed for the isolation of PC fibrils without the prior treatment with crude α-amylase. This procedure employed 4% ethylenediamine tetra acetate (EDTA) pH 7.4 followed by dispersion of PC in dilute acetic acid (Steven, 1967). The content of amino sugars in EDTA PC fibrils is rather higher than in the crude α-amylase prepared PC (Table I), but even so this level is comparable with purified tropocollagen prior to the alcohol fractionation step.

It seems clear that an understanding of the chemistry involved in the conversion of monomeric tropocollagen to the native fibrils may be achieved by studying highly purified collagen fibrils such as PC which can be prepared in an undegraded form. It is also conceivable that PC fibrils could be employed in the preparation of materials which might be used for tissue replacement.

The biological age of a tissue greatly influences the type of PC fibrils which are obtained after crude α-amylase or EDTA extraction procedures. For example young calf extensor tendon and foetal human Achilles tendon yield PC fibrils which are very swollen in dilute acetic acid and which are difficult to collect after neutralisation by rotation of a metal spatula; the fibrils are better collected by gentle centrifugation. These young PC fibrils appear in the electron microscope to be less compact than aged fibrils, and show large numbers of protofibrils which have unwound from the PC fibrils during acetic acid extraction. The young PC fibrils appear similar to HCl treated PC fibrils obtained from mature tendon (Plate 3).

TABLE II

Isolation of Polymeric Collagen Fibrils from Various Connective Tissues

Type	Tissue	Species	Procedure	Yield of polymeric collagen (%)
(A)	Bladder	B	Acetic acid	90
	Intestinal submucosa	H.B.	Acetic acid	90-100
(B)	Tendon	H.B.	α or EDTA	90-100
	Ligament	B	α	80-90
	Sclera	H.B.	α or EDTA	90
	Cornea	H.B.	α or EDTA	90
	Aorta	B	α	90
	Skin	H.B.	α or EDTA	80-90
(C)	Intervertebral disc	H	α	40
	Articular cartilage	H	α	10
(D)	Intercostal cartilage	H	α	2
	Decalcified bone	H.B.	α or EDTA	0

H indicates adult human tissue and B indicates 3-year-old bovine tissue; α indicates prior treatment with crude bacterial α-amylase; EDTA indicates prior treatment with EDTA.

Different connective tissues within the same subject vary enormously in their functions, the compositions of their proteins and protein polysaccharide complexes and also in their abilities to yield PC fibrils after treatment with either crude α-amylase or EDTA. I would like to discuss some of these differences observed in the tissue listed in Table II and offer some suggestions as to why some tissues do not readily yield PC fibrils.

In the simplest connective tissues which we have examined, to date, no pretreatment is necessary. Homogenized and salt extracted bovine bladder, when extracted with 0.2 M acetic acid, yields almost all its collagen as dispersed

PC fibrils. This collagen is highly pure by amino acid analysis and it would appear that the fibrils in the original bladder were very loosely held by the interfibrillar matrix. In a similar manner human intestinal submucosal collagen can be prepared by salt and acetic acid extraction from postmortem material. These PC fibrils are highly purified and possess remarkable stability towards solubilisation during autoclaving. Submucosal PC fibrils can be autoclaved at neutral pH for 12 hr at 30 lbs/sq. in. with the formation of only 6% soluble gelatin (Steven, Jackson, Schofield and Bard, 1969a). It may well be that immediately after death the enzymes of the submucosal cells release the PC fibrils in a manner similar to crude bacterial α-amylase. In the case of bovine intestinal submucosa, obtained from a freshly slaughtered animal, it is extremely difficult to strip off the submucosal cells from the collagen layer of the intestine. On the other hand, if the tissue is allowed to stand at 20°C for 12 hr, the submucosal cells can easily be removed and the PC fibrils extracted in acetic acid without pretreatment with crude α-amylase.

It is worth noting that both bovine and human tendon and skin will not yield PC fibrils after standing for several days at 20°C; a pretreatment with the enzyme or EDTA is necessary. Good yields of PC fibrils can be obtained from the following tissues: tendon, skin, ligamentum nuchae, aorta, sclera, cornea and knee joint synovial membrane after crude α-amylase or EDTA pretreatment. The salt extraction procedure is a particularly important first step when the EDTA procedure is used for skin PC.

The third group of tissues yield very limited amounts of PC fibrils after EDTA or crude α-amylase pretreatment, for example intervertebral disc and articular cartilage yield 40% and 10% PC respectively. In each case the tissue swells well in acetic acid but does not readily release PC fibrils into a dispersion. The unextracted PC remains firmly associated with sulphated polysaccharide (Steven, Jackson and Broady, 1968; Steven, Broady and Jackson, 1969b).

This situation is even more pronounced in intercostal cartilage from which 2% PC can be obtained. Very recent work from this laboratory indicates that the presence of the sulphated proteoglycan complexes present in both the disc and cartilage prevent the dispersion of PC fibrils in dilute acetic. The PC can be released from the glycosaminoglycan by digestion with trypsin at 37°C for 1 hr. The failure of the crude α-amylase to release PC from these tissues compared to the ease with which PC can be extracted after the subsequent trypsin digestion, would again suggest that the crude α-amylase does not depend for its action on a protease.

EDTA-decalcified human bone appears to be a very special type of collagen. After a series of pretreatment involving EDTA, crude α-amylase and trypsin, the decalcified bone does not swell significantly in 0.2 M acetic aicd and no PC fibrils could be dispersed from this material. The method of alternate freezing and thawing (Glimcher, Katz and Travis, 1965) for the isolation of collagen was also found to be useless with this material. The results of this survey of the connective tissues are presented in Table II.

If we then consider the problems of isolating PC fibrils, four separate stages are involved:

(1) thorough washing of the tissue with NaCl and NaH_2PO_4 pH 5.3;

(2) pretreatment with either crude bacterial α-amylase or with EDTA;

(3) swelling of the treated tissue with 0.2 M acetic acid; and

(4) dispersion of PC fibrils in 0.1 M acetic acid followed by isolation.

ACKNOWLEDGEMENT

I wish to thank Dr. J.A. Chapman of the Biophysics Unit, (Rheumatism Research Centre, Manchester) for the electron micrographs presented in Plates 1, 2 and 3.

REFERENCES

Chapman, J.A. and Steven, F.S. (1966). In Biochemie et Physiologie du Tissu Conjonctif, p. 265. Ed. by Comte, P. Lyon.

Drake, M.P., Davison, P.F., Bump, S. and Schmitt, F.O. (1965). Biochemistry 4, 181.

Glimcher, M.J., Katz, E.P. and Travis, D.F. (1965). J. Ultrastructural Res. 13, 163.

Grant, M.E. and Jackson, D.S. (1968). Biochem. J. 108, 587.

McClain, P.E. (1969). Nature 221, 184.

Muzaffar, T.Z. (1968). M.Sc. Thesis, University of Manchester.

Nishihara, T. (1962). Japanese Patent 9295/62.

Nishihara, T and Miyata, T. (1962). Collagen Symposium 3 Collagen Society of Japan. 84.

Rubin, A.L., Drake, M.P., Davison, P.F., Pfahl, D., Speakman, P.T. and Schmitt, F.O. (1963). Biochemistry 4, 181.

Steven, F.S. (1962). Ann. Rheumatic Dis. 23, 300.

Steven, F.S. (1965). Biochem. Biophys. Acta 97, 465.

Steven, F.S. (1966). Biochem. Biophys. Acta 130, 190, 196, 202.

Steven, F.S. (1967). Biochem. Biophys. Acta 140, 532.

Steven, F.S., Broady, K. and Jackson, D.S. (1969b). Biochem. Biophys. Acta 175, 225.

Steven, F.S. and Jackson, D.S. (1967). Biochem. J. 104, 534.

Steven, F.S., Jackson, D.S. and Broady, K. (1968). Biochem. Biophys. Acta 160, 435.

Steven, F.S., Jackson, D.S., Schofield, J.D. and Bard, J.B.L. (1969a). Gut 10, 484.

Veis, A. (1969). This book, p.279.

MATURATION RELATED CHANGES OF THE PROTEIN MATRIX OF BONE

Ch. M. Lapiere and B.V. Nusgens

Bone is a very heterogenous connective tissue in which most of the collagen fibres are calcified. The architecture and the metabolism of such a tissue is related with the homeostasis of calcium in the body fluid and the requirement of bone as a structural framework. These two functions are made possible by three highly synchronized basic mechanisms, synthesis, maturation and degradation of the collagen and the mineral salts. These processes lead to the formation of a complex tissue in which the various units have different structure, composition, properties and rate of metabolism.

Bone is made of blood vessels around which the collagen fibres are orderly arranged, trapping the cells which produce them. The mineral is initially deposited in the light bands of the collagen fibrils (unstained areas on electron microscopic pictures)(Fitton Jackson, 1957) and the number of crystals increases with time in maturing bone (Quinaux, 1968). A continuous process of remodeling, tunneling of mature bone and deposition of new mineralizing tissue, introduces a great deal of heterogeneity at the tissue level. Compact bone is formed of units (osteons or lamellae) displaying various degrees of mineral density (Davies and Engstrom, 1954). Using tetracycline labeling or isotope tracing with bone-seeking elements, these various units of bone have been shown to display different levels of metabolic activity (McLean and Rowland, 1963; Frost, 1969). It would not be surprising that the different properties of these units of bone are a possible consequence of a modification of their composition at the molecular level.

As for any other connective tissue, the ideal fractionation technique would be one that permits the isolation of the collagen fibrils and the additional compounds which determine their structure and properties. We want to show that density fractionation is the procedure which allows the closest approach to this goal, as compared with other methods used for bone fractionation. It will be demonstrated that obvious changes in the structure, metabolism, composition and properties of the protein matrix of a mineralizing tissue occurs during the process of maturation.

I TECHNIQUES FOR FRACTIONATING BONE

All the methods for preparing or fractionating the organic matrix of a mineralized connective tissue depend on one or the other or a combination of the three basic operations: selective removal, fractionated solubilization and density fractionation.

a. Selective removal of the mineral components of the tissue, using diluted acids or chelating agents, ethylenediamine tetra-acetic acid (EDTA), is a frequently used technique in the preparation of samples of the organic matrix of bone. It must be kept in mind that the decalcifying solution of bone contains free amino acids, nucleotides and a certain amount of peptides.

b. Fractionated solubilization is not a very useful technique for studying bone. Except for the bone of newborn rats (Mills and Bavetta, 1966; Kao, Vernier and McGavack, 1965) and lathyritic animals (Tanzer and Gross, 1964; Miller, Martin, Piez and Powers, 1967) no significant amount of native collagen can be collected by extraction. Complete and intact polypeptides ("native gelatin") can be extracted from bone after denaturation of the collagen. The yield is low in normal bone and much larger in lathyritic animals. Bone collagen seems to be highly cross-linked, therefore explaining its low degree of extractibility in normal animals (Miller et al., 1967). The various polypeptides collected from chick bone have been shown to be similar in amino acid composition to those extracted from various other connective tissue in the same animal (Piez et al., 1969). The extent of lysine hydroxylation which initially is high, decreases with advancing age to values found in the collagen of other tissues (Miller et al., 1967).

c. Density fractionation as compared to other procedures is less disruptive in regard to the relationship between the organic and the mineral components of the calcified tissue. Considered at the tissue level, bone is composed of a mosaic of units of various degrees of mineralization as demonstrated by microradiography (Rowland, Jowsey and Marshall, 1959). A technique (Herman and Richelle, 1961) has been devised to fractionate such a tissue into samples of identical degree of calcification by sedimentation in organic solvents of suitable density. Similar results can be obtained by microdissection of individual osteons (Ascenzi and Fabry, 1959) but this technique is much too time consuming.

Using the density fractionation technique in rats, Richelle, Onkelinx and Aubert (1966) and Richelle (1967) have described bone as a population of connective structures undergoing progressive mineralization. Correlated with[^{45}Ca] blood kinetics they have defined that the age of a particle of bone is directly related to its specific gravity.

The technique of Herman and Richelle (1961) has been slightly modified to allow a better recovery of the fractionated samples. It has been applied to the study of the organic matrix of the diaphyseal bone of the rat. All the long bones from the legs are collected and after two extractions in ethanol, they are completely freed of the adhering muscle, tendon and periosteum. The diaphyses are collected between the lines of insertion of the periarticular muscles, the medulla is removed and the cortical is ground in a steel mortar until the particles pass through a 70-mesh screen. They are further reduced to a finer powder (size 5 to 10 μ measured with a microscope) by passing twice through a specially designed grinder formed of two conical carborundum surfaces turning at high speed in a cooled chamber.

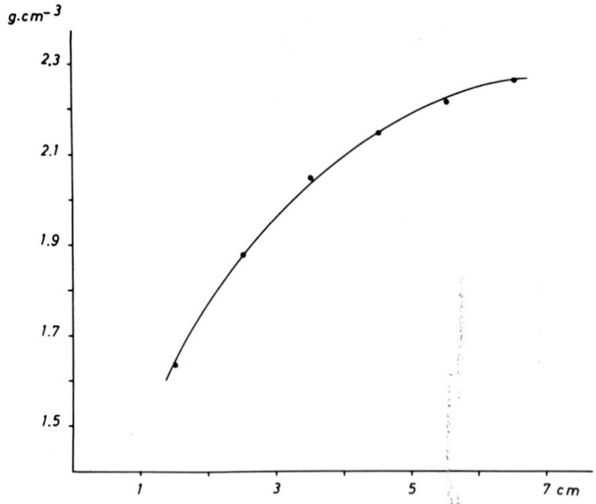

Fig. 1. Variation in specific gravity of the mixture of bromoform and toluene (gxcm^{-3}) as a function of the length of the tube (cm).

A continuous gradient of a mixture of bromoform and toluene is prepared in 35-ml polyallomer centrifuge tubes fitting the swinging bucket rotor (SW25) of a Spinco ultracentrifuge. The density of the gradient as a function of the length of the tube is illustrated in Fig. 1. The shape of the gradient has been determined in such a way that the lightest fractions which are less abundant would be concentrated in the rapidly increasing part of the gradient. More detail in the heaviest and more abundant fraction can be obtained in the slowly increasing denser part of the gradient. The overall specific gravity of the fluid to be used, the mixture of bromoform and toluene, depends on the specific gravity of the samples of bone to be analysed. It can be calculated using the data of Biltz and Pellegrino (1969) or the data of Rowland et al. (1959) reporting the concentration of apatite per unit volume in bone of various animal species.

Between 100 mg and 750 mg of the powdered bone are uniformly laid down through a screen on the top of the gradient. It is covered with 3 mm of distilled water. After 30 min of centrifugation at 10,000 rpm, the bone particles are equilibrated in the gradient.

The floating layer of material at the junction between the water and the organic solvent is removed and referred to as the fraction lighter than 1.50 g cm^{-3} (<1.50) and the organic gradient is collected by aspiration from the top, in fractions of the following specific gravity in g cm^{-3}, 1.50 to 1.86, 1.87 to 2.05, 2.06 to 2.19 and heavier than 2.19. A volume of ethanol is added to each fraction and the bone particles are collected by centrifugation. After washing twice with ethanol the bone samples are dried in air at room temperature. The recovery varies between 92 and 96%.

II THE HETEROGENEITY OF BONE

A. TISSUE STRUCTURE

The growth curve of the diaphyseal bone of female Wistar rats between the ages of 6 weeks and 2 years is presented in Fig. 2. The distribution of the density fractions of bone from young animals, growing rapidly and older animals growing more slowly is detailed in Table I. It is obvious that the compact bone of the youngest animals contains more of the fractions of the lowest densities and less of the heaviest fractions than the bone of the eldest animals. There is no more apparent variation in distribution between the two eldest groups. The occurrence of 90% of the bone in the fraction of high specific gravity in the eldest animals corresponds well with the microradiographic aspect of the diaphyseal bone of such rats (Fig. 3). It is obvious that there is little variation in the density of the various units, lamellae and pseudo haversian osteons, as opposed to what can be seen in the bone from other animal species (Rowland et al., 1959).

The technique of density fractionation has also been used for studying human bone with a gradient ranging from 1.4 to 2.2 gr cm^{-3}. The distribution of the density fractions of the cortical bone of adult man is quite similar to that of adult rat but in the spongiosa the proportion of the lightest fractions is much larger.

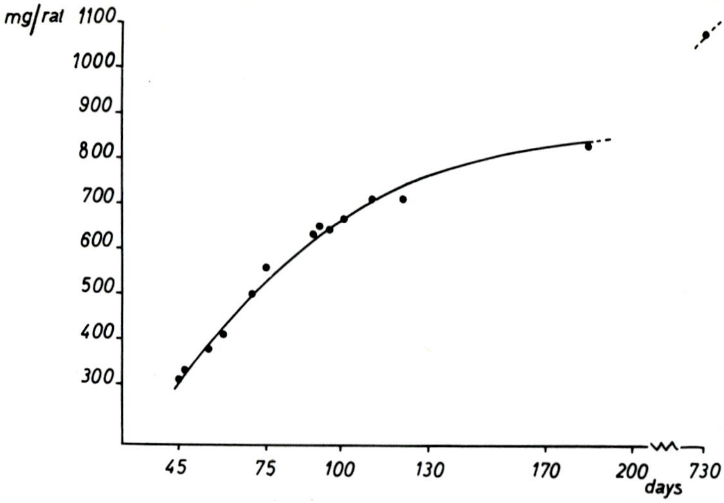

Fig. 2. Weight of cortical bone from the legs of rats (mg/rat) ranging in age from 45 to 730 days (days).

TABLE I

Fractionated Diaphyseal Bone Ponderal Distribution as a Function of Age*

AGE (days)	<1.50	1.50 to 1.86	1.87 to 2.05	2.06 to 2.19	>2.19
45	1.29	1.09	17.8	78.0	1.4
75	0.72	0.97	15.4	80.6	2.4
90	0.57	0.10	17.9	78.1	3.4
110	0.28	0.07	8.5	84.1	7.1
175	0.41	0.07	0.52	91.1	7.9
195	0.47	0.11	0.53	92.1	6.8

*All the values are expressed in percent of the total amount of bone recovered after density fractionation.

In the rat and probably in other animal species, the age of the animals is therefore a factor responsible for some variation in the overall composition of bone at the tissular level. There also exist differences in the

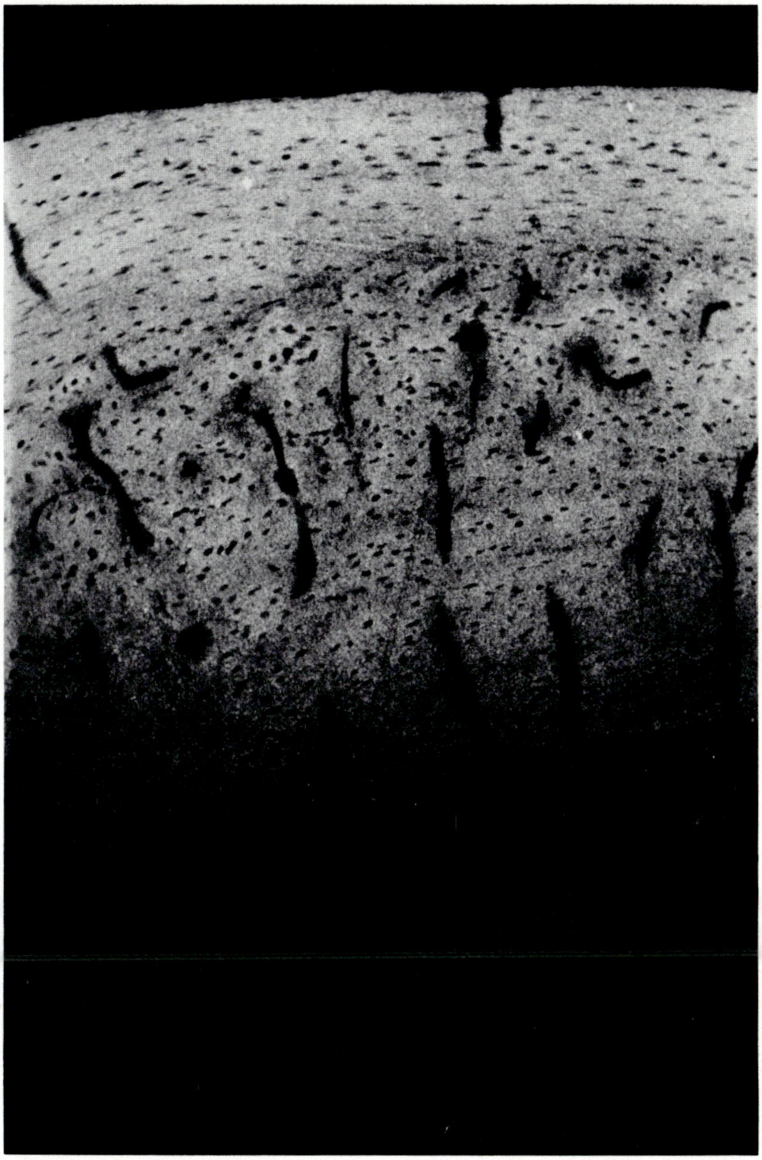

Fig. 3. Microradiograph of a transverse section in the cortex of a femur of a one year old rat. Note the presence of dense bone and some kind of osteons. Microradiograph was made by Dr A. Dhem, Louvain.

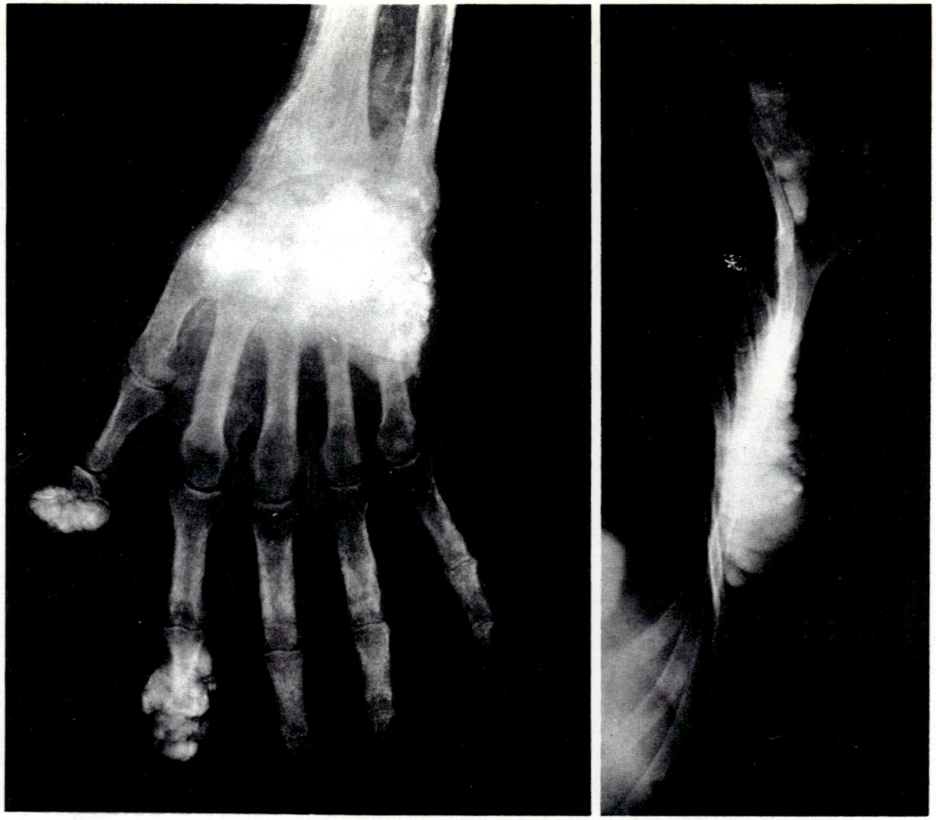

a) b)

Fig. 7.a,b. X-ray photograph of the right hand (a) and the left side of the thorax (b) of a patient suffering from tumoral calcinosis. Note the presence of large calcified subcutaneous masses and the arterial calcifications in the blood vessels of the hand.

structure of bone when comparing animal species and in the same animal when comparing bones of various texture. These variations in the structure of bone as defined by the specific gravity of their basic units, correspond to different rates of metabolism and changes in composition and properties.

B. METABOLISM

1. The rate of synthesis, degradation and maturation of the collagen matrix of bone has been measured in rats of various ages. As described earlier (Lapiere et al., 1966), in young growing female rat, only one out of seven collagen molecules synthesized in cortical bone is used for building up the mineralized connective tissue. A large proportion of the newly synthesized collagen as expected, is initially located in the least calcified fraction. With time passing and mineralization progressing, the peak of labeled molecules is found in fractions of increasing specific gravity. When a precursor of the collagen and labeled calcium arc injected simultaneously the maturation of the collagen matrix defined by its increase in specific gravity, parallels that of the calcium.

Some of the labeled collagen is deposited in already heavily mineralized fractions but it is rapidly removed. Such a turnover of the collagen, depending probably on the metabolic activity of the osteocytes, accounts for a large part of the early degradation of this protein in growing bone.

As demonstrated further, only the uncalcified or lesser calcified collagen fibres of non-demineralized bone are susceptible to degradation by bacterial collagenase. Fractionated bone labeled in vivo for 2 or 48 hr with $[^3H]$proline and then treated with collagenase, released a large proportion of its $[^3H]$hydroxyproline containing material as illustrated in Fig. 4. The susceptibility of the labeled collagen diminishes with increasing density. The proportion of label released from bone of animal injected for 48 hr is larger than after 2 hr. The susceptibility of the collagen to collagenase lysis and the high proportion

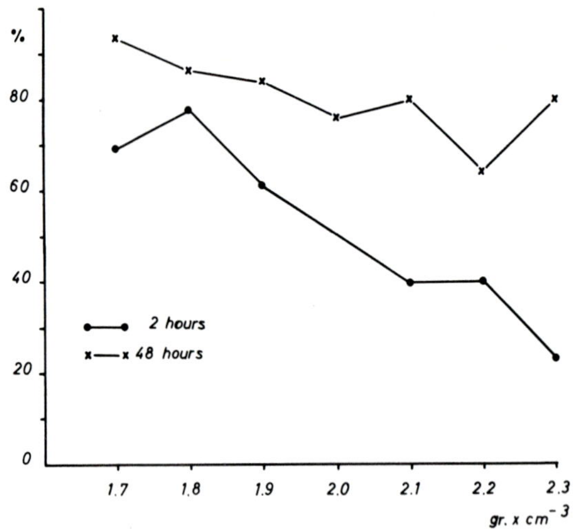

Fig. 4. The[^{3}H]hydroxyproline released by collagenase is expressed in percent (%) of the[^{3}H]hydroxyproline contained in nondemineralized bone fractions obtained at various specific gravities (g cm^{-3}). For explanation, see text.

of[^{3}H]hydroxyproline removed indicate the occurrence of nonmineralized newly synthesized molecules in all the density fractions. The lower proportion of the labeled collagen susceptible to collagenase after two hr is probably due to its intracellular location.

When fractionated bone labeled by[^{3}H]proline injected 2 or 48 hr before collection of the samples is demineralized in diluted acid, in the cold, the proportion of the[^{3}H]hydroxyproline extracted and dialyzable is larger in the densest fraction after 48 hr and greater after 48 hr than after 2 hr (Fig. 5).

Since the newly synthesized collagen is rapidly transformed in dialyzable peptides it can be assumed that it is degraded shortly after its synthesis. Such a situation occurs mainly in the bone fractions of high specific gravity.

2. If a nucleating substance is required for initiating the crystallisation of the calcium salts in bone, a phosphorus bound to the organic part of the matrix seems to be a valid candidate. It could be found in a fraction of bone displaying a high turnover rate for collagen and organic phosphorus.

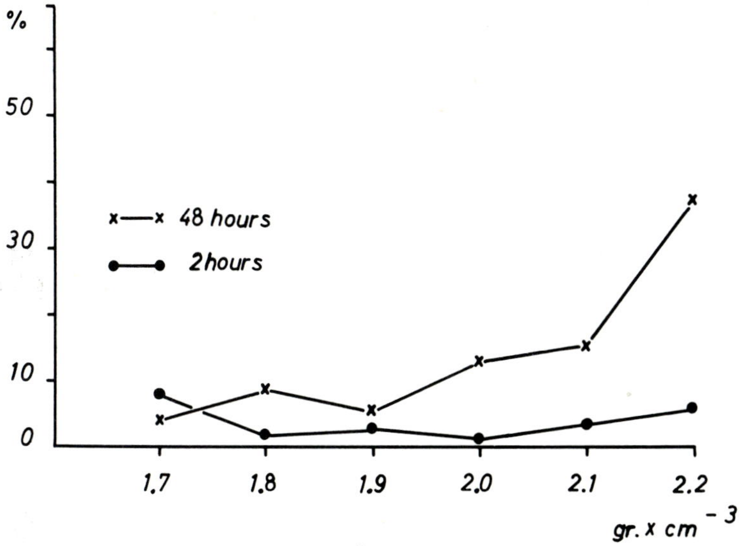

Fig. 5. The dialysable [^{3}H]hydroxyproline is expressed in percent (%) of the ^{3}H hydroxyproline contained in fraction obtained at increasing specific gravities (g cm^{-3}). For explanation see text.

TABLE II

Specific Radioactivity of [^{32}P]and [^{3}H]Hydroxyproline in Fractionated Bone

Isotope	Tissue Fraction	Time between administration of isotope and death of the animal: 2 hours L*	M*	H*	48 hours L	M	H
[^{32}P]	EDTA extract	265	387	76	251	459	101
	Collagenase peptides	72	302	168	146	553	119
	Residue	777	535	195	1199	1068	437
[^{3}H]Hypro	EDTA extract	2599	1705	1479	1379	1236	337
	Collagenase peptides	622	469	32	1008	1449	100
	Residue	6558	6144	472	5860	2878	1399

*L stands for the fraction of low specific gravity up to 1.86 g cm^{-3}, M for medium 1.87 to 2.05 and H for high, above 2.06 g cm^{-3}.

Bone labeled in vivo with [^3H]proline and [^{32}P], for 2 and 48 hr, was fractionated and the density fractions were demineralized in EDTA at neutral pH, extracted in organic solvents to remove phospholipids and in 8 M urea saturated in NaCl at 100°C to remove nucleic acids, before being submitted to enzyme degradation with bacterial collagenase. The specific radioactivity of the phosphorus and the hydroxyproline were determined in each of the subfractions. The results are reported in Table II.

The highest value of specific radioactivity of the hydroxyproline and the phosphorus in the residue after collagenase treatment indicates the occurrence of newly synthesized collagen which is protected from the action of the enzyme. It could represent intracellular polypeptides which are associated with a phosphorus of high specific radioactivity. Little labeled phosphorus is associated with the collagen peptides of the fraction of low density although it is obvious from the specific radioactivity of the hydroxyproline of this fraction that it contains some of the extracellular newly formed collagen. The EDTA extract contains collagen fragments arising from the degradation of a certain proportion of the recently synthesized hydroxyproline. Some labeled phosphorus might be associated with peptides of the kind reported by Leaver and Shuttleworth (1966) but the bulk of it arises from the inorganic phosphate composing the mineral phase of bone. Little can be said about its rate of labeling except that the lightest fractions (L and M) are more labeled than the densest one (H).

From these observations on the rate of turnover of various compounds it can be concluded that the different parts of the bone matrix as well as the inorganic component of bone fractionated by gradient density display a rate of metabolic activity which is inversely related to their specific gravity. The progression of mineralization represents, therefore, an index of a process of maturation characterized in part by a reduction of the rate in the turnover of various components.

TABLE III

The Proteins in the Various Density Fractions of Bone

N°	Specific gravity at which frations were separated g cm^{-3} range	mean	Total protein mg g^{-1}	% extracted in EDTA	Protein (noncollagen) mg cm^{-3}	Collagen mg cm^{-3}
0	<1.50	1.41	438	8.8	297	321
1	1.50 to 1.86	1.68	314	7.7	182	346
2	1.87 to 2.05	1.96	238	6.3	107	359
3	2.06 to 2.19	2.12	175	3.3	33	338
4	>2.19	2.25	165	3.3	42	329

C. PROTEIN COMPOSITION

Beside collagen, each of the gradient density fractions contains a certain amount of amino acids and peptides which can be partially extracted in the EDTA solution used for decalcifying the samples.

In Table III, the amount of protein (noncollagen) and collagen is reported in milligram per unit volume (cm^3) of the various specific gravity fractions for the bone of 50-day-old rats. These data are calculated from the values of the amino acids contained in the EDTA extracts and the decalcified protein matrices hydrolysed in 6 N HCl for 24 hr under nitrogen at 108°C. The analyses were performed in a "Unichrom" Beckman amino acid analyzer using an adaptation of the single column procedure of Miller and Piez (1966) for the M 82 spherical resin of Beckman, Munich. Decalcification of the bone fraction is made by extraction in the cold using 0.1 M sodium EDTA, pH 7.5, in an amount equal to twice that of the calcium in the sample. The EDTA extract is filtered through a 0.45 μ Millipore filter and acidified to pH 1 by HCl. After removing the precipitated EDTA the samples are dried and hydrolysed.

The proportion of protein (noncollagen) extracted

TABLE IV

Amino Acid Composition of Decalcified Bone Fractions
(Residues per 1000 residues)

	FRACTIONS				
	0	1	2	3	4
Hydroxyproline	53	66	76	89	85
Aspartic acid	74	62	53	49	51
Threonine	38	30	23	20	23
Serine (a)	52	45	40	36	38
Glutamic acid	90	82	77	72	76
Proline	77	102	117	121	122
Glycine	191	260	310	320	321
Alanine	93	101	105	102	104
Half cystine	8	3	2	1	-
Valine (b)	45	36	29	24	25
Methionine (c)	16	7	7	6	5
Isoleucine	27	21	15	12	13
Leucine	67	49	36	30	30
Tyrosine	18	10	7	5	5
Phenylalanine	28	20	12	14	14
Hydroxylysine	5	9	11	11	11
Lysine	52	36	26	27	24
Histidine	17	9	4	10	7
Arginine	49	51	50	51	46

The number of the fraction is that of Table III.
(a) - not corrected for loss during hydrolysis.
(b) - not corrected for incomplete release.
(c) - including methionine sulfoxides.

with EDTA and the amount of protein in milligram per cm^3 are larger in the lightest fraction and diminish with increasing specific gravity. Contrary to that observation, the quantity of collagen per cm^3 does not vary significantly with the specific gravity of the sample.

The loss of polypeptidic material accompanying the collagen as a function of increasing calcification is vious from the observation of the amino acid composition of the decalcified protein matrix (Table IV). The amount of hydroxyproline, proline, glycine and hydroxylysine increase up to maximum values, which are close to those found in purified collagen. The reduction of the proportion of acidic amino acids, threonine and serine, valine and leucine and the aromatic compounds as well as the complete elimination of cystine indicates that polypeptides rich in these amino acids are eliminated. It could be some of these compounds which are extracted in EDTA but not all of them as we do not find cystine in the extract (Table V). Furthermore the decalcifying solution contains several unknown ninhydrin positive compounds (X1 to X5) which are not present in the decalcified matrix. X1 is not retarded on the column and could be among other compounds, cysteic acid, phosphoserine or phosphothreonine, X2 elutes shortly after phosphoethanolamine, X3 is a compound which gives an absorption maximum at 570 mμ in the ninhydrin reaction and is eluted between proline and glycine. X4 has the same chromatographic behaviour as lysinonorleucine and X5 elutes shortly after ornithine. It could be significant that the concentration of X2 increases in the extract with increasing specific gravity.

In general, the amino acid composition of the fractions obtained with EDTA extraction shows a progressive change from the light fraction (0) to the heaviest one (4). It is possible that the fractions represent a mixture of one or more peptide components rich in glycine, alanine, glutamic acid and X2 (Table V).

From the isotope studies it can be concluded that the densest bone is approximately 1 month older than the bone of the lowest specific gravity, in 50-day-old rats. The densest bone would have been formed at age 20 days and the lightest one at 50 days. Although there are differences in the overall proportion of hydroxylysine the samples when corrected for the presence of noncollagen proteins, we find no modification in the proportion of this hydroxylated amino acid in the collagen. Rat bone in this respect does not seem to be comparable to chicks

TABLE V

Amino Acid Composition of the EDTA Extract of Fractionated Bone

(Residues per 1000 Residues)

	FRACTIONS				
	0	1	2	3	4
X1 (a)	7	18	26	31	35
X2 (a)	31	47	94	139	138
Hydroxyproline	-	tr	20	39	tr
Aspartic acid	86	94	71	61	56
Threonine	50	39	37	29	18
Serine (b)	59	55	56	50	45
Glutamic acid	111	142	152	112	115
Proline	47	45	43	47	47
X3 (a)	13	24	14	30	12
Glycine	136	209	189	177	307
Alanine	87	72	81	83	83
Half cystine	-	tr	tr	-	-
Valine (c)	56	36	29	28	26
Methionine (d)	17	5	6	1	6
Isoleucine	31	16	15	14	12
Leucine	69	41	34	27	30
Tyrosine	5	13	2	5	2
Phenylalanine	25	16	9	8	8
Hydroxylysine	-	tr	tr	tr	tr
X4 (a)	-	-	-	26	9
X5 (a)	9	20	14	27	16
Lysine	81	59	53	28	11
Histidine	21	17	22	16	5
Arginine	59	32	33	22	19

The number of the fraction is that of Table III.
(a) - calculated with reference values of the next amino acid - see text.
(b) - uncorrected for loss during hydrolysis.
(c) - uncorrected for incomplete release.
(d) - includes methionine sulfoxides.

where the hydroxylation of lysine diminishes with aging (Miller et al., 1967). In rat bone collagen, the hydroxylation of lysine is twice as abundant than in the collagen of the skin or the tail tendon and, therefore, it is similar in this respect to the youngest chick bone collagen.

D. ENZYME DEGRADATION

There has been much controversy over whether or not decalcification of bone precedes the removal of the matrix. The various degrees of mineralization of the fractions obtained after gradient density fractionation provide us with a tool to study the effect of mineralization on the enzyme susceptibility of the collagen in non-demineralized bone. In these studies we have used a purified bacterial collagenase at slightly alkaline pH (7.2) in order to avoid changes in the mineral crystals associated with the matrix.

a) The decalcified collagen matrix of any of the density fractions is equally susceptible to bacterial collagenase. It is lysed to dialysable peptides up to 90%.

b) In absence of decalcification, 80% of the collagen matrix of the least mineralized fractions is lysed to dialysable peptides by an excess of bacterial collagenase. The most mineralized bone fractions are only slightly broken down by the enzyme. The density fractions between these two extremes are lysed to an extent which is inversely related to their degree of calcification (Fig. 6) with a sharp transition around a specific gravity of 2.0 g cm^{-3}.

In this property, enzyme susceptibility, bone is also composed of a population of structures displaying different behaviour. This is due to the presence of the mineral crystals since the decalcified matrix of all the fractions is equally susceptible to the enzyme.

From the results of these experiments one can postulate that mineral removal is required before lysis of the organic matrix when a fully calcified connective tissue is

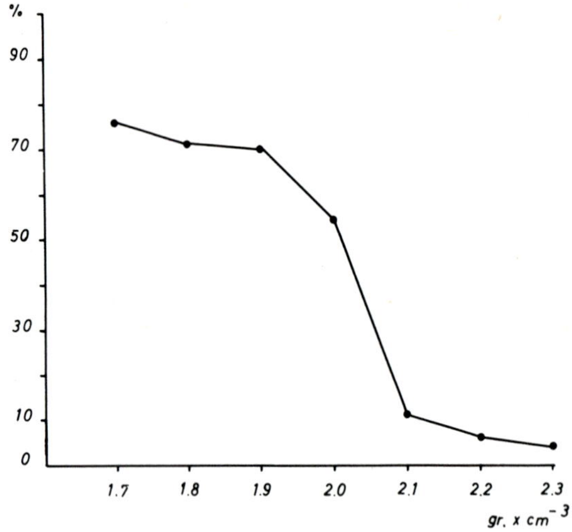

Fig. 6. The proportion (%) of collagen lysed by collagenase is inversely related to the specific gravity (g cm^{-3}) at which the fraction was obtained in nondemineralized bone.

TABLE VI

Comparison of Some Components of an Ectopic Calcification and Bone*

Components	Ectopic calcification	Bone
Organic matter and structural water	31	27
Protein	9	20.2
Collagen	0.1	19.8
Ca	25.9	24.0
P	13.1	11.5
Hexosamines	0.37	0.25
Uronic acids	0.38	-

*All the data are expressed in milligrams per 100 mg of dessicated material.

removed in vivo.

III THE PROTEIN MATRIX OF A DERMAL CALCIFICATION.

The physical and chemical study of the content of a large calcified cystic mass in a patient suffering from a renal failure and secondary parathyroid adenomas provided us with some information on the possible meaning of the non-collagen polypeptide moiety of calcified tissue. The clinical story of this patient (Lapiere, Nusgens, Quinaux and Declercp, (1968) consists mainly in the rapid development of many large dermal calcified masses, calcification of the blood vessels (Fig. 7a and b) and fatal renal failure.

Under local anesthaesia we collected 30 grams of a creamy mixture contained in a fibrous cyst located on the side of the thorax (Fig. 7b). The composition of this product is illustrated in Table VI.

The size of the crystals has been measured by X-ray diffraction and the infrared absorption spectra have been recorded before and after heating at 900°C. Both of these parameters have been found to be very similar to those of the mineral of bone (Table VII).

The suspension of crystals has been fractionated by repeated extractions in cold 0.15 M NaCl and the remaining crystals were divided into two fractions of low (L) and high (H) specific gravity by gradient density fractionation. The major proportion of the organic material (75%) sediments with the crystals.

The amino acid composition of the polypeptides extracted with the saline and those associated with the crystals seems to be related one to the other as can be seen from the data of Table VIII. The main difference lies in the absence of cystine in the material extracted with saline while this amino acid and also methionine are present or more concentrated in the heaviest fraction (H). Various ninhydrin positive compounds non-retarded on the column (X1) or eluting with the amino acids (Xs), some similar to those found in the EDTA extract of bone, were

TABLE VII

Comparison of Some Physical Parameters of the Crystals of an Ectopic Calcification and Bone

	Ectopic calcification	Bone
Crystal size (1)	± 250 Å	± 250 Å
Calcium salts (2)	Ca carbonate apatite β TCP after heating	Ca carbonate apatite β TCP after heating
Ca/P	1.99	2.07

(1) - measured by the width of the (002) X-ray diffraction band with the technique of Quinaux (1968).

(2) - results from the infrared absorption spectra - β TCP = β tricalcium phosphate (Quinaux, 1968).

also present in significant amounts.

The amino acid composition of the polypeptides associated with the crystals is clearly incompatible with the presence of a significant amount of collagen or elastin. Since we know that collagen is not susceptible to enzyme degradation in a fully calcified tissue, the heavy fraction displaying a degree of calcification larger than that of the most calcified fraction of human bone, it is highly improbable that it has served as a nucleating agent and was lysed after the formation of the crystals. We can conclude, therefore, that crystals similar to those in bone can be formed in the absence of collagen. We suggest that the polypeptide moiety that is associated with the mineral salts represents the nucleating and/or the regulating substances.

IV DISCUSSION

The maturation of the collagen in soft connective tissue introduces changes in the structural relationship of the molecules in the fibres. The formation of inter-

TABLE VIII

Aminoacid Composition of the Protein in an Ectopic Calcification

(Residues per 1000 residues)

	FRACTIONS		
	S*	L*	H*
X1 (a)	3	5	1
Hydroxyproline	tr	tr	tr
Aspartic acid	125	118	114
Threonine	70	61	61
Serine (b)	75	72	70
Glutamic acid	136	143	139
Proline	64	64	57
Glycine	71	74	70
Alanine	104	87	85
Half cystine	-	-	26
Valine (c)	90	68	65
Methionine (d)	1	tr	10
Isoleucine	29	32	34
Leucine	113	97	100
Tyrosine	3	2	5
Phenylalanine	6	4	10
Hydroxylysine	-	tr	tr
Lysine	61	85	73
Histidine	tr	25	23
Arginine	23	43	43
Xs (a) (e)	26	20	14

(a) - calculated with reference values of the next neighbor aminoacid.
(b) - uncorrected for loss during hydrolysis.
(c) - uncorrected for incomplete release.
(d) - including methionine sulfoxides.
(e) - sum of unknown ninhydrin positive compounds eluting between hydroxyproline and arginine.
*S stands for the saline extract, L for the fraction of low specific gravity and H for the heaviest fraction.

molecular covalent crosslinks cooperates with this modification to reduce the extractibility of native molecules. Such a progressivity in the maturation of the collagen does not seem to occur in bone. In opposition to what is found in soft connective tissue under normal conditions, crystals of calcium salts are deposited inside of the collagen fibrils of bone and the load of mineral per unit amount of collagen increases as a function of the maturation of the tissue. Depending upon these two features a technique different from that used for soft connective tissues had to be devised in order to study maturation-related changes in the protein matrix of bone.

We described in detail the procedure for fractionation of bone in homogenous samples of calcified structure of similar degree of mineralization. Such fractions are related to the process of maturation of the organic matrix since we have shown that the bulk of the isotope labeled collagen is deposited as a fraction of low specific gravity undergoing a progressive calcification, shifting the location of the labeled molecules in fractions of increasing density. Due to the deposition of the calcium salts, some properties of the protein matrix are modified. This modification can be the result of an indirect effect viz. the collagen matrix is no longer susceptible to enzyme degradation because of the presence of crystals, or a direct effect viz. the modification of the noncollagen polypeptidic material associated with the collagen fibres.

The amount of collagen per cm^3 of newly formed poorly calcified or fully calcified bone is identical in all the fractions within experimental errors. In the youngest fraction of bone, that of low specific gravity, the proportion of noncollagen polypeptides in the protein matrix is much larger than in the fully calcified bone. The amino acid composition of these associated peptides is somewhat similar to that of the material extracted in EDTA. The change in amount of noncollagen protein matrix as a function of increasing calcification is represented by a large variation in the mass of these polypeptides. The difference between the two lowest consecutive density fractions might be due to the presence of blood vessels, free cells and various non-osseous constituents in the lowest density fraction since it contains all the structures which are not calcified. Such an explanation does not hold for the further reduction in protein concentration between the little and the more heavily calcified structures. This loss progresses as the mineralization of the calcifying structures.

Assuming that 50% of the volume of fully calcified bone is occupied by the mineral crystals (Robinson and Stuart, 1957; Biltz and Pellegrino, 1969) when a cm^3 of newly formed noncalcified bone matrix becomes completely mineralized it looses a space equal to one half of a cm^3 containing around 200 mg of protein. Such a high protein concentration, 400 g/liter is much too large to represent serum proteins of the extracellular fluid. Thus the deposition of the mineral crystals occurs in a compartment of high protein concentration, probably some structural proteins which are degraded during maturation. These "structural components" might initiate or regulate the deposition of minerals in the calcified tissue, while the amount of collagen fibres, per unit volume of tissue space, remains constant.

Since we have shown that under pathological conditions in the human, crystals similar to those found in bone are formed in the absence of collagen, we feel that such a protein or peptide material might be related to mineral nucleation and/or the regulation of crystals growth and remodelling which occur in bone (Quinaux and Richelle, 1967). It seems to be required to explain the process of calcification in bone when knowing that the basic fibrous collagen molecules seems to have an amino acid sequence similar to that found in noncalcified connective tissue (Piez et al., 1968) and taking into consideration the fact demonstrated by Glimcher, Hodge and Schmitt, 1957, showing the calcifiability of purified collagen isolated from various noncalcified connective tissues.

REFERENCES

Ascenzi, A. and Fabry, C. (1959). J. Biophys. Biochem. Cytol. 6, 139.

Biltz, R.M. and Pelligrino, E.D. (1969). J. Bone & Joint Surg. 51A, 456.

Davies, H.G. and Engstrom, A. (1954). Exp. Cell Res. 7, 243.

Frost, H.M. (1969). Calc. Tiss. Res. 3, 211.

Glimcher, M.J., Hodge, A.J. and Schmitt, F.O. (1957). Proc. Nat. Acad. Sci. 43, 860.

Herman, H. and Richelle, L. (1961). Bull. Soc. Chim. Biol. 43, 273.

Fitton Jackson, S. (1957). Proc. Roy. Soc. (London) B146, 270.

Kao, K.Y.T., Vernier, C.M. and McGavack, T.H. (1965). Proc. Soc. Exptl. Biol. Med. 119, 584.

Lapiere, Ch.M., Nusgens, B., Quinaux, N. and Declercp, A. (1968). Arch. Belges Dermat. Syphil. 24, 153.

Lapiere, Ch.M., Onkelinx, C. and Richelle, L.J. (1966). In Biochimie et Physiologie du Tissu Conjonctif. Ed. by Comte, P. Sté Ormeco et Imprimerie du Sud-Est à Lyon, Publ. 505.

Leaver, A.G. and Shuttleworth, C.A. (1966). Archs Oral Biol. 11, 1209.

McLean, F. and Rowland, R.E. (1963). In Mechanisms of Hard Tissue Destruction. A.A.A.S. 371.

Miller, E.J., Martin, G.R., Piez, K.A. and Powers, M.J. (1967). J. Biol. Chem. 242, 5481.

Miller, E.J. and Piez, K.A. (1966). Anal. Biochem. 16, 320.

Mills, B.G. and Bavetta, L.A. (1966). J. Gerontol. 21, 449.

Piez, K.A., Bladen, H.A., Bornstein, P., Butler, W.T., Kang, A.H., Lane, J.H. and Miller, E.J. (1968). Brookhaven Symp. Biol. 21, 345.

Quinaux, N. (1968). Thesis, University of Liège.

Quinaux, N. and Richelle, L.J. (1967). Israel J. of Med. Sci. 3, 677.

Richelle, L.J. (1967). Thesis, University of Liége.

Richelle, L.J., Onkelinx, C. and Aubert, J.P. (1966). In 3d European Symposium on Calcified Tissues. Ed. by Fleisch, H., Blackwood, J.J. and Owen, M. Springer Verlag, Publ. 123.

Robinson, R.A. and Stuart, R.E. (1957). J. Bone and Joint Surg. 39-A, 167.

Rowland, R.E., Jowsey, J. and Marshall, J.H. (1959). Radiation Research 10, 234.

Tanzer, M.L. and Gross, J. (1964). J. Exp. Med. 119, 275.

COMPARATIVE STUDIES ON THE CHEMISTRY AND CHAIN STRUCTURE OF COLLAGEN

E. Kulonen and J. Pikkarainen

There is no reason why collagen should be an exception from the evolution of proteins. However, the number of the acceptable mutations is much more restricted by the rigid secondary structure than in globular proteins. As a protein collagen is "young" when compared to most of the intracellular proteins, which also has limited the possible variation.

We wish to summarize our work on the comparative aspects on the chemistry of collagen (Pikkarainen and Kulonen, 1965; Pikkarainen, Rantanen and Kulonen, 1966; Pikkarainen and Kulonen, 1967; Pikkarainen, 1968; Pikkarainen et al., 1968). It was based on and partly inspired by previous knowledge on the composition of collagen (Eastoe and Leach, 1958; Gross, 1963; Eastoe, 1968), which has been related especially with the thermal stability of collagen (Gustavson, 1956; Josse and Harrington, 1964; Harrington and Rao, 1967; von Hippel, 1967).

It is generally accepted that every third residue in collagen must be glycine and that the amount of imino acid residues is correlated rather well with the thermal stability of collagen, assessed either as the denaturation or as the shrinking temperature. Thermal stability is related to the body temperature of the species both in the vertebrates and invertebrates (Nordwig, 1968). There is a certain lower limit in the content of imino acids, necessary to keep collagen as a helix at 0°C (von Hippel and Wong, 1963). The lowest imino acid content and denaturation temperatures are recorded in ice-fish, which live in almost ice-cold water (Rigby, 1968). We believe that during adaptation to higher body temperatures there are several independent evolutionary lines in collagen, each pointing toward a higher imino acid content. This is an example of a convergent evolution.

Eastoe long ago pointed out (Eastoe, 1957) that the number of hydroxy amino acid residues is constant in most collagens, but this fact has been disregarded in structural considerations and in model-building. This issue also has been clouded by the fact that collagen of certain worms has an exceptional amount of hydroxyl groups both as hydroxyproline and as serine and threonine (Maser and Rice, 1962). Rigby (1967) suggested that there was some inverse correlation between the thermal stability and serine content.

I AMINO ACID COMPOSITION

The findings mentioned above were confirmed by our studies on collagen extracted with acidic buffers and purified exhaustively by repeated precipitations. The charge profile of reconstituted SLS particles under the electron microscope, prepared by one of us (J.P.) in Prof. Kühn's laboratory, was similar throughout the investigated series (Nordwig and Hayduk, 1967). Bornstein (1968) suggests that variation is possible mostly in the non-helical regions, but their spacing seems to be constant.

We compiled a series of comparisons of amino acid compositions (Table I). The constancy of hydroxy-amino acids is confirmed, with the exception of the earthworm (Lumbricus). The increase of content of imino acids during the course of evolution is especially distinct in the homothermic species. The content of aliphatic hydroxy-amino acids, serine and threonine, complements the imino acids fairly closely. The amino acids mentioned: proline, serine and threonine, plus alanine, differ in the genetic code by the first letter only, so that single base mutations can produce these changes. These amino acids take approximately the same space in the secondary structure, and the position of the

TABLE I

Amino Acid Contents of Collagen from Various Animals

Group of amino acids	Man	Monkey	Pig	Chick	Frog	Flounder	Dogfish	Rayfish	Hagfish	Lamprey	*Loligo*	*Mytilus*[5]	*Lumbricus*	*Metridium*
Hydroxy amino acids[1]	143	136	154	148	148	152	146	170	165	152	159	163	290	180
Serine+threonine	49	47	53	46*	78	85	71	101	98	81	70	86	136	86
Imino acids	222	225	223	212*	167	166	171	145	154	173	150	147	164	137
Imino acids+Ser+Thr+Ala	374	382	387	385	367	371	361	343	368	375*	312	321	397	295
Nonpolar amino acids[2]	653	673	650	648	655	656	642	611	651	647*	614	597	509	563
Acidic amino acids[3]	115	104	118	120	117	105	114	114	109	116*	154	158	150	162
Basic amino acids[4]	88	91	86	87	83	90	101	108	78	89	93	85	51	107

[1]Hypro+Thr+Ser+Tyr+Hylys; [2]Pro+Gly+Ala+Val+Met+Ileu+Leu+Phe; [3]Asp+Glu; [4]Hylys+Orn+Lys+His+Arg; [5]byssus-threads

*The asterisks indicate marked differences between the adjacent groups. The contents are expressed as residues/1000. The data are based on the amino acid analyses by Pikkarainen (1968) and Pikkarainen et al. (1968), except those on man, monkey and *Loligo* (unpublished data).

hydroxyl group is rather similar. Table II shows the same comparison extended to imino acids and thermal stability. The ratio of imino acids to the sum of serine and threonine is the most sensitive index of this evolutionary trend (Fig. 1). It would be expected from these conclusions that proline is hydroxylated preferentially in such positions of the peptide chain which carried the hydroxyl of serine or threonine at the earlier stages of development.

There is no difference between invertebrates and vertebrates in the hydroxy or imino acids but a characteristic dissimilarity can be located in the acidic amino acids (Table I). The amino acid composition suggests that the complementary amino acid would be alanine or, at least a nonpolar amino acid. Whether the amino acid compositions can be related to the capacity to form bone remains to be studied. Collagen of certain lower animals, for example the sea anemone (Metridium), contains abundant hydroxylysine, but generalizations cannot be made. The presence of cystein is common in invertebrate collagen.

We tried to assess the overall differences between the amino acid composition of collagen of various species. This was done by totaling the differences observed within every

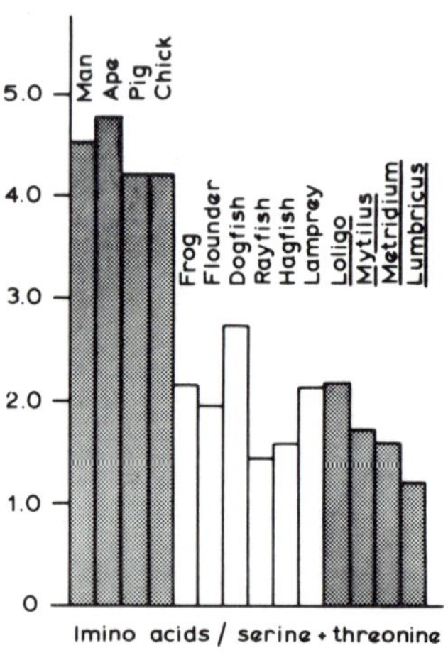

Fig. 1. Ratio of imino acids to serine+threonine in collagens from various species.

TABLE II

Relation of Hydroxy and Imino Acids to the Thermal Stability of Citrate-soluble Collagen

Origin of collagen	Hydroxyproline	Threonine	Serine	Total Hydroxy residues	Imino acid residues
Rayfish	61	30	71	170	145
Hagfish	62	27	71	165	154
Flounder	63	20	65	152	166
Lamprey	66	23	58	152	173
Lumbricus	151	52	84	290	164
Metridium	70	39	47	180	137
Dogfish	72	25	46	146	171
Loligo	70	26	44	159	150
Frog	65	22	56	148	167
Man	91	18	31	148	222
Chick	99	19	27	148	212

The origins of collagen are listed in order of the increasing T_D-values of collagen. Cf. legend of Table I.

pair of species on each amino acid, but disregarding the hydroxylation of proline and lysine. If the contents of individual amino acids are expressed as residues per thousand, the sum of the differences would be 2000 maximally, if all the amino acids were different. The figure is too small because it does not include the mutually cancelling differences in the amino acid sequence. Nevertheless, we think that it reflects the number of mutations when their total number is low. In many proteins this kind of comparison would be too superficial, but a similar approach has been tried with certain success (Metzger, Shapiro, Mosiman and Winton, 1968). With collagen this procedure seems to produce meaningful results (Table III). The order of amino acid composition follows the morphological taxonomy, as expected. Encouraged by this observation, we attempted to align the species on a plane (Fig. 2) on the basis of

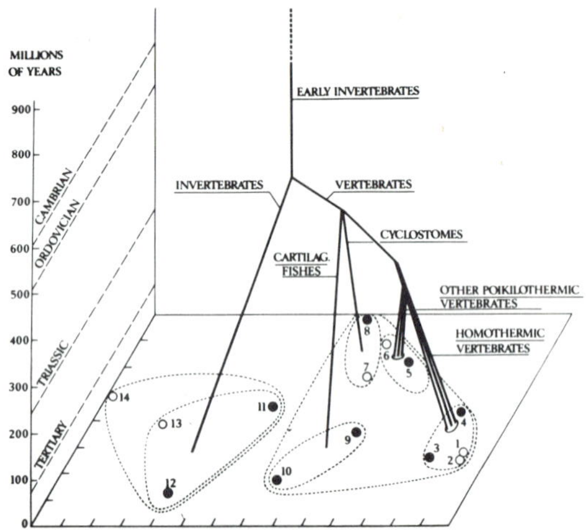

Fig. 2. Summary on the evolution of collagen. The differentiation of the α chains in homothermic and certain poikilothermic vertebrates is indicated. The location of the species on the horizontal plane is based on the differences in the amino acid compositions as explained in the text. Key to numbering: 1 man, 2 monkey (Cercopithecus), 3 pig, 4 chick, 5 frog, 6 flounder, 7 lamprey, 8 hagfish, 9 dogfish, 10 rayfish, 11 squid, 12 sea mussel (Mytilus), 13 sea anemone (Metridium), 14 earthworm (Lumbricus).

TABLE III

Differences in the Amino Acid Composition of Collagen from Various Species

(Cf. legend of Table I.)

Species	Man	Monkey	Pig	Chick	Frog	Flounder	Dogfish	Rayfish	Hagfish	Lamprey	Loligo	Mytilus*	Lumbricus	Metridium
Man	-	-	-	-	-	-	-	-	-	-	-	-	-	-
Monkey	41	-	-	-	-	-	-	-	-	-	-	-	-	-
Pig	43	45	-	-	-	-	-	-	-	-	-	-	-	-
Chick	76	83	71	-	-	-	-	-	-	-	-	-	-	-
Frog	166	162	165	142	-	-	-	-	-	-	-	-	-	-
Flounder	200	191	195	170	62	-	-	-	-	-	-	-	-	-
Dogfish	142	146	127	114	116	134	-	-	-	-	-	-	-	-
Rayfish	196	220	205	214	180	182	108	-	-	-	-	-	-	-
Hagfish	240	233	241	226	104	72	170	170	-	-	-	-	-	-
Lamprey	166	169	165	138	54	60	94	166	96	-	-	-	-	-
Loligo	186	210	207	208	150	182	136	136	178	148	-	-	-	-
Mytilus*	247	273	246	273	234	282	197	163	276	250	151	-	-	-
Lumbricus	278	312	275	292	238	271	230	199	268	255	214	180	-	-
Metridium	276	294	269	282	259	290	196	181	297	266	137	132	213	-

*Byssus-threads

differences in amino acid composition, and assuming that these differences are proportional to the number of mutations in collagen. The differences had to be adjusted to fit into a network; this was done with an electronic computer by minimizing the sum of squares of the necessary changes expressed proportionally. In this way we obtained "coordinates" for 8 species (shown by black dots on the horizontal plane in Fig.2). The others were fitted by dividers with reference to the nearest computer-calculated points. It is the advantage of this presentation that more comprehensive evolutionary schemes could be constructed, with time as the third axis. Collagen of the earthworm (Lumbricus), occupies a special position on the "map" and it may not belong to this scheme at all but to another family of collagens. We also tried to include data available from the literature. Unfortunately, the results were not consistent, which partly is accounted for by analytical differences.

The same procedure as demonstrated in Table III was applied to specific groups of amino acids, for example, on aliphatic hydroxy-amino acids (Table IV) to demonstrate the gap between the homo- and poikilothermic animals. The difference between vertebrates and invertebrates is shown analogously on the basis of the acidic amino acids (Table V).

It is our belief, the evolution of collagen did not necessarily concur with the evolution of other chemical constituents or with the morphological features. Thus, classifications cannot be based on a single morphological characteristic or protein. For example, hagfish and lamprey differ in collagen more than expected from the morphological similarity. The evolutionary pattern of the various parameters is quite diffuse, especially within the group of bony fishes.

II CHAIN STRCUTURE

Analogous comparative calculations were applied to the various chains of tropocollagens, relying entirely on published values of the amino acid composition (Table IV). (Pikkarainan and Kulonen, 1969)

TABLE IV

Differences in the Contents of Serine+threonine in Collagens from Various Species

(Cf. legend of Table I)

Species	Man	Monkey	Pig	Chick	Frog	Flounder	Dogfish	Rayfish	Hagfish	Lamprey	*Loligo*	*Mytilus**	*Lumbricus*	*Metridium*
Man	-	-	-	-	-	-	-	-	-	-	-	-	-	-
Monkey	2	-	-	-	-	-	-	-	-	-	-	-	-	-
Pig	4	6	-	-	-	-	-	-	-	-	-	-	-	-
Chick	3	1	7	-	-	-	-	-	-	-	-	-	-	-
Frog	29	31	25	32	-	-	-	-	-	-	-	-	-	-
Flounder	36	38	32	39	7	-	-	-	-	-	-	-	-	-
Dogfish	22	24	18	25	7	14	-	-	-	-	-	-	-	-
Rayfish	52	54	48	55	23	16	30	-	-	-	-	-	-	-
Hagfish	49	51	45	52	20	13	27	3	-	-	-	-	-	-
Lamprey	32	34	28	35	3	4	10	20	17	-	-	-	-	-
Loligo	21	23	17	24	8	15	1	31	28	11	-	-	-	-
*Mytilus**	37	39	33	40	8	1	15	16	13	5	16	-	-	-
Lumbricus	87	89	83	90	58	51	65	35	38	55	66	51	-	-
Metridium	37	39	33	40	8	1	15	16	13	5	16	0	51	-

*Byssus-threads.

TABLE V

Differences in the Contents of Acidic Amino Acids in Collagens from Various Species

(Cf. legend of Table I.)

Species	Man	Monkey	Pig	Chick	Frog	Flounder	Dogfish	Rayfish	Hagfish	Lamprey	Loligo	Mytilus*	Lumbricus	Metridium
Man	-	-	-	-	-	-	-	-	-	-	-	-	-	-
Monkey	12	-	-	-	-	-	-	-	-	-	-	-	-	-
Pig	3	15	-	-	-	-	-	-	-	-	-	-	-	-
Chick	5	17	2	-	-	-	-	-	-	-	-	-	-	-
Frog	2	14	1	3	-	-	-	-	-	-	-	-	-	-
Flounder	10	2	13	15	12	-	-	-	-	-	-	-	-	-
Dogfish	1	11	4	6	3	9	-	-	-	-	-	-	-	-
Rayfish	1	11	4	6	3	9	0	-	-	-	-	-	-	-
Hagfish	6	6	9	11	8	4	5	5	-	-	-	-	-	-
Lamprey	1	13	2	4	1	11	2	2	7	-	-	-	-	-
Loligo	39	51	36	34	37	49	40	40	45	38	-	-	-	-
Mytilus*	43	55	40	38	41	53	44	44	49	42	4	-	-	-
Lumbricus	35	46	32	30	33	45	36	36	41	34	5	9	-	-
Metridium	47	58	44	42	45	57	48	48	53	46	8	4	12	-

*Byssus-threads.

TABLE VI

Differences in the Amino Acid Composition of the Different Chains in Collagens of Various Species

Species	$\alpha 1$ vs. $\alpha 2$	$\alpha 1$ vs. $\alpha 3$	$\alpha 2$ vs. $\alpha 3$
Calf	126	53	82
Chick	124	23	129
Cod	76	36	60
Species	**$\alpha 1$ vs. $\alpha_{Myx.}$**	**$\alpha 2$ vs. $\alpha_{Myx.}$**	**$\alpha 3$ vs. $\alpha_{Myx.}$**
Mammals	262	240	265
Birds	256	212	259
Bony fishes	146	119	104

Piez, Eigner and Lewis, 1963; Bornstein and Piez, 1964; Heidrich and Wynston, 1965; Piez, 1965; François and Glimcher, 1967a,b; Paz, Salazar and Gaite, 1967.
$\alpha_{Myx.} = \alpha$ chain of collagen from hagfish (Myxine glutinosa).

Even if the data of various authors differ considerably, we believe that some conclusions can be drawn. The chains developed divergently, but $\alpha 3$ chain resembles $\alpha 1$ more than $\alpha 2$ chain. The collagen of mammals and birds differs more from hagfish collagen than does collagen from bony fishes. During the course of evolution there was a tendency toward development of stable forms, as indicated by the increasing ratio of imino acids to serine+threonine, which is higher in the $\alpha 1$ and $\alpha 3$ chains than in the $\alpha 2$ chain. The $\alpha 1$ and $\alpha 3$ chains are more stable than $\alpha 2$ which is reflected also in their higher thermal stability (Hollmén and Kulonen, 1964) and in the slower metabolic turnover (Heikkinen and Kulonen, 1968).

This divergent development suggests a triple-helix composed of similar chains in the ancestral collagen analogous to the evolution of myoglobin and hemoglobin. Indeed, the results of gel electrophoresis and column chromatography on carboxymethyl cellulose suggest that the chains in the available soluble collagens from invertebrates—lamprey, hagfish, rayfish and dogfish—have only

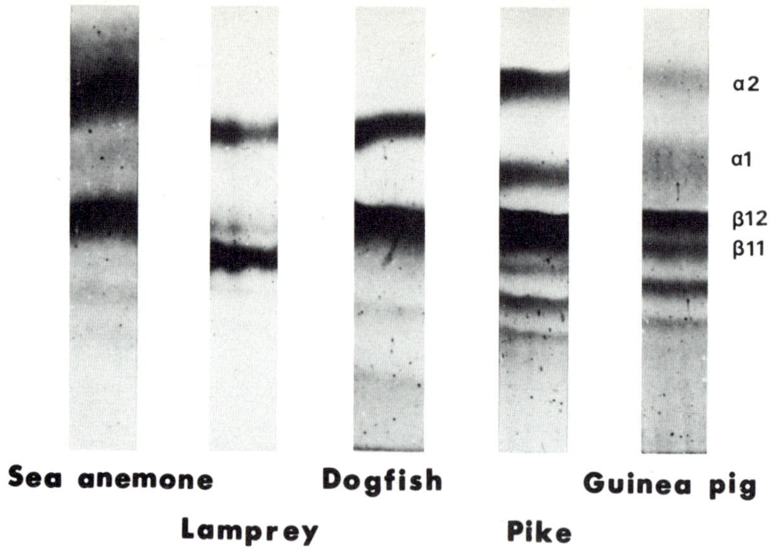

Fig. 3. Starch-gel electrophoretic patterns of denatured citrate-soluble body-wall collagens from various species.

one electrophoretically-distinguishable α component (Fig.3). The higher animals from reptiles upwards all have two or three α components with the corresponding β components. The collagens of bony fishes are variable in this respect. The analysis is obscured by the simple degradation of the fish collagens, which makes analysis of the components uncertain. In the gel electrophoresis pattern of lamprey collagen there is a faint band which could be interpreted as α1 chain. We must consider the possibility that minor amounts of another α chain are present.

Taking into account the knowledge of amino acids we summarised our ideas in Fig. 2, with some reservations about bony fishes.

III STABILITY AND CROSS-LINKING

The more highly developed vertebrates seem to have greater efficiency in forming cross-linked collagen that is resistant to solvents. The rate of the gelatinization of insoluble skin collagen of higher species is slower with minimal heating (Table VII) although we should be cautious in drawing conclusions because of the different metabolic

TABLE VII

Solubilization of Insoluble Vertebrate Skin Collagen

Species	Extracted* at		Residue
	+40°	+65-90°	
Cow	0.5	10.9	88.6
Calf	2.7	76.0	21.3
Guinea pig, adult	9.2	74.9	15.9
Guinea pig, growing	4.2	91.2	4.6
Chick	6.0	72.5	21.5
Snake	2.7	32.3	65.0
Toad	16.9	73.7	9.4
Burbot	69.3	24.1	6.6
Pike	78.4	17.7	3.9
Hagfish	55.9	26.9	17.2
Lamprey	89.9	7.5	2.6

*Into 0.01 M sodium acetate buffer, pH 4.8, in percent of total insoluble collagen (Pikkarainen, 1968).

turnovers of the fractions. Heikkinen (1968) has shown that the 80°C-soluble fraction of insoluble rat collagen contains associated substances different from those in the respective 40°C-soluble fraction. The differences between the species (Table VII) may depend on the associated substances. The existence of a biphasic temperature-shrinkage curve in fish collagens (Pikkarainen et al., 1966) indicates weaker crosslinks, which are hidden by the strong crosslinks in collagens of higher species. This may have a structural basis either in the cross-linking groups or in the accessory substances in the insoluble collagenous fibres. A good example on the effect of the noncollagenous substances is the byssus-threads of the sea mussel (*Mytilus*), which have the thermal shrinking point at about 90°C whereas the skeleton collagen of the same animal shrinks at about 55°C.

Nothing is known about the lysine cross-links during the course of the evolution.

IV DISCUSSION

Judging from the thermal stability and for that matter from the imino acid content, of collagen, there has been a similar but independent natural selection process in worms and in vertebrates. Qualities other than thermal shrinkage and imino acid content are quite different. In the development of the animals with high and constant body temperature the improvement of the thermal stability of collagen is one of the decisive factors, although there are numerous enzyme proteins which also denature just above the body temperature of mammals and birds. Preliminary work from our laboratory indicates that during fever an excess of hydroxyproline is excreted.

What was the original collagen? Presumably it contained every third residue of glycine in common with elastin and silk proteins (Rudall, 1968). Furthermore, there may have been one hydroxyl for every six residues, abundantly acidic and other polar amino acids, and enough imino acids to maintain the helix form even at temperatures near zero. We may speculate that there was originally a tripeptide Gly-X-Y, which was multiplied a thousand-fold; the resulting peptide chain was able to form the collagen-fold and the triple-helix.

What benefit does the organism derive from differentiation of the three chains? Veis, Anesey and Mussell (1967) have proposed a special role for the $\alpha 2$ chain in the formation of the fibrous structure. Is it too farfetched to speak of eventual intramolecular specialization between the chains (Table VIII) in determination of stability, in cross-linking, in intermolecular organization or in the bone formation?

The report given by Dr. Miller during this symposium on the single-chain collagen from the sternal cartilage of chicken is very exciting to us, because in our scheme the cartilaginous fishes are the most advanced species having single-chain collagen, whereas many bony fishes have differentiated chains. The present scheme (Fig. 2) applies to

TABLE VIII

Comparison of the Chains in Collagen

Thermal stability	α1, α3 > α2
Formation of quaternary structure	α2 decisive
Aldehyde content	α1 = α2
Sensitivity to β-APN	α1 > α2
Carbohydrate content	α1, α3 > α2
Content of bound phosphorus	α2 > α1, α3

Hollmên and Kulonen, 1964; Veis et al., 1967; Rojkind and Juarêz, 1966; Glimcher and Krane, 1968.

fibrous collagen. We suggest that the collagen of ectodermal origin (e.g. from basement membrane) may belong to a different system, along with worm-cuticle collagen.

ACKNOWLEDGEMENTS

Institutional support from the U.S. Department of Agriculture, Foreign Research and Development Division, and from Emil Aaltonen Foundation (J.P.) is gratefully acknowledged.

REFERENCES

Bornstein, P. (1968). Science 161, 592.

Bornstein, P. and Piez, K.A. (1964). J. Clin. Invest. 43, 1813.

Eastoe, J.E. (1957). Biochem. J. 65, 363.

Eastoe, J.E. (1968). In Treatise on Collagen, vol. I, p. 1. Ed. by Ramachandran, G.N.Academic Press, London.

Eastoe, J.E. and Leach, A.A. (1958). In Recent Advances in Gelatin and Glue Research, p. 173. Ed. by Stainsby, G. Pergamon Press, London.

François, C.J. and Glimcher, M.J. (1967a). Biochim. Biophys. Acta 133, 91.

François, C.J. and Glimcher, M.J. (1967b). Biochem. J. 102, 148.

Glimcher, M.J. and Krane, S.M. (1968). In Treatise on Collagen, vol. 2-B, p. 67. Ed. by Gould, B.S. Academic Press, London.

Gross, J. (1963). In Comparative Biochemistry. A Comprehensive Treatise, vol. 5, p. 307. Ed. by Florkin, M. and Mason, H.S. Academic Press, New York.

Gustavson, K.H. (1956). The Chemistry and Reactivity of Collagen. Academic Press, New York.

Harrington, W. F. and Rao, N. V. (1967). In Conformation of Biopolymers, vol. 2 , p. 513. Ed. by Ramachandran, G.N. Academic Press, London.

Heidrich, H.-G. and Wynston, L.K. (1965). Z. physiol. Chem. 342, 166.

Heikkinen, E. (1968). Acta Physiol. Scand. Suppl. 317.

Heikkinen, E. and Kulonen, E. (1968). Biochim. Biophys. Acta 160, 464.

von Hippel, P.H. (1967). In Treatise on Collagen, vol. 1, p. 253. Ed. by Ramachandran, G.N. Academic Press, London.

von Hippel, P.H. and Wong, K.-Y. (1963). Biochemistry 2, 1387.

Hollmén, T. and Kulonen, E. (1964). Biochim. Biophys. Acta 93, 655.

Josse, J. and Harrington, W.F. (1964). J. Mol. Biol. 9, 269.

Maser, M.D. and Rice, R.V. (1962). Biochim. Biophys. Acta 63, 255.

Metzger, H., Shapiro, M.B., Mosimann, J.E. and Winton, J.E. (1968). Nature 219, 1166.

Nordwig, A. (1968). Mitteilungen aus der Max-Planck-Gesellschaft, 5, 316.

Nordwig, A. and Hayduk, U. (1967). J. Mol. Biol. 26, 351.

Paz, M.A., Salazar, M.E. and Gaite, E.E. (1967). Arch. Biochem. Biophys. 119, 485.

Piez, K.A. (1965). Biochemistry 4, 2590.

Piez, K.A., Eigner, E. A. and Lewis, M.S. (1963). Biochemistry 2, 58.

Pikkarainen, J. (1968). Acta Physiol. Scand. Suppl. 309.

Pikkarainen, J. and Kulonen, E. (1965). Acta Chem. Scand. 19, 280.

Pikkarainen, J. and Kulonen E. (1967). Scand. J. Clin. Lab. Invest. 19, Suppl. 95, 40.

Pikkarainen, J. and Kulonen, E. (1969). Nature 223, 839.

Pikkarainen, J., Tantanen, J. and Kulonen, E. (1966). In Biochimie et Physiologie du Tissu Conjonctif, p. 303. Ed. by Compte, Ph. Lyon.

Pikkarainen, J. Rantanen, J., Vastamäki, M., Lampiaho, K., Kari, A. and Kulonen, E. (1968). Eru. J. Biochem. 4, 555.

Rigby, B.J. (1967). Nature 214, 87.

Rigby, B.J. (1968). Nature 219, 166.

Rojkind, M. and Juárez, H. (1966). Biochem.Biophys. Res. 25, 481.

Rudall, K.M. (1968). In Treatise on Collagen, vol. 2-A, p. 83. Ed. by Gould, B.S. Academic Press, London.

Veis, A. Anesey, J. and Mussell, S. (1967). Nature 215, 931.

COMPARATIVE BIOCHEMICAL STUDIES OF COLLAGEN

P. Bornstein and A.H. Kang

Collagen serves a wide variety of structural functions in diverse anatomic locations and consequently the macromolecular organization of the protein is dependent upon its tissue of origin. The extent to which such differences are mediated by tissue-specific variations in the collagen molecule itself, or by the association of collagen with other macromolecules to form structural complexes, remains unknown. This brief discussion will examine the differences between rat skin and tail tendon collagen which have thus far been observed and touch upon their possible significance. Certain interspecies variations in collagen structure will also be considered. The latter approach, as shown by studies of other proteins, may reveal those features of the molecule which are relatively invariant and therefore essential to the basic structure and function of the protein, as well as regions which are more susceptible to the type of evolutionary structural changes which can lead to modifications in function.

It is now apparent that the covalent structure of a protein is dependent not only on the nature of the structural gene coding for its underlying polypeptide sequence, but also on a number of subsequent modifications. These include the alteration of amino acid side chains, addition of carbohydrates and prosthetic groups, intramolecular rearrangements, and limited proteolysis. Collagen undergoes an unusually large number of these modifications, raising the possibility that the biogenesis of a collagenous matrix is partially controlled by reactions which occur after the formation of the peptide chain and which may vary in activity from tissue to tissue. A corollary of this supposition is that disordered collagen structure and function can result from metabolic derangements which frequently accompany disease states.

I RESULTS AND DISCUSSION

The hydroxylation of proline and lysine in peptide linkage are reactions which are unique, or almost unique, to collagen (see papers by Udenfriend and Prockop in this volume). Small differences in the contents of these amino acids in collagens from different tissues of the same species have been reported by several authors. An opportunity to examine this question in some detail arose with the preparation of cyanogen bromide (CNBr) fragments of the α chains of rat skin and tail tendon collagen (Bornstein and Piez, 1966; Bornstein, 1967). It was observed that α1-CB2, a peptide containing 36 amino acids located near the NH_2-terminus of the α1 chain, differed in skin and tendon only in the contents of proline and hydroxyproline. The skin peptide contained 7 prolyl and 5 hydroxyprolyl residues whereas the tendon peptide contained 9 prolyl and 3 hydroxyprolyl residues. When the complete amino acid sequences of the two peptides were determined, it was shown that in both instances six prolyl residues (all in the third position in collagen triplet, Gly-X-Y) were hydroxylated to a varying extent and that hydroxylation was incomplete in each position. The overall degree of hydroxylation was greater in the skin peptide (Table I).

It is now known that, at least in rat skin collagen, incomplete hydroxylation of prolyl residues occurs elsewhere in the α chain (Bornstein, unpublished observations). However, the degree of hydroxylation in other regions of the tendon α chain must equal or exceed that in skin since the hydroxyproline content of the two collagens is similar. While the existence of incomplete hydroxylation of prolyl residues is consistent with recent suggestions regarding the mechanism of action of collagen proline hydroxylase

TABLE I

Molar Fractions of Hydroxyproline in Each of Six Positions at Which Prolyl Residues are Susceptible to Hydroxylation in Peptides α1-CB2 from Rat Skin and Tail Tendon Collagen

Position	Skin	Tendon
9	0.9	0.9
12	0.8	0.6
15	0.9	0.9
24	0.5	0.3
27	0.9	0.2
30	0.9	0.2
Total	4.9 (4.9)	3.1 (3.0)

The figures in parentheses indicate the hydroxyproline contents (in residues per peptide) obtained by amino acid analysis of the entire peptide.

(see Prockop, this volume), the functional significance, if any, of differing degrees of hydroxylation of specific prolyl residues is unknown.

Recently the hydroxyproline content of tail tendon α1-CB2 was shown to increase and approach that of the skin peptide after incubation with an in vitro hydroxylating system prepared from rat skin (Rhoads, Udenfriend and Bornstein, 1969). A similar incubation of the skin peptide resulted in only a small increase in hydroxyproline content. Studies to localize the additional hydroxyprolyl residues are in progress, but these preliminary experiments suggest that in vitro, as well as in vivo, hydroxylation is limited to prolyl residues in position three in the collagen triplet.

3-Hydroxyproline is a minor constituent of both rat tail tendon and skin collagen, but its content in tendon is several times greater than that in skin (Piez, Eigner and Lewis, 1963). Hydroxylation at position 3 of proline bears a resemblance to the pattern of formation of 4-hydroxyproline in that fractional residues of 3-hydroxyproline are found in peptides derived from tail tendon collagen (Bornstein, 1969). However, the position of 3-hydroxyproline with respect to glycine in the repetitive collagen sequence, and its function, if any, are unknown.

Differences in the degree of hydroxylation of lysine in collagens are more striking and may represent a means for modulating the function of the protein. Thus, the collagen of glomerular basement membrane contains an unusually high proportion of hydroxylysine and a high carbohydrate content (Kefalides and Winzler, 1966; Spiro, 1967). The attachment of glucosyl-galactose units to hydroxylysine may be expected to affect the structure and function of the collagen; conceivably the hydroxylation and glycosylation of lysyl residues play a role in the regulation of interchain cross-linking since both lysyl and hydroxylysyl residues are known to participate in the formation of these cross-links (Bornstein and Piez, 1966; Bailey and Peach, 1968).

The comparison of other CNBr-produced peptides of rat skin and tail tendon collagen revealed that whereas most of the peptides were similar, if not identical, in chromatographic behavior and amino acid composition (apart from differences related to the hydroxylation of proline and lysine) distinct differences existed in peptides which could be related to the NH_2-terminal end of the α1 chain (Bornstein, 1969). The data, summarized in Fig. 1, indicate that the tendon α1 chain contains the additional tetrapeptide PCA-Met-Ser-Tyr at its NH_2-terminus (PCA, pyrrolidone-5-carboxylic acid). The significance of the additional sequence on the tendon chain is at present unclear. In view of the existence of an identical or homologous sequence in human and chicken skin collagen (Fig. 1) and in chicken bone collagen (Miller, Lane and Piez, 1969), it is possible that the α1 chain of rat skin collagen also contains the missing tetrapeptide, but that it is removed by limited proteolysis either in vivo or during extraction and purification of the protein. The existence of such an alteration in the α1 chain of rat skin collagen in vivo may be of physiologic significance. There is now ample evidence that the NH_2-

Rat Skin					Gly-	Tyr-	Asp-	Glu-	Lys-	Ser-	Ala-	Gly-	Val-	Ser-	Val-	----	Pro-	Gly-	Pro-	Met-
Rat Tendon	PCA-	Met-	Ser-	Tyr-	Gly-	Tyr-	Asp-	Glu-	Lys-	Ser-	Ala-	Gly-	Val-	Ser-	Val-	----	Pro,	Gly,	Pro,	Met-
Human Skin	PCA,	Leu,	Ser,	Tyr,	Gly,	Tyr,	Asp,	Glu-	Lys-	Ser-	Thr-	Gly-	Gly-	Ser,	Val,	Ile,	Pro,	Gly,	Pro,	Met-
Chicken Skin	PCA-	Met-	Ser-	Tyr-	Gly-	Tyr-	Asp-	Glu-	Lys-	Ser-	Ala-	Gly-	Val-	Ala-	Val-	----	Pro-	Gly-	Pro-	Met-
	1	2	3	4	5	6	7	8	9	10	11	13	13	14	15	16	17	18	19	20

Fig. 1. Amino acid sequences at the NH_2-terminal ends of the α1 chains of four collagens. A tentative order of the amino acids separated by commas has been inferred on the basis of homology.

Rat Skin	PCA-Tyr-----Ser-Asp-Lys-------Gly-Val-Ser-Ala-Gly-Pro-Gly-Pro-Met-
Human Skin	PCA,Tyr,----Gly,Asp,Lys-------Gly,Val,Gly,Leu,Gly,Pro,Gly,Pro,Met-
Chicken Skin	PCA-Tyr-Asp-Pro-Ser-Lys-------Ala-Ala-Asp-Phe-Gly-Pro-Gly-Pro-Met-
	1 2 3 4 5 6 7 8 9 10 11 12 13 14 15

Fig. 2. Amino acid sequences at the NH_2-terminal ends of the $\alpha 2$ chains of three collagens. A tentative order of the amino acids separated by commas has been inferred on the basis of homology. Two deletions have been inserted between position 6 and 7 to maximize the homology with the $\alpha 1$ chain.

terminal region of collagen plays a critical role in interchain cross-linking. Relatively minor modifications in this region of the protein may therefore exert a considerable influence on a prime function of collagen, i.e. the formation of stable polymeric aggregates.

The existence of PCA as the NH_2-terminal residues in the α1 and α2 chains of collagen (Figs. 1 and 2) is of interest in view of the role which such an amino acid might play in the initiation of protein synthesis in higher organisms. However, the possibility that PCA results from the subsequent cyclization of a glutaminyl residue has not been excluded (see Bornstein, 1969, for discussion).

While the rat proteins remain the best defined collagens, detailed structural studies including some sequence determinations have now been extended to chicken skin (Kang, Piez and Gross, 1969; Kang, Igarashi and Gross, 1969), chicken bone (Miller, Lane and Piez, 1969; Lane and Miller, 1969) and human skin (Bornstein, 1968) collagens. These studies indicate that the helical regions of the α chains, characterized by the presence of hydroxyproline and a content of one-third glycyl residues, are relatively invariant. Indeed, the degree of structural identity of the helical regions in the collagens of these three species equals or exceeds that of several globular proteins, even when the restriction imposed by the requirement for glycine in every third position is taken into account. Thus, the compositions of human and rat skin α1-CB2 are identical, and chicken α1-CB2 differs only by a single amino acid substitution (alanine in place of serine) in 36 amino acids. The degree of identity in composition of α1-CB3 (150 amino acids) is approximately 98% and 94% (excluding the identical glycine content) when the rat and human, and rat and chicken peptides, respectively, are compared. It seems likely that the aggregation of collagen and its association with other connective tissue macromolecules require intermolecular interactions which severely limit the number of amino acid substitutions which the function of the protein can accommodate.

On the other hand, the NH_2-terminal regions of collagen chains, while clearly homologous, display a somewhat greater degree of variability, particularly in α2 (Figs. 1 and 2). Since these amino acid sequences cannot form a triple helix, it is probable that these regions have evolved to perform specialized functions such as cross-linking of collagen chains, which permit a non-helical conformation. Substitutions at the NH_2-terminus of the collagen molecule may therefore represent a means by which evolutionary changes in function can occur.

The greater variability of the NH_2-terminal region of collagen is reflected in the finding that limited proteolytic digestion with chymotrypsin, which specifically removes non-helical NH_2-terminal sequences from the protein, (Bornstein, Kang and Piez, 1966) results in the loss of most of the species-specific antigenicity of collagen (Davison, Levine, Drake, Rubin and Bump, 1967). It has recently been shown by hemagglutination and hemagglutination inhibition reactions that the antigenicity of rat skin collagen resides largely in the NH_2-terminal region of the α2 chain (see Michaeli, this volume). Similar findings have been obtained using precipitin reactions in gels (Lindsley, Mannik and Bornstein, in preparation). Since the animals immunized in the above studies were rabbits, it is probable that differences between rat and rabbit collagen exist at the NH_2-terminus of the α2 chain. This supposition is consistent with the greater variability apparent at the NH_2-terminus of the α2 chain in rat, human and chicken collagens (Fig. 2), as compared with homologous sequences in the corresponding α1 chains (Fig. 1).

ACKNOWLEDGEMENT

Supported by National Institutes of Health Grants AM 11248 and AM 3564, National Science Foundation Grant GB 6079, and a RGK Foundation Grant.

REFERENCES

Bailey, A.J. and Peach, C.M. (1968). Biochem. Biophys. Res. Commun. 33, 812.

Bornstein, P. (1967). Biochemistry 6, 3082.

Bornstein, P. (1968). Science 161, 592.

Bornstein, P. (1969). Biochemistry 8, 63.

Bornstein, P., Kang, A.H. and Piez, K.A. (1966). Biochemistry 5, 3803.

Bornstein, P. and Piez, K.A. (1966). Biochemistry 5, 3460.

Davison, P.F., Levine, L., Drake, M.P., Rubin, A. and Bump, S. (1967). J. Exp. Med. 126, 331.

Kang, A.H., Igarashi, S. and Gross, J. (1969). Biochemistry 8, 3200.

Kang, A.H., Piez, K.A. and Gross, J. (1969). Biochemistry 8, 1506.

Kefalides, N.A. and Winzler, R.J. (1966). Biochemistry 5, 702.

Lane, J.M. and Miller, E.J. (1969). Biochemistry 8, 2134.

Miller, E.J., Lane, J.M. and Piez, K.A. (1969). Biochemistry 8, 30.

Piez, K.A., Eigner, E.A. and Lewis, M.S. (1963). Biochemistry 2, 58.

Rhoads, R., Udenfriend, S. and Bornstein, P. (1969). Fed. Proceed. 28, 408.

Spiro, R.G. (1967). J. Biol. Chem. 242, 1915.

A COMPARISON OF CHICK BONE AND CARTILAGE COLLAGENS: EVIDENCE FOR A UNIQUE TYPE OF α1 CHAIN IN CARTILAGE COLLAGEN

Edward J. Miller and Victor J. Matukas

Previous studies from our laboratory have led to the characterization of the chick bone collagen molecule at the level of the cyanogen bromide (CNBr) peptides derived from the individual α chains of the molecule (Miller, Martin, Piez and Powers, 1967; Lane and Miller, 1969; Miller, Lane and Piez, 1969a). These studies indicate that the monomeric bone collagen molecule is comprised of two identical α1 chains and one α2 chain. Since many vertebrate cartilages normally calcify and are replaced by bone during development, the studies on bone collagen were extended to cartilage collagen which prior to this time has not been the subject of detailed biochemical investigations. This presentation describes the procedures found useful in characterizing the soluble collagen extracted from cartilage and presents evidence indicating that although a proportion of cartilage collagen is identical to that of bone, cartilage contains yet another type of collagen which is probably unique to cartilaginous structures.

I EXTRACTION OF CARTILAGE COLLAGEN

Cartilaginous sterna were removed from 3-week-old normal chicks as well as those which had been made lathyritic by the addition of β-amino proprionitrile (βAPN) to the diet (Miller et al., 1967). The sterna were dissected free of soft tissue and bone and sliced manually into small pieces with a scalpel blade. The cartilage slices were then sequentially extracted at 4°C for 3 days each in 1.0 M NaCl (0.05 M Tris, pH 7.5) and 0.5 M acetic acid. In Table I, data are presented on the solubility characteristics of the sternal cartilage collagen in these two solvents commonly used for the extraction of native collagen. It is readily seen that neutral salt solutions as well as dilute acetic acid are almost totally ineffective as solvents for the collagen in cartilage from control animals. In this regard, the cartilage collagen of the young chick resembles that of chick bone (Miller et al., 1967) and that of human articular and costal cartilages (Miller,van der Korst and Sokoloff 1969b) which have also been shown to be extremely resistant to solubilization in these solvents. If on the other hand, crosslinking of collagen is inhibited by the administration of βAPN, a significant proportion of the cartilage collagen can be solubilized. It is noteworthy that although 0.5 M acetic acid is a very effective solvent for collagen in most soft tissues, we have found it to be a very poor solvent for cartilage collagen even when used prior to 1.0 M NaCl which, as indicated in Table I, removes up to 15% of the total cartilage collagen. These results indicate that at low pH, the affinity of positively-charged collagen molecules for the anionic groups on the proteoglycans (PG) in cartilage is sufficiently great that removal of the collagen molecules from the bulk of the tissue is effectively prevented. However, in neutral salt solution at high ionic strength, these interactions are reduced allowing collagen and PG molecules to pass into solution.

II PURIFICATION AND CARBOXYMETHYL CELLULOSE CHROMATOGRAPHY OF CARTILAGE COLLAGEN

Collagen purification procedures previously applied to collagen extracted from chick bone (Miller et al., 1967) proved to be of little value when dealing with extracts of cartilage collagen. The chief difficulty appeared to be offered by the large proportion of PG in the cartilage

TABLE I

Extractability of Sternal Cartilage Collagen

Solvent	Percent of total tissue collagen solubilized: Control	Lathyritic
1.0 M NaCl, pH 7.5	<1	15
0.5 M acetic acid	0	0

extracts. Consequently, when collagen was precipitated from the cartilage extract, sufficient PG was coprecipitated to prevent resolubilization of the precipitate in acidic solvents and excluded the possibility of chromatographing the extracted collagen on carboxymethyl (CM) cellulose at low pH and at an initial low ionic strength (Piez, Eigner and Lewis, 1963). A purification procedure was, therefore, developed in which the initial steps (Table II) were designed to remove contaminating PG from the extract. During this procedure, amino acid analyses of the precipitated CPC-PG complex revealed that less than 1% of the extracted collagen was precipitated by the addition of CPC to the solution.

TABLE II

Purification of Cartilage Collagen Extracted with 1.0 M Sodium Chloride, pH 7.5

Adjust pH to 8.0, NaCl concentration to 0.2 M.
Titrate solution with 0.1 M cetyl pyridinium chloride (CPC) in 0.2 M NaCl.
Cool solution to 2°C.
Centrifuge at 100,000 x g for 1 hr.
Continue purification of collagen in supernatant as previously outlined for acid-soluble bone collagen (Miller et al., 1967).

In Fig. 1 is depicted a CM-cellulose chromatogram of heat-denatured sternal cartilage collagen extracted with 1.0 M NaCl at pH 7.5 and purified before application to the column in the manner described above. Planimetry of the

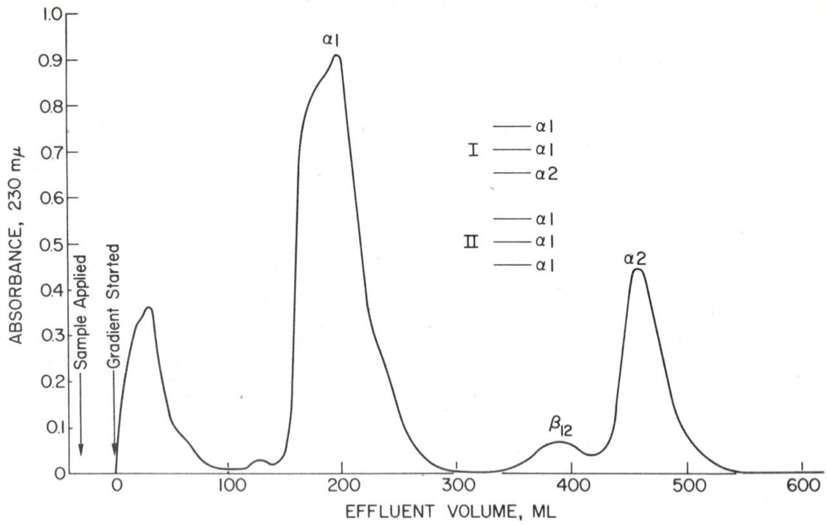

Fig. 1. CM-Cellulose elution pattern of cartilage collagen. Conditions for chromatography have been described (Miller et al., 1969). The material eluted as the forepeak at the beginning of the gradient is noncollagenous.

curves indicated that all of the collagen contained in the extract had chromatographed as the observed components. In comparison with CM-cellulose chromatograms of soluble bone collagen (Miller et al., 1967), the chromatogram of the soluble cartilage collagen has several interesting features. Similar to the collagen extracted from bone, this collagen contains only a small proportion of β-components as would be expected for a neutral salt-soluble collagen from a tissue of lathyritic animals. In contrast to the soluble collagen from chick bone, we routinely observed that the α1 to α2 ratio in soluble cartilage collagen is greater than 2:1 and approaches a value of 3:1 as depicted in Fig. 1. In addition, there is obvious chromatographic heterogeneity in the α1 fraction of cartilage collagen suggesting that the α1 fraction represents a mixture of at least two different types of α1 chains.

III CNBr CLEAVAGE OF CARTILAGE COLLAGEN α CHAINS

In order to gain further information concerning the

cartilage collagen α chains, the separated α1 and α2 fractions were cleaved with CNBr and the resulting peptides were chromatographed on phospho- and CM-cellulose as previously described (Miller et al., 1969a; Lane and Miller, 1969). In this manner, it was possible to demonstrate that the α2 chain of cartilage collagen is identical to the α2 chain of bone collagen both in terms of amino acid composition and the CNBr peptides derived from the chain (Lane and Miller, 1969). Cleavage of the α1 fraction of cartilage collagen with CNBr, however, gives rise to a series of previously unknown peptides in addition to those formerly observed from the α1 chains of chick bone collagen (Miller et al., 1969a). The new peptides are clearly homologous to those derived from the α1 chains of chick bone collagen although several amino acid substitutions are apparent (Miller and Matukas, 1969). Quantitatively, it was noted that each of the new peptides in the soluble cartilege is related to its homologue by a ratio of approximately 1:2, indicating that about one-third of the total α1 fraction may be accounted for by the presence of a new α1 chain. This relationship is consistent with the CM-cellulose chromatogram (Fig. 1) which indicates that there is an excess of one equivalent of α1 chains in the cartilage collagen extract.

IV DISCUSSION

The results of this study clearly indicate the presence in chick sternal cartilage of a new collagen chain which is not presented in collagen extracted from bone of the species. Recent studies on the CNBr peptides derived from chick skin α1 (Kang, Piez and Gross, 1969) indicate that chick bone and skin collagens are identical and no evidence for the presence of an additional α1 chain similar to that found in cartilage collagen extracts was obtained. In order to differentiate the new α1 chain found in cartilage collage, we propose that this α1 chain be designated "Type II", and that the α1 chain common to bone, skin and cartilage be designated "Type I." Studies on the cartilaginous growth plates of embryonic chick tibiae indicate that theα1

(Type II) chain is present in this tissue as well, suggesting that synthesis of the new chain is prevalent in cartilaginous structures. Expression of an additional structural gene for collagen synthesis in cartilages may be of significance both in regard to differentiation and function of the tissues, although sufficient data are not available to assess the relative importance of the many macromolecular species found in cartilage. Also, it is possible that the α1 (Type II) chain is present in the collagen of other as yet unexamined tissue as well as cartilage.

The α1 (Type II) chain in cartilage collagen should not be considered an α3 chain as identified in cod fish skin collagen (Piez, 1965). As pointed out above, the presence of the α1 (Type II) chain represents an excess of α1 chains over that required for triple-chained molecules. The quantitative relationship between the chains found in soluble cartilage collagen is: 2 α1 (Type I): 1 α1 (Type II): 1α2. It is therefore possible that cartilage collagen is a mixture of two different collagen molecules, one having the chain structure $[\alpha 1 \text{ (Type I)}]_2 \alpha 2$, identical to the molecules of bone and skin, and the other comprised of three identical chains $[\alpha 1 \text{ (Type II)}]_3$ as diagrammatically illustrated in Fig. 1. Although the studies reported here on the soluble collagen from sternal cartilage indicate that approximately one-quarter of the cartilage collagen is comprised of the α1 (Type II) chain, examination of the CNBr peptides of insoluble cartilage collagen after extraction with neutral salt solutions indicates that the α1 (Type II) chain actually represents approximately two-thirds of the total mass of collagen in sternal cartilage and 90% of the collagen in the cartilaginous growth plates of embryonic chick tibiae. The reason why molecules containing the α1 (Type II) chain are not extracted in proportion to their content in the tissue is, at present, unclear although it may be related to the degree of intermolecular cross-linking or to some unusual relationship with PG molecules in the cartilage. In any event, these results with regard to the large proportion of the α1 (Type II) chain in these cartilages indicate that some of the molecules would of necessity have the chain structure [α1 (Type II) $]_3$. It is of interest to note that the collagen molecules of some lower vertebrates and invertebrates appear to be comprised of a single type of α chain (Pikkarainen, 1968; Pikkarainen, et al., 1968) and therefore synthesis of the α1 (Type II) chain in cartilages may represent a modern manifestation of a "primitive" collagen.

REFERENCES

Kang, A.H., Piez, K.A. and Gross, J. (1969). Biochemistry 8, 1506.

Lane, J.M. and Miller, E.J. (1969) Biochemistry 8, 2134.

Miller, E.J., Martin, G.R., Piez, K.A. and Powers, M.J. (1967). J. Biol. Chem. 242, 5481.

Miller E.J., Lane, J.M. and Piez, K.A. (1969a). Biochemistry 8, 30.

Miller, E.J., van der Korst, J.K. and Sokoloff, L. (1969b). Arth Rheum. 12, 21.

Miller, E.J. and Matukas, V.J. (1969). Proc. Natl. Acad. Sci. (U.S.) (In press.)

Piez, K.A., Eigner, E.A. and Lewis, M.S. (1963). Biochemistry 2, 58.

Piez, K.A. (1965). Biochemistry 4, 2590.

Pikkarainen, J. (1968). Acta Physiol. Scand. Suppl. 309.

Pikkarainen, J., Rantanen, J., Vastamaki, M., Lampiaho, K., Kari, A. and Kulonen, E. (1968). European J. Biochem. 4, 555.

LOCALIZATION OF CHEMICAL AND STRUCTURAL FEATURES ON THE COLLAGEN MOLECULE

Karl A. Piez, Edward J. Miller, Joseph M. Lane
and William T. Butler

The determination of the complete amino acid sequence of a protein usually requires the preparation and isolation of peptides of a size suitable for study. After each peptide has been sequenced, the sequence of residues in the protein is known if the order of the peptides can be established. In the case of the collagen molecule this is a particularly difficult task since each of the three α chains in the molecule contains about 1000 amino acids and there are generally two kinds of α chains, α1 and α2 (Piez, 1967). The problem has been approached by the use of cyanogen bromide (CNBr) cleavage at methionyl residues. It has been possible to isolate 6-10 peptides (per chain) from CNBr digests of the α1 and α2 chains of rat skin and tendon and chick bone and skin collagen (Butler, Piez and Bornstein, 1967; Bornstein, 1969; Miller, Lane and Piez, 1969; Kang, Piez and Gross, 1969; Fietzek and Piez, 1969; Lane and Miller, 1969). In each case the peptides account for all of the amino acids and all of the weight of the chain. A tentative order for the peptides in the α1 chain has been suggested (Piez et al., 1968). We present evidence here which confirms this order with one correction.

Since the collagen molecule is rod-like with the three polypeptide chains parallel and wound in a regular helix around the axis with a known residue repeat (Ramachandran, 1967), the placement of a chemical feature in the amino acid sequence permits its localization on the collagen molecule. The resulting model has considerable relevance to an understanding of function since the primary property of the collagen molecule is its interaction with itself in a very specific manner to produce a collagen fibril under physiologic conditions. Furthermore, certain features of the collagen molecule can be observed in the electron microscope which will permit the comparison of chemical and visual findings. We show here some preliminary examples of this type of analysis.

I ORDER OF CNBr PEPTIDES

The isolation and characterization of the CNBr peptides from the α1 chain of several collagens has been described (Butler et al., 1967; Bornstein, 1969; Miller et al., 1969; Kang et al., 1969) and the monenclature has been discussed (Miller et al., 1969).* The α1 chains from rat skin and tendon collagen appear to have identical primary structures except for the absence of four amino acids at the N-terminal end of the α1 chain of rat skin collagen and other alterations such as hydroxylation and aldehyde formation that must occur after the amino acids are assembled. The same conclusion holds for the α1 chains of chick skin and bone collagen except that there are no missing residues at the N-terminal end. Furthermore, the rat and chick collagen bear a close homology (Piez et al., 1968); very similar CNBr peptides can be isolated from each. The only major difference is that α1-CB6 from the rat is represented by two peptides α1-CB6A and α1-CB6B, from the chick, consistent with the presence of an extra methionyl residue in the

*The nomenclature includes the chain designation (α1 or α2), CB for CNBr, and a number assigned according to the order of elution from an ion exchange column using the peptides from rat skin collagen as the standard, e.g. α1-CB2. Where a fragment contains an uncleaved methionine, thus representing two adjacent CNBr peptides, the double peptide is designated by the two peptide numbers separated by a dash, e.g. α1-CB (4-5). Where an extra methionine is present in a collagen, when compared to rat skin collagen as the reference, the two peptides that arise from CNBr cleavage are identified by A and B, e.g. α1-CB6A and α1-CB6B.

α1 chain of the chick collagen. Therefore the α1 chains of these four collagens can be considered together for purposes of ordering the CNBr peptides.

The order of the peptides has been determined from a variety of evidence. Since CNBr cleavage converts methionine to homoserine which appears as the C-terminal residue on each peptide except the C-terminal peptide and α1-CB6 contains no homoserine, α1-CB6 must be C-terminal. In the case of chick collagen, α1-CB6B contains no homoserine and is therefore C-terminal. α1-CB6A must immediately preceed α1-CB6B since the two together are clearly homologous by molecular weight and amino acid composition to α1-CB6 (Miller et al., 1969).

The presence in CNBr digests of products of incomplete cleavage permits the isolation of fragments containing a methionyl residue and therefore representing two adjacent CNBr peptides. From the isolation and characterization of α1-CB(0-1) and α1-CB(1-2) it has been shown that α1-CB0, 1, and 2 are N-terminal and have the order 0-1-2. These data have been published (Bornstein and Piez, 1966; Bornstein, Kang and Piez, 1966a; Bornstein, 1966b; Miller et al., 1969; Kang et al., 1969). α1-CB(3-7) and α1-CB(4-5) have also recently been isolated (Piez, Miller, Lane and Butler, 1969). That α1-CB4 precedes α1-CB5 is shown by the existence of an overlap peptide isolated from an enzymatic digest containing the C-terminal two residues of α1-CB4 and the N-terminal residues of α1-CB5 in the same sequence as in the individual peptides (Butler and Cunningham, 1966). The identification is unequivocal since the overlap peptide contains O-glucosyl-galactosyl hydroxylsine which occupies the N-terminal position of α1-CB5 and represents the only position in the α1 chain of rat skin collagen containing a significant amount of carbohydrate (Butler et al., 1967). The order of the peptides in α1-CB(4-5) has been confirmed by N-terminal analysis. Glycine was shown to be the N-terminal of α1-CB4 but not of α1-CB5 (see Butler, this book, p.149).

That α1-CB7 immediately precedes α1-CB6 is shown by a comparison of the CNBr peptides with the products produced by the action of tadpole collagenase on native collagen. This enzyme cuts through all three chains of the collagen molecule one-quarter of the way in from the C-terminal end producing a C-terminal piece from α1 that by composition and molecular weight (Kang, Nagai, Piez and Gross, 1966) must consist of α1-CB6 plus a portion of α1-CB7 (Piez et al., 1968). The isolation of α1-CB(3-7), discussed above, requires that α1-CB3 and 7 be adjacent, and since 7 precedes 6, 3 must precede 7. The order in the C-terminal portion of the α1 chain is then 3-7-6 or 3-7-6A-6B in the case of the chick collagens.

The position of α1-CB8 has been determined by renaturating the peptide to form a shortened, collagen-like molecule and comparing the segment-long-spacing (SLS) form with the SLS form of whole collagen by electron microscopy (Piez et al., 1968). This comparison is possible since alternate charged and uncharged regions along the molecule can be seen after appropriate staining as a band pattern which is unique throughout the length of the molecule. The pattern is clearly visible since the collagen molecules in the SLS form lie side-by-side in bundles. The bands produced by renatured α1-CB8 could be uniquely matched to a portion of the pattern of whole collagen lying between the positions of α1-CB0, 1 and 2 at the N-terminal end and α1-CB3, 7 and 6 at the C-terminal end. A calculation based on the number of residues in each peptide and the known residue repeat suggested (Piez et al., 1968) that there were small spaces preceding and following α1-CB8 of a size sufficient for α1-CB4 and 5. It is now clear that a cumulative error, corresponding to an underestimation by a few percent of the size of α1-CB3, 7 and 6, was present since the isolation of α1-CB(4-5) indicates that the two peptides must be adjacent. Furthermore, Rauterberg and Kuhn (1968) have renatured α1-CB8, 3, 7 and 6 and have shown from the SLS patterns that they have the order 8-3-7-6. They have also isolated a fragment identified as α1-CB(8-3) by electronmicroscopy and amino acid composition which rules out any possibility that a small peptide such as α1-CB4 or 5 could lie between α1-CB8 and 3 (Kuhn, personal communication). By deduction α1-CB4 and 5 must then precede α1-CB8 giving a complete order for the α1 chain of the rat collagens of 0-1-2-4-5-8-3-7-6. In the case of the chick collagens, 6A-6B replaces 6. The four missing residues in the α1 chain from rat skin collagen include the residues comprising α1-CB0 (a dipeptide, pyrrolidonecarboxyl homoserine) and the first two residues of α1-CB1 (Bornstein, 1969).

When the amino acid sequences of the individual peptides are placed in order there should result an unbroken series of triplets of the form gly-x-y, where x and y represent any amino acid, if it can be assumed that the helical structure (which requires triplets) is continuous and if the order is correct. The sequences of α1-CB1 and 2 from rat skin collagen have been published (Kang, Bornstein and Piez, 1967; Bornstein, 1967) and the sequences of α1-CB4 and 5 have been recently completed (Butler, unpublished data). Except for the region including α1-CB0 and part of α1-CB1 which is nonhelical (Piez et al., 1968), the prediction of an unbroken series of triplets is correct for the N-terminal region through α1-CB5. This is a reasonable test of the correctness of the order since α1-CB1, 2 and 5 end in full triplets (homoserine is in the third position) while α1-CB4 does not (homoserine is in the second position). In addition, Edman degradation of α1-CB8 indicates that it starts with a full triplet (glycine in N-terminal). Data are also available (Butler, unpublished data) to test the order of α1-CB3 and 7 in the same manner. α1-CB3 ends with homoserine in position 2 of the triplet and α1-CB7 begins with the sequence hyp-gly.

II LOCALIZATION OF FEATURES

It is then possible to represent the α1 chain in a linear fashion with the CNBr peptides plotted according to their correct order and relative size. This plot is shown

TABLE I

CNBr Peptides from the α1 Chain of Rat Collagen

Peptide	M	Residues	Length (Å)
α1-CB0	243*	2	6
α1-CB1	1726*	17	49
α1-CB2	3325*	36	104
α1-CB4	4461*	47	136
α1-CB5	3813*	37	107
α1-CB8	24800	275	798
α1-CB3	13800	153	443
α1-CB7	24800	275	798
α1-CB6	17000	188	545
Total	94000	1030	2990

*Calculated for the region of the α1 chain represented by the peptide including, in the case of α1-CB5, the carbohydrate.

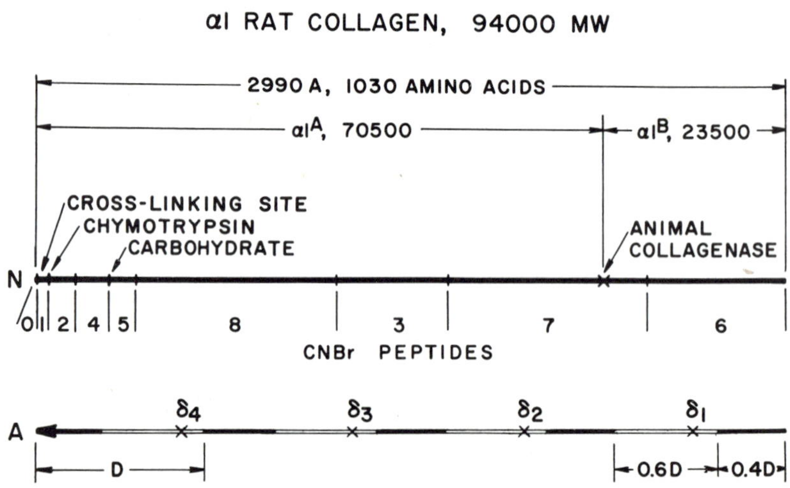

Fig. 1. A representation (above) of the α1 chain of rat collagen showing the position and relative size of the CNBr peptides and other features. The arrow (below) shows a representation of the collagen molecule derived by electronmicroscopy of native and SLS forms. See text.

in Fig. 1 together with other known features of the chain, including the cross-linking site near the N-terminal end of the chain where the lysyl residue in position 9 is a precursor of an aldehyde which can react to form cross-links (Piez et al., 1968; Piez, 1968), the place where chymotrypsin cleaves the nonhelical cross-link region from the native molecule (Bornstein et al., 1966a, b), the location of the carbohydrate at the N-terminal end of α1-CB5 (Butler et al., 1967), and the position within α1-CB7 where animal collagenase initiates cleavage of native collagen yielding, from the α1 chain, two pieces, $\alpha 1^A$ and $\alpha 1^B$ (Kang et al., 1966).

Also shown in Fig. 1 for comparison is a representation of the collagen molecule derived from electronmicroscopy of the native and SLS forms (Hodge, 1967). The molecule, with ends designated A and B corresponding to the N- and C-terminal ends (Kang et al., 1966), respectively, is staggered in the native fibril in a regular fashion to produce a repeat of length D (about 680 Å). Since the molecule has a nonintegral length of 4.4D, "overlap" (Fig. 1, filled portions) and "hole" (open portions) regions occur in the fibril. The δ bands are prominent bands seen in stained preparations of the SLS and native forms and are useful for orientation. The number of known chemical features are still too few for an extensive comparison with structure as seen by electronmicroscopy. However, it can be seen that the crosslinking site is in an overlap region where crosslinking would be more efficient and the carbohydrate is in a hole region where its relatively bulky size may be more readily accommodated. As more chemical information becomes available it will be possible to make a more complete comparison possibly including a comparison of amino acid sequence with the band pattern produced by specific staining agents.

III SUMMARY

The order of the peptides obtained by cyanogen bromide cleavage of the α1 chain of rat and chick collagen has been determined. This will permit amino acid sequencing of the entire chain. Since collagen can be represented as a linear molecule with a uniform residue repeat, the positions of specific amino acid residues and other features can be established.

REFERENCES

Bornstein, P. (1967). Biochemistry 6, 3082.

Bornstein, P. (1969). Biochemistry 8, 63.

Bornstein, P. and Piez, K. A. (1966). Biochemistry 5, 3460.

Bornstein, P., Kang, A. H. and Piez, K. A. (1966a). Proc. Nat. Acad. Sci. U.S. 55, 417.

Bornstein, P., Kang, A. H. and Piez, K. A. (1966b). Biochemistry 5, 3803.

Butler, W. T. and Cunningham, L. W. (1966). J. Biol. Chem. 241, 3882.

Butler, W. T., Piez, K. A. and Bornstein, P. (1967). Biochemistry 6, 3771.

Fietzek, P. P. and Piez, K. A. (1969). Biochemistry 8, 2129.

Hodge, A. J. (1967). In Treatise on Collagen. I. Chemistry of Collagen, ch. 4. Ed. by Ramachandran, G. N. Academic Press, New York.

Kang, A. H., Nagai, Y., Piez, K. A. and Gross, J. (1966). Biochemistry 5, 509.

Kang, A. H., Bornstein, P. and Piez, K. A. (1967). Biochemistry 6, 788.

Kang, A. H., Piez, K. A. and Gross, J. (1969). Biochemistry 8, 1506.

Lane, J. M. and Miller, E. J. (1969). Biochemistry 8, 2134.

Miller, E. J., Lane, J. M. and Piez, K. A. (1969). Biochemistry 8, 30.

Piez, K. A. (1967). In Treatise on Collagen. I. Chemistry of Collagen, ch. 5. Ed. by Ramachandran, G. N.

Piez, K. A. (1967). In Treatise on Collagen. I. Chemistry of Collagen, ch. 5. Ed. by Ramachandran, G. N. Academic Press, New York.

Piez, K. A. (1968). Ann. Rev. Biochem. 37, 547.

Piez, K. A., Bladen, H. A., Lane, J. M., Miller, E. J., Bornstein, P., Butler, W. T. and Kang, A. H. (1968). Brookhaven Symposia in Biology 21, 345.

Piez, K. A., Miller, E. J., Lane, J. M. and Butler, W. T. (1969). Biochem. Biophys. Res. Communs. (In press).

Ramachandran, G. N. (1967). In Treatise on Collagen. I. Chemistry of Collagen. Ch. 3. Ed. by Ramachandran, G. N. Academic Press, New York.

Rauterberg, J. and Kuhn, K. (1968). FEBS Letters 1, 230.

HELIX FORMATION IN COLLAGEN-LIKE SYNTHETIC POLYPEPTIDES

J. Engel

For the physical chemist who wishes to understand the detailed interatomicinteractions which stabilize the structure of collagen, or who would like to learn about the mechanism of its conformational transition, the collagen molecule is a very complex system. Model peptides which have a collagen-like structure but of a simple, known sequence containing only a small number of different amino acid residues offer an obvious simplification of the problem. Moreover, it is quite easy to make systematic changes in the chemical properties of such model peptides. For example, the chain length may be varied in order to study the influence of the size of the molecules on stability. Also, the effect of amino acid substitutions or of changes in the sequence of amino acid residues can be readily studied.

One of the simplest polypeptides, poly-L-proline, has been studied extensively as a model for collagen. (Harrington and von Hippel, 1961a,b; Katchalski, Berger and Kurtz, 1963; Mandelkern, 1967). In this review this polypeptide will serve to illustrate some general properties of cooperative transitions in linear biopolymers and the role of solvent polymer interactions.

Poly-L-proline can exist in a helical conformation, the so-called polyproline II helix, in which all the peptide bonds are in the *trans*-configuration. It is this conformation which is found in the individual helices which make up the collagen triple-helix. Hydrogen bonds cannot participate in the stablization of the polyproline II helix because polyproline does not contain hydrogens at the peptide nitrogens. Its stabilization comes mainly from the strong steric restrictions which are imposed by the proline rings. Solvent-polymer interactions must, however, also play a role in the stabilization. This follows from the observation of a second type of helix, the so-called polyproline I helix, which has all peptide bonds in the cis-configuration. This helix is stable in certain organic solvents, whereas the polyproline II helix is stable in water and other hydrogen bond donors. Strassmair, Engel and Zundel (1969) were able to show that these solvent molecules bind to the peptide CO-groups of polyproline, via hydrogen bonds. The binding is much better when the CO-groups are in the II helix than when they are in the I helix. The molecular explanation can be found in the varying accessibility of the carbonyl groups in the two conformations. In the II helix they are much more exposed to the solvent than in the I helix. The experimental proof for the preferential binding to form II comes from infrared measurements of the streching vibrations of the CO-groups. (Strassmair, Knof and Engel, 1969). When trifluoroethanol binds to the peptide CO-group of poly (O-acetyl-hydroxy-L-proline) in form II, a new band appears which belongs to the hydrogen-bonded CO-group (Fig. 1). The shift of the CO band is the same for the peptide CO and for the fully exposed CO-group of the acetyl group. When the polymer is in the I conformation, however, only a small amount of alcohol binds to the peptide CO, whereas the binding to the acetyl group remains the same. Water shows a similar preferential binding to the II helix. According to the law of mass action, a solvent will always shift the equilibrium between two conformations toward that conformation for which the solvent has the higher binding constant. This would explain the high stability of polyproline II in water, without the need of assuming a special bridge-like arrangement of the water molecules between the CO groups.

In this context an important question arises. What change in free energy is necessary for a complete conversion of one conformation into another via a cooperative

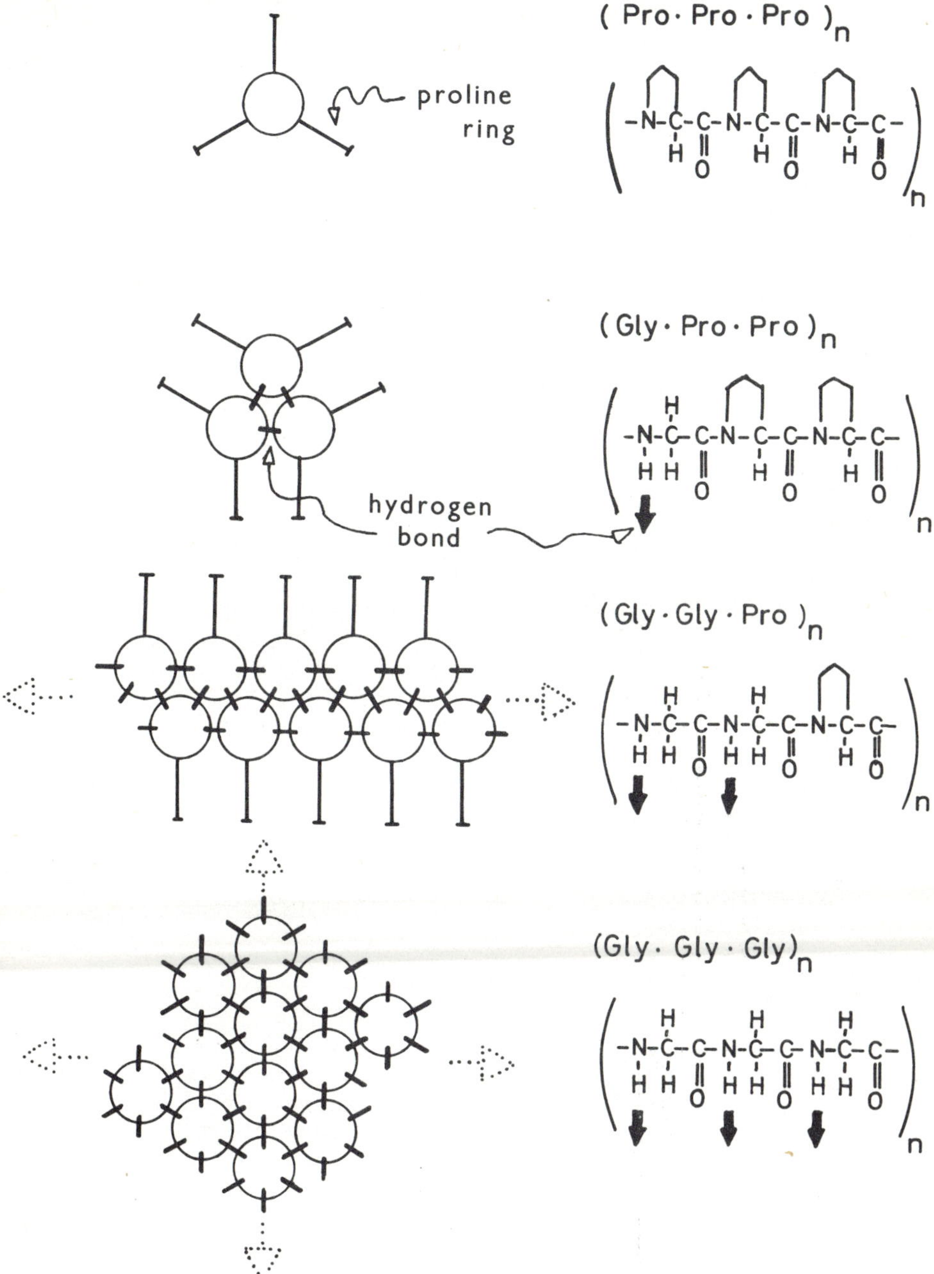

Fig. 1. Greatly simplified diagrams of the conformations of polypeptides with the sequences (Pro-Pro-Pro)$_n$, (Gly-Pro-Pro)$_n$, (Gly-Gly-Pro)$_n$ and (Gly-Gly-Gly)$_n$. The view is always down the helix axis. Helices of the polyproline II type are shown as rings, proline rings as long lines and hydrogen bonds as short lines. The number of proline rings and hydrogen bonds shown corresponds to one tripeptide unit in each helix.

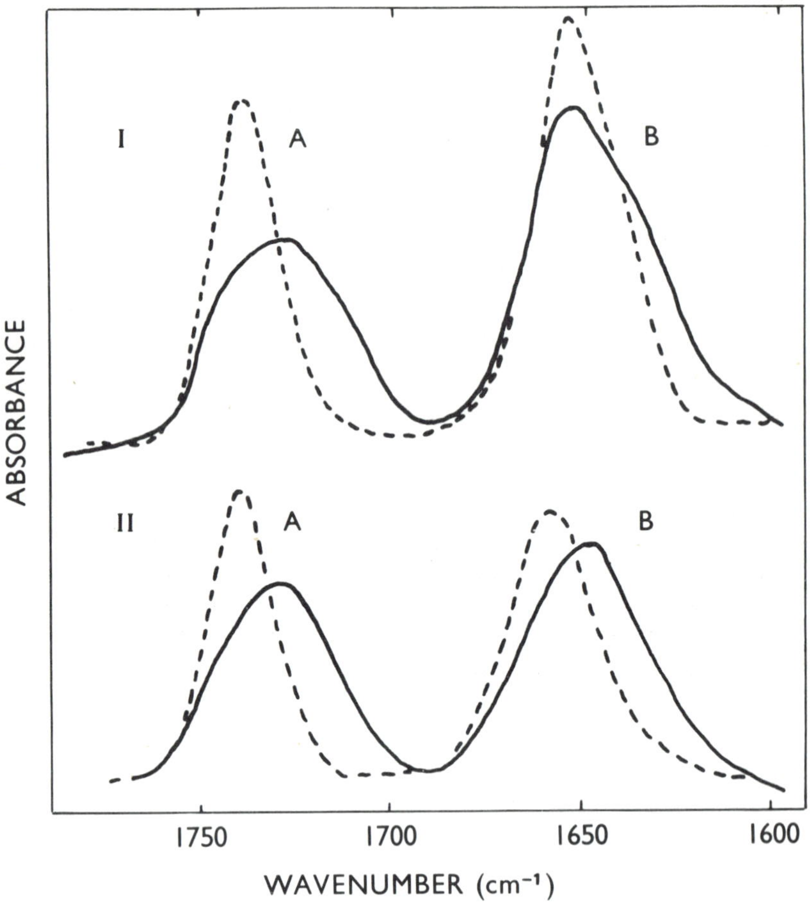

Fig. 2. Stretching vibration of the acetyl-CO-group (A) and the peptide-CO-group (B) of (O-acetyl Hyp)$_{100}$ in the I conformation (I) and the II conformation (II) in chloroform (---) and in 36% (v/v) trifluoroethanol (5 M) in chloroform (——).

transition? The polyproline I$\rightleftarrows$II transition (Steinberg, Harrington, Berger and Sela, 1960; Gornick, Mandelkern, Diorio and Roberts, 1964; Engel, 1967; Ganser, Engel, Winklmair and Krause, unpublished data) and the triple helix $\rightleftarrows$ random coil transition (Veis, 1964; Harrington and Rao, 1967) are cooperative. This means that each residue has a tendency to maintain or reproduce the conformational state of its neighbors. It is a general property of cooperative transitions that an extremely small excess free energy of one of the conformations may be sufficient for a complete stabilization of this form (Engel and Schwarz, 1969).

The equilibrium constant of a cooperative transition is determined by an apparent free energy which is a first approximation is Z-times larger than the real difference of the free energies of the competing conformations. The so-called cooperative length Z is the average length of uninterrupted sequences of residues in identical conformational states at the midpoint of the transition and for very long chains (Poland and Scheraga, 1967). For the polyproline I$\rightleftarrows$II transition Z=360 and a free energy chang of only 0.1 kcal/mole (which in this instance is added by the perferential binding of solvent) is sufficient for a 95% conversion between the two helical forms (Ganser et al, unpublished data). Without cooperatively, under the same induced charge of free energy the equilibrium would be only slightly altered.

It is important to note that similar considerations must be taken into account in any discussion of the stability of the collagen triple helix, or of the various triple-helical structures which have been proposed. Here again, a very small imbalance between all forces affecting the competing conformations (hydrogen bonds, van der Waals forces, hydrophobic interactions, polymersolvent interactions, entropy of the coiled state, etc.) can be sufficient for a complete stabilization of one conformation.

What happens when every third residue in poly-L-proline is substituted by glycine. The sterical stabilization is partially removed because freely rotatable groups are introduced by the glycine residues. In compensation, however, the NH groups of the glycine residues can form hydrogen bonds with peptide CO groups of neighboring chains. Because there are three residues per turn in the polyproline II helix, all of these NH groups will be at one side of the helix. Furthermore, this side of the helix is naked, because glycine does not have side chains. Therefore, three polyproline II helices can come so close together that hydrogen bonds can form and the triple helix is created. Figure 2 shows the triple helix of $(\text{Gly-Pro-Pro})_n$ but for reasons of clarity in this paper the sequence of the polytripeptides will always be written with glycine in the first position. $(\text{Pro-Gly-Pro})_n$ and $(\text{Gly-Pro-Pro})_n$ differ only in the end residues, which for larger chain lengths have little or no influence.

By substituting a second glycine for proline, $(\text{Gly-Gly-Pro})_n$ is formed; it was discovered by Traub and Yonath (1966) that the polyproline-II structure is maintained but the saturation of all possible hydrogen bonds leads to an arrangement of the helices in a double-layered sheet. The large number of hydrogen bonds which are possible in polyglycine leads to an unlimited aggregation of polyproline-II helices in two dimensions (Harrington and von Hippel, 1961 a,b). Having obtained a general understanding of the concerted action of hydrogen bonding and steric effects, we can discuss the triple helix in more detail.

Within the framework of the general concept of the triplehelical arrangement which was first proposed by Ramachandran and Kartha (1955), three detailed structures have been proposed which all fit the X-ray data obtained from collagen. They differ in the arrangement of the hydrogen bonds connecting different chains (Rich and Crick, 1961).

one-bonded collagen I structure $N_1\ H \rightarrow O_1$
one-bonded collagen II structure $N_1\ H \rightarrow O_1$
two-bonded Ramachandran structure $N_1\ H \rightarrow O_3$
and $N_2\ H \rightarrow O_2$

if there is an amino acid residue in position 2 (Ramachandran and Sasisekharan, 1965). The indices indicate the positions of the amino acid residues (Gly, X, Y, hold positions 1, 2, 3, in $(Gly\text{-}X\text{-}Y)_n$).

The model peptides offer four advantages for a decision, based on X-ray analysis, as to which proposed structure is the correct one.

1. The X-ray patterns show more detail because the repeating units are exactly identical.

2. The known chemical formula permits an exact calculation of the intensities which are to be expected for the proposed structures.

3. Exact steric models can be built and tested to see whether they fit into the unit cell which is derived from the X-ray data.

4. The X-ray structures of polytripeptides which possess the chemical ability to form a second hydrogen bond per tripeptide unit can be compared with those which can form only one hydrogen bond per unit.

Traub et al. (1969) were able to determine the structure of (Gly-Pro-Pro)$_n$ with high precision. It is similar to the collagen II structure of Rich and Crick (1961) and shall be termed the Traub helix. All other proposed structures are clearly excluded. It is, however, still possible that a two-bonded structure of the Ramachandran type might be formed in those cases where the chemical possibility for formation of a second hydrogen bond exists. In order to check this, the structures of polytripeptides containing the sequence Gly-Ala-Pro or Gly-Pro-Ala were compared (Traub and Yonath, 1967; Traub et al. 1969). In the first instance a second hydrogen bond is possible, and in the latter it is not, because the NH group in position 3 points out of the triple helix. The result (Table I) is that in all instances in which the triple helix is formed it is of the Traub type, whether the chemical potential for a second hydrogen bond exists or not. This indicates that the enthalpy gain which would proceed from the second hydrogen bond does not compensate for bad steric contacts existing in the Ramachandran two-bonded structure.

Before discussing the conformational stability of the model peptides in solution, we should consider the accessibility of the CO groups in the triple helix to solvent binding. In the collagen II or Traub helix, the CO groups are nicely exposed to the solvent, but this is not the case for the two-bonded Ramachandran helix. We have found that one molecule of water per tripeptide unit is very tightly bound to (Gly-Pro-Pro)$_n$. It is not removed by P_2O_5 in a dessicator. We have seen from studies with space-filling models that one water molecule per tripeptide unit fits very nicely between the CO groups of adjacent chains. This idea, which was also discussed by Harrington and von Hippel (1961b), who, however, postulate water bridges within single chains was worked out in detail by Ramachandran, Doyle and Blout (1968). These authors also discuss a second water bridge of the type NH-water-CO. In solution, all of these highly ordered arrangements of the water molecules appear improbable from the point of view of entropy. However, as was mentioned earlier, the mere binding of water without the

TABLE I

Model peptides*	Structure in the solid state (X-ray) (references 1-4)	Melting temperatures of peptides of various chain lengths (n) in different solvents			
		°C	solvent	n	References
(Gly-Pro-Pro)$_n$ ↓	One-bonded triple helix	~70	water	→∞	5
(Gly-Pro-Ala)$_n$	One-bonded triple helix	<0	water	60	6
		<	ethylene glycol: water 2:1		7
		~45	water	~160	8.0
(Gly-Pro-Ala-Gly-Pro-Pro)$_n$ ↓ ↓	One-bonded triple helix	49	water	2n=48	4
(Gly-Ala-Pro-Gly-Pro-Pro)$_n$ ↓ ↓ ↓	One-bonded triple helix	32	water	2n=48	4
(Gly-Ala-Ala-Gly-Pro-Pro)$_n$ ↓ ↓ ↓	One-bonded triple helix				
(Gly-Ala-Pro-Gly-Pro-Ala)$_n$ ↓ ↓ ↓	One-bonded triple helix				
(Gly-Pro-Hyp)$_n$ ↓	One-bonded triple helix				
(Gly-Ala-Pro)$_n$ ↓ ↓	One-bonded corrugated sheet	0	trifluoro-ethanol	~24	
(Gly-Gly-Pro)$_n$	Double-layered sheet of polyproline-II helices	60	1.4 M acetic acid		

The arrows indicate NH groups which are capable of participating in hydrogen bonds in a triple-helical structure. References: 1) Andreeva, Esipova, Millionova, Rogulenkova and Shibnev (1967); 2) Traub and Yonath (1966); 3) Traub and Yonath (1967); 4) Traub et al. (1969); 5) Engel (1966); Engel et al. (1966); 6) Oriel and Blout (1966); 7) Brown et al. (1969); 8) Heidemann and Bernhardt (1968a); 9) Heidemann and Bernhardt (1968b).

formation of water bridges will stabilize a structure with exposed CO groups.

Concerning the conformation of the polytripeptides in solution, it is known for some of them from measurements of circular dichroism and optical rotary dispersion that they are most probably triple-helical under helix stabilizing conditions (Engel, 1967; Brown, Carver and Blout, 1969; Heidemann and Bernhardt, 1968 a,b). These methods do not supply us with the same structural details which one obtains from the X-ray data. One can only say that the optical properties of the model peptides in solution are very similar to those of collagen. Therefore, it is possible that antiparallel single chain triple helices of the type discussed by Ramachandran et al. (1968) exist in solution. This type of structure would explain the finding that the molecular weight of $(Gly\text{-}Pro\text{-}Pro)_n$ does not drop to one-third of its initial value during the triple helix to coil transition (Egnel, Kurtz, Katchalski and Berger, 1966). This transition may be followed optically. It is strongly dependent on the chain length, which offers proof of the cooperative nature of the transition. The melting temperatures (temperatures at the midpoint of the transition curves T_m) have to be extrapolated to very long chain lengths in order to permit a comparison with the value for the large collagen molecule. The value obtained by extrapolation is about 70° C. According to the method of preparation, our material has a broad molecular weight distribution which also influences the width of the transition. Sakakibara, Kishida, Kikuchik Sakai and Kakiuchi (1968) recently obtained much narrower size distributions of $(Gly\text{-}Pro\text{-}Pro)_n$ which show much sharper transitions. The melting temperature, however, seems to be in the same range as before. For $(Gly\text{-}Pro\text{-}Ala)_n$ of long chain length (n= about 160) Heidemann and Bernhardt (1968a, b) have obtained a melting temperature of about 45°C. Brown et al. (1969) observed the melting of a fraction with lower molecular weight (n = 60) of the same polymer at a temperature which was lower than 0°C. (For a summary of all published melting data, see Table I.) Both polytripeptides,

$(Gly\text{-}Pro\text{-}Pro)_n$ and $(Gly\text{-}Pro\text{-}Ala)_n$ contain one hydrogen bond per tripeptide unit, so that the decrease of the melting temperature with decreasing proline content is most likely due to the loss of steric stabilization. In thermodynamic terms, the entropy gain which takes place when a residue is transferred from the helical conformation to the random coil is much higher for amino acid residues which do not have the steric restrictions of the proline or hydroxyproline residues.

As pointed out by Rao and Harrington (1966). See also Harrington and Rao, 1967),

$$Tm = \frac{\Delta H}{\Delta S_{imino} + \Delta S_{amino}}$$

ΔS_{imino} (ΔS_{amino}) = entropy change due to a transfer of proline and hydroxyproline (all other amino acids) residues from the triple helix to the coiled state. The entropy change of the triple helix $\rightleftarrows$coil transition is designated as H. Harrington and Rao (1967) have made the assumption that the entropy change for the proline and hydroxyproline residues is zero. With this assumption the melting temperature of $(Gly\text{-}Pro\text{-}Ala)_n$ should be about 170°C lower than that of $(Gly\text{-}Pro\text{-}Pro)_n$. In spite of the limited accuracy of the experimental data, this seems not to be the case. This shows that the entropy change for the proline residues is not zero and/or that ΔH depends on the sequence and not only on the number of hydrogen bonds.

The melting temperatures of the model peptides $(Gly\text{-}Pro\text{-}Ala\text{-}Gly\text{-}Pro\text{-}Pro)_n$ and $(Gly\text{-}Ala\text{-}Pro\text{-}Gly\text{-}Pro\text{-}Pro)_n$ with equal chain lengths are almost the same. (Traub et al., 1969). This again is a strong indication that a second hydrogen bond per tripeptide unit which is possible for the second peptide is either not formed or does not add stability to the triple helix.

REFERENCES

Andreeva, N.S., Esipova, N.G., Millionova, M.I., Rogulenkova, V.N. and Shievnov, V.A. (1967). In

Conformation of Biopolymers, Vol. 2, p. 469. Ed. by Ramachandran, G.N. Academic Press, London.

Brown, III, F.R., Carver, J.P. and Blout, E.R. (1969). J. Mol. Biol. 39, 307.

Engel, J. (1966). Biopolymers 4, 945.

Engel, J. (1967). In Conformation of Biopolymers, Vol. 2, p. 483. Ed. by Ramachandran, G.N. Academic Press, London.

Engel, J., Kurtz, J., Katchalski, E. and Berger, A (1966). J. Mol. Biol. 17, 255.

Engel, J. and Schwarz, G. (1969). Angew. Chemie (In press).

Gornick, F.,Mandelkern, L., Diorio, A.F. and Roberts, D.F. (1964). J. Am. Chem. Soc. 86, 2549.

Harrington, W.F. and von Hippel, P.H. (1961a). Adv. Protein Chem. 16, 1.

Harrington, W.F. and von Hippel, P.H. (1961b). Arch. Biochem. Biophys. 92, 100.

Harrington, W.F. and Rao, N.V. (1967). In Conformation of Biopolymers, p. 153. Ed. by Ramachandran, G.N. Academic Press, London.

Heidemann, E. and Bernhardt, H.W. (1968a). Nature 220, 1326.

Heidemann, E. and Bernhardt, H.W. (1968b). Leder 19, 281.

Katchalski, E., Berger, A. and Kurtz, J. (1963). In Aspects of Protein Structure, p. 205. Ed. by Ramachandran, G.N. Academic Press, London.

Mandelkern, L. (1967). In Poly-α-Amino Acids, p. 675. Ed. by Fasman, G.D. Marcel Dekker, New York.

Oriel, P.J. and Blout, E.R. (1966). J. Am. Chem. Soc. 88, 2041.

Poland, D. and Scheraga, H.A. (1967). In Poly-α-Amino Acids, p. 391. Ed. by Fasman, G.C. Marcel Dekker New York.

Ramachandran, G.N., Doyle, B.B. and Blout, E.R. (1968). Biopolymers 6, 1771.

Ramachandran, G.N. and Kartha, G. (1955). Nature 176, 593.

Ramachandran, G.N. and Sasisekharan, V. (1965). Biochem. Biophys. Acta 109, 314.

Rao, N.V. and Harrington, W.F. (1966). J. Mol. Biol. 21, 577.

Rich, A. and Crick, F.H.C. (1961). J. Mol. Biol. 3, 483.

Sakakibara, S., Kishida, Y., Kikuchi, Y., Sakai, R. and Kakiuchi, K. (1968). Bull. Chem. Soc. Jap. 5, 1273.

Steinberg, I.Z., Harrington, W.F., Berger, A., Sela, M. and Katchalski, E. (1960). J. Am. Chem. Soc. 82 5263.

Strassmair, H., Engel, J. and Zundel, G. (1969). Biopolymers (In press).

Strassmair, H., Knof, S. and Engel, J. (1969). Z. Physiol. Chem. (In press).

Traub, W. and Yonath, A. (1966). J. Mol. Biol. 16, 404.

Traub, W. and Yonath, A. (1967). J. Mol. Biol. 25, 351.

Traub, W., Yonath, A. and Segal, D.M. (1969). Nature 221, 914.

Veis, A. (1964). The Macromolecular Chemistry of Gelatin. Academic Press, New York.

STRUCTURAL FEATURES OF COLLAGEN AS DETERMINED THROUGH THE USE OF HYDROLYTIC ENZYMES

Howard B. Bensusan

Although several investigators have used single hydrolytic enzymes to reduce the collagen chains to polypeptide fragments, only two laboratories have used a combination of enzymes in an attempt to approach a complete enzymic hydrolysis. Grassman, Hannig and Nordwig (1963) used a combination of pepsin, trypsin, chymotrypsin, leucine aminopeptidase, and carboxypeptidases A and B. Seifter, Gallop and Franzblau (1961) tried a combination of collagenase, prolidase, and leucine aminopeptidase. In both cases the peptide fragments obtained were quite large. This paper describes the products of an enzymic hydrolysis which results in the liberation of 70-80% of the residues as free amino acids.

Insoluble, acid-soluble, and salt-soluble bovine-skin collagen and ichthyocol were treated with collagenase and the product was then treated according to the method of Hill and Schmidt (1962) using papain, prolidase, and leucine aminopeptidase. The final mixture was dialyzed and the dialyzate was concentrated in vacuo. Analyses of the products were carried out on the 0.6 x 140-cm column of the Technicon Amino Acid Analyzer with the 21-hr gradient system. A typical elution diagram is shown in Fig. 1. A stream-splitting device was used to collect various fractions. These fractions were then analyzed quantitatively after acid hydrolysis. The unresolved fraction of serine, threonine, glutamine, and asparagine was isolated, acid hydrolyzed, and the individual constituents were determined by amino acid analysis. Pyrrolidone-5-carboxylic

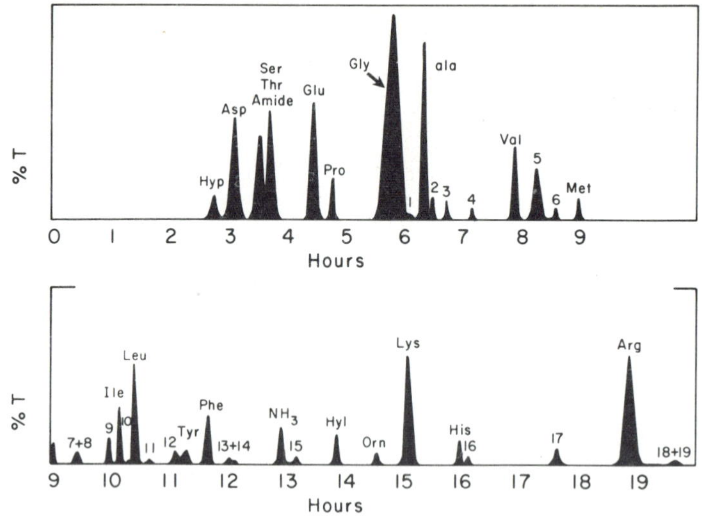

Fig. 1. Elution diagram of a typical enzymic digest. The ordinate is plotted as percent transmission in order to accentuate the numbered peptide peaks.

acid (PCA) was isolated from a fractional sample by passage through a short column of Dowex-50, adsorption on a short column of Dowex-1, and elution with HCl. It was determined as glutamic acid after acid hydrolysis. The peptide fraction was separated on a 1.2 x 140-cm column of Bio-Gel P2 and was fractionated on a 1.2 x 140-cm column of Dowex-50, x8. The fractions were desalted on short Dowex-50H^+ columns and the sequence determinations were carried out by the usual procedures.

Of the 18 peptides isolated, 15 were tripeptides having the general sequence Gly-Pro-X or Y-Hyp-Gly and 2 were tetrapeptides having the sequence Gly-Pro-Pro-Gly and Gly-Pro-Hyp-Gly. The sum of these last two peptides and the isolated Gly-Pro-Hyp amounted to an average of 40 μM per chain in bovine-skin collagen and 32 μM per chain in ichthyocol, in good agreement with the number estimated by Josse and Harrington (1964) from their probability calculations. Twelve of these 17 peptides have already been found in the sequence of the α1 chain (Bornstein, 1967; Butler, this book, p.149). Only the peptides Gln-Hyp-Gly, Ile-Hyp-Gly,

Gly-Pro-Val, Gly-Pro-Ile, and Gly-Pro-Phe remain to be accounted for. The remaining peptide had the tentative sequence of Gly-(Gln, Hyp, ε-Lys) as shown by the presence of dansyl-Gly and α-dansyl-Lys following dansylation and acid hydrolysis. This peptide is reminiscent of the peptide N^{ε}-(Gly-Glu)-Lys isolated by Mechanic and Levy (1959) from partial acid hydrolyzates of collagen. This peptide is being investigated further.

A complete analysis of the enzymic digest of insoluble collagen, as one example, is given in Table I. The amount of each amino acid occurring in the peptides was determined. When these values were added to the content of each of the free amino acids, the total content of each amino acid and the total amino acid content could be calculated. These values are given in the second column. Using this value of the total amino acid content, the number of residues of each of the free amino acids could be determined on the basis of their amount per collagen chain (1000 total residues). These values are shown in the first column. The total amount of the free amino acids from the first column as compared with the total amino acid content from the second column shows that the enzymic hydrolysis of this sample was about 70% complete. Since the relative amount of each amino acid is not very sensitive to errors in the total amount, we determined the amino acid composition and total amount of the amino acids in acid hydrolyzates of aliquots of the dialyzed enzymic hydrolyzate. These values are given in the third column. The addition of the free and peptide-bound amino acids in the second column agrees within experimental error with the amino acid content after acid hydrolysis of the enzyme hydrolyzate. The data obtained from acid hydrolyzates of insoluble collagen without enzymic treatment are given in the last column.

With the exception of a small amount of glutamine-containing peptides, all of the glutamic acid and glutamine appear to be accounted for as free residues in the enzymic hydrolyzates. A breakdown of the individual values for all 4 collagen samples is given in Table II. Since none of the

TABLE I

The Amino Acid Composition of Enzymic Hydrolyzates of Insoluble Collagen

	Amino acid content (residues/1000 total residues)			
	Enzyme hydrolyzate			Original
	Free*	Free + Peptide	Acid hydrolyzate	Acid hydrolyzate
Hydroxyproline	41.2	98.4	93.8	93.1
Aspartic acid	46.9	46.9	48.1	47.2
Threonine	13.0	13.0	18.3	15.4
Serine	27.6	34.4	42.0	36.0
Glutamic acid	71.5	73.6	65.0	71.3
Proline	33.1	108	120	121
Glycine	221	323	329	325
Alanine	106	126	115	112
Valine	23.2	24.7	22.5	16.9
Methionine	5.9	5.9	7.2	7.6
Isoleucine	11.3	13.1	11.4	9.9
Leucine	24.3	25.6	23.8	28.4
Tyrosine	3.3	3.3	3.8	3.7
Phenylalanine	10.5	12.5	12.3	14.2
Lysine	22.8	26.0	27.3	30.2
Histidine	3.7	3.7	3.8	3.7
Arginine	48.4	53.6	49.4	52.3
Hydroxylysine	5.5	6.1	6.9	7.1
Ornithine	1.6	1.6	1.4	1.0
Total μMoles	8.60	11.95	12.15	

*The total number of micromoles of the free amino acids plus the number of micromoles of amino acids in the peptides (last entry in the second column) was used to calculate the residues of each free amino acid per 1000 total residues.

enzymes used in the hydrolysis procedure are known to be capable of hydrolyzing γ-glutamyl bonds, these results appear to be contrary to those of Gallop, Seifter, Lukin and Meilman (1960) and Franzblau, Gallop and Seifter (1963), who, on the basis of the results of a series of chemical reactions, suggested that there are a minimum of 20 γ-glutamyl linkages in collagen. This apparent discrepancy was then investigated.

Preliminary experiments with model peptides showed

that the enzymes used in the enzymic hydrolysis were incapable of hydrolyzing the γ-glutamyl peptide linkage in γ-glutamyl alanine, γ-glutamyl glutamic acid, or glutathione. These results do not eliminate the possibility that the enzymes might hydrolyze these linkages in the polypeptide or protein. In order to test this possibility, the free carboxyl groups of ichthyocol gelatin were alanylated by the treatment of the protein with L-alanine methyl ester and 1-ethyl-3-dimethylaminopropyl carbodiimide (EDC) according to the method of Hoare and Koshland (1967). Thus, if there are γ-glutamyl linkages in the gelatin which can be hydrolyzed by the enzyme mixture, their hydrolysis and the hydrolysis of the alanine methyl ester groups attached to the free α- and γ-carboxyl groups should liberate all the glutamic acid. On the other hand, if all the glutamyl residues are involved in α-linkages, and if the enzymes are unable to hydrolyze the γ-linked alanine methyl ester groups, no free glutamic acid should be liberated in the enzymic hydrolyzates.

The alanylation experiment was carried out as outlined above. Acid hydrolysis of a control and the alanylated sample showed an excess of 81 alanine groups in the latter sample which is in reasonable agreement with the sum of glutamic acid and aspartic acid content (Table II). Enzymic hydrolysis of the control and alanylated samples showed that 49 residues of free glutamic acid were liberated from the control sample but only 2.6 residues were liberated from the alanylated sample. Therefore, it was concluded that the enzyme mixture was incapable of hydrolyzing γ-glutamyl linkages and that at least 95% of the glutamic acid residues are involved in normal α linkages.

A further demonstration that the glutamic acid residues in collagen are α linked resulted from the use of the chemical technique developed by Hoare, Olson and Koshland (1968). These authors showed that carboxylic acids treated with hydroxylamine and EDC would first form hydroxamates, which, after further reaction with EDC, would undergo the Lossen rearrangement to give the derivative with the carboxyl group replaced by an amino group. As with the technique developed by Gallop, et al. (1960), an α-linked glutamyl residue should result in the formation of a 2,4-diaminobutyryl residue and a γ-linked glutamyl residue should result in the liberation of succinic acid semialdehyde on acid hydrolysis of the protein so treated. In our experiments using the method of Hoare, et al. (1968), a loss of 24 residues of glutamic acid was accompanied by the formation of 21 residues of 2,4-diaminobutyric acid in acid hydrolyzates of treated ichthyocol and a loss of 15 residues of glutamic acid and the recovery of 15 residues of 2,4-diaminobutyric acid from acid hydrolyzates of treated salt-soluble calf-skin collagen. These results again indicate that most, if not all, of the glutamyl residues in collagen are involved in α linkages.

TABLE II

The Free Dicarboxylic Acids in Enzymic Hydrolyzates of Various Collagens

	Content (residues/1000 amino acid residues)				
	Enzyme hydrolyzate				Original+
	Glu	Gln	PCA	Total*	Total
Insoluble	49.3	18.9	3.3	71.5	71.3
Acid-soluble	42.0	22.0	6.4	72.4	76.0
Salt-soluble	48.4	24.8	4.2	77.4	78.8
Ichthyocol	46.7	16.2	7.2	70.1	70.3
	Asp	Asn		Total	Total
Insoluble	33.2	12.6		45.8	47.2
Acid-soluble	30.9	15.2		46.1	44.6
Salt-soluble	32.5	16.3		48.8	49.6
Ichthyocol	27.5	16.3		43.8	47.0

*Does not include the 0.4-2.6 residues of glutamine remaining in peptides 1 and 14.

+Values from acid hydrolyzates.

ACKNOWLEDGEMENTS

This work was supported by Grants AM01825 and HD00669 from the National Institutes of Health, U.S. Public Health Service.

REFERENCES

Bornstein, P. (1967). Biochemistry 6, 3083.

Franzblau, C., Gallop, P.M. and Seifter, S. (1963). Biopolymers 1, 79.

Gallop, P.M., Seifter, S., Lukin, M. and Melman, E. (1960). J. Biol. Chem. 235, 2619.

Grassman, W., Hannig, K. and Nordwig, A. (1963). Z. Physiol. Chem. 333, 154.

Hill, R.L. and Schmidt, W.R. (1962). J. Biol. Chem. 237, 389.

Hoare, D.G. and Koshland, D.E., Jr. (1967). J. Biol. Chem. 242, 2447.

Hoare, D.G., Olson, A. and Koshland, D.E., Jr. (1968). J. Am. Chem. Soc. 90, 1638.

Josse, J. and Harrington, W.F. (1964). J. Mol. Biol. 9, 269.

Mechanic, G.L. and Levy, M. (1959). J. Am. Chem. Soc. 81, 1889.

Seifter, S., Gallop, P.M. and Franzblau, C. (1961). Trans. N.Y. Acad. Sci. 23, 540.

STRUCTURAL STUDIES IN COLLAGEN

William T. Butler

A systematic chemical dissection of the collagen molecule was begun with rat skin collagen and has been extended to rat tendon, chicken skin and chick bone collagens. The approach to this problem involves fractionation of heat-denatured lathyritic collagen into α chains (Piez, 1967) cleavage of the individual chains at methionyl residues with cyanogen bromide (CNBr) (Bornstein and Piez, 1965, 1966), isolation and characterization of the resultant CNBr peptides (Bornstein and Piez, 1965, 1966; Butler, Piez and Bornstein, 1967; Miller, Lane and Piez, 1969; Fietzek and Piez, 1969; Kang, Piez and Gross, 1969; Lane and Miller, 1969), and determination of the alignment of the peptides in each α chain (Piez et al., 1968). Eight CNBr peptides with unique compositions and sizes were shown to account for all the weight and amino acids of the α1 chain of rat skin collagen (Butler et al., 1967). These CNBr peptides are a reasonable size for further chemical studies. The amino acid sequences of the first two peptides from the N-terminal end of α1 (residues 1 through 51 of rat skin) have been reported (Kang, Bornstein and Piez, 1967; Bornstein, 1967). In a continuation of the chemical characterization of the CNBr peptides of α1, the amino acid sequences of CNBr peptide 3 (α1-CB4) and 4 (α1-CB5) are reported here. In addition, the probable identity of a hydroxylamine (NH_2OH)-sensitive bond in one of the CNBr peptides of α1 is indicated.

I SEQUENCE STUDIES

α1-CB4 is a basic peptide containing 47 amino acids and representing residues 52 through 98 of the α1 chain of rat skin collagen. Its probable amino acid sequence is indicated in Fig. 1. Briefly, the conclusions depicted are based on the following observations:

A. Cleavage of α1-CB4 with trypsin (at positions 3-4, 11-12, 27-28 and 36-37) liberated five peptides. The totals of their amino acid compositions agreed exactly with the composition of α1-CB4. Partial amino acid sequences for these five tryptic peptides were determined by Edman degradation (Schroeder, 1967; Konigsberg, 1967).

B. When α1-CB4 was cleaved with collagenase a large number of peptides were observed. The compositions and partial sequences (Edman degradations) of three of these peptides (representing residues 10-18, 34-36, and 40-45) provided additional sequence information.

C. Proteolysis of α1-CB4 with pepsin produced two fragments containing 17 and 30 amino acids. Eight steps of Edman degradation of the latter gave the amino acid sequence of residues 18-27 of α1-CB4.

D. Twelve steps of Edman degradation of α1-CB4 indicated the alignment of the first three tryptic peptides and verified conclusions concerning the amino acid sequence of this area of α1-CB4, which had been derived from studies on these three peptides. The presence of homoserine in a fourth tryptic peptide established that it was derived from the C-terminal end of α1-CB4 (residues 37-47) and deductively that the remaining peptide represented residues 28-36 of α1-CB4.

The structure for α1-CB4 which is depicted in Fig. 1 should be considered tenative, since in some cases the sequence depends upon the assumption that glycine is found in every third position. Further studies involving the proteolysis of individual tryptic peptides are being conducted in order to provide additional evidence concerning this

GLY-PRO-ARG-GLY-PRO-HYP-GLY-PRO-HYP-GLY-LYS-ASN-GLY-ASP-ASP-
1 5 10 15

GLY-GLX-ALA-GLY-LYS-PRO-GLY-ARG-HYP-GLY-GLN-ARG-GLY-PRO-HYP-
20 25 30

GLY-PRO-GLN-GLY-ALA-ARG-GLY-LEU-HYP-GLY-THR-ALA-GLY-LEU-HYP-GLY-HSE
35 40 45

Fig. 1. The amino acid sequence of α1-CB4.

structure.

The amino acid sequence of α1-CB5 is depicted in Fig. 2. This peptide has recently been shown to be CNBr peptide 4, representing residues 99 to 135 of the α1 chain of rat skin collagen (Piez, Miller, Lane and Butler, 1969). The conclusions shown in Fig. 2 are based on the following observations and experiments:

A. Cleavage of α1-CB5 with chymotrypsin yielded a small hexose-containing peptide of 6 amino acids and a larger one containing the remainder to the amino acids of α1-CB5, including the homoserine. The larger peptide was cleaved at its two lysyl residues to produce three smaller peptides of 7,9 and 15 amino acids. The sum of the amino acids in the four above peptides agreed exactly with the composition of α1-CB5, and were thus judged to represent its complete sequence.

B. The amino acids sequences of the four peptides were established by further proteolysis with bacterial collagenase

HYL-GLY-HIS-ARG-GLY-PHE-SER-GLY-LEU-ASP-GLY-ALA-LYS-
/ 5 10
O
/
GAL
/
GLC GLY-ASN-THR-GLY-PRO-ALA-GLY-PRO-LYS-GLY-GLU-HYP-
15 20 25

GLY-SER-HYP-GLY-GLU-ASN-GLY-ALA-HYP-GLY-GLN-HSE
30 35

Fig. 2. The covalent structure of α1-CB5.

or with pepsin.

C. The results from several experiments provided information concerning the alignment of these four peptides from α1-CB5. The hexose-containing peptide produced by hydrolysis with chymotrypsin (see above) was from the N-terminal of α1-CB5 (encompassing residues 1-6) since it contained phenylalanine and no homoserine. The peptide of 15 amino acids represents the C-terminal of α1-CB5 (residues 23-37) since it contained homoserine. When α1-CB5 was hydrolyzed with trypsin without prior hydrolysis at the phenylalanyl bond by chymotrypsin, a new peptide containing 9 amino acids was found. It was identical with the heptapeptide (see above) except for additional residues of glycine and phenylalanine at its NH_2- terminus. This peptide must be an overlap between the N-terminal hexose-containing peptide and the heptapeptide. The latter was therefore judged to be peptide 2 (residues 7-13) of α1-CB5 and, by deduction the nonapeptide 3, (residues 14-22), in the alignment.

D. The carbohydrate of α1-CB5 was shown to consist of ~1 mole each of galactose and glucose per mole of peptide, by paper chromatography and by determinations with glucose and galactose oxidases. The glycosidic linkage to hydroxylysine and the sequence of the sugars is assumed from previous studies (Butler and Cunningham, 1966; Cunningham and Ford, 1968) since the unusual amino acid sequence about the hydroxylysine is identical to that of a glycopeptide from guinea pig skin collagen.

The structure of the collagen molecule is generally thought to be composed of alternating nonpolar regions containing relatively large amounts of the imino acids, proline and hydroxyproline, and of polar regions having relatively few imino acids (Gallop and Seifter, 1966). The amino acid sequence of α1-CB5 (Fig. 2) illustrates this phenomenon since imino acids do not occur among the first 17 of its amino acids but are relatively rich in the latter half of its sequence. The imino acid-rich portion of α1-CB5 is however, not void of charged amino acids, for residues of lysine (position 22) and of glutamic acid (position 24) are found adjacent to proline and hydroxyproline, respectively. This principle is illustrated to a more limited extent by the amino acid sequence of α1-CB4, which has a higher concentration of more evenly distributed proline and hydroxyproline.

The occurrence of five arginyl residues within a span of less than 50 amino acids (positions 54-102 of α1) is indicitive of an area heavily staining with phosphotungstic acid and thus, of a broad band (at least 150 Å) visible under the electron microscope. It will be interesting to see if future conclusions concerning the amino acid sequence of collagen can be related to findings with electron microscopy (Piez et al., 1969).

Previous studies by Grassman and coworkers (see Hannig and Nordwig, 1967) indicated that a number of the lysyl and arginyl bonds of collagen could not be cleaved with trypsin. Indirect evidence was presented that the peptide bonds in question involved prolyl or hydroxyprolyl residues bound to the basic amino acids. Two of the peptide bonds of α1-CB4 involving lysine or arginine which could not be cleaved by trypsin were identified as Lys-Pro and Arg-Hyp bonds (positions 20-21, and 23-24 of α1-CB4, respectively) verifying these earlier conclusions.

II THE IDENTITY OF A HYDROXYLAMINE-SENSITIVE BOND IN COLLAGEN

The demonstration that denatured samples of collagen will react with nucleophiles such as hydrazine (NH_2NH_2) or hydroxylamine (NH_2OH) has lead to the proposal that the α chains of collagen are not continuous polypeptide chains but are composed of subunits linked by "ester or ester-like bonds", of an unknown nature (Gallop, Blumenfeld and Seifter, 1967).

I have recently found that one of the relatively small CNBr peptides from α1 will react with NH_2OH to yield

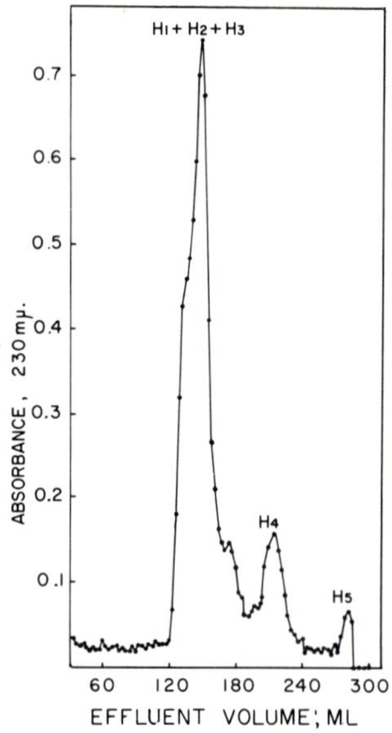

Fig. 3. Partial separation of the products of cleavage of α1-CB3 with NH_2OH by gel filtration on a 1.8 x 140 cm column of Sephadex G-50. Elution was with 0.1 M acetic acid.

apparently specific products. This peptide, α1-CB3, composed of 149 amino acids is derived from the central portion of α1. After cleavage with 0.72 M NH_2OH at pH 9.5 and 37°C for 7 or 24 hr, the products were partially separated by gel filtration on Sephadex G-50 (Fig. 3). Four products have been observed and partially characterized. Their compositions and sizes indicate that two bonds, rather near the COOH-terminus of α1-CB3 were cleaved during the reaction (Butler, 1969). Approximately one-half of the material (H1, Fig. 3) was uncleaved. In a control sample where NH_4HCO_3 was substituted for NH_2OH, no degradation took place, indicating that the reaction is not merely a result of the relatively high pH.

Experiments were designed to isolate a small peptide containing an intact NH_2OH-sensitive bond. One of the products of NH_2OH cleavage of α1-CB3, H4 (see Fig. 3) contained 29 amino acids including one residue each of homoserine and lysine. The presence of the lysine suggested

TABLE I

Amino acid compositions of some products of NH_2OH or trypsin cleavage of α1-CB3.*

Amino acid	H4	T1	H4-T1	T4
	(residues per peptide)			
Hydroxyproline	4	3	1	1
Aspartic acid	3	1	2	4
Threonine	1	1	0	0
Serine	1	1	0	0
Homoserine	1	1	0	0
Glutamic acid	2	2	0	0
Glycine	10	7	3	4
Alanine	5	3	2	2
Leucine	1	1	0	0
Lysine	1	0	1	1
Total	29	20	9	12

* See the text concerning nomenclature.

that the products of trypsin hydrolysis of α1-CB3 might give more information about the area containing the NH_2OH-sensitive bonds. One of the peptides released from α1-CB3 after its hydrolysis with trypsin,T1, contained homoserine, but no lysine, in a total of 20 amino acids; thus, it represents the portion of α1-CB3 C-terminal to the lysine of peptide H4. The difference in the compositions of peptides H4 and T1 (Table I), which represents the composition of H4 N-terminal to its lysine, indicates that the tryptic peptide bearing the intact NH_2OH-sensitive bond must have at least two residues each of aspartic acid and alanine and one of lysine. Of the five lysine-containing tryptic peptides of α1-CB3 only one peptide, T4, fulfilled these compositional requirements. Peptide T4 contained 12 amino acids, including four of aspartic acid, two of alanine and one of lysine (Table I). The composition of T4, therefore suggested that it contained an intact NH_2OH-sensitive bond, cleavage of which had produced H4. To further test this hypothesis, peptide T4 was treated with NH_2OH in the usual manner and the products partially separated by gel filtration on a Sephadex G-10 column. A substantial proportion of T4 was indeed degraded to smaller molecules eluting at volumes greater than untreated T4.

In order to identify one of the NH_2OH bonds of α1-CB3, chemical studies employing the Edman reagent were performed on the appropriate peptides. The PTH amino acids following Edman degradations were identified by thin-layer chromatography. In addition the amino acid compositions of residual peptides of T4 were determined following each step of Edman degradation. The following partial sequences were indicated by these experiments:

NH_2-terminums of α1-CB3:	Gly-Phe-Hyp-Gly-Pro-,
NH_2-terminus of H4:	Gly-Ala-Hyp-,
Peptide T4:	Gly-Asn-Asn-Gly-Ala-Hyp-(Gly_2, Asx_2, Ala)-Lys.

Since a new NH_2-terminus was liberated by the treatment of α1-CB3 with NH_2OH, as indicated by the non-identical NH_2-terminii of α1-CB3 and H4, the bond in question was a peptide bond. The observation that the amino acid sequences at positions 4-6 of peptide T4 and of 1-3 of H4 are identical further strengthens the conclusion that peptides T4 and H4 are from the same site in α1-CB3 and indicates that the bond being cleaved by NH_2OH is an Asn-Gly (peptide) bond.

A second bond (presumably a peptide bond) located near this Asn-Gly bond was cleaved at a slower rate during the reaction of α1-CB3 with NH_2OH. This conclusion is based on the composition and size of peptide H5 (see Fig. 3) as well as the sizes of products of cleavage of peptide T4 with NH_2OH (judged by their positions of elution from Sephadex G-10). Since two additional residues of aspartic acid (or asparagine) reside in this portion of the α1-CB3 (see the analysis for peptide T4, Table I), the amino acid sequence about the second site of attack by NH_2OH may be identical or similar to that of the first (i.e. the Gly-Asn-Asn-Gly sequence). These tentative conclusions are therefore in partial agreement with those of Gallop et al. (1967) who have noted the nucleophilic attack (by NH_2OH or NH_2NH_2) upon a special set of bonds in collagen which are found as pairs (i.e. two bonds are in close proximity). The data presented here, however, suggest that the bonds in question are peptide bonds, and therefore that α chains are not composed of "subunits", but are in fact continuous polypeptide chains.

In studies involving cleavage of calf skin collagen with NH_2OH, Volpin, Hörmann and Kühn (1968) have presented evidence that one of the bonds cleaved by the nucleophile was in the central portion of α1. My observations are in agreement with their results, since α1-Cb3 represents a peptide segment from the middle of α1.

REFERENCES

Bornstein, P. (1967). Biochemistry 6, 3082.

Bornstein, P. and Piez, K.A. (1965). Science 148, 1353.

Bornstein, P. and Piez, K.A. (1966). Biochemistry 5, 3460.

Butler, W.T. (1969). J. Biol Chem. 244, 3415.

Butler, W.T. and Cunningham, L.W. (1966). J. Biol. Chem. 241, 3882.

Butler, W.T., Piez, K.A. and Bornstein, P. (1967). Biochemistry 6, 3771.

Cunningham, L.W., and Ford, J.D. (1968). J. Biol. Chem. 243, 2390.

Fietzek, P.P. and Piez, K.A. (1969). Biochemistry 8, 2129.

Gallop, P.M., Blumenfeld, O.O. and Seifter, S. (1967). In Treatise on Collagen, vol. 1, p. 339. Ed. Ramachandran, G.N. Academic Press (Inc.) Ltd., London.

Gallop, P.M. and Seifter, S. (1966). In The Proteins, vol. 4, p. 153. Ed. Neurath, H. Academic Press (Inc) Ltd., New York.

Hannig, K. and Nordwig, A. (1967). In Treatise on Collagen, vol. 1, p. 73. Ed. Ramachandran, G.N. Academic Press (Inc.) Ltd., London.

Kang, A.H., Bornstein, P. and Piez, K.A. (1967). Biochemistry 6, 788.

Kang, A.H., Piez, K.A. and Gross, J. (1969). Biochemistry 8, 1506.

Konigsberg, W. (1967). In Methods in Enzymology, vol. 11, p. 461. Ed. Hirs, C.W.H. Academic Press (Inc.) Ltd., New York.

Lane, J.M. and Miller, E.J. (1969). Biochemistry 8, 2134.

Miller, E.J., Lane, J.M. and Piez, K.A. (1969). Biochemistry 8, 30.

Piez, K.A. (1967). In Treatise on Collagen, vol. 1, p. 207. Ed. Ramachandran, G.N. Academic Press (Inc.) Ltd., London.

Piez, K.A., Bladen, H.A., Lane, J.M., Miller, E.J., Bornstein, P., Butler, W.T. and Kang, A.H. (1968). Brookhaven Symp. Biol. 21, 345.

Piez, K.A., Miller, E.J., Lane, J.M. and Butler, W.T.(1969). Science (in press).

Schroeder, W.A. (1967). In Methods in Enzymology, vol. 11, p. 351. Ed. Hirs, C.W.H. Academic Press (Inc.) Ltd., New York.

Volpin, D., Hörmann, H. and Kühn, K. (1968). Biochim. Biophys. Acta 168, 389.

THE CLEAVAGE OF COLLAGEN WITH HYDROXYLAMINE

Helmut Hörmann and Dino Volpin

Gallop, Seifter and Meilman (1959) have found that collagen can be degraded by hydroxylamine. During the treatment of soluble collagen 18 moles of protein-bound hydroxamic acid are formed (Hörmann, 1960, 1962), which may originate from the bonds cleaved by the reagent. Suitable conditions for degradation are 0.72 M hydroxylamine in 4 M LiCl, pH 9.5. Under these conditions formation of hydroxamic acid is almost finished after 7 hr at 40°C.

In the present study the fragments obtained by treatment of citrate-soluble collagen from calf skin with hydroxylamine were chromatographed on CM-Cellulose (Volpin, Hörmann and Kuhn, 1968; Heidemann and Heinrich, 1968). Almost identical separation patterns were observed for the degradation mixtures of collagen or of purified α1-chains (Fig. 1). The same holds for electrophoretic separations on acrylamide gel. Obviously, the distinct fractions of the reaction mixture originate from the α1-chains. The α2-chains probably are degraded less specifically and to a greater extent resulting in fractions hidden in the background of the separation pattern.

After rechromatography the major fractions IV and V of the eluate were shown to be homogeneous compounds by electrophoresis on acrylamide gel. Fraction VI contained several components. Some of them exhibiting a high molecular weight, were removed by gel filtration over Sephadex G-100. The resulting fractions of lower molecular weight could be resolved on CM-cellulose into two fragments (Fractions VIa and VIb). Fraction VIa and VIb also originated from the α1-chains as shown by electrophoretic comparison of the two purified fractions with a degradation mixture of the α1-chains on acryl-

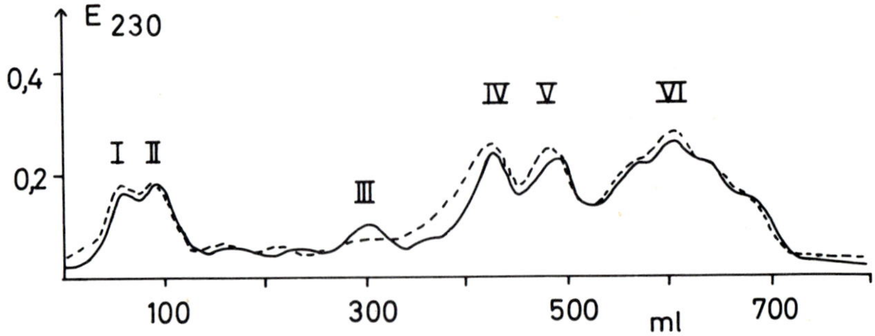

Fig. 1. Chromatographic fractionation of hydroxylamine treated collagen (————) and α1-chains (- - -) on CM-cellulose. 0.04 M sodium acetate, pH 4.8; gradient: 0 → 0.06 M NaCl.

amide gel.

By means of an electronmicroscopic procedure developed by Rauterberg and Kuhn (1968) fractions IV, V, VIa and VIb could be allocated to the corresponding regions of the collagen molecule. The fragments were renatured to triple helices, precipitated as segment fragments with ATP and correlated with segments of undegraded collagen according to their electronmicroscopic cross-striation (Fig. 2).

Fractions IV and V appeared to be long chain degradation products from the B-end of the α1-chains. Peptide V was shorter than peptide IV. Some short piece at the B-end was missing.

Fraction VIa and VIb gave rise to segment fragments corresponding to a molecular weight of the single chains of 22,000 (VIa) and 24,000 (VIb) respectively. Segments of VIb correspond to a region which was already covered by the longer fractions IV and V. Obviously, VIb was derived from these fractions by further degradation. On the other hand, fraction VIa was allocated to a region immediately following fractions IV or V on the A-side.

Between fractions VIa and VIb there is a gap corresponding to a peptide of a molecular weight of 19,000. On the A-side of collagen there is still a region of 850 Å not covered by isolated fragments of the α1-chains. The single peptide chains of this part should have a molecular weight of 28,000 corresponding to approximately 300 amino acid residues.

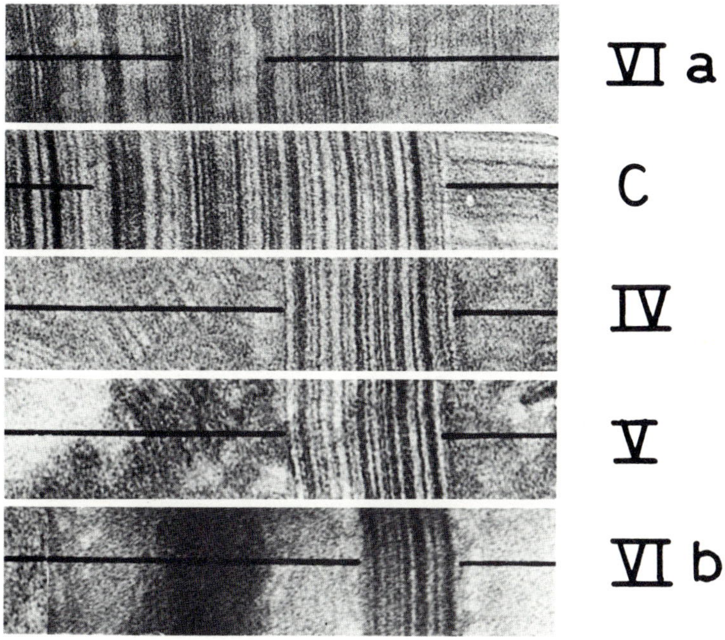

Fig. 2. Segments of collagen (C) and of renatured fragments IV, V, VIa and VIb. Siemens Elmiskop I at 80 kV.

From the amino acid composition of the individual fractions published elsewhere (Volpin and Hormann, 1968, and unpublished data) the corresponding molecular weights were calculated. Agreement with the electronmicroscopic data was achieved, if one assumes that fractions IV and V contain two methionine residues each and fractions VIa and VIb only one methionine residue (Table I). The methionine content of the various fractions determined in this way is in accord with the distribution of methionine residues along the α1-chains as shown by Rauterberg and Kuhn (1968). In the α2-chains the methionine residues are distributed in quite another manner (compare Stark and Kuhn, 1968).

Fractions II and III could not be allocated so far with certainty by means of electronmicroscopy. Fraction II was also present in degradation products of the α1-chains. Fraction III seems to be unstable and was not always found in reaction mixtures. Both fragments were purified to electrophoretically homogeneous compounds, although their bands were diffuse to some extent. Assuming that these two fractions contained one methionine residue each, one can calculate from the amino acid composition (Volpin and Hormann, unpublished data) a molecular weight of 19,600 for II and of 21,250 for III, respectively. Estimation in the ultracentrifuge by the method of Yphantis (1960) resulted in a molecular weight of 17,300 for III. The amino acid composition of the two fractions was very similar. We, therefore, suggest that these two fractions belong to the same region of the α1-chains, fraction II originating from fraction III by limited degradation. Since there is only one methionine residue present, we conclude that they contain the peptide chain from the gap between fractions VIa and VIb. They cannot be derived from the A-terminal sequence of the α1-chains, because in this region three methionine residues are concentrated (Rauterberg and Kuhn, 1968).

Fraction II, III, IV and V contain one hydroxamic acid residue each as determined with the iodine method (Yashphe, Halpern and Grossowicz, 1960) and the indole method (Seifter, Gallop, Michaels and Meilman, 1960) (Table I). Obviously, the

TABLE I

Molecular Weight and Hydroxamic Acid Content of Peptides Isolated from Hydroxylamine Treated Collagen

Fragment	Molecular Weight: Electron microscope	Amino acid analysis	Sedimentation equilibrium	Hydroxamic Acid Moles per mole*: Iodine	Indole
II	--	19,600	--	0.82	1.2±
III	--	21,250	17,300	0.82	1.1±0.2
IV	47,000	48,200	45,200	1.12	1.3
V	45,000	45,300	42,000	1.03	1.2
VIa	22,000	20,500	34,000	0.52 (0.86⁺)	0.6 (1.0⁺)
VIb	24,000	23,000	37,700	0.44 (0.73⁺)	0.47 (0.9⁺)

*Calculated for molecular weight estimated from amino acid analysis.

⁺Calculated for molecular weight estimated by sedimentation equilibrium.

hydroxamic acid was derived from the carboxyl group originally involved in the bond split by hydroxylamine. In fraction VIa and VIb only about 0.5 moles of hydroxamic acid were present calculated for a molecular weight as estimated from the electronmicroscopic length of their segments. On the other hand, the molecular weight determined in the ultracentrifuge (Yphantis, 1960) was about twice the value obtained by electronmicroscopic investigations. We, therefore, suggest that these two fractions are subject to dimerisation, one hydroxamic acid being involved in this reaction and lost.

The results presented show clearly that hydroxylamine splits the α1-chains of calf skin collagen at some distinct linkages. The reaction results in peptide fragments with an approximate weight of 20,000. Besides the specific cleavage one cannot exclude an unspecific degradation, especially of some more sensitive regions, e.g. near the A-end or the α2-chains.

ACKNOWLEDGEMENTS

We are indebted to Professor K. Kühn for discussion, advice and equipment and to Mrs. H. Wiedmann for technical assistance with the electronmicroscope.

Gallop, P.M., Seifter, S. and Meilman, E. (1959). Nature, 183, 1659.

Heidemann, H. and Heinrich, W. (1968). Leder 19, 176.

Hörmann, H. (1960). Leder 11, 173.

Hörmann, H. (1962). Leder 13, 79.

Rauterberg, J. and Kühn, K. (1968). FEBS Letters 1, 230.

Seifter, S., Gallop, P.M., Michaels, S. and Meilman, E. (1960). J. Biol. Chem. 235, 2613.

Stark, M. and Kühn, K. (1968), European J. Biochem. 6, 534.

Volpin, D. and Hörmann, H. (1968). Zt. Physiol. Chem. 349, 1231.

Volpin, D., Hörmann, H. and Kühn, K. (1968). Biochim. Biophys. Acta 168, 389.

Yashphe, J., Halpern, Y.S. and Grossowicz, N. (1960). Analytical Chemistry 32, 518.

Yphantis, D.A. (1960). Ann. N.Y. Acad. Sci. 88, 586.

CYANOGEN BROMIDE AND COLLAGENASE DERIVED PEPTIDES FROM THE α1 CHAIN OF CALF SKIN COLLAGEN: THEIR LOCALIZATION WITHIN THE CHAIN BY ELECTRON MICROSCOPIC METHODS

J. Rauterberg, K.von der Mark, F. Rexrodt and K. Kühn

Tkocz and Kühn (1969) recently reported that isolated α1 and α2-chains from calfskin collagen can form molecules with the triple-helical structure of the native collagen molecule. We can now show that this also applies to fragments of the α1 and α2 chains. The fragmentary collagen molecules produced in this way can be precipitated with ATP to long spacing fragments as can be done with native collagen molecules. From the cross-striation pattern of these segments information can be drawn about the position of the peptide within the whole chain.

I POSITION OF THE NON-DIALYSABLE PEPTIDES DERIVED FROM CYANOGEN BROMIDE DIGESTION OF CALFSKIN-α1

We used the method of Butler, Piez and Bornstein (1967) to prepare cyanogen bromide (CB) peptides of α1 chains of calfskin collagen. Calfskin collagen was used because of its greater tendency to renature compared to rat skin collagen. (Tkocz and Kühn, 1969).

Figure 1 shows the separation of the CB-peptides on CM-cellulose. Peaks a and c represent smaller dialysable peptides whereas peak b, d and e are non-dialysable. At first we tried to form triple helices from peaks b, d and e without further purification.

The renaturation process was done as follows: The salt

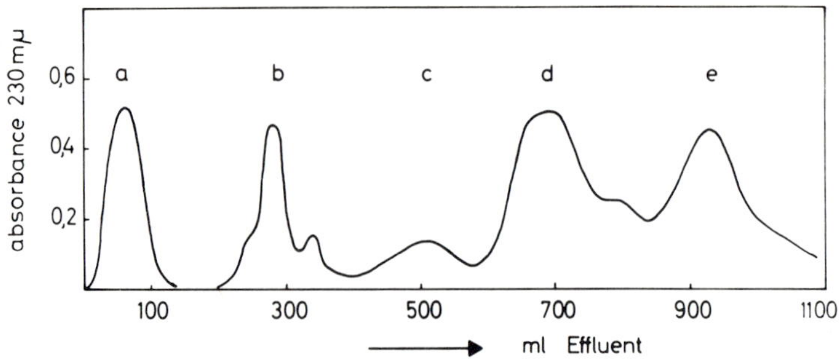

Fig. 1 Chromatography of the products of CB cleavage of α1 from acid soluble calfskin collagen on CM-cellulose (Whatman CM 32) at pH 3.6. Linear gradient from 0.02 M sodium citrate--0.04 M NaCl (pH 3.6) to 0.02 M sodium citrate--0.14 M NaCl over a volume of 1600 ml.

free lyophilised peptide was dissolved in citrate buffer of pH 3.7 and denatured by warming to 40°C. The solution was cooled stepwise starting at 18°C. The optical rotation was also measured at the same time. When the increase in optical rotation obtained a practicable rate, that means a rate at which the median value between the denatured and native state would be reached within 2 days, the solution was allowed to stay at this temperature for 2 or 3 days. This procedure was followed in order to bring about renaturation at as high a temperature as possible, because the tendency to form non-specific aggregates at the low cost of native triple helical structure increases at lower temperatures. A part of the solution was then dialysed against 0.05% acetic acid and then against 0.4% ATP solution. It is again important that the formation of SLS was brought about by dialysis against ATP solution and not by addition of ATP, as in the former case a slow precipitation is guaranteed. The precipitated segments were positively stained with phosphotungstic acid and with uranyl acetate before examination in the electron microscope.

Treatment of the solution with pepsin at renaturation temperature before dialysis against acetic acid aids the production of "segment long spacing" fragments (SLS) with well defined cross-striations. Randomly aggregated structures formed during renaturation are more susceptible to

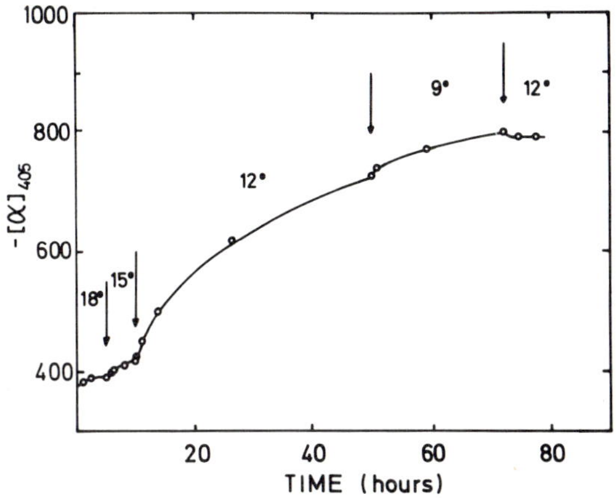

Fig. 2. The increase in negative specific optical rotation during renaturation of peak e. Solution in 0.225 M citrate buffer pH 3.6; concentration 1 mg/ml. Optical rotation was measured at 405 mμ.

attack by proteases than the triple helical native structures and therefore are broken down to dialysable peptides. The substrate-enzyme ratio was 10:1. To exclude the possibility that the pepsin treatment produces shorter fragments, it is of course necessary to form SLS from solutions not pretreated with pepsin. The CB-peptides in both cases, however, showed SLS segments of equal length.

Figure 2 shows the increase in negative optical rotation from peak e on renaturation. The optimum renaturation temperature is obtained at as low a temperature as 12°C. After 2 days the temperature was lowered again by 3°C, when a further slight increase in negative optical rotation was obtained. Rewarming the solution to 12°C had only a slight effect.

The SLS fragments obtained from the renaturation of CB-peptides are shown in Fig. 3 on the left hand side. Fraction b and e show one type of segment, while fraction d yields two types of segments indicating the presence of two different peptides in the fraction. The right side of the picture shows the coordination of these SLS fragments with normal SLS from ASC. Figure 4 gives a schematic representation of the positions of the SLS from CB-peptides within

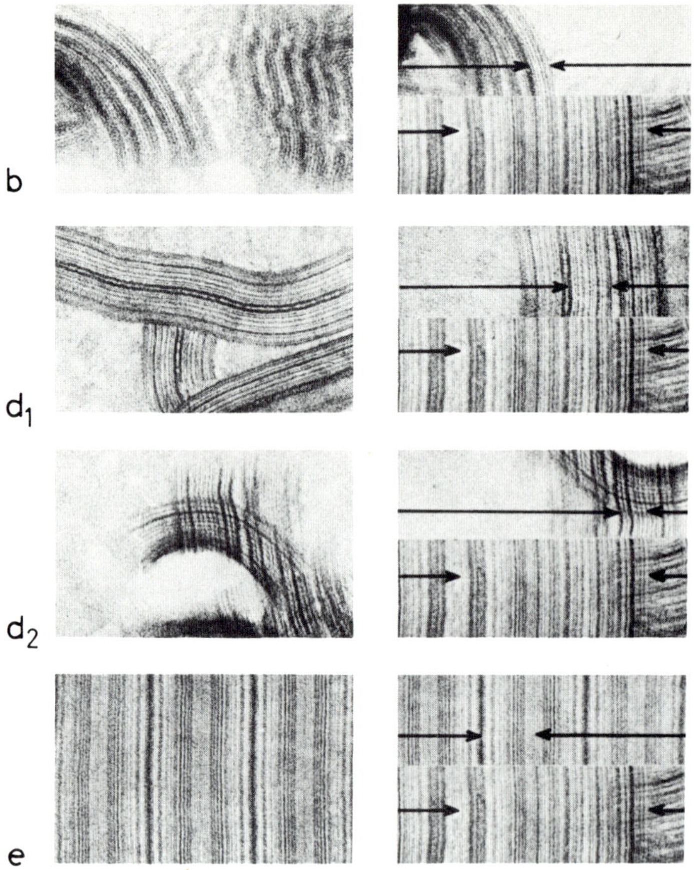

Fig. 3. Left hand side: Long spacing segments obtained from the non-dialysable CB-peptides after renaturation in citrate buffer pH 3,7. The segments tend to end-to-end aggregation on one end (d 1 and d 2) or on both ends (b and e). For preparation and staining of the segments see text on the right hand side: Correlation of the CB-peptide segments with a segment from native collagen molecules, 2900 Å in length. The arrows indicate the ends of individual segments.

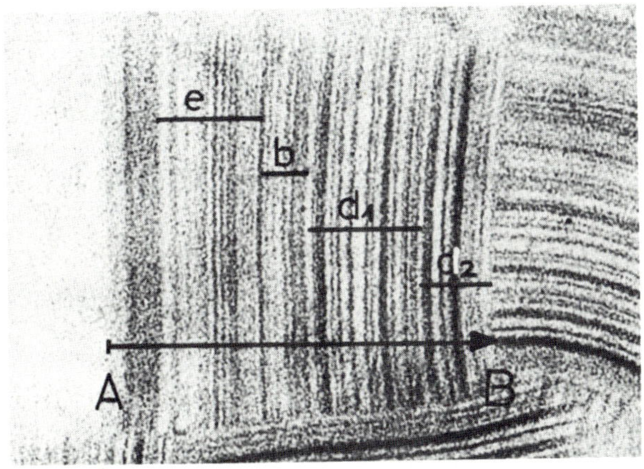

Fig. 4. Position of the non-dialysable CB-peptides.

a normal SLS.

It is seen that d 2 corresponds to the B-end of the molecule, followed by d 1, b and finally e. A fragment of about 350 Å at the A-end does not correspond to any of the renatured peptides. It is likely that the smaller peptides obtained by CB cleavage are localised in this region. The rest of the molecule is made up only from the four bigger peptides. A comparison of the size and the amino acid composition with the data given by Piez and co-workers (Butler, Piez and Bornstein, 1967) for the CB peptides of rat skin collagen shows that there is no essential difference and that the nomenclature proposed by the Piez group can also be applied to the CB-peptides of calfskin-α1:

Fraction	b	corresponds	to	CB 3
"	d 1	"	"	CB 7
"	d 2	"	"	CB 6
"	e	"	"	CB 8

II ISOLATION OF OVERLAPPING PEPTIDES

From the electron microscopic study, it is not possible to state whether smaller CB-peptides are also localized in between the renatured peptides just illustrated. This could be checked by isolation of overlapping peptides.

An incompletely cleaved peptide could be isolated by rechromatography of peak e. Figure 5 shows rechromatography on CM-cellulose at pH 4.8 in a sodium acetate buffer. The adjacent peaks β,γ,δ and ε show after renaturation SLS segments identical with those obtained from peak e. Peak α yielded segments long spacing fragments which showed that this peptide is made up from peptides e and b (CB 8 and CB 3).

Figure 6 gives a comparison of the imcompletely cleaved fragment with a normal SLS. The amino acid analysis shows, that this peptide contains equal amounts of methionine and homoserine. It is then certain, that the CB-peptides b and e include no smaller peptides. Further peptides which overlap with CB-peptides could be produced on treatment of native collagen with collagenase; a method introduced by

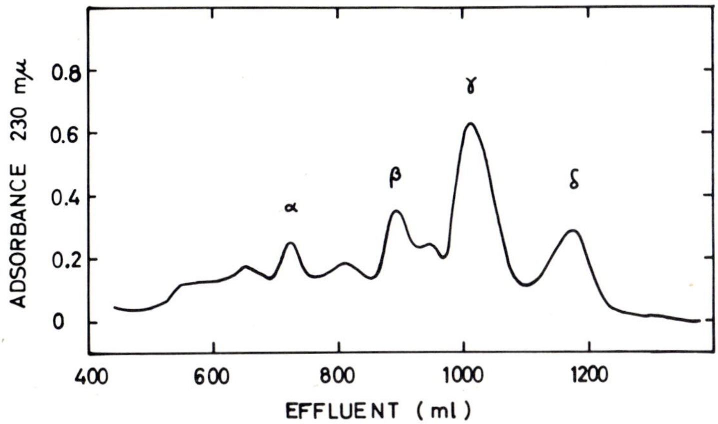

Fig. 5. Rechromatography of peak e on CM-cellulose at pH 4.8. Elution was in 0.02 M sodium acetate (pH 4.8) with a linear gradient from 0.02 M to 0.1 M NaCl over a volume of 1800 ml.

Stark and Kühn (1968). At low temperatures, collagenase attacks native collagen molecules from both the ends. Certain regions are relatively less labile and are cleaved only very slowly. This results in the formation of considerable quantites of molecular fragments of definite length.

The results of collagenase treatment are summarized schematically in Fig. 7. The fragments of 1250 Å and 780 Å length could be isolated in considerable quantities. The single chains are subsequently isolated by chromatography on CM-cellulose. The 780Å-long fragment overlaps the CB peptides d 1 and d 2 (CB 7 and CB 6). The amino acid analysis of the α1 chain of this peptide (780-α1) shows only one methionine per chain, meaning that there is only one cleavage point in this peptide.

The 1250 Å fragment overlaps 3 CB-peptides: d 1 (CB 7), part of b (CB 3) and d 2 (CB 6). The amino acid analysis of 1250-α1 chain provided 2 methionines. This means, there is no smaller CB-peptide between b and d 1, as also between d 1 and d 2. Finally the amino acid analysis of the CB-peptide d 2 (CB 6) gives no homoserine showing that this peptide forms the carboxyl end of the α1 chain.

It is thus seen that the other smaller CB-peptides must be situated at the 350 Å long region at the A end, from which

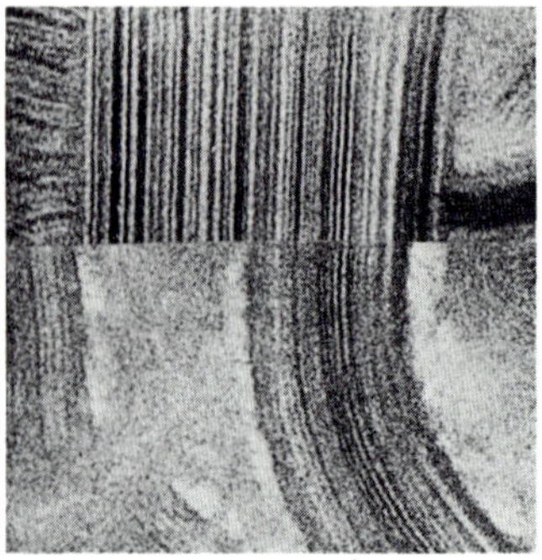

Fig. 6. Comparison of a SLS from incompletely cleaved CB-peptide e-b (CB 8 -3) with a normal SLS.

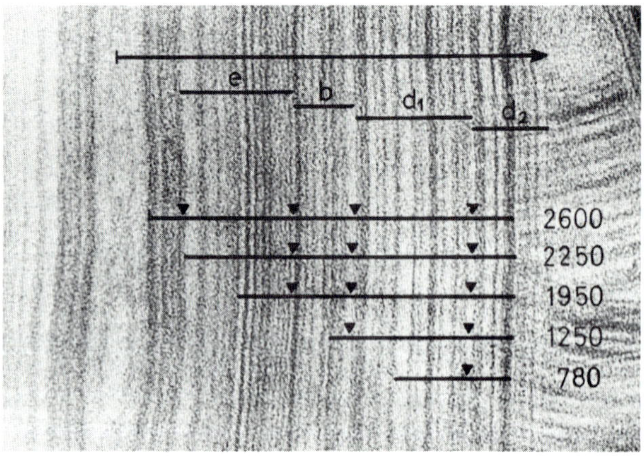

Fig. 7. Position of the non-dialysable CB-peptides of α1 and of the fragments derived from the collagenase treatment of native acid soluble collagen. The positions of methionines in the α1 chains of these fragments are marked.

no ordered structures can be formed on renaturation.

III CYANOGEN BROMIDE CLEAVAGE OF COLLAGENASE DIGESTION DERIVED FRAGMENTS

It is possible to get a further series of α1-peptides by CB cleavage of fragments derived from collagenase digestion of native collagen. Their location along the length of the molecule can be ascertained again by renaturation and precipitation of SLS and also partly by amino acid analysis. (The C-terminal peptide contains no homoserine.)

CB cleavage of α1-780 and α1-1250 has been carried out. Figure 8 shows the position of the fragments which we have isolated. α1-780 was cleaved into two peptides, named α1-780 CBC and α1-780 CBN. We could split up the α1-1250 into 3 peptides: a carboxyl-end peptide--this was found to be identical with α1-780 CBC; a central peptide, identical with CB d 1 (CB 7) obtained by CB cleavage of α1, and α1-1250 CBN. All the expected peptides could be isolated and with the exception of α1-1250 CBN could be renatured and formed into SLS fragments. The α1-1250 CBN cannot be precipitated after renaturation in this manner because of its small length. Figure 9 gives a comparison of segments derived from the renatured CB-peptides of α1-780 and of SLS from untreated collagen.

As shown by Stark and Kühn (1968) the α1 components in the fragments obtained by collagenase treatment resolve into two constituents, which vary significantly in their running velocity in disc-electrophoresis and in CM-cellulose chromatography. The amino acid analysis however, shows a close similarity, so that the terminology "α1" and "α3" which was introduced by Stark and Kühn (1968) may not be very suitable; one might speak more correctly of two variants of α1. With the help of CB-cleavage of these two α-components of the 780 Å long fragment, it is possible to show that the difference between the two must be localized in a distinct small region.

As illustrated in Fig. 10 in disc-electrophoresis only

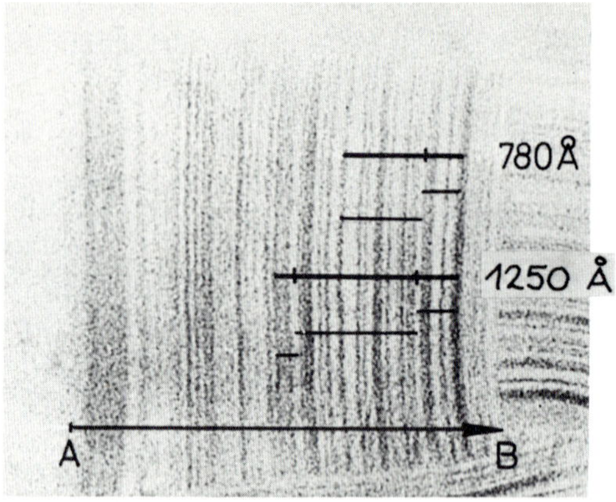

Fig. 8. Position of the CB-peptides derived from α1-780 and α1-1250 collagenase fragments.

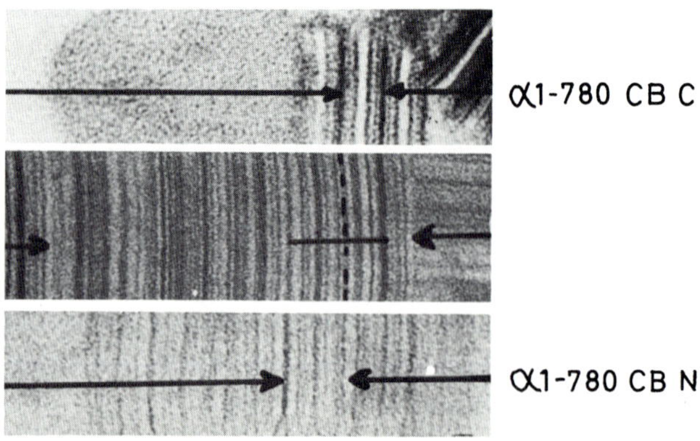

Fig. 9. Comparison of electronmicrographs of segments derived from renatured CB peptides of α1-780 and of SLS from untreated collagen.

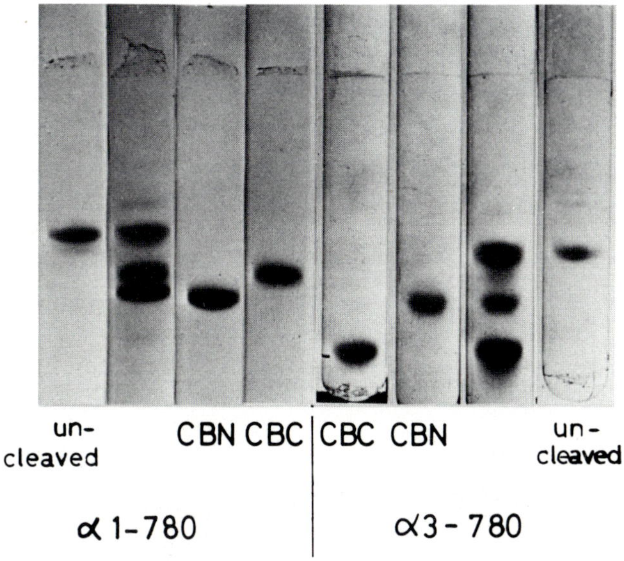

Fig. 10. Disc-electrophoresis of the cyanogen bromide digestion of α1-780 and α3-780. Disc-electrophoresis was carried out as described by Stark and Kühn (1968).

the C-terminal peptides move with different velocities whereas the N-terminal peptides have the same mobilities. The difference between both variants should therefore be located in the C-terminal CB peptide of α1-780 and α3-780. Within these peptides the difference between "α1" and "α3" also seems to be limited to short amino acid sequences. In the paper-electrophoresis of the tryptic peptides, shown in Fig. 11 there can be seen only one additional spot in the region of the basic peptides in case of "α3".

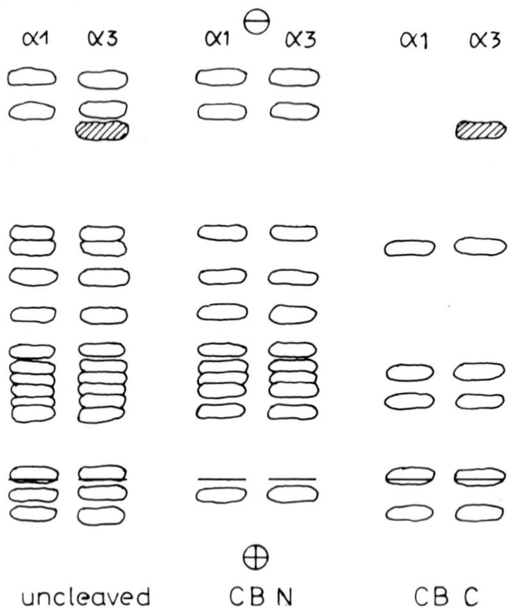

Fig. 11. Paper-electrophoresis of the tryptic peptides from α1-780 and α3-780 and their CB-peptides. Electrophoresis was carried out at 100 V/cm on Whatman No 1 in 0.2 M pyridine acetate.

ACKNOWLEDGEMENTS

This work was supported by the Deutsche Forschungsgemeinschaft.

REFERENCES

Butler, T., Piez, K.A. and Bornstein, P. (1967). Biochemistry 6, 3771.

Stark, M. and Kühn, K. (1968). Europ. J. Biochem. 6, 534.

Tkocz, C. and Kühn, K. (1969). Europ. J. Biochem. 7, 454.

ALDEHYDES AND ALDEHYDE DERIVATIVES IN COLLAGEN

Paul M. Gallop, Olga O. Blumenfeld and Mercedes A. Paz

In 1965, a number of years after our initial observation that aldehyde functions are present in tropocollagen (Blumenfeld, Paz and Gallop, 1963; Gallop, 1964), Rojkind, (Rojkind, Blumenfeld and Gallop, 1964, 1966), in our laboratory isolated, from a collagenase digest of this protein a peptide containing an aldehyde in the form of a 2,4-dinitrophenylhydrazone derivative. The aldehydic compound resembled an aldol (β-hydroxyaldehyde), and was located in close proximity to the blocked amino-terminus of a collagen chain. The suggestion was made that an aldehyde might be important in crosslinking of tropocollagen as part of the maturation process in which tissue collagen is formed. This was confirmed shortly afterwards by Bornstein and Piez (1966). Furthermore, these workers demonstrated that in an α-chain a particular lysyl residue is converted to one of α-amino adipic acid-δ-semialdehyde and that the aldol derivative might be due to a condensation of two residues of this aldehyde on adjacent α-chains. Such a compound, in a reduced form, was first isolated and characterized in elastin by Franzblau and Lent (1968) and subsequently in collagen, where it is present in much smaller quantities, by Paz et al. (1969).

To facilitate the isolation of the aldehydic compounds from collagen we first introduced the use of tritiated sodium borohydride in order to reduce the compounds to labeled derivatives stable to acid or base hydrolysis. Mass spectrometry was used to identify compounds present in small amounts, and postulated structures were verified in some cases by organic synthesis.

Valuable contributions from the laboratories of many investigators, several of whom will offer summaries of their work at this meeting, have brought a rapid advance in our understanding of the structural features and maturation processes of collagen and elastin. In this discussion, we shall present some of our own observations, correct a serious error we have made, hopefully obviate similar difficulties for other workers, and finally discuss certain still unresolved and potentially important questions dealing with structural features of collagen.

I SODIUM BOROHYDRIDE REDUCTION PRODUCTS DERIVED FROM CARBONYL COMPOUNDS IN COLLAGEN

In Fig. 1 are depicted some of the compounds involved in maturation of collagen and elastin. The isolation of ε-hydroxynorleucine, the $NaBH_4$-reduced product of α-amino adipic acid δ-semialdehyde (α-AASA), can be accomplished best after alkaline hydrolysis (2 N NaOH, 105°C, 20 hr), as shown by Franzblau and Lent (1968). After acid hydrolysis (6 N HCl, 105°C, 22 hr), about 70% of the ε-hydroxynorleucine is converted to ε-chloronorleucine which, upon treatment with base or with Dowex-1 (OH^-), is converted to pipecolic acid (Gallop, Blumenfeld, Henson and Schneider, 1968). This compound was previously isolated by us as part of fraction N_2 obtained by column chromatography of the neutral amino alcohols on IR-120 (Gallop et al, 1968). The isolation of the reduced aldol compound of two residues of α-AASA also requires alkaline hydrolysis as shown by Franzblau and Lent (1968).

Lysinonorleucine and dehydrolysinonorleucine have so far been found only in elastin (Franzblau, Sinex, Faris and Lamadis, 1965), whereas dehydrohydroxylysinonorleucine has been recently shown by Bailey and Peach (1968) to be present in insoluble collagen. The first suggestion of the presence of Schiff bases in intact collagen was by Tanzer and Mechanic (1968).

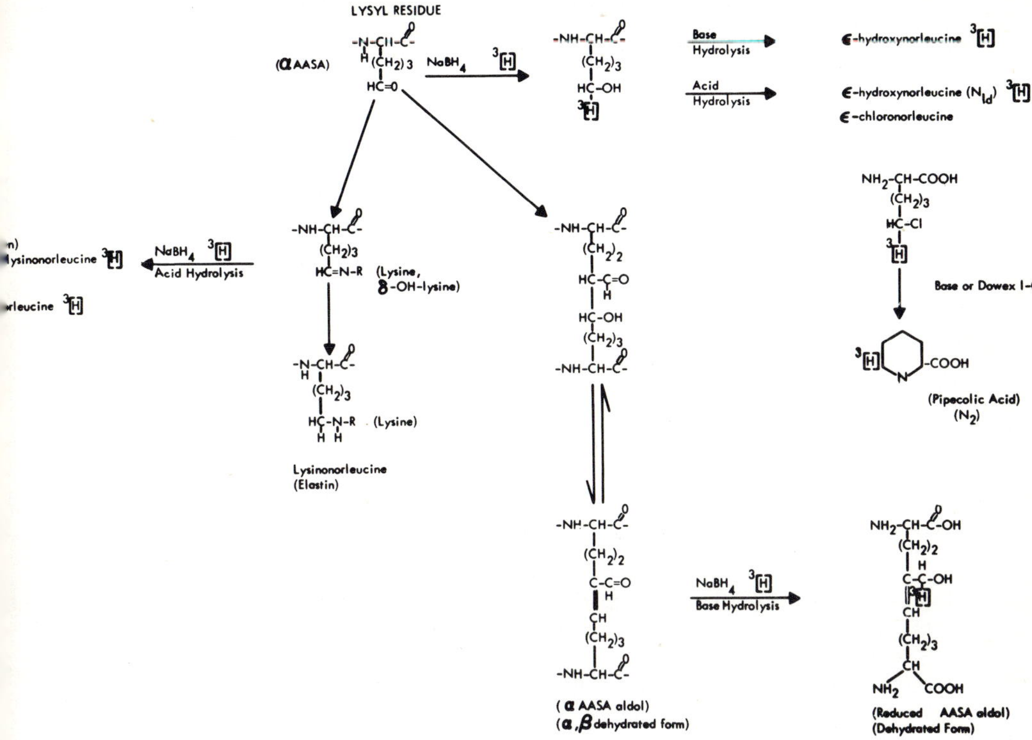

Fig. 1. Residues of α-amino adipic acid δ-semialdehyde (α-AASA) derived from lysyl residues can be detected by sodium borohydride reduction and base hydrolysis as ε-hydroxynorleucine. Acid hydrolysis yields some ε-hydroxnorleucine (N_{1d} in Gallop et al., 1968) and mainly ε-chloronorleucine which on base hydrolysis with Dowex 1(OH^-) treatment yields pipecolic acid (N_2 in Gallop et al., 1968).

In elastin there exist crosslinks that involve a Schiff base between α-AASA and a lysyl side chain (dehydrolysinonorleucine) as well as the corresponding reduced Schiff base (lysinonorleucine). This compound has not been found in collagen although a Schiff base crosslink between α-AASA and hydroxylysine has been demonstrated in insoluble collagen. The Schiff bases can be reduced with tritiated sodium borohydride and labeled.

In elastin and to a much lesser extent in collagen two residues of α-AASA to an aldol which dehydrates to form an α,β unsaturated crosslinking compound which can be labeled with tritiated sodium borohydride and isolated after base hydrolysis.

In an early report (Blumenfeld and Gallop, 1966), we described the isolation from $NaBH_4$-treated collagen of two reduced compounds, one apparently an aminohexenol and the other its dimer, suggesting a crosslinking function. These

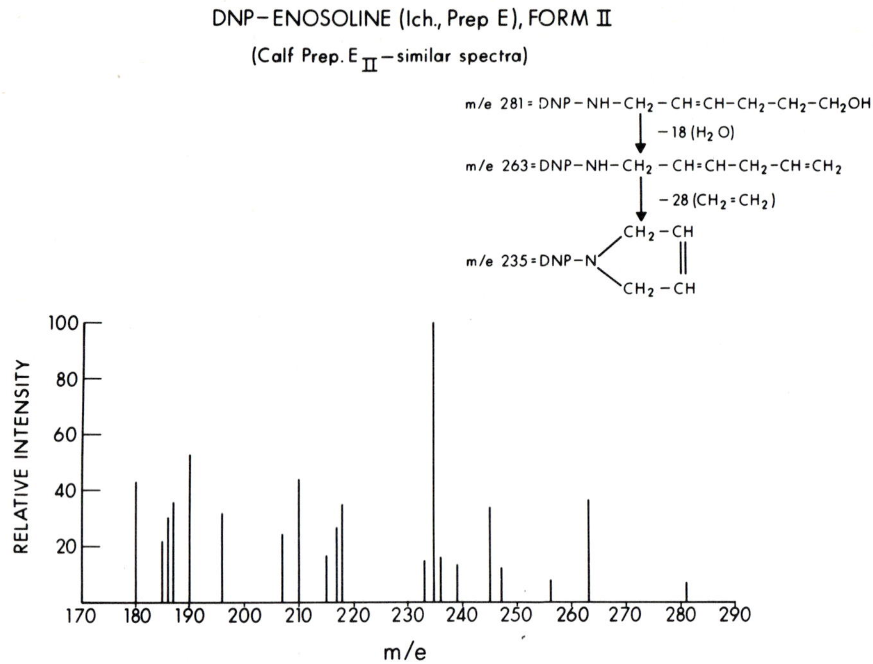

Fig. 2. Mass spectrum of DNP-enosoline form II isolated from the B fraction of sodium borohydride reduced ichthyocol or calf skin acid extracted tropocollagens. The base peak at M^+235 is apparently derived from the loss of 18 (H_2O) and 28 ($CH_2= CH_2$) from the parent ion of M^+281. Such a 46 loss (18 and 28) is found in many aliphatic alcohols. The absence of a strong M^+ 196 (DNP - NH^+ = CH_2) suggests a double bond in an allylic position. The suggested although unconfirmed structure as pictured is N-DNP-6 aminohex-4-en-1-ol.

compounds were isolated as the DNP-amino alcohols; their mass spectra were determined and are given in Figs. 2 and 3. The first of the compounds (termed enosoline) appears to be a 6-aminohexenol and could possibly be derived from a 6-aminohexenal (termed enosaline) in the protein. Earlier we had suggested that the double bond could be in the 2 position, but attempted confirmation of structure by organic synthesis showed that the position of the double bond is uncertain. As a first step we decided to synthesize 6-DNP-aminohex-2-enol. The synthesis is instructive, and accordingly is summarized in Fig. 4. Following the procedure of Hoaglin and Hirsh (1949), DNP-aminobutyraldehyde diethyl acetal and ethyl vinyl ether are coupled in th

MASS SPECTRUM OF Di-DNP-(DIENOSOLINE)

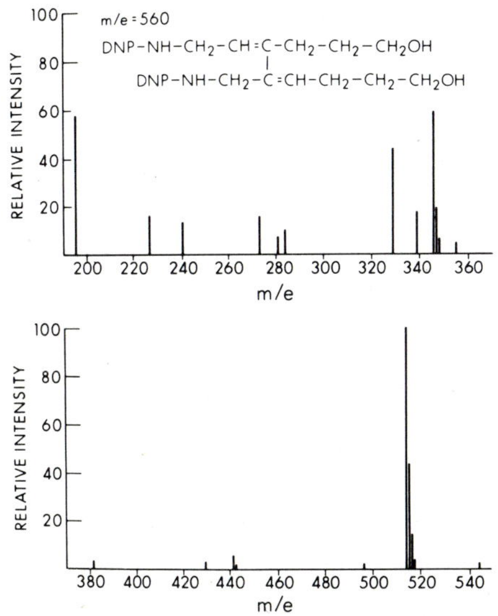

Fig. 3. Mass spectrum of di-DNP dienosoline pictured as two crosslinked enosolines. The large peak at M/e 514 is probably derived from a parent of M^+560 by a loss of 46(18 + 28) as in DNP enosoline (M^+ at 542 is also present). The parent ion is probably at M^+560 (281 x 2 - 2H). If two enosalines (M^+279 as the DNP compound) condensed by an aldol condensation to form a dimer (M^+558) and the one aldehyde group were then reduced with $NaBH_4$ the final mass of the DNP compound would be 560. Alternatively, and as pictured above, two enosalines (M^+279 as the DNP compound) could oxidatively condense (-2H) to form dienosaline (M^+556 as the di-DNP compound) and the reduction of the dialdehyde could form dienosoline (M^+560 as the di DNP compound).

presence of BF_3 and anhydrous ether. The product one should expect, shown in brackets, is not obtained, but an expulsion of ethanol occurs with formation of the depicted ring compound. The latter is indicated by the mass spectrum obtained and by occurrence of an absorption maximum at 370 mμ. Absorption at this wavelength is typical of DNP-N-CH (-CH) whereas absorption at 348 mμ is typical of the DNP-NH-CH compounds. Upon mild acid hydrolysis of the acetal, β-elimination occurs to form the α, β-unsaturated aldehyde, a reaction analogous to the α, β-dehydration of

SYNTHESIS OF DNP-ISOENOSOLINE I.

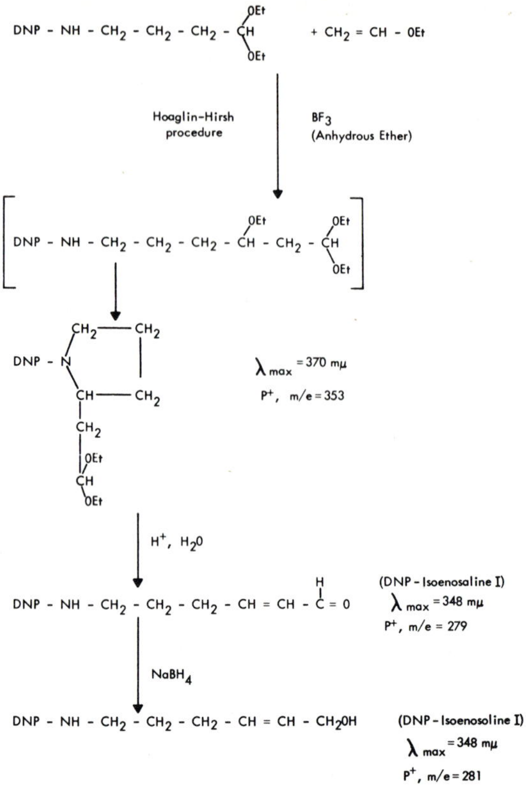

Fig. 4. The ethyl acetal N-DNP 4-aminobutyraldehyde and ethyl vinyl ether are coupled, and after spontaneous elimination of the β-ethoxy group, N-DNP pyrollidine 2-ethanol di ethyl acetal is isolated (λmax = 370 mμ, P^+, m/e = 353). After mild acid hydrolysis (0.1 N HCl in 50% dioxane: H_2O) N-DNP-6 aminohex-2-enal (DNP-Isoenosaline I) is obtained, λ max 348, P^+, m/e = 279. The formation of the α,β unsaturated aldehydes is typical of β-amino or β-hydroxy substituted aldehydes. Reduction of the α,β unsaturated aldehyde yield mainly the α,β unsaturated alcohol N-DNP-6-aminohex-2-enol (DNP-Isoenosoline I) λmax, 348 m , P^+, m/e = 281. Some double bond reduction occurs to form N-DNP-6-amino-hexan-1-ol, P^+, m/e = 283.

aldol compounds such as occurs in the aldol present in collagen and elastin. Reduction of the α,β-unsaturated aldehyde with $NaBH_4$ gives mainly the α,β-unsaturated alcohol (M^+281), although some evidence of double bond reduction is seen (M^+283) in the mass spectrum of the final product (Fig. 5). The partial reduction of the double bond of the unsaturated aldehyde with $NaBH_4$ should be noted and

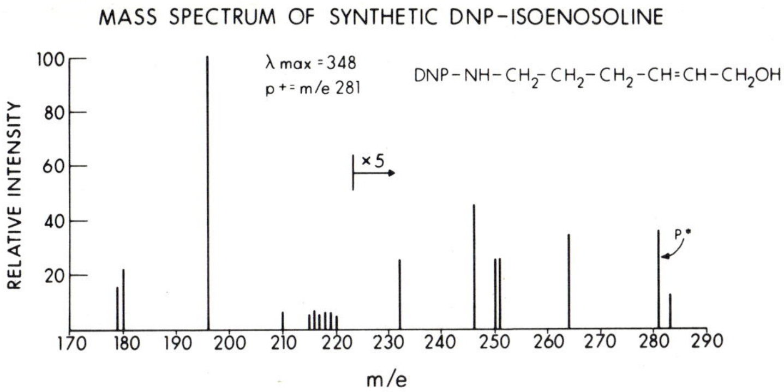

Fig. 5. Mass spectrum of synthetic N-DNP-6 aminohex-2-en-1-ol, P^+, m/e = 281 with a trace of N-DNP-6 aminohexan-1-ol- obtained by reduction of the corresponding α-β unsaturated aldehyde with $NaBH_4$. The base peak m/e, 196 ($DNP\text{-}\overset{+}{\underset{H}{N}} = CH_2$) is typical of such compounds. A loss of 18 (H_2O) is seen at m/e, 263 but m/e, 235 found in DNP enosoline is not seen. The spectrum of isolated DNP-enosoline is clearly not very similar to this spectrum suggesting a different position for the double bond, as discussed in legend of Fig. 2.

may be an important side reaction in studies on aldehydes present in the structural proteins. The cracking pattern of this compound (DNP-isoenosoline) is dissimilar to that of the isolated DNP-enosoline. Synthesis of other DNP-aminohexenols with the double bond in other positions is contemplated so that we may gain understanding of the structure of the compounds isolated from reduced collagen.

II α-AMINO ALCOHOLS: PRODUCTS OF SIDE REACTIONS OF SODIUM BOROHYDRIDE REDUCTION

When denatured collagen is reduced with tritiated sodium borohydride, one finds, in addition to small amounts of reduction products of the carbonyl compounds mentioned above, much higher levels of tritiated α-amino alcohols. Over the past years we have expended considerable effort in isolation and characterization of these compounds. Because determination of their specific activities appeared to indicate that they were mainly one-fold reduced, we concluded that they had arisen from α-amino aldehydes on the protein, and not from side reaction reductions of amino acid residues in the polypeptide backbone. If they were α-amino alcohols derived from side reactions, they would be two-fold reduced (Blumenfeld and Gallop, 1966; Gallop et al., 1968). However, the origin of these compounds continued to disturb us, and we recently re-investigated the problem using sodium borodeuteride. The mass of an α-amino alcohol isolated from the protein reduced with sodium borodeuteride would reveal unequivocally whether the compound was one-fold or two-fold reduced. When such an experiment was carried out with collagen, determinations of mass in the mass spectrometer indicated that some of the α-amino alcohols isolated, namely glycinol, α-alaninol, α-aspartol, serinol and threoninol were indeed two-fold reduced and derived from undesirable side reactions involving peptide bond reduction and conversion of an acyl group to an alcohol.

The specific activities of DNP-α-amino alcohols isolated from various preparations of collagen treated with tritiated sodium borohydride are listed in Table IV of our previous publication (Gallop et al, 1968). In most cases they appear to be one-fold reduced although, in individual experiments, reduced compounds of lower or higher specific activity than one were obtained ("0.8-to 1.4-fold" reduced). These compounds had been separated either by (a) column chromatography, in which case each peak was rechromatographed on a column and its specific activity corrected for an observed isotope effect; or (b) a fractionation by means of column chromatography followed by two-dimensional chromatography on thin layers of silica gels and subsequent elution. Now, having more recently established by mass spectrometry of the deuterated DNP-compounds that the products were in fact two-fold reduced, we re-investigated the method for determination of the specific activity that had been used for tritiated compounds. For purposes of reduction, we used tritiated borodeuteride (the carrier used in the dilution of $NaB(^3H)_4$ was sodium borodeuteride). The resultant tritiated, deuterated DNP-α-amino alcohols were isolated by column chromatography and more rigorously purified by two-dimensional thin layer chromatography of each peak. Evidently the isotope effect due to tritium when the carrier compounds contained deuterium as contrasted with that when the carriers contained normal hydrogen (^1H) was minimal, and the extent of reduction could be estimated more accurately. In one experiment the reduction of the isolated compounds was estimated as follows: O,N-di-DNP-glycinol, 1.8; O,N-di-DNP-serinol, 1.1; O,N-di-DNP-threoninol, 1.9; N-DNP-glycinol, 1.9; N -DNP-alaninol, 2.1; N-DNP-threoninol, 2.4; N-DNP-serinol, 2.2; (a value of 1.0 would indicate origin of the alcohol by reduction of an aldehyde function, a value of 2.0 by reduction of an acyl function). We conclude that these new values, now consistent with values obtained from mass spectral data, are due to a more thorough elimination of impurities by the combined chromatography as used, and to the minimization of the errors due to isotope effects during the chromatographic purifications.

The origin of the α-amino alcohols was established in yet another way. Denatured collagen was reduced with sodium borohydride, hydrolyzed with acid (6 N HCl, 105°C, 22 hr), and the hydrolysate subjected to oxidation with periodate. α-Amino alcohols formed would give rise to formaldehyde. Formaldehyde was then converted to the 2,4-dinitrophenylhydrazone; this was isolated and purified by thin layer chromatography, and examined by mass spectrometry. The mass of 2,4-DNP-formaldehyde hydrazone is 210, that of the monodeutero compound, 211, and that of the dideutero compound, 212. Table I shows the likely origin of these parent ions. Acetaldehyde 2,4-DNP-hydrazone (M224) was also isolated; this compound could arise from threonine, threoninol, or α-alaninol. The level at 211 was, of course, corrected for that fraction of 211 due to the additional mass of naturally occurring carbon 13. The level of 211, when 212 is present, was corrected for a 4.6% (^1H) hydrogen

TABLE I

Origin of 2,4-DNP-Hydrazones of Acetaldehyde and Formaldehyde isolated after Periodate Oxidation of an Acid Hydrolysate of Collagen previously reduced with Deuterated Sodium Borohydride

	M^+210	M^+211	M^+212	M^+224
Threonine	-	-	-	+
Serine	+	-	-	-
Hydroxylysine	+	-	-	-
Glycinol (if one-fold reduced)	+	+	-	-
Glycinol (if two-fold reduced)	+	-	+	-
Other α-amino alcohols*				
(one-fold reduced)	+	+	-	+
(two-fold reduced)	+	-	+	+
Other one-fold reduced compounds+	?	+	-	?
Other two-fold reduced compounds	?	-	+	?

*α-alaninol and threoninol would yield acetaldehyde and monodeutero (one-fold reduced) or di-deutero (two-fold reduced) formaldehyde; serinol would yield formaldehyde and mono- or di-deutero formaldehyde.

+For example, the reduced alcohol derived from α-amino, δ-hydroxy adipic acid semialdehyde would yield monodeutero formaldehyde.

content present in the $NaBD_4$ by use of a factor of 2 x 4.6%. The 212 was also corrected for the [^{13}C] content of the 211 peak. All these corrections of mass were determined from experiments in which suitable model compounds were reduced with $NaBD_4$, followed by periodate oxidation of the reduced compounds and subsequent isolation of the 2,4-dinitrophenyl-hydrazones of formaldehyde and acetaldehyde. Thus, reduced glucose yields a derivative of formaldehyde (210) and mono-deuteroformaldehyde (211); reduced fucose yields derivatives of monodeuteroformaldehyde (211) and acetaldehyde (224); and alanine ester after reduction to α-alaninol yields dideuteroformaldehyde (212) and acetaldehyde (224).

It should be noted that, in these experiments, the ratio of dideutero to monodeutero 2,4-dinitrophenyl formal-dehyde hydrazone, or the corrected peak intensity ratios at masses 212 to 211 indicate the ratio of actual amounts of two-fold (side reaction) to one-fold (carbonyl reduction) reduced α-amino alcohols present. In reduced denatured collagen after acid hydrolysis the ratio found is 3:1; in $NaBH_4$ reduced trypsin, where two-fold reduced amino alcohols are produced, no significant 211 peak is present after correction. It is also noteworthy that this ratio was increased to 10:1 in the basic fraction (B) isolated from a hydrolysate denatured, reduced collagen (Gallop et al., 1968) by chromatography on Dowex 1 (OH^-); this fraction contains the basic α-amino alcohols, glycinol, α-alaninol, serinol, threoninol and lysinol. This suggests that the major amount of the two-fold reduced compounds is in this fraction. Accordingly, most of the one-fold reduced, periodate-sensitive compounds contain carboxyl groups and are retained on Dowex-1 (OH^-); they are eluted in the neutral (N) and acidic (A) fractions (Gallop et al., 1968).

Accordingly, it should be emphasized that if 100 mg of denatured collagen, reduced with tritiated sodium borohydride, incorporates non-exchangeable tritium to the extent of 14 μmoles of one-fold reduced equivalents (calculated by use of a one-fold reduced standard), in fact only about 2 μmoles of truly one-fold reduced compounds are present. This follows from the fact that the incorporation of tritium indeed occurs by two-fold and one-fold reductions, and the resultant ratio of products of these reductions is about 3:1. The value of 2 μmoles per 100 mg of collagen is more consistent with the total aldehyde, direct and indirect, measured by the spectrophotometric procedure of Paz et al. (1965). Of course reduced compounds which are not periodate-sensitive are neglected in this calculation and there may be as much as 1 μmole of these.

We suggest that the concurrent and simultaneous use of tritiated sodium borodeuteride and tritiated sodium borohydride for reduction of collagen not only will tend to eliminate ambiguities about the origin of isolated reduced compounds but will also greatly aid in the interpretation of the mass spectral data.

The new findings, however, do not completely explain certain other experimental data. As previously reported, from unreduced collagen treated appropriately with 2,4-dinitrophenylhydrazine, we also separated 2,4-DNP-osazones with side chains suggesting an origin from α-amino aldehydes identical with those inferred from the reduction experiments. However, the amounts of DNP-osazones obtained were much lower than those of corresponding tritiated α-amino alcohols isolated after reduction with tritiated sodium borohydride. The origin of these osazones remains obscure.

III INDIRECTLY REACTIVE ALDEHYDES IN COLLAGEN

Of special concern to us over the years has been seemingly "hidden" carbonyl functions in collagen. These appear to be aldehyde intermediates or derivatives that become detectable by reaction with carbonyl agents or reduction with borohydride after the collagen is treated with selected nucleophilic reagents. These carbonyl functions are present in addition to the aldehyde components or Schiff base derivatives that can be detected or labeled more directly. The quantitation of the indirectly reactive carbonyl functions is difficult, and requires careful control and knowledge of the limitations of a specific agent used for their exposure. The bonds ruptured in the course of exposure have been designated as "ester-like" or imide in that they are easily and specifically cleaved by hydroxylamine, hydrazine or mild base under conditions at which peptide bonds are stable. For example, vinyl esters ($R\text{-}CH{=}CH\text{-}OC{\lessgtr}^{O}_{R}$) or acylals (esters involving an acyl linkage to an aldehyde function) would react in this manner. Penicillin is a particularly interesting example of a compound containing a labile amide which reacts as an aldehyde following nucleophilic cleavage. The 6-aminopenicillanic acid portion of the molecule contains an N,S-acetal, the nitrogen atom of which is engaged also in a β-lactam formation:

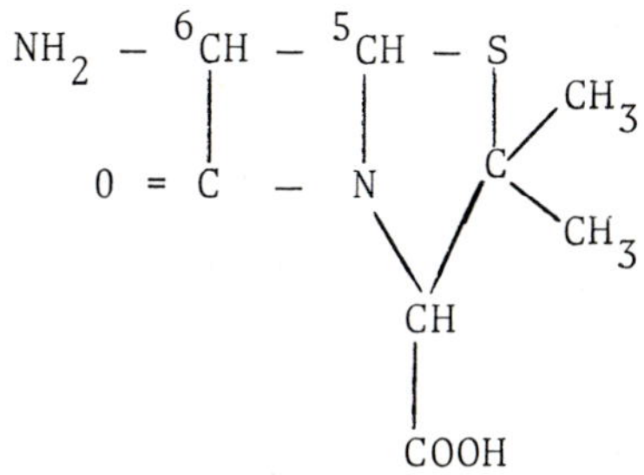

If the very labile β-lactam is cleaved, the thiazolidine ring can be easily opened by various agents to give aldehyde derivatives at carbon atom No. 5.

In collagen, after digestion with collagenase, "ester-like" bonds remain intact. The number of these bonds in peptides was determined by their conversion to acyl hydrazides by reaction with dilute aqueous hydrazine under standard selective conditions (Blumenfeld and Gallop, 1962); excess hydrazine was then removed by treatment with benzaldehyde and extraction with organic solvents. Dr. Gerald Lovinger, in our laboratory, has isolated several peptides containing the "ester-like" functions from collagenolytic digests of α1 chains of ichthycol. One of these ($S_{III}PC_{B1}$) isolated by gel filtration on Sephadex (Peak III) (Fig. 6) followed sequentially by chromatography on phosphocellulose and high voltage electrophoresis had the composition: H_2N-gly-(pro_2, gly_{4-5}, ala_2, $hypro_1$,asp_2). This composition resembles that of aggregated hydrazide peptides obtained by Blumenfeld and Gallop (1962) after cleavage of collagen. Other peptides isolated by Lovinger are similar in composition and all contain aspartic acid and/or asparagine.

Another of these aspartic acid containing peptides isolated by Lovinger could be selectively cleaved with hydrazine to yield a product that reacted as an aldehyde with benzothiazolone hydrazone (Paz et al., 1965). The amount of aldehyde exposed corresponded to the degree of

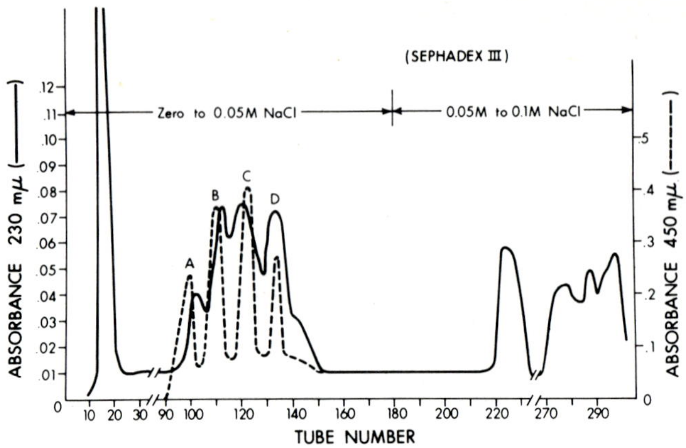

Fig. 6. Separation, on phosphocellulose, of a Sephadex fraction (III) containing ester-like bonds (from a collagenase digest of α1 chains of ichthyocol). Four fractions are obtained which contain ester-like bonds as assayed by 1 M hydrazine treatment and the formation of peptide bound hydrazide. Most other collagenase peptides do not contain bound hydrazide upon treatment with 1 M hydrazine under the conditions employed.

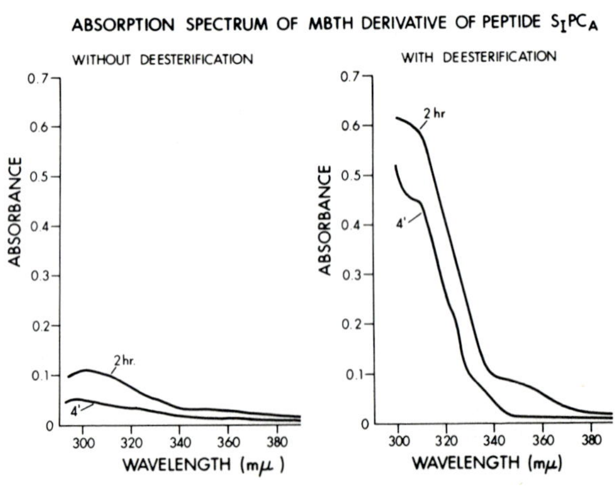

Fig. 7. A peptide from a collagenase digest of α1 chains of ichthyocol containing ester-like bonds purified by Sephadex and Phosphocellulose chromatography. The peptide releases aldehyde after hydrazine deesterification. The released aldehyde is measured spectrophotometrically with MBTH showing the correspondence between "ester-like" bonds and "indirectly reactive" aldehydes.

of "ester-like" bonds (Fig. 7).

The observations of Lovinger suggest that the indirectly reactive aldehyde may in fact be an acylal type of ester or N-acetal involving an aspartic or asparagine residue. The preliminary observations of Butler and of Bornstein, reported at this meeting, that only partial cleavage of peptides, sensitive to hydroxylamine, probably occurred when this reagent was used can be shown not to be in conflict with aldehydic attachments to the aspartyl residues; indeed, this may be responsible for the lability of these bonds to nucleophilic attack. Our observations over the years have shown that treatment of collagen with hydrazine causes aldehydes to be exposed but remain bound to the protein, although similar treatment with hydroxylamine does not result in an increase in protein-bound aldehydes. This is an area where much remains to be done, since virtually nothing is yet known of the nature of the indirectly reactive aldehydes or other indirectly reactive carbonyl compounds in collagen.

In summary, we have traced the concept of the role and nature of some aldehydes involved in the crosslinking of collagen chains and molecules, stressing the methodology we have introduced for these studies. Also, we have shown that the α-amino alcohols, previously reported by us as derived from aldehyde constituents of collagen, are in fact mainly side-products of the reductive cleavage of peptide bonds. A methodology (free of side-reactions) which could be used to quantitatively identify and label all the carbonyl compounds in denatured collagen (where the labile Schiff bases would probably not be stable) is still required. The use of tritiated borohydride in view of the side reactions must be judicious and probably is best reserved for studies in native collagen. However, criteria now exist for distinguishing peptide side reactive reduction from true carbonyl or Schiff base reductions.

REFERENCES

Bailey, R. J. and Peach, C. M. (1968). Biochem. Biophys. Res. Commun. 33, 812.

Blumenfeld, O. O., Paz, M. A. and Gallop, P. M. (1963). Fed. Proc. 22, No. 2.

Blumenfeld, O. O. and Gallop, P. M. (1962). Biochemistry 1, 947.

Blumenfeld, O. O. and Gallop, P. M. (1966). Proc. Nat'l Acad. Sci., U.S. 56, 1260.

Bornstein, P. and Piez, K. A. (1966). Biochemistry 5, 3460.

Franzblau, C., Sinex, F. M., Faris, B. and Lamadis, R. (1965). Biochem. Biophys. Res. Commun. 21, 575.

Franzblau, C. and Lent, R. W. (1968). Brookhaven Symp. Biol. 21, 358.

Gallop, P. M. (1964). Biophys. J. 4,(1), Part 2, 79.

Gallop, P. M., Blumenfeld, O. O., Henson, E. and Schneider, A. L. (1968). Biochemistry 7, 2409.

Hoaglin, R. I. and Hirsh, D. H. (1949). J. Am. Chem. Soc. 71, 3468.

Paz, M., Blumenfeld, O. O., Rojkind, M., Henson, E. Furfine, C. and Gallop, P. M. (1965). Arch. Biochem. Biophys. 109, 548.

Paz, M. A., Lent, R. W., Faris, B., Franzblau, C., Blumenfeld, O. O. and Gallop, P. M. (1969). Biochem. Biophys. Res. Commun. 34, 221.

Rojkind, M. Blumenfeld, O. O. and Gallop, P. M. (1964). Biochem. Biophys. Res. Commun. 17, 320.

Rojkind, M. Blumenfeld, O. O. and Gallop, P. M. (1966). J. Biol. Chem. 241, 1530.

Tanzer, M. L. and Mechanic, G. (1968). Biochem. Biophys. Res. Commun. 32, 885.

THE CARBOHYDRATE OF COLLAGENS

Robert G. Spiro

Although it has been known for some time that collagens have carbohydrate associated with them (Grassman and Schleich, 1935; Grassman, Hörmann and Hafter, 1957; Gross, Dumsha and Glazer, 1958; Blumenfeld, Paz, Gallop and Seifter, 1963) it is only in recent years that they have become firmly established as members of the glycoprotein family, and that the carbohydrate-peptide linkages in some of them have been elucidated.

The fibrillar collagens from vertebrate sources contain only a small amount of carbohydrate which usually constitutes less than 2% of the weight of the protein. The purification of these collagens from the other carbohydrate-rich polymers present in connective tissue therefore tends to pose a major problem, often making it difficult to assess the precise chemical relationship of the carbohydrate found in these preparations to the peptide portion of the molecules. Nevertheless, interest in the carbohydrate was stimulated by various proposals that the sugars in collagen may play an important role as cross-linking agents (Harding, 1965).

In contrast to these fibrillar vertebrate collagens, there are a large number of proteins which are members of the collagen family and which contain a substantially greater amount of carbohydrate, in the range of 10 to 15% of their weight. These include collagens from various invertebrate sources (Gross et al., 1958) and the group of very specialized collagens which are represented by basement membranes.

The carbohydrate-rich collagens present an attractive subject to the glycoprotein chemist. We directed our attention in particular to basement membranes because of the important physiological role which they play in such locations as the renal glomerulus and the serious consequences which result from alterations in their structure in pathological states.

Although our work on the basement membranes will be described in some detail in another chapter of this book (Spiro, 1969a) reference to certain aspects of these studies will be made in this presentation because of the close parallel between the structural features of the carbohydrate of these membranes and those of the fibrillar collagens. The structural studies of the carbohydrate units have been greatly facilitated by the high carbohydrate content of the membranes.

The carbohydrate composition of two basement membranes and two fibrillar collagens is shown in Table I, and indicates that the basement membranes have considerably more

TABLE I

Comparison of the Carbohydrate Composition of Collagens and Related Membranes

Monosaccharide	Ichthyocol (carp)*	Tendon collagen (bovine)*	Glomerular basement† membrane (bovine)	Anterior lens capsule‡ (bovine)
	Residues per 1000 total amino acid residues			
Glucose	1.1	1.2	16.4	38.8
Galactose	1.4	2.2	20.3	40.0
Mannose	0.3	0.8	5.2	3.7
Hexosamines	0.5	2.3	11.5	5.3
Sialic acids	0.06	0.2	4.3	0.4
Fucose	0.05	0.2	1.6	2.0
Hexuronic acid	0.1	0.5	---	0.4

*Data taken from Spiro (1969b).

†Data taken from Spiro (1967c).

‡Data taken from Fukushi and Spiro (1969).

carbohydrate than the collagens; the anterior calf lens capsule, for example, has 11.2% of its weight as sugar residues while ichthyocol contains only 0.7% of its weight as carbohydrate. It may be noted moreover that the insoluble tendon collagen has more carbohydrate than ichthyocol, the citrate-soluble collagen. In all of the proteins, glucose and galactose are the major components, but the basement membranes, as well as the tendon collagen, have significant amounts of other sugars.

In order to characterize the carbohydrate units occurring in these proteins, the basement membranes and the collagens were extensively digested with proteolytic enzymes (collagenase followed by Pronase) to obtain the carbohydrate units with a minimum number of amino acids attached. The digests were then submitted to gel filtration on Sephadex G-25 in order to separate glycopeptides of varying size from each other and from amino acids and small peptides not containing carbohydrate.

Gel filtration of the collagenase-Pronase digest of the glomerular basement membrane (Fig. 1) gave two glycopeptide peaks. Glycopeptide peak 2, which penetrated the gel, contained as its sugar components, only glucose and galactose, which were present in equimolar amounts. Peak 1, which was excluded from the gel, could be further fractionated on Sephadex G-50 into glycopeptides containing galactose, mannose, hexosamines, sialic acids and fucose but no glucose, and high molecular weight material which contained all of the sugar types present in the original membrane (Spiro, 1967a).

The glycopeptides from peak 2 containing the glucose and galactose were further resolved by ion exchange chromatography on Dowex 50-X2 into a number of fractions, each one of which contained glucose, galactose, and hydroxylysine in the molar ratio of 1:1:1, in addition to a limited number of other amino acids. Molecular weight determinations performed on these glycopeptides by amino-terminal analyses indicated that each contained only a single residue of glucose, galactose, and hydroxylysine and suggested the occurrence of a hydroxylysine-linked disaccharide. The hydroxylysine in

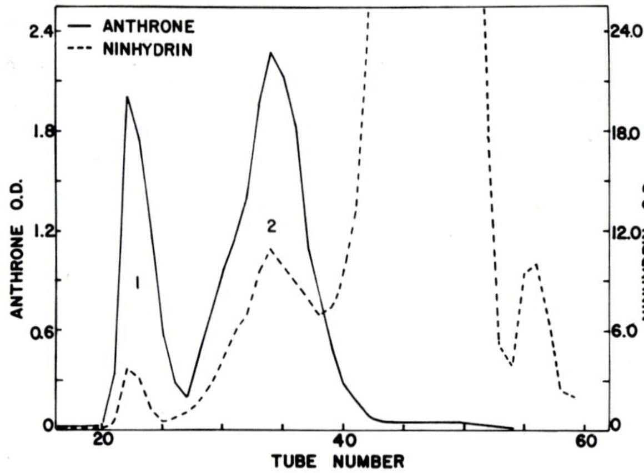

Fig. 1. Gel filtration on Sephadex G-25 of collagenase-Pronase digest of bovine glomerular basement membrane. Elution was carried out with 0.10 M pyridine acetate buffer, pH 5.0. Taken from Spiro (1967a).

these glycopeptides was resistant to destruction by periodate oxidation which indicated that either the hydroxyl group or the adjacent ε-amino group was involved in the glycosidic linkage. Since it was further shown that the ε-amino group was free to react with fluorodinitrobenzene, it was concluded that the disaccharide was linked glycosidically to the hydroxyl group of this amino acid (Spiro, 1967a).

The sequence of the sugars in the disaccharide was studied by graded acid hydrolysis of the glycopeptides. As may be seen in Fig. 2, glucose was released at a more rapid rate than galactose, indicating that it is the sugar in the external position. The rate of release of galactose from the glycopeptides could be markedly increased by prior N-acetylation, which indicated that the positive charge on the ε-amino group of the hydroxylysine hinders the cleavage by acid of the O-glycosidic bond adjacent to it. Partial acid hydrolysis of the N-acetylated glycopeptides, moreover, released a disaccharide with an $R_{lactose}$ of 1.35, which could be isolated in good yield by paper chromatography. This disaccharide consisted of glucose and galactose, with galactose in the reducing position, which confirmed the

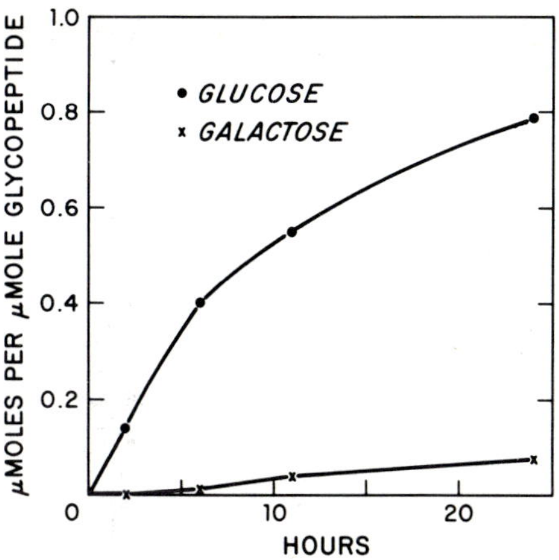

Fig. 2. Release of glucose and galactose from glomerular basement membrane glycopeptides during hydrolysis with 0.10 N sulfuric acid at 100°C. Taken from Spiro (1967b).

sequence suggested by the acid release studies.

Periodate oxidation of the glycopeptides containing glucose and galactose resulted in the rapid and complete destruction of these sugars. Sodium borohydride reduction of the products of periodate oxidation gave glycerol as the only alcohol and therefore indicated that glucose is linked to the C-2 or C-6 of the galactose. Galactose oxidase treatment of the glycopeptides resulted in the complete destruction of the galactose by oxidation at C-6, thereby showing that C-2 of the sugar is involved in the linkage of the glucose. Methylation of the glycopeptides yielded tetramethylglucose and 3,4,6-trimethylgalactose, further demonstrating that the linkage of the glucose is to C-2 of the galactose. The anomeric configuration of this linkage was shown to be α by treatment of the disaccharide with α- and β-glucosidases (Spiro, 1967b).

Because of the alkali stability of the glycosidic linkage to hydroxylysine, it was feasible to isolate the disaccharide unit attached to this amino acid in almost quantitative yield after alkaline hydrolysis (2 N NaOH, 105°C, 24 hr) of the basement membrane or of the glycopeptides (Spiro, 1967b). The resulting glucosylgalactosyl-

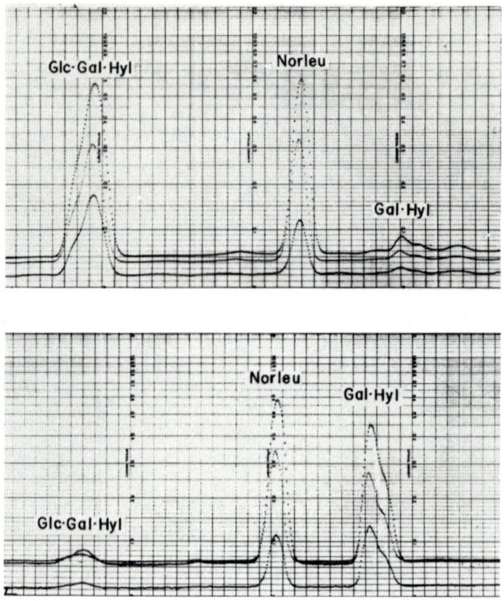

Fig. 3. Elution from amino acid analyzer (Technicon) of hydroxylysine-linked carbohydrate isolated from glomerular basement membrane, before (upper) and after (lower) partial acid hydrolysis (0.10 N H_2SO_4, 100°C, 28 hr). Glucosylgal-actosylhydroxylysine (Glc-Gal-Hyl) and galactosylhydroxy-lysine (Gal-Hyl) are shown relative to norleucine standard. The asymmetry of these peaks is due to the presence in both of these compounds of the diastereoisomers of hydroxylysine. Taken from Spiro (1967b).

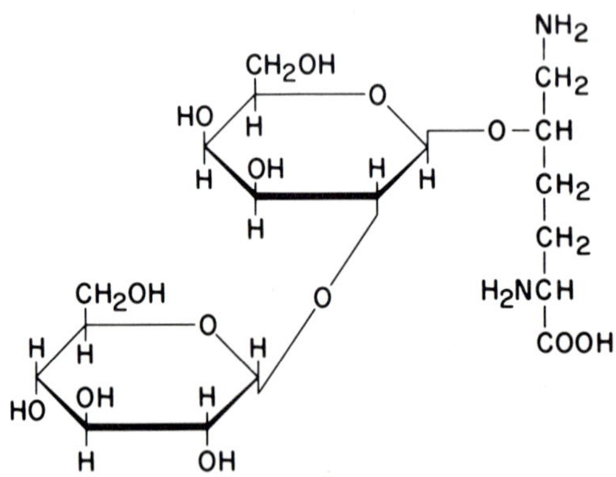

Fig. 4. Structure and peptide attachment of the disaccharide unit of the glomerular basement membrane (2-O-α-D-glucopyranosyl-O- -D-galactopyranosylhydroxylysine). Taken from Spiro (1967b). The disaccharide units of the lens capsule (Spiro and Fukushi, 1969) and of ichthyocol (Spiro, 1969b) have been shown to have the same structure.

hydroxylysine could be shown to appear as a new component in the elution diagram from the amino acid analyzer. It could be separated from the amino acids present in the hydrolysate by gel filtration or preparative paper chromatography. Mild acid hydrolysis of the isolated glucosylgalactosylhydroxylysine released the glucose preferentially and permitted the isolation of galactosylhydroxylysine (Fig. 3). The anomeric configuration of the linkage of the galactosylhydroxylysine was shown to be β from the observation that the N-acetylated derivate of galactosylhydroxylysine was split by β-galactosidase from E. coli but was resistant to cleavage by coffee bean α-galactosidase.

A representation of the structure of the disaccharide and its peptide attachment is shown in Fig. 4. The occurrence of a glycosidic linkage adjacent to a free amino group, as in the attachment of this disaccharide unit to the peptide chain, is an unusual occurrence in nature. This unit can be selectively removed by a single Smith degradation, which serves to uncover the specific hydroxylysine residues involved in the carbohydrate attachment (Spiro, 1967b). Quantitative analysis of the alkaline hydrolysate of the basement membrane on the amino acid analyzer has indicated that essentially all of the hydroxylysine-linked carbohydrate is present as this disaccharide and that about 78% of the hydroxylysine residues of the basement membrane are glycosidically substituted. The hydroxylysine-linked disaccharide, however, only accounts for about 50% of the weight of the carbohydrate of the basement membrane. The remaining carbohydrate is present as a heteropolysaccharide unit which will be discussed in another chapter of this book (Spiro, 1969a).

While we were finding this hydroxylysine-linked disaccharide of the basement membrane, Butler and Cunningham (1966) were involved in a study of guinea pig skin tropocollagen and reported the occurrence of what appeared to be a similar carbohydrate unit linked to hydroxylysine. This prompted us to survey a large number of vertebrate collagens in order to determine whether hydroxylysine-linked carbohydrate units were a common structural feature of the collagen family. It was also important to prepare sufficient glycopeptides from one of these collagens to work out the detailed structure of the collagen unit, which had not yet been established, so that a comparison could be made with the unit from the basement membrane (Spiro, 1969b).

The glycopeptides obtained after collagenase-Pronase digestion of bovine tendon collagen received our first attention. Gel filtration of this digest on Sephadex G-25 (Fig. 5) indicated the presence of two major glycopeptide peaks followed by a large peak containing peptide material. The sialic acid was limited to the first peak which emerged with the void volume of the column. This peak also contained all of the other sugar types present in the collagen. The second glycopeptide peak, which penetrated the gel, contained as its monosaccharide components only galactose and glucose. It was divided into several fractions, all of which contained larger quantities of galactose than glucose, with the galactose to glucose ratio increasing with the greater penetration of the glycopeptides into the gel (Fig. 5). This finding was in marked contrast to the basement membrane, where the ratio of galactose to glucose in this peak was one to one (Spiro, 1967a). After alkaline hydrolysis of the tendon collagen glycopeptides it was possible to show that the high ratio of galactose to glucose was due to the presence of galactosylhydroxylysine and glucosylgalactosylhydroxylysine in varying proportions, with the peptides containing the galactosyl unit tending to penetrate the gel more deeply than those containing the disaccharide.

Alkaline hydrolysis was also performed on the tendon collagen without prior proteolytic digestion. After separation of the hydroxylysine-linked carbohydrate from such a hydrolysate by preparative paper chromatography, it was placed on the amino acid analyzer (Fig. 6) and was shown to contain significant amounts of galactosylhydroxylysine in addition to the glucosylgalactosylhydroxylysine, in contrast to the basement membranes, where this fraction contained essentially only glucosylgalactosylhydroxylysine.

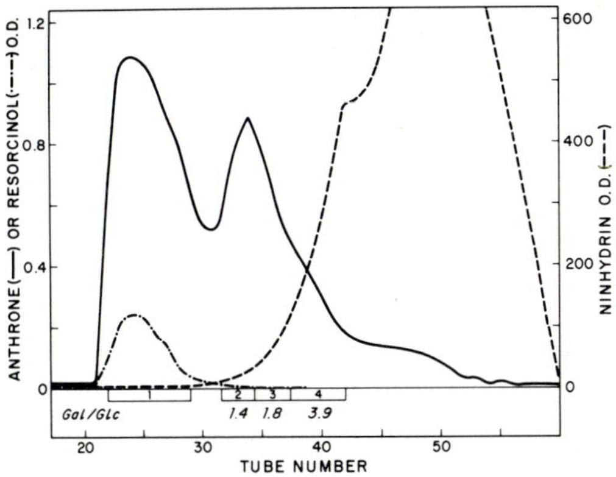

Fig. 5. Gel filtration on Sephadex G-25 of collagenase-Pronase digest of bovine tendon collagen. Elution was performed with 0.1 M pyridine acetate, pH 5.0. Diagram shows hexose analyses by the anthrone method, sialic acid by the resorcinol method, and peptide by the ninhydrin method. Numbered areas designate tubes which were pooled for study. The ratio of galactose to glucose (Gal/Glc) is given for the fractions of the second glycopeptide peak. Taken from Spiro (1969b).

Several other vertebrate collagens were examined for hydroxylysine-linked carbohydrate units by analyzing their alkaline hydrolysates on the amino acid analyzer. Up to 10 mg of protein could be placed on the analyzer (Fig. 7) and varying amounts of glucosylgalactosylhydroxylysine could be detected and quantitated. The galactosylhydroxylysine content of these proteins could be determined on the amino acid analyzer after separation from the free amino acids by preparative paper chromatography. The information about the hydroxylysine-linked carbohydrate of some of the collagens and basement membranes examined is presented in Table II. It may be noted that the basement membranes contain considerably greater amounts of hydroxylysine-linked carbohydrate units than the fibrillar collagens. Moreover, in the membranes a greater percentage of the hydroxylysine residues are involved in glycosidic linkages than in the collagens. The hydroxylysine-linked carbohydrate of the membranes moreover occurs almost exclusively in the form of disaccharide units, while in the collagens a substantial number of units occur in the form of single galactose residues.

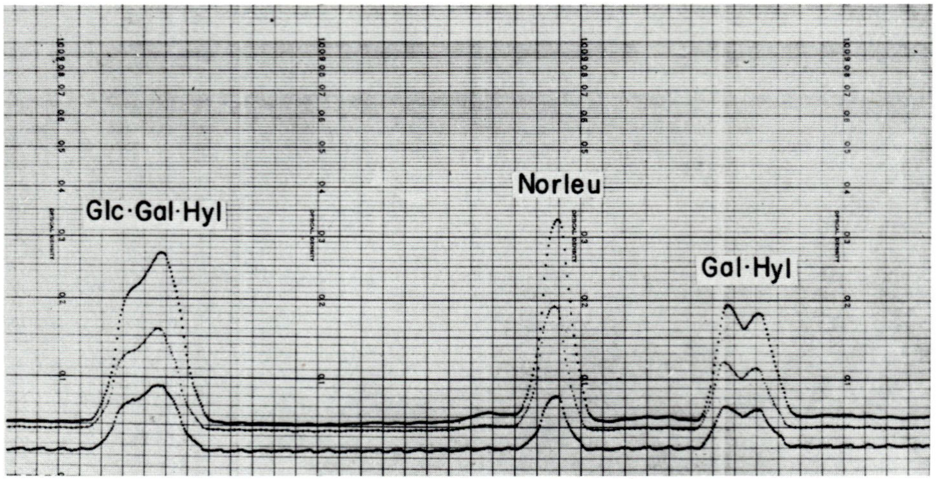

Fig. 6. Elution diagram from amino acid analyzer (Technicon) of the hydroxylysine-linked carbohydrate isolated from bovine tendon collagen after alkaline hydrolysis. Glucosylgalactosylhydroxylysine (Glc-Gal-Hyl) and galactosylhydroxylysine (Gal-Hyl) are shown in relation to the norleucine standard. Both of these peaks contain the diastereoisomers of these compounds.

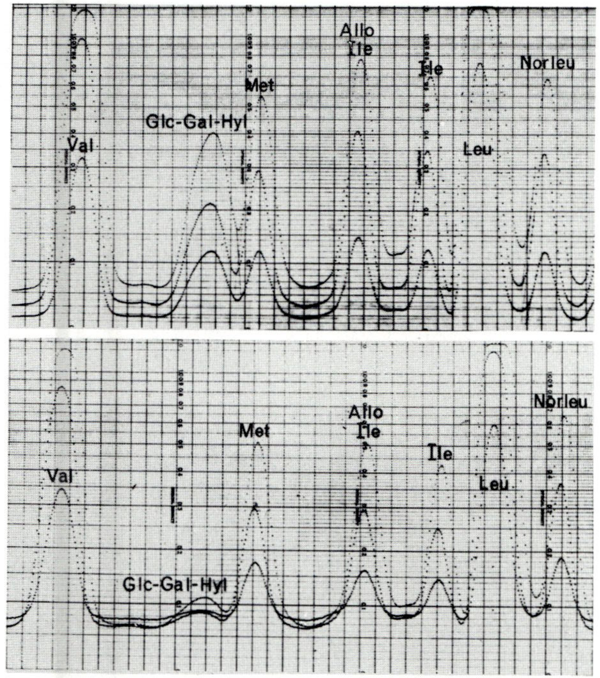

Fig. 7. Portions of elution diagrams from the alkaline hydrolysates of two collagens on amino acid analyzer (Technicon) showing glucosylgalactosylhydroxylysine (Glc-Gal-Hyl) content. Upper calf cornea collagen (9.95 mg); lower rabbit sclera collagen (7.38 mg). Taken from Spiro (1969b).

TABLE II

Hydroxylysine-Linked Carbohydrate of Collagens and Basement Membranes

Protein	Total number of carbohydrate units linked to hydroxylysine	Total hydroxylysine	Hydroxylysine involved in linkage of carbohydrate units	Distribution of carbohydrate between disaccharide and monosaccharide units	
				Glc-Gal-Hyl	Gal-Hyl
	Units/1000 amino and residues	Residues/ 1000 amino acid residues	(%)	(%)	(%)
Collagens*					
Rat skin, citrate-soluble	1.3	7.6	17	56	44
Calf skin, citrate-soluble	2.3	8.7	26	54	46
Ichthyocol (carp)	1.4	11.2	13	83	17
Bovine Achilles tendon	1.8	12.6	14	64	36
Rabbit sclera, citrate-insoluble	1.0	7.3	14	63	37
Rabbit cornea, citrate-insoluble	5.8	10.4	56	60	40
Membranes:					
Bovine glomerular basement membrane+	17.3	22.3	78	97	3
Bovine anterior lens capsule‡	37.5	44.8	84	94	6

*Data taken from Spiro (1969b).
+Data taken from Spiro (1967b).
‡Data taken from Spiro and Fukushi (1969).

It is of interest to speculate on what effect this variation in the density of substitution of the carbohydrate units may have on the overall structure of the proteins. The density of the carbohydrate units varies from one per 1000 amino acid residues in scleral collagen to 27 per 1000 amino acid residues in lens capsule (Table III). It appears that collagens isolated from such tissues as skin, tendon, swim bladder, and sclera, which have wide fibrils with distinct 640 Å banding have the smallest number of these hydroxylysine-linked carbohydrate units. The basement membranes, which show the least organization and no fibrillar structure under the electron microscope have by far the largest number of hydroxylysine-linked carbohydrate units, while the corneal collagen, which contains intermediate amounts of hydroxylysine-linked carbohydrate units, has narrow fibrils although these possess 640-Å banding.

The question arises as to what role the hydroxylysine-linked carbohydrate units play and why there is such a wide variation in their number. No evidence has been obtained that they are directly involved in crosslinking the peptide

TABLE III

Density of O-Glycosidically-Linked Carbohydrate Units in Various Collagens and Related Membranes

Protein	Number of amino acid residues per carbohydrate unit	Amino acid involved in linkage
Scleral collagen (rabbit)	1,000	Hydroxylysine
Swim bladder collagen (carp)	716	Hydroxylysine
Tendon collagen (bovine)	556	Hydroxylysine
Corneal collagen (rabbit)	173	Hydroxylysine
Glomerular basement membrane (bovine)	58	Hydroxylysine
Anterior lens capsule (bovine)	27	Hydroxylysine
Cuticle collagen (earthworm)	43	Threonine and serine

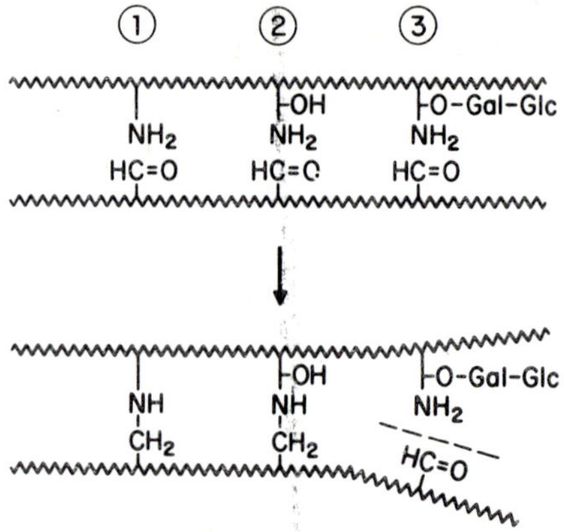

Fig. 8. Representation of the postulated effect which glycosylation may have on crosslink formation between lysine derivatives. See text for discussion.

chains. It is possible, however, that they could play a role in crosslinking in an indirect manner by modifying lysine residues so that they could not participate in the type of crosslinks which have been reported to occur in collagens and elastins (Piez, 1968). A hypothetical manner in which the hydroxylysine-linked carbohydrate units may regulate crosslinks involving lysine residues is shown in Fig. 8, which portrays three ways in which lysine residues or modifications thereof can react with the aldehyde group derived from another lysine (after epsilon deamination). Scheme 1 shows the reaction of lysine to form lysinonorleucine (Franzblau, Sinex, Faris and Lampidis, 1965), but could equally apply to the aldol condensation of two aldehydes formed by oxidative deamination of two lysine residues (Bornstein and Piez, 1966). Scheme 2 shows the modified lysine, that is, hydroxylysine, reacting to form hydroxylysinonorleucine, which has recently been described by Bailey and Peach (1968) to occur in the labile Schiff base form in rat-tail tendon collagen. Scheme 3 shows a further modified lysine, which is both hydroxylated and glycosylated. It is not known whether this derivative can take part in the condensation with an aldehyde or for that matter whether it can undergo oxidative deamination.

It is conceivable that steric or other hindrances imposed on this lysine by the carbohydrate group may make this lysine residue unavailable for crosslink formation. Studies performed on the glomerular basement membrane, where there are a very large number of glycosylated hydroxylysine residues, have produced no evidence so far for the occurrence of substantial amounts of a possible glucosylgalactosylhydroxylysinonorleucine component. The amount of glucosylgalactosylhydroxylysine found after alkaline hydrolysis was the same whether the native or sodium borohydride reduced membrane was studied. It is of interest that in the glomerular basement membrane, which is so highly glycosylated, disulfide bonds appear to serve as a major crosslinking agent between the peptide chain.

In order to carry out detailed structural investigations on the disaccharide unit from a fibrillar collagen, the glycopeptides containing glucose and galactose obtained after collagenase-Pronase digestion of ichthyocol were used (Spiro, 1969b). It was convenient to use this collagen for these studies since it contains a particularly high percentage of hydroxylysine-linked carbohydrate in the disaccharide form (Table II). This made it possible to isolate glycopeptides which contained only the disaccharide unit and were essentially free of the monosaccharide. Using the same methods previously employed for the study of the disaccharide of the glomerular basement membrane, including methylation, periodate oxidation, graded acid hydrolysis, and enzymatic treatment, it could be shown that the structure of the unit was identical to that found in the basement membrane, namely, 2-_O_-α-_D_-glucosylgalactose and that this was linked by a β-glycosidic bond to hydroxylysine. Studies carried out on the disaccharide unit of the lens capsule have also shown this identical structure (Spiro and Fukushi, 1969).

Little is yet known about the carbohydrate units of the large number of invertebrate collagens, many of which are rich in carbohydrate. Recent work on the sea cucumber has shown that in this organism hydroxylysine-linked carbo-

TABLE IV

Comparison of the Composition of Earthworm Cuticle and Calf Skin Collagens

Component	Earthworm cuticle collagen	Calf skin collagen*
	Residues per 1000 amino acid residues	
Glycine	318	320
Alanine	98	112
Valine	17	20
Isoleucine	16	11
Leucine	29	25
Proline	7.1	138
Phenylalanine	5.7	13
Tyrosine	1.5	2.6
Serine	87	36
Threonine	50	18
Hydroxyproline	179	94
Hydroxylysine	0.5	7.4
Lysine	18	27
Histidine	1.1	5.0
Arginine	25	50
Aspartic acid	60	45
Glutamic acid	84	72
Amide	96	46
Methionine	1.3	4.3
Half-cystine	0.8	--
Galactose	59.9+	2.3
Glucose	--	1.2

*Amino acid data for calf skin collagen taken from Piez and Gross (1960).

+In addition to galactose small amounts of glucosamine, galactosamine, fucose, xylose, and mannose were found in all earthworm cuticle collagen preparations.

hydrate of the same type as occurs in the vertebrate collagen is present (Jeanloz, Bhattacharyya and Roberts, 1969).

Collagen from the earthworm cuticle contains carbohydrate units of a quite different type, both in composition and peptide linkage. Earthworm cuticle collagen obtained by sodium chloride extraction was found to be very high in hydroxyproline and essentially free of hydroxylysine (Table IV), in agreement with the work of Josse and Harrington (1964). In comparison with calf skin collagen, it is high not only in hydroxyproline (two times as much) but contains also approximately two and a half times as much serine plus threonine. The major sugar component of this collagen is galactose, and no glucose is present.

Work in our laboratory (Spiro and Bhoyroo, unpublished data) in agreement with the work of Lee and Lang (1968) has shown that most of the galactose is linked to serine or threonine residues and can be released from the protein by mild alkaline treatment, through the process of β-elimination. While disaccharide units are the predominant form in which the galactose occurs in this collagen, our studies indicate that substantial amounts of monosaccharides, trisaccharides, and higher molecular weight galactose oligosaccharides also occur attached to the protein by alkali labile linkages.

Approximately 18 residues of threonine and 5 residues of serine per 1000 amino acid residues are involved in the linkage of these galactose units and are specifically destroyed by mild alkaline treatment. The density of the carbohydrate units of the earthworm cuticle collagen is approximately 43 units per 1000 residues (Table IV), which falls into the same order as found for the vertebrate basement membranes.

After collagenase and Pronase digestion of the earthworm cuticle collagen, we have been able to separate several small molecular weight galactose-containing glycopeptide fractions by gel filtration on Sephadex G-25, as well as a higher molecular weight fraction which contains small amounts of other sugars present in this collagen, including fucose, xylose, mannose, glucosamine, and galactosamine (Spiro and Bhoyroo, unpublished data). Further purification of the galactose-containing glycopeptides was achieved by chromatography on Dowex 50-X2. The elution diagram for the group of glycopeptides which penetrated the Sephadex G-25 gel most deeply is shown in Fig. 9. The analyses of these glycopeptides expressed as molar ratios to the sum of serine and threonine are given in Table V. Treatment of these glycopeptides with mild alkali has shown that not all of the serine and threonine is involved in the glycopeptide linkages. Consequently the

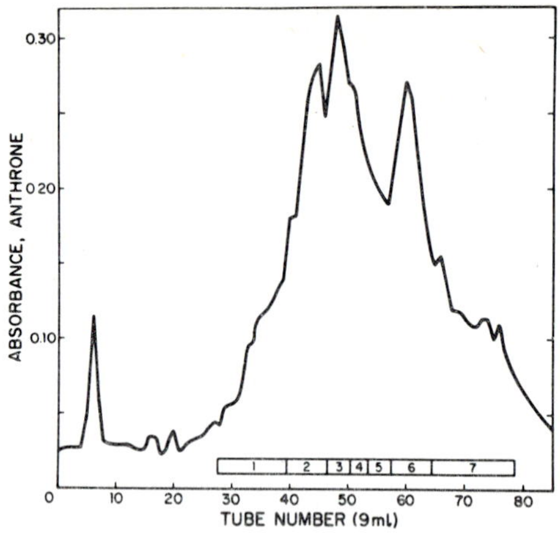

Fig. 9. Chromatography on Dowex 50-X-2 of small molecular weight glycopeptides from collagenase-Pronase digest of earthworm cuticle collagen. Column size was 0.9 x 135 cm and elution was achieved with 0.05 M pyridine formate buffer, pH 3.0. Numbered areas designate tubes which were pooled for study.

TABLE V

Composition of Glycopeptides from Earthworm Cuticle Collagen*

Component	Sephadex G-25 peak+	Dow 50 fractions						
		1‡	2	3	4	5	6	7
Galactose	0.62	1.41	1.26	1.30	1.20	1.45	1.47	0.9
Serine+threonine	1.00	1.00	1.00	1.00	1.00	1.00	1.00	1.0
Serine	0.58	0.57	0.58	0.63	0.58	0.57	0.61	0.4
Threonine	0.42	0.43	0.42	0.37	0.42	0.43	0.39	0.5
Glycine	1.65	1.22	1.06	1.05	1.09	1.34	1.19	1.5
Hydroxyproline	0.66	0.54	0.44	0.50	0.49	0.75	0.53	0.6
Alanine	0.38	0.32	0.39	0.24	0.27	0.40	0.36	0.3
Aspartic acid	0.54	0.16	0.10	0.14	0.19	0.30	0.29	0.5
Glutamic acid	0.25	0.18	0.12	0.19	0.11	0.20	0.23	0.1

* All values expressed as molar ratios relative to serine plus threonine.

\+ This fraction contains the lowest molecular weight glycopeptides obtained by gel filtration of the collagenase-Pronase digest.

‡ The numbers refer to fractions designated in Fig. 9.

number of residues of galactose per glycopeptide is higher than indicated by the molar ratio given in this table. These glycopeptides, from the earthworm cuticle collagen, have a limited number of amino acids other than serine and threonine and can be compared to the small molecular weight glycopeptides obtained by collagenase and Pronase digestion of the glumerular basement membrane (Spiro, 1967a). In the earthworm collagen threonine and serine substitute for the hydroxylysine of the basement membrane and digalactose occurs instead of the glucosylgalactose. Furthermore, the carbohydrate-peptide linkage in the basement membrane glycopeptides is exceedingly stable to alkali, while the glycopeptide bonds in the earthworm cuticle glycopeptides are split by mild alkali. It is of interest that despite the very high hydroxyproline content in the cuticle collagen, the hydroxyl group of this amino acid was found not to be involved in glycopeptide bonds. So far no evidence for the involvement of hydroxyproline in glycopeptide linkages has been found in collagens, although a recent report indicates that it may serve as the site of attachment for carbohydrate in the cell walls of plants (Lamport, 1969).

In summary it may be stated that collagens are glycoproteins which contain from less than 1% to close to 15% carbohydrate. In all vertebrate collagens so far studied, a substantial portion of the carbohydrate is present as mono-or disaccharide units linked by a characteristic type of bond to the hydroxyl group of hydroxylysine in the peptide chain. There is great variation among the collagens, both in the extent of hydroxylation of lysine residues and in the extent of their glycosidic substitution. It appears that in the vertebrate collagens, higher carbohydrate content seems to be reflected in a lower degree of morphological organization, as seen under the electronmicroscope. Although the carbohydrate has so far not been directly implicated as a crosslinking agent, it is conceivable that it may play an indirect role in crosslinking by modifying the lysine or hydroxylysine residues involved therein. An unusual form of collagen is found in the earthworm cuticle, where galactose units of varying size are attached to serine and threonine residues.

ACKNOWLEDGEMENTS

This work was supported by grants AM 05363, AM 10482, and HE 11306 from the National Institutes of Health, United States Public Health Service.

REFERENCES

Bailey, A. J. and Peach, C. M. (1968). Biochem. Biophys. Res. Commun. 33, 812.

Blumenfeld, O. O., Paz, M.A., Gallop, P. M., and Seifter, S. (1963). J. Biol. Chem. 238, 3835.

Bornstein, P. and Piez, K. A. (1966). Biochemistry 5, 3460.

Butler, W. T. and Cunningham, L. W. (1966). J. Biol. Chem. 241, 3882.

Franzblau, C., Sinex, F. M., Faris, B., and Lampidis, R. (1965) Biochem. Biophys. Res. Commun. 21, 575.

Fukushi, S. and Spiro, R. G. (1969). J. Biol. Chem. 244, 2041.

Grassman, W. and Schleich, H. (1935). Biochem. Z. 277, 320.

Grassman, W., Hörmann, H., and Hafter, R. (1957). Z. Physiol. Chem. 307, 87.

Gross, I., Dumsha, B., and Glazer, N. (1958). Biochim. Biophys Acta 30, 293.

Harding, J. J. (1965). Adv. Prot. Chem. 20, 109.

Jeanloz, R. W., Bhattacharyya, A. K., and Roberts, G. P. (1969) Z. Physiol. Chem. (In press.)

Josse, J. and Harrington, W. F. (1964). J. Mol. Biol. 9, 269.

Lamport, D. T. A. (1969). Biochemistry 8, 1155.

Lee, Y. C. and Lang, D. (1968). J. Biol. Chem. 243, 277.

Piez, K. A. (1968). Ann. Rev. Biochem. 37, 547.

Piez, K. A. and Gross, J. (1960). J. Biol. Chem. 235, 995.

Spiro, R. G. (1967a). J. Biol. Chem. 243, 1923.

Spiro, R. G. (1967b). J. Biol. Chem. 243, 4813.

Spiro, R. G. (1967c). J. Biol. Chem. 242, 1915.

Spiro, R. G. (1969a). This book, p. 511.

Spiro, R. G. (1969b). J. Biol. Chem. 244, 602.

Spiro, R. G. and Fukushi, S. (1969). J. Biol. Chem. 244, 2049.

THE CARBOHYDRATE CHEMISTRY OF INVERTEBRATE CONNECTIVE TISSUE*

Richard L. Katzman and Roger W. Jeanloz

Soluble and insoluble collagens from a large number of vertebrate sources are glycoproteins which contain a carbohydrate moiety consisting of glucose and galactose (Kuhn, Grassman and Hofmann, 1959; Blumenfeld, Paz, Gallop and Seifter, 1963; Butler and Cunningham, 1966; Spiro, 1967; Kefalides, 1968). Invertebrate collagens, on the other hand are reported to contain relatively large proportions of a wide spectrum of firmly bound sugars, including glucose, galactose, mannose, fucose, ribose, arabinose, glucosamine, galactosamine, and hexuronic acid (Gross, 1963) (See Table I).

We felt that it would be desirable to investigate intensively the chemical structure of the macromolecular components of the connective tissue of a few selected invertebrates. Some of the questions we are attempting to answer are the following ones: How does invertebrate collagen differ chemically from mammalian collagen? What is the structure of the carbohydrate moiety of invertebrate collagens? What acid polysaccharides and glycoproteins are present in invertebrate connective tissue? And finally, what interactions, if any, exist between the collagen and glycoprotein components of invertebrate connective tissue?

The first selected tissue was the body-wall of the common North Atlantic sea cucumber (*Thyone briareus*) from

* Amino sugars LXIII. Publication No. 489 of the Robert W. Lovett Memorial Group for the Study of Crippling Diseases, Harvard Medical School at the Massachusetts General Hospital, Boston, Massachusetts 02114.

TABLE I

Carbohydrate Composition of Some Invertebrate Connective Tissue Components*

	Hexosamine	Hexose	Pentose	Sugars detected by paper chromatography
	(g/100g)			
Thyone body-wall	1.1	3.3	0.6	glc, gal, man,
Thyone body-wall gelatin	0.6	4.4	0.5	ara, fuc, glcN, galN, uronic acid
Metridium body-wall	1.0	8.9	0.9	---
Metridium body-wall limed	0.6	5.1	0.8	---
Metridium body-wall gelatin	0.7	6.7	0.8	---
				glc, gal, man,
Amorphous substance	4.5	13.9	3.5	ara, fuc, glcN
Spongin A collagen	1.8	11.0	2.7	galN, uronic acid,
Spongin B collagen	0.2	4.9	0.5	man, ara, glc, gal

*Gross et al., 1956, 1958; Gross, 1963

TABLE II

Composition of Intact Thyone briareus Body-wall*

Component	g/100 g
Water	89.5-92
Collagen+	6 - 8
Non-collagen protein+	0.7-1.0
Lipid+	0.2- 0.6
Polyfucose sulfate	0.2- 0.25
Chondroitin sulfate	0.25-0.3
Other carbohydrate	0.02-0.04

+Echinoderm body-wall lipid and protein values vary greatly with the seasons (Giese, 1966)

*Katzman et al., 1969; Katzman and Jeanloz, unpublished data the phylum Echinodermata, closely related to Vertebrata. The second tissue was obtained from an animal at the bottom of the evolutionary scale, a tropical marine sponge, *Hippospongia gossypina*. The third tissue was the body-wall of the sea anemone, *Metridium dianthus*, which occupies an intermediate phylogenetic position.

I SEA CUCUMBER (ECHINODERMATA) CONNECTIVE TISSUE

The body-wall of the echinoderm *Thyone briareus*, when scraped free of eipthelium and adhering viscera, has the composition shown in Table II. The body-wall was completely gelatinized by heating in an autoclave at 123°C and neutral pH, and fractionated on DEAE-cellulose into three well-separated peaks (Katzman, Bhattacharyya and Jeanloz, 1969). The first two peaks had amino acid compositions, particularly a glycine content, very similar to that of mammalian collagen; both collagen fractions contained glucose and galactose as the sole carbohydrate residues (Katzman et al., 1969). O-α-d-glucopyranosyl-(1→2)-O-β-D-galactopyranosyl-hydroxylysine was isolated from Thyone collagen (Jeanloz, Bhattacharyya and Roberts, 1969).

A third fraction obtained by DEAE-cellulose chromatography of the gelatin contained 50 per cent of non-collagen protein and 50 per cent of sulfated carbohydrate, predominantly fucose, hexosamine, and hexuronic acid (Katzman et al., 1969). Poly-L-fucose sulfate and an oversulfated chondroitin 6-sulfate (Ch6-S) were isolated from this fraction, after removal of the protein, by ethanol precipitation (Katzman and Jeanloz, 1969). Thyone body-wall also contains small, but significant amounts of mannose, galactose, xylose, glucosamine, and galactosamine, most likely in the form of a neutral glycoprotein. These carbohydrates cannot be separated from the acid polysaccharides by alcohol precipitation unless a prior alkaline hydrolysis (0.5 N, 65°C, 2 hr) is employed.

Since the gelatinization procedure described above

caused a six to ten-fold increase in ninhydrin-reactive groups (Katzman and Jeanloz, unpublished data), it is not possible to exclude the possibility of a covalent linkage between Thyone collagen and the acid polysaccharide or glycoprotein.

II SPONGE (PORIFERA) CONNECTIVE TISSUE (SPONGIN)

Although there has been a great deal of research on the chemistry of the connective tissue of the sponge, it has been directed almost exclusively at the halogenated amino acids of spongin (Roche and Michel, 1951). Very little has been published on the carbohydrate content of spongin. Stary, Tekman and Öner (1956) identified galactose as a component of unfractionated *Euspongia officinalis* spongin by paper chromatography, and subsequently Tekman and Öner (1963) identified xylose in the same sponge. Gross, Sokal and Rougvie (1956) trypsinized *S. graminae* spongin and obtained three morphologically and chemically distinct fractions, determined their carbohydrate content, and unequivocally established the collagen nature of spongin.

Recently we have fractionated *H. gossypina* by the method of Gross et al. (1956) and chemically examined the two major fractions, Spongin B and the amorphous substance. Highly purified Spongin B was found to contain 3.0% galactose, 2.3% glucose, and 0.3% mannose; arabinose was not detected (See Table I). Glucosylgalactosylhydroxylysine was isolated in high yield from Spongin B and shown to be identical to Thyone glucosylgalactosylhydroxylysine by paper and thin-layer chromatography, by rate and extent of oxidation with galactose oxidase, by co-chromatography on the amino acid analyzer, and by optical rotation, $[\alpha]_D^{20}$ +42° (water, *c* 1.2). The per-*O*-acetyl-di-(*N*-benzyloxycarbonyl) methyl ester derivatives of glucosylgalactosyl- and galactosylhydroxylysine were prepared and purified by silica gel chromatography, and are currently being characterized by nuclear magnetic resonance and combined g.l.c.-computer assisted mass spectroscopy.

An acid polysaccharide fraction was isolated from the amorphous substance (see Table I) of H. gossypina following exhaustive proteolysis and alkaline hydrolysis, detergent precipitation, and fractionation by ethanol precipitation. It was found to contain, per mole of arabinose, 0.6 mole of fucose, 0.5 mole of galactose, 0.1 mole of mannose, 0.07 mole of xylose, 0.9 mole of glucosamine, 0.8 mole of hexuronic acid, and 7.2 moles of sulfate. No glucose was detected. Attempts are presently being made in this laboratory to isolate a sulfated arabinose-containing oligosaccharide.

Arabinose is a sugar that is commonly encountered in the polysaccharides from the plant kingdom (Horton and Wolfrom, 1963), but is extremely rare in the animal kingdom. It has been reported to be present in only two other tissues, human brain (Wardi, Allen, Turner and Stary, 1966) and squid liver (Rosenberg and Zamenhof, 1962). Curiously enough, the arabinose from human brain also occurs as a detergent-precipitable polysaccharide.

III SEA ANEMONE (COELENTERATA) CONNECTIVE TISSUE

It was hoped that the connective tissue of Metridium dianthus body-wall (see Table I) could be clearly separated into collagen and non-collagen protein fractions with the techniques employed for Thyone (see Section II). Metridium gelatin, prepared by autoclaving fresh, unextracted tissue, was fractionated to give three peaks (Fig. 1) on DEAE-cellulose, but analysis of the fractions (Table III) gave inconclusive results regarding the nature of the carbohydrate moiety of the gelatin. The first two peaks appeared to be quite pure collagen fractions, with glycine contents close to one-third mole percent; however, sugars other than glucose and galactose were present (Table III). Based on the hydroxylysine and hydroxyproline content, Peak 3 was approximately two-thirds collagen and one-third of a non-collagen protein, and contained, in addition, relatively large pro-

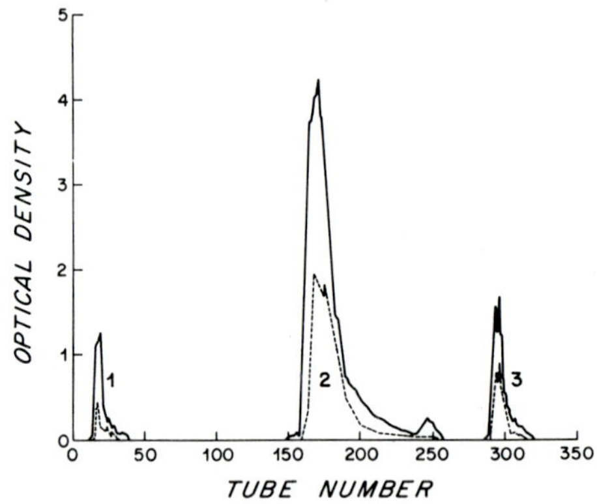

Fig. 1. Chromatography of Metridium gelatin (1.88 g) on a DEAE-cellulose column (12.3 cm^2 x 42 cm). The column was eluted with a linear NaCl gradient at pH 4.8. Peak 1 eluted with water; Peak 2 eluted at approximately 0.1 M NaCl; Peak 3 eluted at 0.4 M NaCl. Protein was estimated by 230 nm absorbancy (———); carbohydrate with anthrone (---------). Yields of Peaks 1,2, and 3 were 0.20 g, 1.26 g, and 0.19 g, respectively. The overall recovery, by weight, after removal of NaCl by dialysis, was 88%.

portions of fucose and hexosamine (Table III).

Metridium gelatin was then proteolyzed and fractionated on Bio-Rad P-2, essentially as described by Butler and Cunningham (1966). The anthrone-positive peak was quantitatively recovered and filtered on Bio-Rad P-4 (Fig. 2), to give two distinct carbohydrate peaks, A and B. Peak A, a heteropolysaccharide, contained all the fucose, xylose, mannose, and hexosamine present in the unfractionated gelatin, and a considerable amount of the glucose, but only traces of the galactose. Its amino acid composition (Table IV) is not typical of collagen. Thus, if the heteropolysaccharide is covalently linked to the tropocollagen molecule (and we suspect it may be), the linkage must occur via an intervening non-collagen protein or peptide. We are presently fractionating Metridium gelatin in the hope of

TABLE III

Composition of Metridium Gelatin Fractions from DEAE-Cellulose Chromatography (see Fig. 1)

Component*	Gelatin	Peak 1	Peak 2	Peak 3
3-Hydroxyproline	8.0	9.0	8.5	6.0
4-Hydroxyproline	50	58	59	38
Aspartic acid	83	63	77	107
Threonine	41	38	36	52
Serine	53	52	56	49
Glutamic acid	94	83	94	118
Proline	60	60	57	70
Glycine	331	335	344	221
Alanine	66	66	65	68
Cysteine	2.6	0.2	0.6	9.6
Valine	33	33	34	36
Methionine	7.0	3.3	4.6	7.7
Isoleucine	23	20	20	39
Leucine	32	32	30	42
Tyrosine	4.8	2.8	3.5	11.3
Phenylalanine	8.2	6.4	7.1	14.5
Hydroxylysine	23	28	26	16.7
Lysine	23	29	21	37
Histidine	3.2	4.9	3.1	8.0
Arginine	54	76	54	47
Fucose	0.5	0.15	0.3	2.15
Glucose	4.3	3.6	4.3	2.05
Galactose	4.1	3.7	4.5	1.6
Mannose	0.3	0.06	0.35	0.34
Xylose	0.08	0.01	0.04	0.23
Arabinose	0.005	0.001	0.005	0.1
Hexosamine	1.2	0.34	1.05	4.8
Sialic acid	0	---	---	0
Hexuronic acid	0	---	---	0
Sulfate	<0.05	---	---	0

*Amino acids expressed as moles/1000 moles of amino acid. Carbohydrate and sulfate expressed as g/100 g dry weight.

establishing such a linkage.

Peak B (Fig. 2) contained only glucose and galactose in equimolar amounts, and from this fraction glucosylgalactosylhydroxylysine was isolated and is being characterized (see Section II) by NMR and mass spectroscopy.

The most striking feature of the chemistry of Metridium connective tissue is undoubtedly the lack of acid polysaccharides containing hexuronic acid, sialic acid, or sulfate (Table III). This absence cannot be simply ascribed to the primitive evolutionary state of Metridium, since the sponge

TABLE IV

Amino Acid Composition of Fraction A from P-4 Filtration of Metridium Digest*

Aspartic acid	0.3
Threonine	1.0
Serine	0.4
Glutamic acid	0.5
Proline	0.6
Glycine	0.6
Alanine	0.7
Valine	0.2
Isoleucine	0.1
Hydroxyproline	trace
Hydroxylysine	trace
All Others	<0.07

*Moles/mole threonine

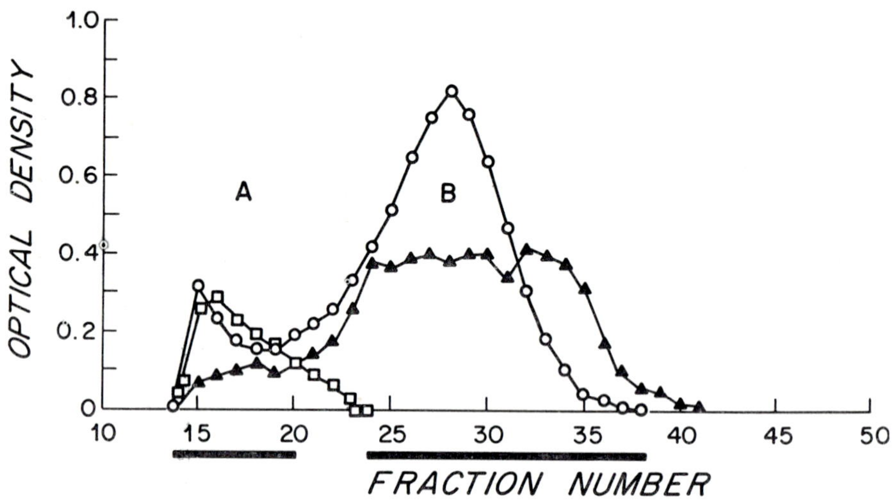

Fig. 2. Gel filtration of Metridium digest (see text) on Bio-Rad P-4 column (12.3 cm^2 x 57 cm), eluted with 0.05 N ammonium formate. Amino acid was measured with the ninhydrin reagent (open triangles); carbohydrate with anthrone (open circles); fucose with the sulfuric acid-cysteine reaction (open squares). The fractions indicated by the heavy bars were pooled and dialyzed to give Peaks A and B, respectively. The recovery of carbohydrate from the original gelatin was 84%, determined as the galactose-equivalents (anthrone) in Peaks A and B.

contains an acid polysaccharide, and is a far more primitive animal. To the best of our knowledge this is the first reported example of a collagenous tissue that does not contain an acid polysaccharide. The current hypotheses on the roles of acid polysaccharides in collagen fibril formation, wound healing, and the calcification process may have to be modified or abandoned in view of this finding.

IV CONCLUSIONS

Glucosylgalactosylhydroxylysine is apparently widely distributed throughout the animal kingdom as the carbohydrate moiety of collagen. Thus far, no other carbohydrate moiety has been found. Earthworm cuticle collagen (Watson, 1958) contains no hydroxylysine, but it does contain α-D(1→2) linked disaccharides of D-galactose (Lee and Lang, 1968; Muir and Lee, 1969) which are very similar structurally to the glucosylgalactosyl unit.

Whereas a considerable phylogenetic substitution of amino acids may take place (with the possible exception of glycine), the glucosylgalactosylhydroxylysine unit appears to be invariant. This invariance suggests that an important biological role exists for this unit. Eylar (1965) has proposed that the carbohydrate moiety of glycoproteins exists exclusively to facilitate export of the molecule from the cell. The existence (indeed the persistence) of an identical carbohydrate moiety, attached to a closely related group of proteins existing throughout the animal kingdom, is consistent with Eylar's theory. It is also possible that the carbohydrate unit has some indirect, but important, influence on the crosslinking reaction of collagen.

Whether or not collagen may have an additional heteropolysaccharide moiety, a question which is central to this discussion, is extremely difficult to answer at present. An invertebrate connective tissue such as that of Metridium, where no acid polysaccharide is present, and where the amount of heteropolysaccharide is one order of magnitude greater than that which is present in most mammalian tissues may provide the ideal system for answering this question.

The phylogenetic distribution of acid polysaccharides in connective tissue appears to be quite sporadic, and is in sharp contrast to the invariance of the glucosylgalactosylhydroxylysine unit of collagen, suggesting that the acid polysaccharides may have had independent biogeneses (Katzman and Jeanloz, 1969). Thus far, we have no evidence to suggest that there may be a covalent linkage between acid polysaccharide and collagen in any invertebrate tissue we have examined.

ACKNOWLEDGEMENTS

We thank Drs. S. Gardell, J. Gross, R. Spiro and D. Swann for advice and discussions. This work has been supported by grants AM-03564 and CA-18166-01 from the National Institutes of Health, U.S. Public Health Service.

REFERENCES

Blumenfeld, O.O., Paz, M.A., Gallop, P.M. and Siefter, S. (1963). J. Biol. Chem. 238, 3835.

Butler, W.T. and Cunningham, L.W. (1966). J. Biol. Chem. 241, 3882.

Eylar, E.H. (1965). J. Theoret. Biol. 10, 89.

Giese, A.C. (1966). In Physiology of the Echinoderms, p. 780. Ed. by Boolootian, R.A. Wiley, New York.

Gross, J. (1963). In Comparative Biochemistry, vol. 5, p. 307. Ed. by Florkin, M. and Mason, H.S. Academic Press, New York.

Gross, J., Dumsha, B. and Glazer, N. (1958). Biochim. Biophys. Acta 30, 293.

Gross, J., Sokal, Z. and Rougvie, M. (1956). J. Histochem. Cytochem. 4, 227.

Horton, D. and Wolfrom, M.L. (1963). In Comprehensive Biochemistry, vol. 5, p. 185. Ed. by Florkin, M. and Stotz, E.H. Elsevier, Amsterdam.

Jeanloz, R.W., Bhattacharyya, A.K. and Roberts, G.P. (1969). Z. Physiol. Chem. (In press).

Katzman, R.L., Bhattacharyya, A.K. and Jeanloz, R.W. (1969). Biochim. Biophys. Acta 184, 523.

Katzman, R.L. and Jeanloz, R.W. (1969). Science (In press).

Kefalides, N.A. (1968). Biochemistry 7, 3103.

Kühn, K., Grassmann, W. and Hofmann, V. (1959). Z. Natureforsch. 146, 436.

Lee, Y.C. and Lang, D. (1968). J. Biol. Chem. 243, 677.

Muir, L. and Lee, Y.C. (1969). Data presented at Meeting of the Glycosaminoglycan-Glycoprotein-Glycolipid Group, Philadelphia, Penn., May 26.

Roche, J. and Michel, R. (1951). In Advances in Protein Chemistry, p. 253. Ed. by Anson, M.L., Edsal, J.T. and Bailey, K. Academic Press, New York.

Rosenberg, E. and Zamenhof, S. (1962). J. Biochem. (Tokyo) 51, 274.

Spiro, R.G. (1967). J. Biol. Chem. 242, 4813.

Stary, Z., Tekman, S. and Öner, N. (1956). Biochem. Z. 328, 195.

Tekman, S. and Öner, N. (1963). Nature 200, 77.

Wardi, A.H., Allen, W.S., Turner, D.L. and Stary, Z. (1966). Arch. Biochem. Biophys. 117, 44.

Watson, M.R. (1958). Biochem. J. 68, 416.

CARBOHYDRATE-RICH SOLUBLE COLLAGEN OF THE BOVINE CORNEAL STROMA

Zacharias Dische

The highly organized collagen, as isolated from the tendon or skin (Grassman et al., 1957), was shown to contain between 0.5 and 1% hexose, in form of glucosylgalactosyl disaccharide units (Cunningham Ford and Segrest, 1967). It has been shown on the other hand, that the collagen present either in non-fibrillar basement membranes (Dische, 1964; Spiro, 1967) or in thin non-striated fibrils as in the central part of the vitreous (Matoltsy. 1952; Dische and Zelmenis, 1955) contains a much higher proportion of hexose consisting of galactose and glucose. There is also evidence that the fine fibrils (reticulin) of adolescent human kidneys contains about 4% hexose (Windrum, Kent and Eastoe, 1955), suggesting the presence of a higher proportion of hexose than is found in fully organized collagen fibrils. Collagen fibrils appearing in connective tissue at an early state of the embryonal development appear as fibrils either without any characteristic periodicity or with an abnormal periodicity of 210 Å (Randall, 1954). Such fibrils were also found in tissue cultures of fibroblasts which start to produce the intercellular matrix (Fitton Jackson, 1965). This suggests the possibility that the higher content of hexose is characteristic for collagen present in tissues in an unorganized state or in a state of lower degree of organization, and that this form of collagen may represent the precursor of the fully organized collagen fibrils. The avascularity of the cornea and its lack of significant amounts of elastic and nerve fibers make it appear as particularly suitable for the investigation of this problem. The corneal stroma contains fibrils of a diameter of 250 to 300 Å. Preliminary experiments carried out in 1962 in our laboratory showed indeed that the corneal stroma from which glycosaminoglycans were removed by extraction with 10% $CaCl_2$ contained a relatively larger percent of hexose than other tissues (Dische and Robert, 1962). A study was therefore undertaken in our laboratory to determine the nature of this hexose.

I EXPERIMENTAL PROCEDURE

A. TISSUE EXTRACTION

Corneal stroma was prepared from eyes of freshly slaughtered steers by scraping off the epithelium and the endothelium of the excised corneas. The corneas were swollen overnight at 4°C in saline, and cut in a tissue slicer into an anterior, medial, and posterior part. Only the first two were investigated to eliminate the presence of the carbohydrate of the Descemet's membrane (Dohlman and Balazs, 1955). The corneas were then homogenized and extracted with 0.16 M NaCl solution (pH 6-7) for 24 hr at 4°C with shaking and in the presence of suitable combination of antibiotics which prevented bacterial growth in the samples. After the extraction, the suspension was centrifuged on the Model L Spinco Centrifuge for 1 hr at 20,000 rpm. The supernatant was dialyzed overnight against running tap water and then for 48 hr in several times changed distilled water. A fine precipitate appeared which was collected by centrifugation. It contained collagen and glycosaminoglycans and will be referred to as extractable collagen fraction A. The once extracted residue was rehomogenized and re-extracted the same way as before. This procedure was repeated four to six times. The extracted residue was extracted repeatedly with 10% $CaCl_2$ adjusted with tris-citrate buffer to pH 8. The solubilized material was precipitated by dialysis against distilled water. This sample is referred to as Extracted Fraction B. Finally in some experiment the $CaCl_2$ extracted residue was rehomogenized and extracted with 5 M guanidine HCl. The solubilized material was dialysed against distilled water and the precipitate collected. This sample will be designated as Extracted Fraction C. The residues of the stroma which remained insoluble after the various extractions is designated as Insoluble Fractions B and C.

B. ANALYTICAL PROCEDURES

The collagen extracted with saline, $CaCl_2$ and 5 M guanidine hydrochloride as well as the insoluble residue were solubilized either by digestion with a 0.065% solution of high purity collagenase (Worthington) in M/50 Tris buffer containing $CaCl_2$ during 16 hr at room temperature (with addition of $CHCl_3$ 1 hr after the start of the digestion), or by extraction with 5% TCA for 30 min at 90°C. The TCA extracts were neutralized, freed from TCA by dialysis and then treated with collagenase (Clostridium hystoliticum, Worthington). As all extracts, particularly those with saline solution, contained various amounts of acid glycosaminoglycans and possibly of glycoproteins, the determination of the hexose linked to collagen was carried out in the following way. Each collagenase digest was dialyzed in an equal or double volume of distilled water, and the dialyzate which was shown to contain hydroxyproline but no significant amounts of hexosamine, was analyzed. The retentate was then dialyzed exhaustively against running and distilled water and the analysis of hexose and hydroxyproline was carried out on these two fractions separately. The concentration of hydroxyproline in the dialyzed fluid corresponded to 71-96% of the total concentration of hydroxyproline in the preparation. As the retentate contained all of the hexosamine of the preparation, the hexosamine and hexuronic acid content was determined in this fluid in addition to the hydroxyproline and hexose content. The hexose-bound hexosamine was calculated from the excess of hexosamine over the amount corresponding to hexuronic acid assuming a one to one ratio of hexosamine to hexuronic acid. In the case of the retentate obtained by treatment of the insoluble collagen, the ratio of hexose to hexose-bound hexosamine was assumed to be 1:1 (as in keratan sulfate), whereas for the retentate obtained from extractable collagen, it was assumed to be 0.6 as in the mannose-containing, sulfated glycoprotein of the stroma (Dische, unpublished data). The values obtained for hexose not bound to hexosamine are therefore maximum values in the first case and minimum values in the second case. The collagen present was then calculated by multiplying the hydroxyproline content by 7.46, since the collagen of the corneal stroma shows a normal content of hydroxyproline. The results of these determinations are listed in Table I. In the dialyzate obtained from all fractions of extractable collagen, the hexose content of collagen was found to be between 2.1 and 5.8%, whereas in the dialyzates obtained from the insoluble collagen, the hexose content varied between 1.08 and 1.67%. The content of collagen-linked hexose in the nondialyzable fragments exclude the possibility that the difference in the hexose content between extractable and insoluble collagen is due to a difference in the mode of distribution of the hexose units in the two collagen molecules. Determinations of the nitrogen content of both types of collagen showed that the difference in hexose content cannot be related to a difference in hydroxyproline content.

The soluble collagen could be derived from keratocytes, from the interfibrillary matrix or from collagen fibrils. To decide between the first two and the third localization, we compared, in one experiment, the amounts of collagen and of hexosamine extracted in six consecutive 0.16 M NaCl extractions and in a second experiment the extraction of these two compounds in four consecutive NaCl extractions, followed by a $CaCl_2$ extraction.

The data are listed in Table II. As can be seen

TABLE I

Hexose Content of Various Fractions of Collagen of Corneal Stroma Expressed in Percent of the Collagen Content

Exp. No.	Fraction*	Solubilization of collagen	Hexose in the dialyzable portion of the collagen digest	Hexose in the nondialyzable portion of the collagen digest	Hydroxyproline in dialysate (% of total hydroxyproline)
I	Extractable fraction A	collagenase	3.3		71
	Extractable fraction B	collagenase	5.75		
	Extractable fraction C	collagenase	5.80	3.3	81
	Insoluble fraction B	collagenase	1.26	8.5	95
	Insoluble fraction C	collagenase	1.30	6.15	94
II	Insoluble fraction B	collagenase	1.05	8.2	80
	Insoluble fraction B	5% TCA at 90° for 30'	1.19		96
	Extractable fraction B	5% TCA	4.1	8	84
III	Insoluble fraction C	collagenase	1.21	8.7	94.5
	Extractable fraction C	collagenase	2.08	10.5	92

*See text for explanation.

TABLE II

Comparison of Amounts of Hydroxyproline and Hexosamine Extracted by Consecutive Extractions with M 0.16 NaCl and 10% $CaCl_2$

Exp.	No.	Extraction	Hydroxyproline extracted (mg)	Hexosamine extracted (mg)	Weight ratio hydroxyproline to hexosamine
II	a.	3^d and 4th NaCl extract of Extractable Fraction A	1.30	4.42	3.4
	b.	5th and 6th NaCl extract of Extractable Fraction A	0.39	1.64	4.1
	c.	1st $CaCl_2$ extract of Extractable Fraction B	1.92	5.75	3.0
IV	a.	1st and 2nd NaCl extract of Extractable Fraction A	5.1	23.1	4.6
	b.	3^d and 4th NaCl extract of Extractable Fraction A	0.89	4.05	4.48
	c.	5th and 6th NaCl extract of Extractable Fraction A	0.36	2.2	6.0

the amounts of both substances extracted decline sharply in consecutive NaCl extracts to a low, fairly constant value and then increased about 7-fold, when $CaCl_2$ was applied for the first time. In experiment II and IV the ratio of collagen to hexosamine extracted is nearly identical for all extractions. The glycosaminoglycans of the stroma are known to be localized in the interfibrillary spaces. The constant ratio of collagen and glycosaminoglycans extracted during various extractions seems difficult to understand without assuming that both types of compounds have the same localization. This conclusion is further supported by the recent finding, in our laboratory, that calf cornea contains several times as much extractable collagen per unit dry weight than does steer cornea. In calf cornea the collagen fibrils already present have definitive form and optical properties, but new fibrils are also formed continually.

ACKNOWLEDGEMENTS

This investigation was supported by Grant NB 07033 of the National Institute of Neurological Diseases and Stroke, National Institutes of Health and the grant CA-02075 of the National Cancer Institute.

REFERENCES

Cunningham, L.W., Ford, J.D. and Segrest, J.P. (1967). J. Biol. Chem. 242, 2570.

Dische, Z. (1964). In Involvement of Small Blood Vessels in Diabetes, p. 201. Ed. by Siperstein et al. Am. Inst. Biol. Sci., Washington.

Dische, Z. and Robert, L. (1962). Fed. Proc. 21, 172.

Dische, Z. and Zelmenis, G. (1955). Arch. Ophthalmol. 54, 528.

Dohlman, C.H. and Balazs, E.A. (1955). Arch. Biochem. 57, 445.

Fitton Jackson, S. (1965). In Structure and Function of Connective and Skeletal Tissue, p. 156. Ed. by

Tristram et al. Butterworth, London.
Grassmann, W., Hofmann, U., Kuhn, K., Harmann, H., Endres, H. and Wolf, K. (1957). In Connective Tissue Symposium, p. 157. Ed. by Tunbridge, R.E. Blackwell, Oxford.
Matoltsy, A.G. (1952). J. Gen. Phys. 36, 29.
Randall, J.T. (1954). Nature 179, 853.
Spiro, R.G. (1967). J. Biol. Chem. 242, 1923.
Windrum, G.M., Kent, P.W. and Eastoe, J.E. (1955). Brit. J. Exp. Pathol. 36, 49.

CHEMICAL AND PHYSICAL PROPERTIES OF STRUCTURAL GLYCOPROTEINS

A.M. Robert, B. Robert and L. Robert

I OPERATIONAL DEFINITION OF "STRUCTURAL GLYCOPROTEINS"

Glycoproteins extractable with urea-mercaptoethanol were isolated from the TCA-insoluble residue of the fibrous stroma of several different connective tissues such as cornea, sclera (Robert, and Dische, 1963; Robert and Robert, 1967); aorta, heart valve (Moczar, Moczar and Robert, 1967; Moczar and Robert, 1969); skin tendon, cartilage, synovial membrane and others (Robert, Robert and Moczar, 1966).

The method of isolation applied to all of these tissues is the same:

1) the soluble tissue components are removed by exhaustive extraction with 1M $CaCl_2$ buffered to pH 7.5-8.0 with tris-citrate (CTC-extract);

2) the water-washed insoluble fibrous stroma is heated in TCA 0.15 M to 90°C to remove fibrous collagen (TCA-extract);

3) the water-washed residue is extracted with 8 M urea and then with 8 M urea 0.1 M in mercaptoethanol under nitrogen (urea and urea-SH-extract);

4) elastin is found in the urea-insoluble residue. Fraction 3, the urea extract, contains the structural glycoproteins. "Keratoglycosaminoglycan" was used by the authors as a preliminary denomination for the structural glycoprotein (SGP) of cornea (Robert, Parlebas and Robert, 1963). In order to avoid confusion in the nomenclature, however, in this paper the general name structural glycoproteins of the cornea (SGPC) or aorta (SGPA) will be used.

II CHEMICAL AND PHYSICAL PROPERTIES OF STRUCTURAL GLYCOPROTEIN

SGP-s can be further purified by delipidation in chloroform-methanol (2:1), water-washing at 40°C and redissolved in 8 M urea (Moczar and Robert, 1969). The urea extract from cornea was purified by alcohol fractionation and gel filtration. (Fig. 1 shows a gel filtration of 50% alcohol precipitate eluted with pyridine-urea 4 M from a Biogel-P-100 column. A major peak is eluted slightly behind the dextran blue, followed by some minor components. In free electrophoresis, the SGPC showed only one boundary. The homogeneity of this preparation was confirmed by the analysis of the fringe pattern obtained by high speed sedimentation equilibrium (Robert, 1969), giving a molecular weight of 78,000. The urea-mercaptoethanol-extract showed a fringe pattern on sedimentation equilibrium, indicating the presence of two components--one of 34,000 (about 80% of the substance), and one of 78,000 (about 20% of the substance). This indicates the existence of a subunit structure held together bydisulfide bridges. The amino acid analysis of several SGPC preparations indicates the presence of 1 to 5disulfide bridges between the subunits.

Tables I and II give some of the physical and chemical properties of purified structural glycoprotein preparations from beef cornea and pig aorta. The presence of two peaks on the sedimentation velocity diagrams and on the free boundary eletrophoresis diagram at acid pH (Robert and Robert, 1967) indicates a partial splitting in subunit of the SGP-preparations.

The sugar and amino acid composition of the cornea and aorta preparations are quite different. SGPC contains significantly higher amounts of hexose and hexosamine and the SGPA contains more sialic acid. Their amino acid composition is similar enough to indicate that both proteins are closely related. The most interesting differences are in the hydroxylysine and cystein content (Robert and Comte,

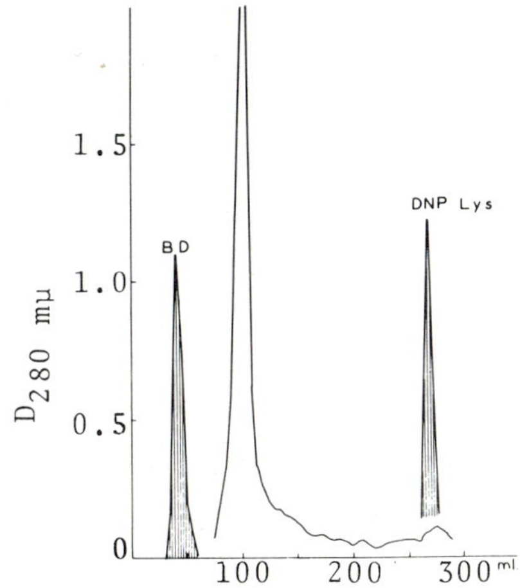

Fig. 1 Elution diagram of a purified corneal structural glycoprotein preparation (SGPC-P-65-3, bovine, 56 mg) from a iogel P-100 column (30 x 420 mm). BD: dextran blue, DNP-Lys dinitrophenyl-lysine (markers). The protein was applied in a pyridine-urea solution and eluted with 0.1 M pyridine, pH 7.0 5 ml. fractions collected.

(1968). The cornea preparation is somewhat richer in dicarboxylic amino acids, glycine and leucine. There are also interesting differences in the composition of the isolated and purified glycopeptides (Moczar, Robert and Moczar, 1968; Moczar, 1968).

III STRUCTURAL GLYCOPROTEINS AND FIBROGENESIS

A close correlation was observed between the proportion of SGP isolated from the fibrous stroma of connective tissue and the ultrastructural characteristic of the fibers. Cornea, for instance, is much richer in SGP than sclera and has thin and regular collagen fibers while those of the sclera are thick, anastomosing and irregular. This finding, together with the variability in hydroxylysine and in sugar, of SGP and also of collagen prompted us to propose a hypothesis for the SGP as a regulatory factor in fibrillo-genesis (Robert and Robert, 1967). It was proposed that the hydroxylation of lysine and the glycosylation of hydroxylysine could sterically prevent the form-

TABLE I

Some Physical and Chemical Properties of Structural Glycoprotein Preparations from Calf Cornea and Pig Aorta

	Cornea(1) (calf)	Aorta(2) (pig)
Sedimentation velocity (10 to 15 mg.ml, pH 7.5 tris buffer) (59.780 + pm 20°C)	S_1 : 0.78 S_2 : 3.03	S_1 : 0.9 S_2 : 5.5
Molecular weight (sedimentation equilibrium)	78,000 (34,000) (3)	--
Electrophoretic mobility	-3.75 cm^2/V/ac	--
Isoelectric pH	5.9	--
Protein content	88	94
Hexoses	6.7	2.1
Hexosamine	2.2	2.9
Fucose	0.42	traces
Sialic acid	0.04-0.6	0.5-1.0
Sulfate	0.94	none

Chemical data are given as % on a dry weight basis.

(1) Preparation P-65-3, from Robert and Robert (1967).

(2) Lipid-extracted urea extract (chloroform-methanol) washed with water and redissolved in urea [fraction U_S; see Moczar (1968), and Moczar and Robert (1969)].

(3) In the presence of mercaptoethanol, the urea extract gave a molecular weight of 34,000 (Robert, 1969).

ation of lysine cross-links between adjacent peptide chains. The chemical composition and the molecular weight of SGPC, suggests a subunit structure consisting of one polypeptide chain of 34,000 molecular weight with one or two large glycopeptide portions of about 2000 to 3000 molecular weight, or with more oligosaccharide chains of a lower molecular weight. Some hydroxylysine glycosides are also present in SGP preparations (Moczar, Moczar and Robert, 1969), but the

TABLE II

Amino Acid Composition of Purified Structural Glycoproteins from Calf Cornea and Pig Aorta

	cornea(1)	Aorta(2)
Allo OH-Lys	3.8	1.3
OH-Lys	7.6	
Lys	44.2	57.2
His	15.9	22.3
Arg	59.8	45.8
OH-pro	--	--
Asp	102.1	89.8
Thréo	50.9	54.4
Ser	59.3	56.5
Pro	56.6	52.1
Glu	113.2	99.5
Gly	105.3	87.9
Ala	70.1	80.8
Val	86.3	73.9
Cys	15.2	26.7
Meth	10.8	0.7
i-Leu	46.9	43.4
Leu	96.5	76.7
Tyr	17.4	28
Pheala	37.7	31.4
NH_4	94.5	82.6

Results given as residue per 1000 residues.

(1) Preparation P-65-2 (Parlebas, 1969).

(2) Lipid-extracted, water-washed residue of the crude urea extract (Moczar, 1968).

hydrolytic nature of the separation of polymeric collagen from the SGP renders difficult the interpretation of this finding. The oligosaccharide chains of SGP are bulky enough to contribute efficiently to the steric hindrance exerted by the SGP-s on the lateral aggregation and cross-linking of collagen fibers. The detailed mechanism of these interactions in the morphogenetic processes of the intercellular matrix is now being explored in our laboratory.

REFERENCES

Moczar, M. (1968). Glycoprotéines de le trame fibreause de la paroi arterielle. Thesis, Univ. Lille.

Moczar, M. Moczar, E. and Robert L. (1967). Biochem. Biophys. Res. Commn. 28, 380.

Moczar, E., Moczar, M., and Robert, L. (1969). Life Sciences 8 part II, 757.

Moczar, M. and Robert, L. (1969). J. Arterioscler. Res. (In press).

Moczar, E., Robert, L. and Moczar, M. (1968). Europ. J. Biochem. 6, 213.

Parlebas, J. (1969) Etude Chimique et Immunologique d'une nouvelle glycoproteine de la cornée. Thesis, Univ. Paris.

Robert, A.M. (1969). Etude comparative de la massa moléculaire des mucines. Thesis, Ecole Pratique des Hautes Etudes, Paris.

Robert, L. and Comte, P. (1968). Life Sciences 7, part 2, 493.

Robert, L. and Dische, Z. (1963). Biochem. Biophys. Res. Comm. 10, 209.

Robert, L. Parlebas, J. and Robert, B. (1963). C.R. Ac. Sci. 256, 232.

Robert L. and Robert, B. (1967). In Protides of Biological Fluids, vol. 15, p. 143. Elsevier, Amsterdam.

Robert, L., Robert, B. and Moczar, E. (1968). In 4th Conference on the Cystic Fibrosis of the Pancreas (1966), part II, p. 309. S. Karger, Basel.

DISTRIBUTION OF CARBOHYDRATES IN THE INSOLUBLE NETWORK OF CONNECTIVE TISSUE

E. Moczar and M. Moczar

Structural glycoproteins (SGP) are associated to the insoluble collagen fraction of the connective tissues (Robert and Dische, 1965; Robert, Oudea, Zweibaum, Parlebas and Robert, 1965; Robert, Robert and Moczar, 1968). They may be isolated after elimination of the polymeric collagen.

In order to obtain information on the nature and distribution of the carbohydrates other than glycosaminoglycans present in the insoluble tissue components, we made a comparative study of the glycopeptides obtained from the structural glycoproteins and from the whole insoluble stroma of the tissue (Robert and Robert, 1969).

I CARBOHYDRATES IN THE WATER INSOLUBLE FRACTION OF THE CORNEAL STROMA AND MEDIA OF AORTA

Our experiments were carried out on the corneal stroma of several species and on the media of the pig aorta. In the first step, the homogenised connective tissue from which the soluble proteins were removed by extraction with 1 M $CaCl_2$, pH 7.5, was designated as "insoluble stroma". It contains the carbohydrate components in the native state. The glycopeptides were prepared from these residues by successive hydrolysis by collagenase and by pronase, followed by exclusion chromatography on Sephadex G-50 columns.

The elution diagram of the hydrolysate of the dogfish (*Scyliorhinus canicula L.*) cornea is presented as an example in Fig. 1. Two main glycopeptide fractions were

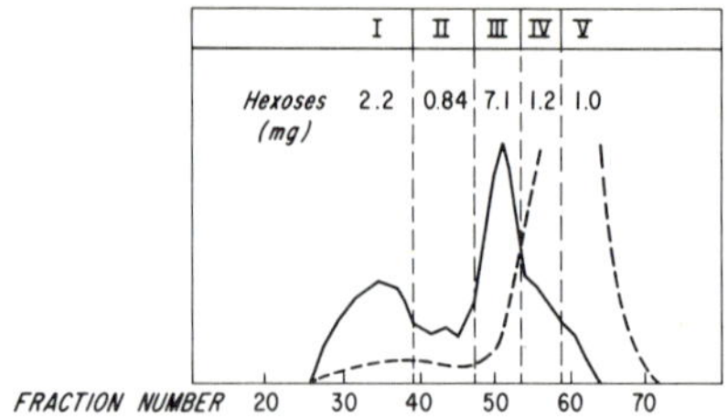

CARBOHYRATE MOIETIES	A	A	B	B	B
GALACTOSE	1	1	1	1	1
GLUCOSE	0.4	1	0.5	0.6	0.5
MANNOSE	3	1	0.1	1.3	1.2
GLUCOSAMINE	3.5	1	0.3	1	1
SIALIC ACID	1				
FUCOSE	+				

Fig. 1. Elution pattern (Sephadex G-50, 100x4 cm) of the glycopeptides from the collagenase-pronase digest of the insoluble stroma of dogfish cornea (Scyliorhinus canicula L.). The molecular ratio of the sugar constituents (related to galactose) and the total hexose content of the fraction are represented in the column above the main fractions. Orcinol, ——; ninhydrin ----.

isolated: 1) a higher molecular weight fraction containing galactose, glucose, mannose and glucosamine as main carbohydrate components; and 2) a lower molecular weight fraction with galactose and galactosido-glucoside chains. The high molecular weight glycopeptide fraction was separated by preparative paper electrophoresis in six main glycopeptides. Ala, Asp, Glu, Gly, Ser and Thr are the predominant amino acid constituents from all these glycopeptides; their sugar composition is presented in Fig. 2.

The low molecular weight fraction was hydrolysed by alkali (Butler and Cunningham, 1966). The Hyl-Gal-Glc and Hyl-Gal were identified by comparison with an authentic sample obtained from Professor Cunningham. The electrophoretic (pH 6.3 and 3.8) and the chromatographic comportment (cellulose thin layers; three different solvents) of the isolated product and of the sample were identical (Moczar, Robert and Moczar, 1968). The proportion of the di- and monosaccharides was determined by densitometry of the electrophoregrams (pH 6.3) by pre-

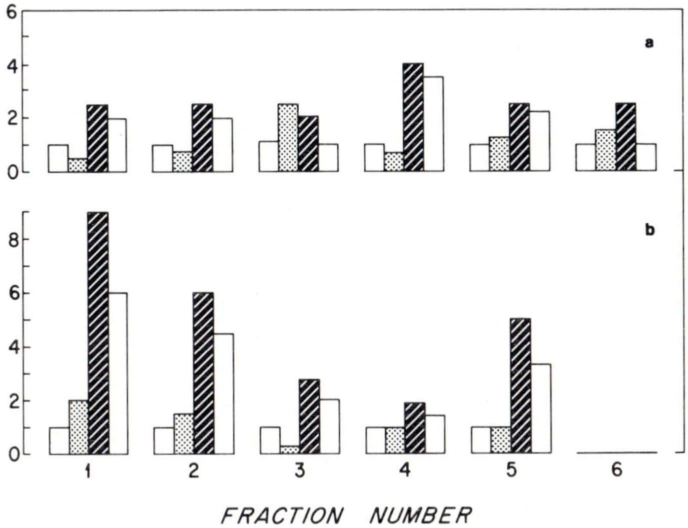

Fig. 2. Ratio of the main sugar constituents in the glycopeptides of the dogfish cornea. a) Glycopeptides isolated by gel filtration and preparative electrophoresis (5000 V, 2 hr, pH 6.4) from the collagenase and pronase digest of the insoluble stroma of dogfish cornea. Fractions 1, 2, 3 and 4 also contain sialic acid and fucose; fractions 3 and 6 contain xylose; fractions 3 and 5 contain hydrox lysine. b) Glycopeptides isolated by gel filtration and high-voltage electrophoresis from the structural glycoprotein fraction of dogfish cornea. Galactose is taken as the unity. Galactose, open squares; glucose, stippled squares; mannose, barred squares; glucosamine, open rectangles on the right.

parative elution of the electrophoretic strips, as well as by the determination of the galactose-glucose ratio of the crude mixtures.

The ratio of the two types of carbohydrate moieties (A, heteropolysaccharide; B, mono- and disaccharide) was calculated from the yield of the crude glycopeptide fractions and from the distribution of the hexoses.

Similar results were obtained from the enzymatic hydrolysates of the insoluble stroma of the pig, rabbit and calf cornea.

In the enzymatic hydrolysate of the pig aorta, some peptidoglycan (glycosaminoglycan) fractions were also isolated well separated from the heteropolysaccharide (A) and the oligo- and monosaccharide (B) containing glycopeptide fractions. However, the proportion of the sugar constituents (galactose, glucose, mannose, glucosamine, fucose, xylose and sialic acid) in the heteropolysaccharide (A) and in the high molecular weight (B) fraction varied from one tissue to another, as did the ratio of the two types of carbohydrate moieties (A and B) (Table I).

II CARBOHYDRATE MOIETY OF THE STRUCTURAL GLYCOPROTEINS

In another series of experiments, the glycoproteins were prepared from the structural glycoprotein fraction of the same tissues. The isolation of the structural glycoprotein fraction consists in the extraction of the polymeric collagen from the insoluble stroma by 0.17 N trichloracetic acid at 90°C (Robert, Parlebas and Robert, 1963; Fitch, Harkness and Harkness, 1955) succeeded by the solubilisation of the residue in 8 M urea. This general extraction principle yields different distribution of the tisse constituents in the various extracts according to the tissue and the animal species. It was noticed in the case of dogfish cornea that after the extraction by the $CaCl_2$ buffer part of the glycoprotein and collagen could even be extracted from the insoluble stroma by using hot water. The residue of the TCA extraction, the crude SGP fraction, is free from hydroxyproline (Robert et al., 1963).

The glycopeptides obtained by the hydrolysis by pronase of the structural glycoproteins were isolated under the same conditions as the glycopeptides obtained from the insoluble stroma. These glycopeptides were analysed and compared to those isolated from the insoluble stroma.

In the digest of the structural glycoproteins, glycopeptides with a heteropolysaccharide sugar moiety (type A) were isolated as the main products accompanied by small quantities of disaccharides linked to Hyl (Table I).

The galactose-mannose ratio is not the same in type A

TABLE I

Ratio of the Carbohydrate Part of the Glycoproteins of the Structural Glycoproteins

Source of glycoprotein	Insoluble Stroma				Structural Glycoprotein		
	Total carbohydrate (%)[‡]	A[*]	-Gal	B[+] -Gal-Glc	Total carbohydrate (%)	A[*]	B[+] -Gal + -Gal-Glc
Calf cornea	1.2	1	7	14	7.5	1	0.8
Rabbit cornea	1.6	1	14	14	7.5	1	0.8
Pig cornea	1.6	1	11	14	8	1	0.8
Pig aorta	2.5	1	4	4	4	1	0.3
Dogfish cornea	5	1	4	7	7	1	0

[*] The A type heteropolysaccharide moiety is taken as unity. The ratios are calculated with an average molecular weight of 2500 for this carbohydrate.

[+] B = galactose and glucosido-galactose moieties linked to hydroxylysine.

[‡] The sum of hexoses and hexosamines.

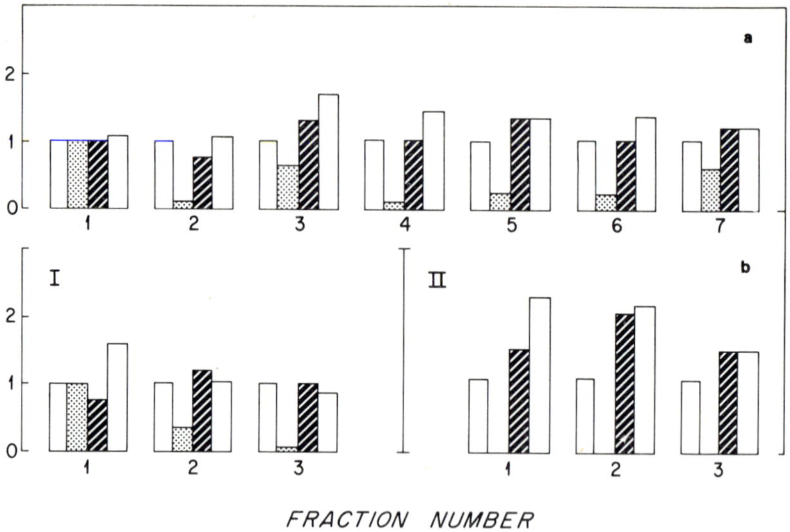

Fig. 3. Ratio of the main sugar constituents in the glycopeptides of the media of pig aorta. a) Glycopeptides isolated by gel filtration and by preparative paper electrophoresis (5000 V, pH 6.4) from the insoluble stroma of the media of pig aorta, digested successively by collagenase and by pronase. b) Glycopeptides isolated by gel filtration and by preparative paper electrophoresis from the pronase digest of the structural glycoprotein fractions of the media of pig aorta. I, water soluble fraction of the SGP; II, urea soluble fraction of the SGP. Galactose is taken as the unity. Galactose, open; glucose, stippled squares; mannose, barred squares; glucosamine, open rectangles on the right.

glycopeptides derived from SGP, and from the insoluble stroma, indicating that during the TCA-treatment part of the galactose could be removed (Fig. 2). The same difference in galactose content was found in the high voltage subfractions of type A glycopeptides of insoluble stroma and of SGP. However, the same amino acids were present in both series of glycopeptides. There is much less variations of the galactose-mannose ratio during the TCA treatment in the glycopeptides obtained from the analogous fractions of the calf cornea and the porcine aorta than in the dogfish cornea (Moczar et al., 1968; Moczar, Moczar and Robert, 1969). Fig. 3 shows the hexose ratios in pig aorta glycopeptides. The Gal:Glc:Man:GlcN ratios were different from those found in dogfish and calf corneas.

The glucosamine-mannose ratio was quite similar in the carbohydrate part of the glycopeptides obtained from SGP and from the insoluble stroma. The terminal sialic acid was quantitatively removed by this TCA-treatment (Moczar, 1968a, b; Kohn, Winzler and Hoffman, 1962). It appears from these results that the composition of the glycopeptides isolated from the A fraction of insoluble stroma and of SGP differs only in its galactose-mannose ratio. This difference is more important in dogfish cornea than in mammalian cornea and aorta.

The nature of the carbohydrate-protein linkage was also investigated in the glycopeptides that contained a heteropolysaccharide moiety, (type A) obtained from dogfish, calf and pig corneas and from the procine aorta. 2-Acetamido-1-(L-β-aspartamido)-1,2-dideoxy-β-D-glucose was identified in the partial hydrolysates of these glycopeptides by comparing the electrophoretic and chromatographic behaviour of the substance (Moczar, 1968a, b) with an authentic sample prepared from ovalbumin (Bogdanov, Kaverzneva and Andrejeva, 1962). This finding permits the conclusion that at least one part of the heteropolysaccharide chain is linked by an aspartamido-glucosaminidic linkage to the protein.

The fact that we could isolate glycopeptides from the insoluble structural glycoproteins in which the protein part does not contain Hyp, would indicate that heteropolysaccharide side chains exist in the insoluble fibrous network of connective tissues which are not linked to collagen. The ratio of the heteropolysaccharide moiety (type A) and the mono- and disaccharidic units (B) in the insoluble stroma and in the structural glycoproteins is shown in Table I. This ratio is very similar in the mammalian corneas studied; however, the galactose to glucosido-galactose ratios are significantly different in the calf and the rabbit corneas. The dogfish cornea and the pig aorta contain less mono- and disaccharide units related to the heteropolysaccharide chains than do mammalian corneas.

It appears from these results that the ratio of the two types of carbohydrate moieties A and B, as well as the ratio of sugar components of the heteropolysaccharide (A) containing glycopeptides, varies according to the origin and organisation of connective tissues (Robert and Robert, 1967).

REFERENCES

Bogdanov, V., Kaverzneva, E. and Andrejeva, A. (1962). Biochem. Biophys. Acta 65, 168.

Butler, W. and Cunningham, L.W. (1966). J. Biol. Chem. 241, 3883.

Fitch, S.M., Harkness, M.L.D. and Harkness, R.D. (1955). Nature 176, 163.

Kohn, P., Winzler, R.J. and Hoffmann, R.C. (1962). J. Biol. Chem. 237, 406.

Moczar, E., Moczar, M. and Robert, L. (1969). Life Sciences 8, Part II, 757.

Moczar, E., Robert, L. and Moczar, M. (1968). European J. Biochem. 6, 213.

Moczar, M. (1968a). Thesis, Faculte des Sciences, Lille.

Moczar, M. (1968b). FEBS Letters 1, 169.

Robert, L. and Dische, Z. (1965). Biochem. Biophys. Res. Comm. 10, 209.

Robert, L., Oudea, P., Zweibaum, A., Parlebas, J. and Robert, B. (1965). In Biochemistry and Physiology of Connective and Skeletal Tissue, p. 406. Ed. by Tristram, G.R. Butterworth, London.

Robert, L., Parlebas, J. and Robert, B. (1963). Comptes-Rendus 256, 323.

Robert, L. and Robert, B. (1967). In Protides of the Biological Fluids, Proceedings of the 15th Colloquium (Bruges, 1967), p. 143. Ed. by Peeters. Elsevier, Amsterdam.

Robert, L. and Robert, B. (1969). This volume, p.665.

Robert, L., Robert, B., and Moczar, E. (1968). In 4th International Conference on Cystic Fibrosis of the Pancreas (Mucoviscidosis) (Berne, Grindelwald 1966), part II, p. 309. Karger, Basel and New York.

THE FORMATION AND STRUCTURE OF INSOLUBLE COLLAGEN

K. Kühn, K. Bräumer, B. Zimmermann and J. Pikkarainen

The macromolecular organization of collagen is adapted to suit the physiological functions of the individual connective tissues, e.g. tendons consist of parallel fibril bundles with a great mechanical stability. The elastic, flexible skin is built up of an interwoven three-dimensional fibrous network and in loose connective tissues the fibrils are arranged as a light network in which other substances are embedded. Thus far it is not known how the formation of the various macromolecular structures takes place and is controlled in the extracellular space. Our knowledge is restricted to the individual fibrils, the smallest structural unit. They are produced by the ordered aggregation of rod-like collagen molecules and later obtain their stability by the formation of covalent intermolecular crosslinks.

This article deals with two problems: (1) the aggregation of the molecules to form fibrils and the influence of proteoglycans in fibril formation and (2) the several intermolecular crosslinks which significantly influence the properties of insoluble collagen.

I FORMATION OF FIBRILS FROM COLLAGEN MOLECULES

Figure 1 shows the arrangement of collagen molecules in the fibrils. The molecules lie parallel to each other and are displaced by one- two- three-fourths of their length, respectively (Schmitt, 1956; Hodge and Schmitt, 1960; Kühn, Grassmann and Hofmann, 1960). Simultaneously they overlap each other by about 300 Å with their ends

(Hodge and Petruska, 1963). This arrangement of the molecules is reflected in the electronmicrographs of the fibrils. The characteristic cross-striation pattern is due to the quarter stagger arrangement of the 2800 Å-long collagen molecules. Because of the overlap of the ends of the molecules, the 700 Å-period is subdivided into a loose and densly packed region. This can be seen after negative staining of the fibrils. The densly packed overlapping region appears as a 300 Å-wide light band in which not as much staining is absorbed as in the rest of the period.

The rod-like body is built of three polypeptide chains which form the triple-helix (Rich and Crick, 1961; Ramachandran and Sasisekharan, 1961). Its characteristic charge-pattern with distinct positive and negative charge-centres is important for the ordered aggregation of the molecules at the neutral pH of the connective tissue. The charge pattern is caused by the arrangement of the polar amino acids in local accumulation of basic or acidic amino acids along the chains (Kühn and Zimmer, 1961). The aggregation of the molecules is controlled by electrostatic forces in such a way that the centres of positive and negative charges of adjacent molecules neutralize one another. This situation is best obtained if the molecules are displaced by a quarter of their length.

Disturbance of the charge-pattern changes the properties of the collagen molecules. They lose their ability to form fibrils of the native type (Rauterberg and Kühn, 1968). Table I shows some examples. In methylated collagen, the carboxyl-groups have lost their negative charge. It is soluble at a neutral pH. In desamidated collagen the amide groups of asparagine and glutamine have been split off. This increases the number of negative charges. In succinylated collagen the positive charges of the amino groups in lysine have been replaced by negative groups. This preparation precipitates at acidic pH. All three derivatives have lost the ability to form fibrils of the native type.

Although the arrangement of the collagen molecules in

TABLE I

Properties of Various Collagen Derivatives

	Groups changed	Change in charge	Carboxyl group per g collagen (from titration curve)(mmole)	Formation of fibrils (5)	Formation of SLS (6)
Acid soluble collagen (1) untreated	-	-	0.81	+	+
Methyl collagen (2)	COOH → $COOOCH_3$	- → 0	0.31	-	-
Desamido collagen (3)	$-CONH_2$ → COOH	0 → -	1.24	-	+
Succinyl collagen (4)	$-CH_2-NH_2$ → $-CH_2NHOC-$ $-(CH_2)-COOH$	+ → -	1.18	-	-

(1) From calfskin
(2) Prepared by treatment with 0.2 N methanolic HCl, 4°C, 24 hr.
(3) Prepared by treatment with 5% NaOH in saturated Na-sulphate, 20°C, 72 hr.
(4) Prepared by treatment of dissolved collagen in 0.2 M Ca-acetate, pH 7.5, with succinyl anhydride.
(5) By dialysis of collagen solution in 0.225 M citrate buffer, pH 3.7, against tap water.
(6) By dialysis of collagen solution in 0.05% acetic acid against 0.4% ATP, pH 3-4.

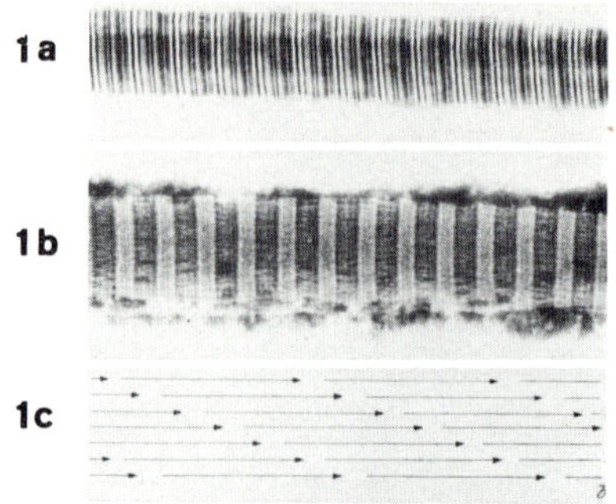

Fig. 1. Electron micrographs of collagen fibrils.
a) Positively stained with phosphotungstic acid and uranyl acetate. Asymmetric cross striation pattern.
b) Negatively stained with phosphotungstic acid at pH7. The lighter bands represent the densely packed 300 Å-long overlapping region of the molecule.
c) Schematic representation of the arrangement of the collagen molecules in the fibrils

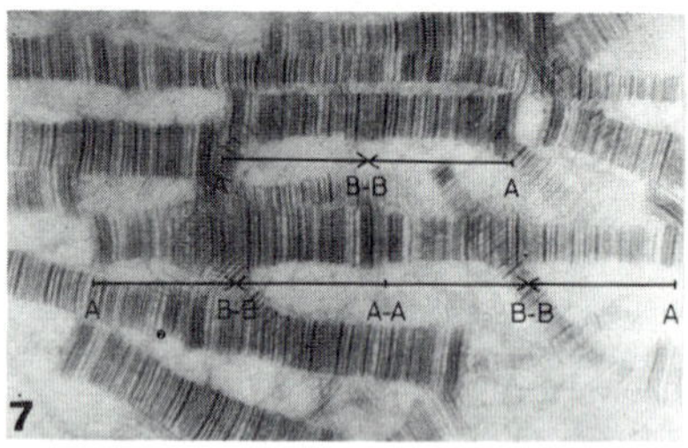

Fig. 7. Segment long-spacing end-to-end polymers prepared from 1% acetic acid extract of calf skin collagen by dialysis against 0.4% ATP-solution at pH 2.8; stained with phosphotungstic acid and uranyl acetate.

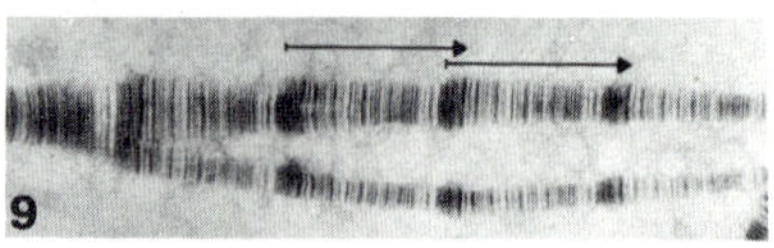

Fig. 9. Segment long-spacing fibrils prepared from achilles tendon collagen (calf) after digestion with pepsin (2 hr at pH 2.0; weight ratio collagen:enzyme, 10:1) by dialysis against 0.4% ATP solution at pH 2.8. Stained with phosphotungstic acid and uranyl acetate. The arrows indicate the overlap and the orientation of the collagen molecules.

the fibril is determined chiefly by the distribution of charges and therefore by the amino acid sequence, there is evidence that other substances can retard, accelerate, or in some way influence the process of fibril formation. A classical example is the formation of the fibrils long-spacing (FLS) (Highberger, Gross and Schmitt, 1950). These fibrils are produced from neutral solutions in the presence of an excess of glycosaminoglycans (GAG) such as hyaluronic acid (HA) and chondroitin sulphate (ChS) (Kühn and Zimmer, 1961). In the electronmicroscope they show a cross-striation period of about 2600 Å with a symmetrical pattern. The collagen molecules are arranged in an antiparallel manner with their ends in register. The fibrils are formed by overlapping the ends of the molecules by 300 Å, as in the native fibrils. The thread-shaped molecules of the glycosaminoglycans have a strong affinity for the collagen molecules, and this results in a different type of aggregation.

Another example is the effect of small amounts of contaminating material that accompanies the soluble collagen during extraction from connective tissue and is very difficult to remove. Impure collagen samples form fibrils of the native type relatively quickly. Upon purification of the collagen samples, the ability of the molecules to aggregate is reduced. Unstructured material and fibrils with unnatural cross-striation pattern are formed, e.g. a band period of 120 Å with no further differentiation (Kühn, Schuppler and Kühn, 1964). These anomalous reformations cannot be the result of badly damaged collagen molecules since the purification effect is reversed by the addition of collagen-free connective tissue extracts.

From these results it can be concluded that some noncollagen substances of the connective tissue influence the aggregation of collagen molecules and regulate the fibril formation in the connective tissue. Consequently we are interested in substances that are able to influence fibril formation in vitro. The following section describes the influence of different proteoglycan fractions from rat skin on the in vitro fibril formation of collagen molecules.

II THE INFLUENCE OF PROTEOGLYCANS FROM RAT SKIN ON THE COLLAGEN FIBRIL FORMATION IN VITRO

A. ISOLATION OF PROTEOGLYCANS (PG) OF RAT SKIN

Rat skin contains a mixture of GAG of about 50% hyaluronic acid (HA), 40% chondroitin sulphate (ChS) and dermatan sulphate (DS), and 10% heparin. The individual GAG fractions possess varying affinities towards the collagen fibril network of the skin. HA seems not to be firmly bound to collagen as it can be readily and completely extracted with a phosphate buffer of physiological pH and ionic strength. By extraction with 2 M NaCl, ChS and heparin can be dissolved, and thereby heparin is extracted quantitatively while a part of ChS is left in the skin. This fraction contains mainly dermatan sulphate which can be extracted with urea solution.

Table II shows the composition of the PG that can be extracted with phosphate buffer and 2 M NaCl solution. In addition to HA, the phosphate extract contains mainly serum proteins, a small amount of non-collagenous connective tissue-specific proteins, and salt-soluble collagen. The high molecular weight HA is then purified by gel chromatography on Sepharose 4-B. The molar ratio of glucuronic acid to glucosamine is 1, and the protein content is 6% by weight.

The NaCl extract contains, in addition to the PG, mainly salt-soluble collagen. By precipitation with ammonium sulphate (10% saturated), collagen, like heparin, is removed without loss of PG. Further purification is carried out by precipitation of PG with cetyl-pyridinium chloride OCPC), or by chromatography on Sephadex G-200.

B. FIBRIL FORMATION IN THE PRESENCE OF HAYLURONIC ACID AND PROTEOGLYCANS

Acid-soluble collagen from rat skin is used to test the effect of PG on fibril formation. Increase in turbidity during incubation of the neutral salt solution of collagen at 23°C is taken as measure of fibril formation (Gross,

TABLE II

Composition of Proteoglycans Isolated from Different Extracts of Rat Skin

	Extracts	Hexosamine: uronic acid (molar ratio)	Protein content (weight %)	Per cent glucosamine total hexosamine
Hyaluronic acid (1)	Phosphate-buffer pH 7.4, Γ/2=0.14	1:0.96	6	100
Proteoglycan (CPC) (2)	2.0 M NaCl	1:0.64	31	42
Proteoglycan (Seph) (3)	2.0 M NaCl	1:0.63	18	28

(1) Isolated from phosphate extract by gel filtration on Sepharose 4-B.

(2) Isolated from NaCl extract. After separation of collagen by ammonsulphate precipitation the PG was purified by CPC precipitation.

(3) Isolated from NaCl extract. After separation of collagen by ammonsulphate precipitation the PG was purified by gel filtration on Sephadex G-200.

1956).

Figure 2 shows the influence of the hyaluronic acid. In the control, fibril formation is completed in 1 hr. HA at high concentrations delays fibril formation considerably; whereas in low concentrations the effect is insignificant.

On the other hand, the effect of PG is considerably greater. In agreement with Toole and Lowther (1968a,b), ChS in high concentrations precipitate collagen at 4°C, which makes it impossible to study fibril formation by the warming of solutions. In the electronmicroscope the precipitate shows only unstructured material and no striated fibrils of the native type can be detected.

To study fibril formation, the concentrations of PG are lowered to such an extent that at 4°C precipitation does not take place. Finally the solution is warmed to 23°C and the turbidity is measured. Figure 3 shows the results

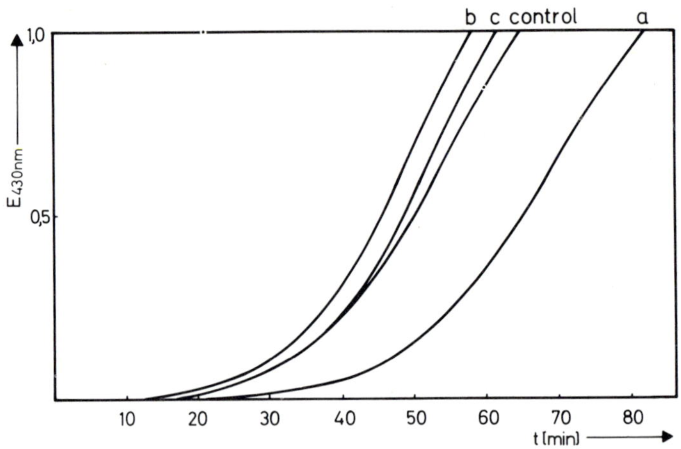

Fig. 2. Effect of HA on the rate of collagen fibril formation. Acid-soluble collagen from rat skin (1 mg collagen/ml) in phosphate buffer pH 7,4 $\Gamma/2$ = 0.14 was warmed at 23°C. Fibril formation was followed by turbidity measurement at 430 mμ. HA in phosphate buffer was added at 4°C immediately before warming. HA concentration in the incubation medium (mg/ml) a) 0.5, b) 0.25, c) 0.125.

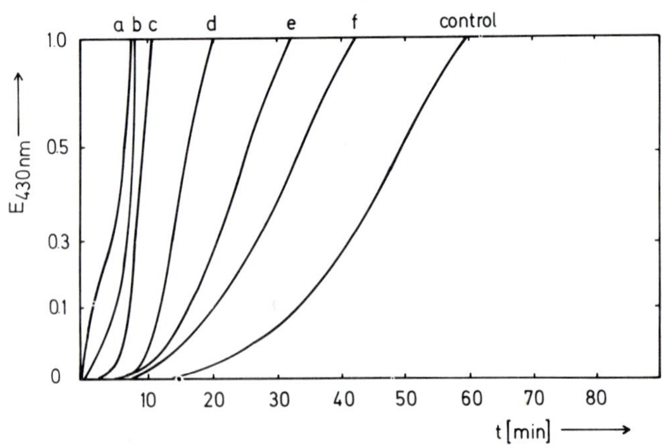

Fig. 3. Effect of PG (CPC-purified) on the rate of collagen fibril formation (for experimental conditions see Fig. 2). Collagen concentration 1 mg/ml. PG concentration (mg/ml) = a) 0.05, b) 0.025, c) 0.006, d) 0.0015, e) 0.0004, f) 0.0002.

obtained with the CPC-purified PG. Even at a ratio of 100:0.02 (w/w) of collagen to PG, an obvious acceleration of fibril formation can be observed. Nucleation and growth-phases are accelerated equally. In each case normal native type fibrils with perfect cross striation patterns are observed.

The ability to influence fibril formation is found to depend on the method of purification. In comparison to the CPC purified complex, PG, purified by gel chromatography, shows a similar effect which is quantitatively different. For example, the ability to form non-specific precipitations at 4°C is more pronounced. Even at a ratio of 100:1 of collagen to PG, the formation of a small amount of a precipitate can be observed. This is seen as a sudden increase of the extinction before warming the solution. The following increase in extinction by warming to 23°C represents the normal fibril formation. A significant acceleration of the nucleation and growth phase, as compared to control, is not observed. In the electronmicroscope unstructured material is seen along with native type fibrils and FLS. On further decrease of the concentration of "Sephadex purified" - PG no precipitation at 4°C occurs, and an acceleration of the fibril formation is apparent. This effect is obviously less in comparison to that obtained from the CPC-purified PG (Fig. 4).

Toole and Lowther (1968a) have shown for the first time that PG, which is firmly attached to the collagen fibrils in vivo, also has a strong affinity towards soluble collagen in vitro. An urea-extracted soluble dermatan sulphate from calf skin precipitates collagen at 4°C, as in our preparations. In both these cases the precipitate does not accelerate the fibril formation. From our results, such PG form suitable nuclei with collagen at very low concentrations only. The answer to the question, whether such PG also control fibril formation in vivo, awaits further investigation.

It is known from the work of Mathews and Decker (1968) that a number of GAG-preparations from different sources form complexes with soluble collagen. However, they do not increase the rate of fibril formation. To the contrary they retard it sometimes, like the PG used in this present investigation. We have also had similar experience with water-extracted PG obtained from the knee joint cartilage of a calf. This means that those soluble PG-collagen complexes are not suitable as nuclei for fibril formation.

III THE COVALENT CROSSLINKS IN COLLAGEN

Following the formation of fibrils, the collagen molecules undergo a linkage process which results in the fibrils becoming progressively less soluble and mechanically more stable. Two different types of covalent bonds are involved in this process: (1) the intramolecular bonds formed between two or three chains of a single molecule and (2) the intermolecular bonds joining the peptide chains of different molecules. The latter are solely responsible for rendering the fibrils insoluble and mechanically more stable. Recently for this investigation three types of intermolecular cross-links have been demonstrated by using the electronmicroscope. Polymerized collagen molecules soluble in acids are used and also the stepwise degradation with pepsin of the highly cross-linked achilles tendon of calf (Kühn, Fietzek and Kühn, 1966).

A. THE END-TO-END LINKAGE

On extracting a connective tissue like calf skin with acids, not only collagen monomers but also a small fraction of polymers go into solution. The higher the swelling capacity of the acid, the greater is the amount of polymers that are dissolved. A good test for the presence of polymers is the concentration-dependence of the reduced viscosity. This is clearly seen in Fig. 5, which shows the reduced viscosities of different collagen extractions from calf skin. The neutral extract is composed solely of monomeric collagen molecules. The concentration dependence of viscosity is very little. With increasing contents of polymers, the viscosity also increases. Its dependence on concentration is most noticeable in a lactic acid extract, which contains the largest amount of polymers.

A better proof for the presence of polymers, as well as their quantitative evaluation, is achieved by gel

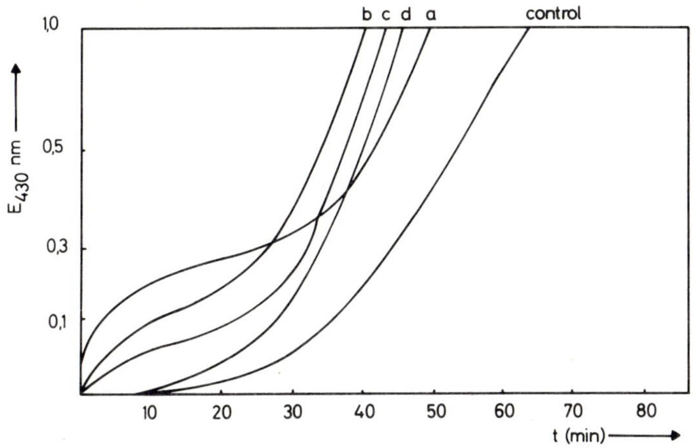

Fig. 4. Effect of PG (purified by Sephadex G-200 chromatography) on the rate of collagen fibril formation. (For experimental conditions see Fig. 2). Collagen concentration 1 mg/ml. PG concentration (mg/ml). a) 0.01, b) 0.005, c) 0.0025, d) 0.00125.

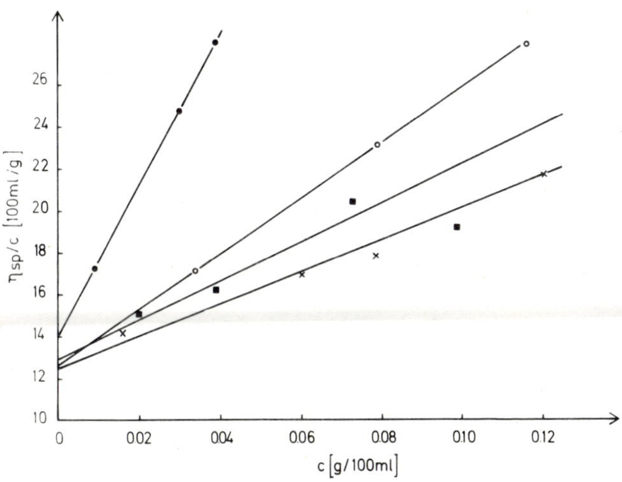

Fig. 5. Dependence of the reduced viscosity of the concentration of different collagen extracts from calf skin (in 1% acetic acid + 0.1 M NaCl, 20°C). Extracted with: x 0.5 M NaCl, pH 8; filled squares, 0.225 M citrate buffer pH 3.7; open circles, 0.1% acetic acid; filled circles, 0.28 M lactic acid.

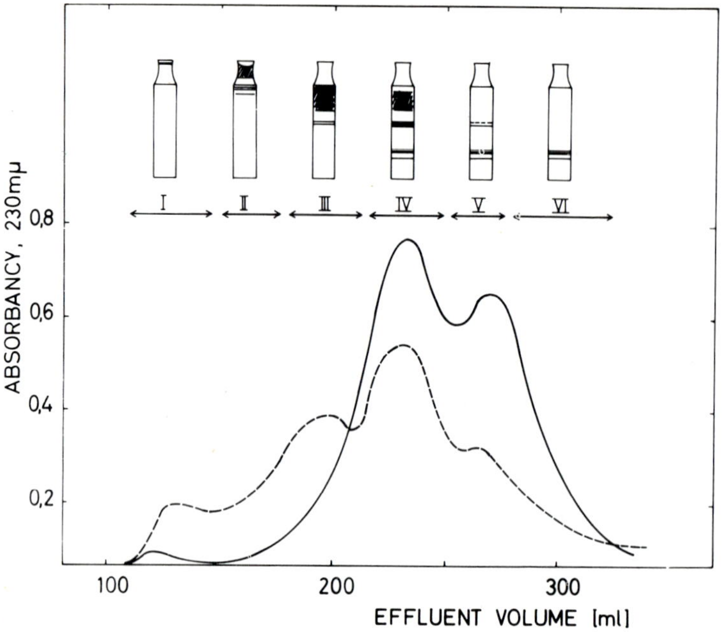

Fig. 6. Gel filtration on Sepharose 4-B and disc electrophoresis of citrate buffer soluble (——) and lactic acid soluble (----) collagen of calf skin. Elution was with 1 M $CaCl_2$ + 0.1 M Na acetate; elution rate 16 ml/hr; temperature 25°C; column 2.5 x 85 cm. Electrophoresis as described by Stark and Kühn (1968).

chromatography of the denatured collagen preparations. Here, the polymers are separated according to their size and molecular weight. The chromatography of a citrate extract and a lactic acid extract from calf skin collagen are compared in Fig. 6. One can clearly see that the lactic acid extract contains a larger amount of polymers than the citrate extract. Fractions 1 and 2 contain the largest polymers which are not able to penetrate the running gel of the disc electrophoresis. The main constituent of fraction 4 is the β-component, whereas, fraction 6 is comprised of α-chains only. Table III shows the amounts of the collagen components in each of the fractions.

The native polymeric collagen molecules can be made visible in the electronmicroscope. By precipitation with ATP, they form SLS-polymers (Fig. 7). The SLS are joined in this case with their same ends--that is BB and AA; dimers and higher polymers containing both BB and AA junctions can

TABLE III

Gel Filtration on Sepharose 4-B of Citrate Buffer Soluble-And Lactic Acid-Soluble Collagen from Calf Skin (Fig. 6)

Distribution of Collagen on the Six Fractions Obtained

Collagen	Fraction					
	I	II	III	IV	V	VI
	(% of total amount)					
Citrate buffer-soluble	1	--	19	35	19	26
Lactic acid-soluble	3	12	27	31	14	13

be observed. The ends of the molecules do not overlap each other more than 30 Å. Therefore the covalent crosslinks should be located at the end regions of the molecules. This is in agreement with the fact that these bonds can easily be split by pepsin. We have designated this type of crosslinks end-to-end bond. The electronmicroscopic observation is in accordance with the polymer content of the extract. The citrate extract with a small amount of polymers shows, in addition to monomeric SLS, dimers with AA and BB bonds. On the other hand, the lactic acid extract shows larger amounts of polymeric SLS consisting of four, five or more end-to-end joint segments.

B. HEAD-TO-TAIL AND SIDE-TO-SIDE BONDS

Two further different types of crosslinks can be located by stepwise pepsin digestion of highly crosslinked achilles tendon of calf (Kühn et al., 1966); this is shown schematically in Fig. 8. The insoluble collagen fibrils of the tendon are crosslinked by side-to-side and by head-to-tail bonds. The quarter-staggered array of the molecules are fixed by the side-to-side bonds. The site of this bond along the length of the molecule is uncertain. Mild pepsin treatment attacks chiefly the side-to-side bonds while the head-to-tail bonds, which are localized in the 300 Å-overlap zones of the molecules, remain intact. If the highly

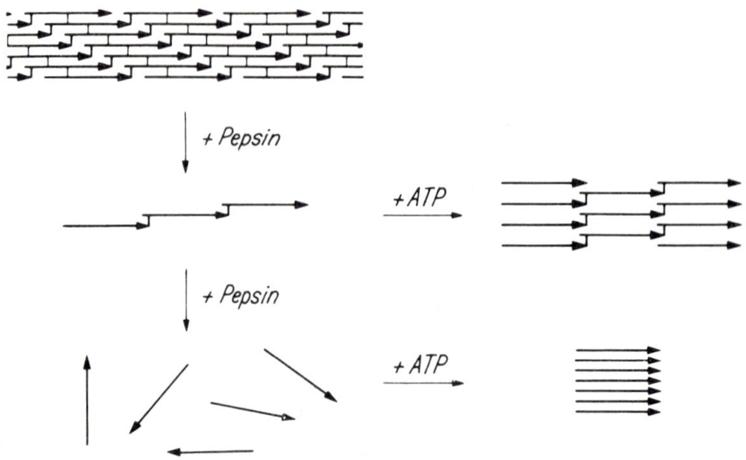

Fig. 8. Scheme for the dissolution of an insoluble collagen fibril into monomer collagen molecules by splitting the intermolecular bonds with pepsin. First step: splitting of the intermolecular side-to-side bonds. Second step: splitting of the intermolecular head-to-tail bonds. Head-to-tail bonds are more resistant to pepsin attack than side-to-side bonds. Head-to-tail bonds are localised in the 300-Å overlap zone of the molecules. Localisation of the side-to-side bond is not known. For clarity these bonds are drawn lightly in the middle of the molecule.

acid-swollen polymers are now treated with ATP under the same conditions as used for the preparation of SLS, then SLS fibrils are obtained. The electronmicrographs clearly show how the collagen molecules with unlike ends overlap about 300 Å (Fig. 9). On the other hand, the same treatment of the acid-swollen preparations, not pretreated with pepsin, give rise to native fibrils in the electronmicroscope. This is because a combination of molecules with their ends in register is hindered by the intact side-to-side bond. Intensive treatment with pepsin also cleaves the head-to-tail bonds.

Figure 10 shows a chromatogram on Sepharose of denatured head-to-tail polymers. For comparison, an acetic acid extract of untreated tendon containing only a few polymers has also been chromatographed. Fractions 1 and 2 contain the larger polymers, fraction 3 mainly the γ- and β-components, while the main constituent of fraction 4 is the α chain. It is surprising to note that such large amounts of α chains are

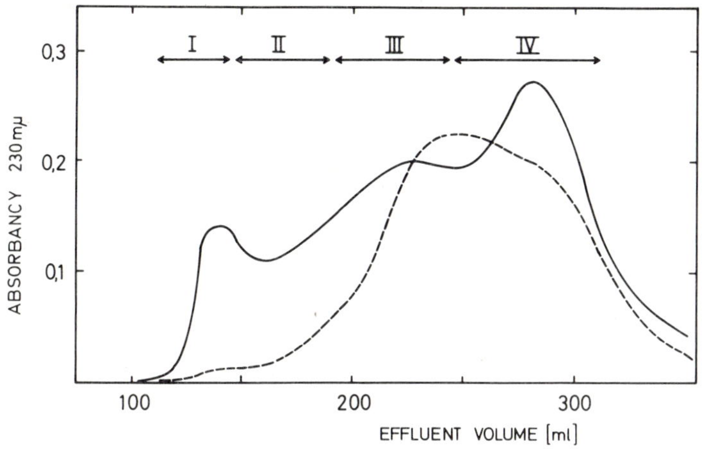

Fig. 10. Gel filtration on Sepharose 4-B of acetic acid soluble collagen and pepsin soluble collagen from calf achilles tendon. (Pepsin digestion: 2 hr at pH 2; weight ratio collagen:enzyme, 10:1). Elution with 1 M $CaCl_2$ + 0.1 M Na acetate + 0.02% Sodium azide; elution rate 16 ml/hr; temperature 25°C; column 2.5 x 95 cm.

TABLE IV

Gel Filtration on Sepharose 4-B of Pepsin-Soluble And Acetic Acid-Soluble Collagen from Calf Achilles Tendon (Fig. 10) Distribution of Collagen on the Four Fractions Obtained

Collagen	Fractions I	II	III	IV
	(% of total amount)			
Pepsin-soluble	4	24	27	45
Acetic acid soluble	-	5	41	55

present in head-to-tail polymers (Table IV). The reason for this seems to be that pepsin cleaves not only the side-to-side bonds but also the end-to-end bonds.

Figure 11 is a schematic drawing showing how the molecules within the fibrils could possibly be held together by all three types of intermolecular crosslinks. In the known two-dimensional scheme for the arrangement of the molecules in the fibril, only the head-to-tail and the side-

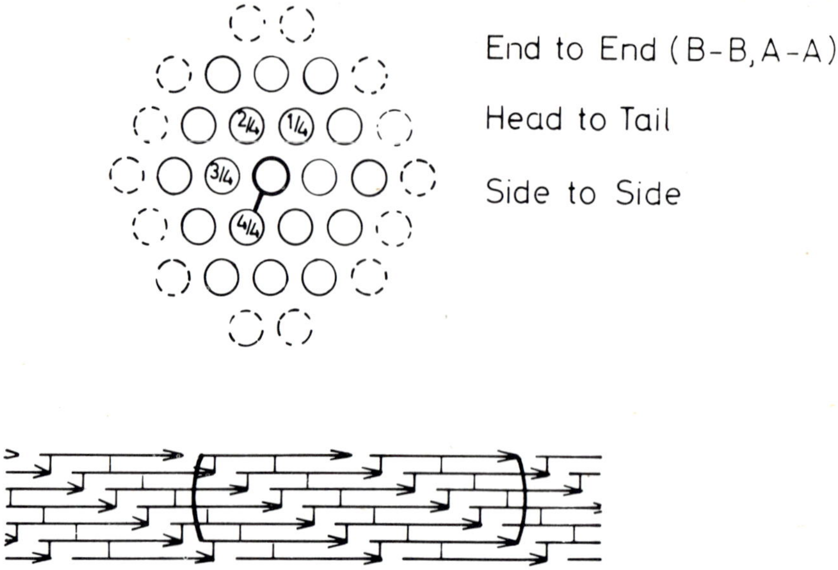

Fig. 11. Scheme of the location of the intermolecular bonds in the insoluble collagen fibril. The end-to-end bonds link neighbouring molecules which are in register across like ends. (Upper part: cross section through a collagen fibril).

to-side bonds can be correctly represented. A three-dimensional picture of the relationship of the molecules one to another is required for a description of the end-to-end bonds. Therefore, a cross-section through a fibril is shown in Fig. 11. A hexogonal arrangement has been chosen for clarity; but other arrangements are also possible. Since each of the molecules is surrounded by six neighbours, each neighbour cannot be shifted by one-, two- or three-quarters with respect to the reference molecule. There are also neighbours arranged parallel and with their ends in register; consequently it is sterically possible for them to be linked across the same ends even in the fibril.

IV STABILIZATION OF INTERMOLECULAR CROSSLINKS THROUGH REDUCTION WITH SODIUM BOROHYDRIDE ($NaBH_4$)

According to Tanzer (1967, 1968), Bailey (1968) and Bailey and Tanzer (1968) reduction by $NaBH_4$ diminishes the solubility of acid-soluble collagen and increases the stability of insoluble collagen. This may be due to the stabilization of the intermolecular crosslinks of the Schiff-base type, which can be converted by reduction with $NaBH_4$ to a secondary amine. The resulting linkage is more stable and is resistant to cleavage by weak acids.

It was thought worthwhile to investigate which of the crosslinkages among the three types mentioned above is labile in acidic conditions and which is stabilized by reduction with $NaBH_4$. The following experiments have been carried out to determine this (Fig. 12). Lyophilized fibrils of the native type from different collagen sources are reduced with $NaBH_4$. First the products are extracted with 1% acetic acid. After centrifugation two fractions are obtained--the supernatant (acetic acid-Sup) and the residue. The acetic acid residues are digested with pepsin for 3 hr at pH 2 (25°C). Again two fractions are obtained--pepsin supernatant and pepsin residue. The quantitative estimation of these four fractions gives a measure of the crosslinks stabilized by reduction with $NaBH_4$. The electron-microscopic investigation after treatment with ATP allows characterization of the types of crosslinks present in each case. Thus the presence of fibrils of the native type in acetic acid residues is proof of the side-to-side crosslinks, and the presence of SLS-fibrils is an indication of head-to-tail bonds.

Table V shows the solubility of neutral salt soluble collagen, citrate-soluble collagen and acetic acid-soluble collagen from rat skin and calf achilles tendon after reduction. The solubility in acetic acid of rat skin collagen decreases from Salt-soluble collagen to acetic acid soluble collagen. While Salt-soluble collagen is 90% soluble, only

TABLE V

Solubility of Rat Skin and Calf Achilles Tendon Collagen After Reduction with Sodium Borohydride in 1% Acetic Acid and After Pepsin Treatment

Source of collagen	Collagen fractions soluble in	Acetic acid Supernatant		Acetic acid Residue		Pepsin Supernatant		Pepsin Residue		Total soluble	
Rat skin	salt	88	(96)	12	(4)	4		8		92	(97)
	citrate	51	(97)	49	(3)	28		21		79	(99)
	acetic acid	21	(90)	79	(10)	58	(7)	21	(3)	79	(97)
Calf achilles tendon	salt	2	(99)	98	(1)	4		94		6	(99)
	citrate	2	(100)	98		6		92		8	(100)
	acetic acid	2	(91)	98	(9)	5	(5)	93	(4)	7	(96)

For scheme of fractionation see Fig. 12.
(The values of the non-reduced controls are given in parentheses).

Fig. 12. Flow Scheme for the investigation of $NaBH_4$-reduced collagen.

Lyophilized fibrils of the native type

Reduction (weight ratio collagen:$NaBH_4$, 30:1, in 0.2 M Na_2CO_3, pH 7.4; 4 hr; 4°C.)

Extraction (with 1% acetic acid for 2 days; 4°C.

Centrifugation (30,000 x g; 2 hr)

→ Acetic acid supernatant

→ Acetic acid residue

Pepsin digestion (collagen:pepsin = 10:1; 25°C; 3 hr; pH 2)

Centrifugation (30,000 x g; 2 hr)

→ Pepsin supernatant

→ Pepsin Residue

(Simultaneously control samples without reduction were investigated).

20% is soluble in the case of acetic acid soluble collagen. A large portion of acetic acid residue is solubilized on treatment with pepsin. The effect of reduction is considerably more in the case of calf achilles tendon collagen. All three preparations are practically insoluble in acetic acid and the short treatment with pepsin has no visible effect. The corresponding control samples are almost completely soluble in acetic acid in all cases.

Table VI shows the results of electronmicroscopic investigations after deswelling of the various preparations with ATP. The control samples that are more than 90% soluble in acetic acid show mainly SLS, as did the starting material. The acetic acid-soluble fraction of the reduced rat skin collagen shows a clear increase in the amount of SLS fibrils. The acetic acid residue from rat skin collagen also contains mainly SLS fibrils. The presence of SLS fibrils is a criterion for the stabilization by reduction of the head-to-tail bonds. Since these crosslinks are only

TABLE VI

Electronmicroscopic Investigation of Reduced Rat Skin and Calf Achilles Tendon Collagen

	$NaBH_4$ reduced	Segment long spacing	Segment long spacing fibrils	Native fibrils	Unstructured material
Rat skin collagen salt-soluble fraction					
Acetic acid supernatant control	-	+	-	-	-
Acetic acid supernatant	+	-	+	-	-
Acetic acid residue	+	(+)	+	-	-
Pepsin supernatant	+	-	+	-	-
Pepsin residue	+	--	+	-	-
Citrate soluble fraction					
Acetic acid soluble fraction	-	+	-		(+)
Acetic acid supernatant	+	+	(+)	-	-
Acetic acid residue	+	-	+	-	(+)
Pepsin supernatant	+	-	+	-	-
Pepsin residue	+	-	+	-	-
Acetic acid soluble fraction					
Acetic acid supernatant control	-	+	(+)		
Acetic acid residue control	-	+	+	-	(+)
Acetic acid supernatant	+	(+)	+	-	(+)
Acetic acid residue	+	(+)	+	(+)	(+)
Pepsin supernatant	+	-	+	-	
Pepsin residue	+	-	+	-	
Calf achilles tendon collagen					
Acetic acid soluble fraction					
Acetic acid residue control	-	+	(+)	-	(+)
Pepsin residue control	-	+	-	-	-
Acetic acid residue	+	-	+	+	+
Pepsin residue	+	+	+	-	(+)

The fractions (see Fig. 12 and Table V) were dialysed against 0.4% ATP; pH 2.8. After application to the sample holder they were stained with phosphotungstic acid and uranyl acetate. - absent; + considerable amounts; (+) traces.

slowly cleaved by pepsin, SLS fibrils are also present in the pepsin treated samples. Fibrils of the native type indicate the presence of side-to-side bonds and can be demonstrated in acetic acid residue from the acid soluble fraction of rat skin collagen only.

The investigations on calf achilles tendon collagen show again clearly the presence of head-to-tail bonds. The Pep-Res of all three fractions (about 90% of the total material consists mostly of SLS fibrils. The acetic acid residue (before treatment with pepsin) shows the presence of not only SLS fibrils and unstructured material, but also normal fibrils of the native type. However, a quantitative estimation with the electronmicroscope is impossible since the insoluble preparations always contain considerable amounts of unstructured material which cannot be clearly classified.

The following conclusions can be drawn from these investigations: soluble collagen molecules contain aldehyde groups or similar functional groups which after the formation of fibrils build up intermolecular crosslinks with the amino or other similar groups of the neighbouring molecules. These linkages are labile under acidic conditions, but can be stabilized by reduction. In the case of rat skin collagen, the number of these groups increases from Salt-SC to acetic acid soluble collagen and stabilized crosslinks are almost exclusively head-to-tail bonds. These are as stable to pepsin treatment as the head-to-tail bonds which are formed in vivo. All collagen fractions extracted from achilles tendon exhibit considerably larger amounts of functional groups which are able to form intermolecular crosslinks. But in this case, side-to-side crosslinks are also found to be present along with the head-to-tail bonds. It is obvious that in all investigated preparations a considerably smaller amount of side-to-side bonds are stabilized in comparison to the head-to-tail bonds. This is probably due to one of the following reasons: (1) during the development of collagen in the extracellular space of connective tissue the functional groups responsible for side-to-side bonds become reactive at a comparatively later stage than those responsible for head-to-tail bonds; or (2) the functional groups of side-to-side and head-to-tail bonds are formed at the same time; however, the side-to-side bonds are less suitable for forming crosslinks with adjacent molecules during fibril formation in vitro.

ACKNOWLEDGEMENTS

This work was supported by the Deutsche Forschungsgemeinschaft.

REFERENCES

Bailey, A.J. (1968). Biochim. Biophys. Acta 160, 447.

Bailey, A.J. and Lister, D. (1968). Nature 220, 280.

Gross, J. (1956). J. Biophys. Biochem. Cytol. 2, 261.

Highberger, J.H., Gross, J. and Schmitt, F.O. (1950). J. Am. Chem. Soc. 72, 3321.

Hodge, A.J. and Schmitt, F.O. (1960). Proc. Nat. Acad. Sci. (USA) 46, 186.

Hodge, A.J. and Petruska, J.A. (1963). In Aspects of Protein Structure, pp. 289-300. Ed. by Ramachandran, G.N. Academic Press, London-New York.

Kühn, K., Fietzek, P. and Kühn, J. (1966). Biochem. Z. 344, 418.

Kühn, K., Grassmann, W. and Hofmann, U. (1960). Naturwiss 47, 258.

Kühn, K., Schuppler, G. and Kühn, J. (1964). Hoppe-Seyler's Z. Physiol. Chem. 338, 10.

Kühn, K. and Zimmer, E. (1961). Z. Naturforschg. 16b, 648.

Mathews, M.B. and Decker, L. (1968). Biochem. J. 109, 517.

Ramachandran, G.N. and Sasisekharan, V. (1961). Nature 190, 1004.

Rauterberg, J. and Kühn, K. (1968). Hoppe-Seyler's Z. Physiol. Chem. 349, 611.

Rich, A. and Crick, F.H. (1961). J. Mol. Biol. 3, 483.

Schmitt, F.O. (1956). Proc. Am. Philos. Soc. 100, 476.

Stark, . and Kühn, K. (1968). Europ. J. Biochem. 6, 534.

Tanzer, M.L. (1967). Biochim. Biophys. Acta 133, 584.

Tanzer, M.L. (1968). J. Biol. Chem. 243, 4045.

Toole, B.P. and Lowther, D.A. (1968a). Arch. Biochem. Biophys. 128, 567.

Toole, B.P. and Lowther, D.A. (1968b). Biochem. J. 109, 857.

LOCALIZATION OF THE ANTIGENIC DETERMINANTS OF COLLAGEN

D. Michaeli, G. R. Martin and E. Benjamini

Collagen has been shown by several workers to be immunogenic (O'Dell, 1968), although the antibody titers obtained were in most cases quite low. In order to study the immunochemical properties of collagen high-titer sera are required; we have found that rabbits injected 3-4 times, at intervals of 10-12 days, with 10 mg collagen emulsified in Freund's complete adjuvant, produced antibodies of sufficiently high titers for our studies.

As antigens, lathyritic salt-soluble rat skin collagen and acid-soluble guinea pig skin collagen were purified according to Piez, Eigner and Lewis (1963). The anti-collagen activity of the sera was assayed either by precipitin reaction (Michaeli et al., 1968) and/or by the passive microhemagglutination reaction (Kettman, Michaeli and Benjamini, unpublished data). The anti-collagen specificity of the antiserum was ascertained by the following criteria: a) no precipitation occurred when antiserum was incubated with collagenase; b) digestion of the immune precipitate with collagenase resulted in the dissolution of the precipitate; c) the expected quantities of hydroxyproline were detected in the precipitate, and d) the expected collagen components were detected in the precipitate when assayed by disc polyacrylamide gel electrophoresis.

Immunological studies on the specificity of the reaction of anti-collagen antisera with collagens of various species revealed a high degree of species specificity. For example, rabbit antisera to guinea pig skin collagen had a hemagglutination titer of 1:4096, a titer to rat skin collagen of only 1:8 and no titer to rabbit skin collagen.

Similarly, rabbit antisera to rat skin collagen had a titer of 1:64,000 with rat skin collagen, but only a titer of 1:32 with guinea pig skin collagen.

Since collagen molecules contain two types of chains we have measured the reactivity of each chain with antisera. The chains were separated and purified as described by Piez et al (1963). The β11 and β12 components of collagen which arise by intramolecular cross linking of collagen were isolated by the same procedures. The immunological activity of the separated chains was assayed by their capacity to inhibit the hamagglutination reaction between collagen-coated sheep red blood cells and the homologous antibodies. Results in Table 1 show that pre-incubation of anti-rat skin collagen with α2 or β12 of rat skin collagen resulted in a marked reduction of the original titer, whereas α1 and β11 caused little or no inhibition. Substantially the same results were obtained with guinea pig skin collagen and homologous antibodies where α2 and β12 were inhibitory whereas α1 and β11 were essentially inactive. The material which does not bind to the CM-cellulose column used for the separation of the chains of guinea pig skin collagen (denoted as "front") was also devoid of activity.

These results indicate that the major antigenic determinants of these collagens reside in the α2 component. This conclusion is also corroborated by the fact that red blood cells coated with α2 or β12 showed essentially the same titers with anti-collagen as that obtained with collagen-coated red blood cells. Red blood cells coated with α1 or β11 showed little or no titer.

In order to further localize the antigenic determinants on the α2 chain of guinea pig skin collagen, the immunological activity of cyanogen bromide fragments of the chain was tested. Cyanogen bromide cleavage and separation of the resulting peptides was performed as described by Bornstein and Piez (1966). The immunological activity of the CNBr fragments was assayed by their capacity to inhibit the hemagglutination reaction between anti-guinea pig skin collagen and red blood cells coated with either guinea pig

TABLE I

Inhibition of Hemagglutination Reaction between Collagen and Anti Collagen with Collagen Polypeptide Chains

Antigen*	Inhibitor+	Titer (reciprocal)
Rat skin collagen	-	64,000
	α1	64,000
	α2	2048-4096
	β11	32,000
	β12	1024
Guinea pig skin collagen	-	4096
	front	4096
	α1	2048
	α2	512-1024
	β11	4096
	β12	256

* Sheep red blood cells were coated with a 0.5 μg/ml collagen solution.

\+ Stock solutions of 10 μg/ml were used.

skin collagen and red blood cells coated with either guinea pig skin collagen or with α2 chain. Only the material which was eluted from the phosphocellulose column in the position that the amino-terminal peptide (α2-CB1) of several different collagens chromatogramed (Bornstein and Piez, 1966; Piez et al., 1968) was inhibitory.

While further work is required to ascertain that it is indeed the amino-terminal position of the α2 chain that is primarily responsible for binding antibody to collagen, it is known that this region in the α1 chain differs in structure and composition from the rest of the collagen molecule. Furthermore, treatment of collagen with proteolytic enzymes can selectively remove these portions of the collagen molecule and reduce their reaction with anti-collagen antibodies (Davison, Levine, Drake, Rubin and Bump, 1967; Steffen, Timpl and Wolff, 1968). That the major antigenic determinants of guinea pig skin collagen are restricted to the α2 chain may be explained by recent studies summarized by Piez et al (1968) which indicated that there are disparities in the amino acid sequence of the amino-terminal portion of α2 different species, whereas the amino-terminal portions on the α1 chains of different species are similar.

REFERENCES

Bornstein, P. and Piez, K. A. (1966). Biochemistry 5, 3460

Davison, P. F., Levine, L., Drake, M. P., Rubin, A. and Bump, S. (1967). J. Exptl. Med. 126, 331.

Michaeli, D., Kamenecka, H., Benjamini, E., Kettman, J. R., Leung, D. Y. K. and Miner, R. C. (1968). Immunochemistry 5, 433.

O'Dell, D. S. (1968). In Treatise on Collagen, vol. 2, p. 311, Ed. by Gould, B.S. Academic Press, London and New York.

Piez, K. A., Bladen, H. A., Lane, J. M., Miller, E. J. Bornstein, P., Butler, W. T. and Kang, A. H. (1968). In Brookhaven Symposia in Biology: Structure Function and Evolution in Proteins, vol. 21, p. 345.

Piez, K. A., Eigner, E. A. and Lewis, M. S. (1963). Biochemistry 2, 58.

Steffen, C., Timpl, R. and Wolff, I. (1968). Immunology 15, 125.

THE MICROFIBRILLAR STRUCTURE OF COLLAGEN AND THE PLACEMENT OF INTERMOLECULAR COVALENT CROSS LINKAGES

A. Veis and R.S. Bhatnagar

The insolubility of mature normal collagens has been ascribed to the presence of a system of covalent intermolecular cross-linkages that, in effect, covert a collagen fiber into an infinite cross-linked network of its monomeric elements (Veis and Cohen, 1956, 1958). Veis and Cohen (1956) concluded that at least two sets of cross-linkages of different chemical character existed, one set within structures which could best be represented as long filaments while the other set were bonds transverse to the filaments and joining them together. The transverse bonds were thought to be more labile, and fewer in number than the internal filament bonds. Direct observation of the intermolecular β_{22} (Bornstein and Piez, 1964) and γ_{III} and γ_{222} polymers (Veis and Anesey, 1965) verified the presence of intermolecular covalent cross-linkages and renaturation studies on γ_{III} and γ_{222} (Veis, Anesey and Mussell, 1967) indicated differing modes of placement of the cross-linkages. Recently, Bailey and his colleagues (Bailey, 1968; Bailey and Lister, 1968; Bailey, Fowler and Peach, 1969) have shown that at least two chemically different intermolecular cross-linkages exist in insoluble collagen.

Upon consideration of the cross-linking patterns and the Hodge-Petruska (1963) model for the packing of the collagen monomer units, Veis et al. (1967) concluded that collagen fibers should not be considered as being constructed of large close-packed aggregates of the axially staggered monomer units. The alternative suggested was to consider an arrangement, called the "limiting microfibril system" in which unit assemblies of 4 or 5 (Smith, 1968) collagen molecules, staggered successively by 1 repeat unit (~700 Å) from the B-end, are suequentially overlapped (Figure 1) to form continuous filaments containing the Hodge-Petruska gaps of ~400 Å along the filament surface. The filaments or limiting microfibrils" are packed together with repeat periods in phase but with no preferred phasing of filament ends, to form the tissue elements, the collagen fibers. The purpose of the present work was to verify the presence of the microfibrils and to begin a study of the placement of the intermolecular cross-linkages relative to the microfibrillar structure.

Steven (1964, 1967) has described several methods for the dispersion of collagen into soluble high molecular weight aggregates without denaturation. Since our aim was to obtain solution or dispersions of the microfibrils with a minimum of hydrolytic or structural degradation, we began by utilizing a modification of these procedures.

I DISPERSION OF INSOLUBLE COLLAGEN

Purified insoluble collagen was prepared from fresh steer skin corium by the method of Veis, Anesey and Cohen (1960). After extraction of the lipids the neutral- and acid-soluble collagens were extracted. The insoluble residue, which served as the starting material in all subsequent studies was lyophilized after extensive washing with cold (~2-4°C) distilled water.

The lyophilized collagen, in the form of small cubes, was rewetted with sterile distilled water, in the ratio of 0.5 g collagen to 10 ml H_2O, and then stirred gently at 25° under sterile conditions for 18-20 hours. The collagen was then cooled to 4° and diluted to 100 ml with acetic acid to give a final acid concentration of 0.2 N. After standing for one hour, the swollen collagen was homogenized in a Waring blendor for 15 minutes. Care was taken to keep the blendor cooled to 4° during this operation.

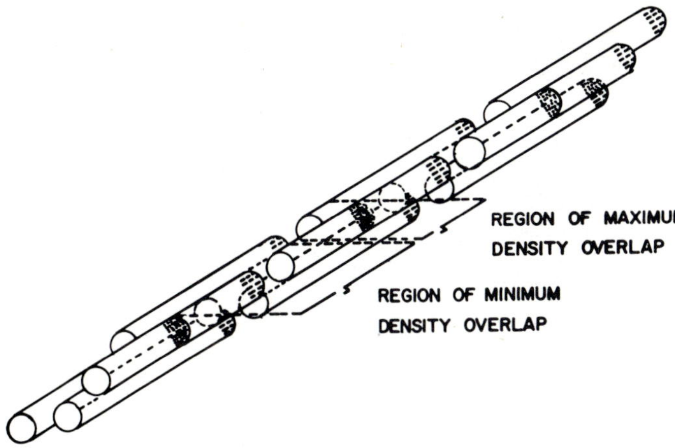

Fig. 1 A schematic representation of a "limiting microfibril" built from Unit assemblies of four monomer collagen units. The region with 0.6 D holes labeled "region of density overlap" is an inter-unit assembly junction region. The maximum density of overlap region is within the unit assembly and is the single region in which all four monomers of the same assembly overlap together.

The suspended collagen was diluted to 1 liter with 0.2 N acetic acid, and this suspension was centrifuged at 15000 x G for 60 minutes in a refrigerated centrifuge. The clear supernatant solution of soluble collagen was the material taken for subsequent examination.

Twenty percent of the initial "insoluble" citrate-extracted collagen was obtained as soluble collagen by this procedure. Control experiemtns in which the single difference was the treatment of the insoluble collagen-H_2O suspension at 4° rather than 25° after rewetting yielded less than 4% of the collagen in solution after the acid homogenization. The treatment at 25° at neutral pH and low ionic strength had the obvious effect of loosening the fiber weave and permitting more extensive subsequent acid swelling. The key factor is the reorientation which takes place within the fibril at 25°.

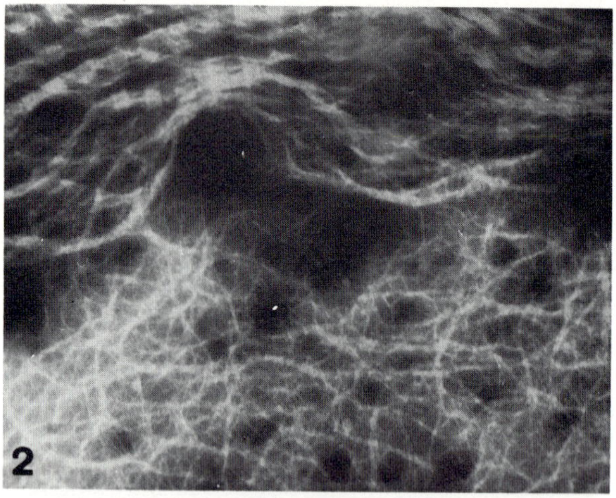
2

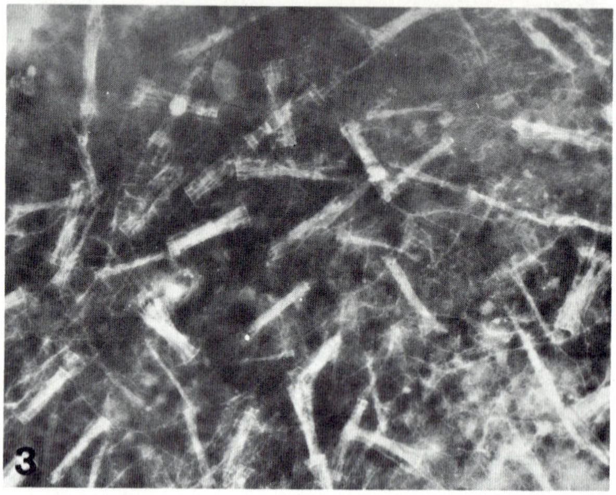
3

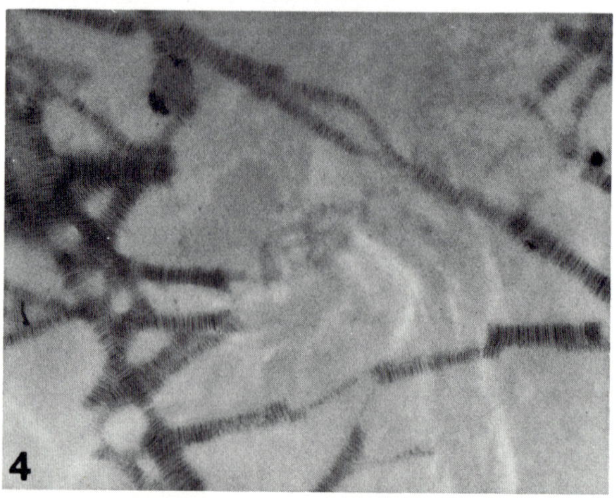
4

Fig. 2 Electron micrograph of the acid solubilized collagen disperion. The solution was dropped directly on the electron microscope grid and negatively stained with 1% PTA at pH 7. The pH was adjusted with NaOH. x 66,000.

Fig. 3 Negatively stained ATP precipitate of the acid solution of collagen. Stained with 1% PTA, pH 7. Note the thin SLS segments embedded in a much larger amount of fine filamentous material. x 75,000.

Fig. 4. Positively stained SLS segments obtained after pepsin depolymerization of the collagen solution. The thin SLS segments line up along filaments which were not depolymerized during the pepsin treatment. Stained with 1% PTA at pH 2.5, followed by saturated uranyl acetate. x 75,000.

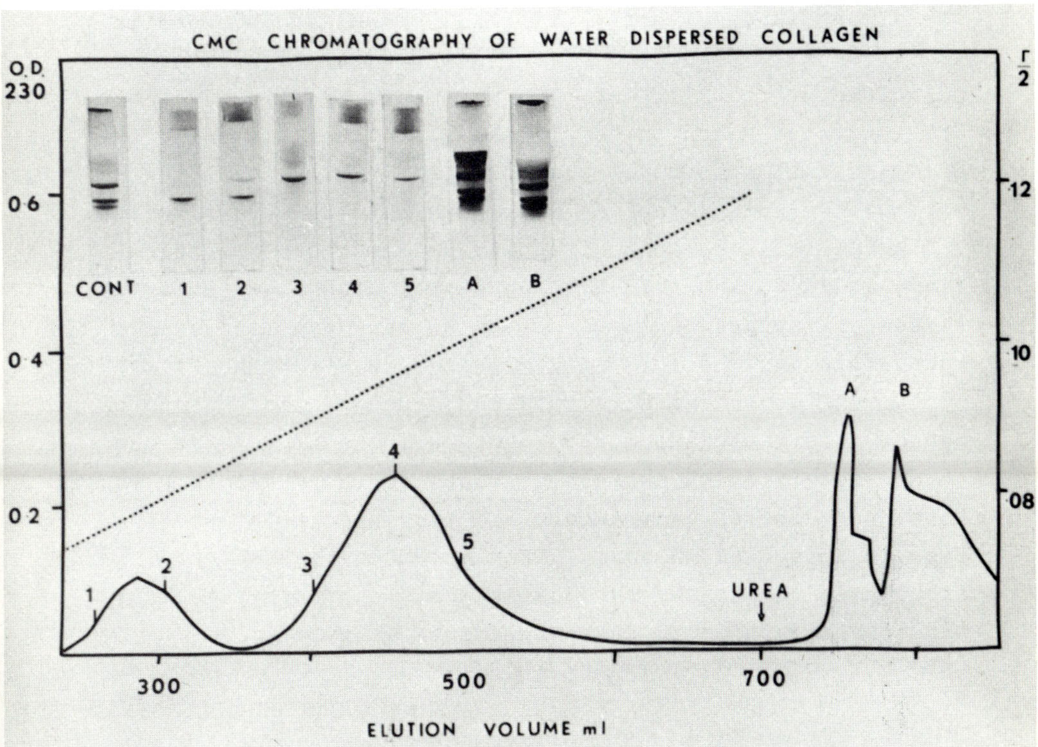

Fig. 5. The CM cellulose chromatography and disc electrophoresis of the soluble collagen. The numbers along the chromatogram correspond to the samples taken for disc electrophoresis. Cont. is the disc pattern of the soluble collagen before chromatography. Chromatography by the procedure of Veis and Anesey (1965), electrophoresis by the procedure of Clark and Veis (1968).

II ELECTRON MICROSCOPIC EXAMINATION OF THE DISPERSED COLLAGEN

Examination of the acid dispersion, after centrigugation but retaining some of the suspended material along with the soluble phase, as in Figure 2. shows that the fibers are unwound into fine filaments with diameters on the order of 30 to 50 Å. The fibers, as visualized with negative staining in Figure 2, are entirely normal in terms of the fine structure of the transverse bands and the band spacings. The loosening of the fiber structure, however, is quite evident. The addition of salt to the acid solution of particle-free centrifuged solutions leads to the formation of normal native fibrils. When ATP is added to salt-free acid solutions of the soluble collagen, the principle product is long thin filaments (Figure 3). Some SLS spools are seen to be aligned along the filaments, indicating that some monomeric collagen is present. Treatment of the acid solutions with pepsin to depolymerize the collagen, followed by addition of ATP to cause precipitation, leads to the formation of larger amounts of SLS. These data suggest that the dissolved collagen is present undenatured in the form of aggregates in which the native staggering of monomers is retained. Hence, the aggregates cannot form in-register SLS segments. The aggregates can be depolymerized (Drake etal., 1966) to the monomers with pepsin and these readily form SLS type precipitates. Even in this case, however, many extended filamentous structures remain and the SLS segments coprecipitate in overlapped fashion on these filaments (Figure 4).

III CHARACTERIZATION OF THE DENATURED SOLUBLE COLLAGEN

The soluble collagen was denatured by heating acid solutions to 60°. The denatured material was then subjected to carboxymethyl cellulose chromatography by the method of Veis and Anesey (1965). Quantitative measurements of recovery showed that of the collagen charged to the column, less than 17% could be recovered, including the material in the urea eluate. Normal acid soluble collagens give yields in excess of 75% upon similar treatment (Veis and Anesey, 1965) and yields decrease as the degree of polymerization increases. The fractionation pattern, Figure 5, also differs from the usual in that β_{12} is the predominant component aside from the urea eluants. Disc electrophoretic analyses by the Clark-Veis (1968) procedure gave essentially the same picture. The urea eluants were greatly enriched in γ-components. As seen in the insets in Figure 5, the amount of material unable to penetrate the spacer gel was greater than that which did distribute through the gel as subunit species. The very small fraction of α- and β-components present in the dispersed collagen indicates that nearly every α-chain must be involved in a cross-linked network.

IV CONCLUSION

The electron microscopic evidence shows that the lyotropic relaxation-acid swelling process separates the fibers into microfibrils with diameters less the 100 Å. Since the dispersion method was not drastic and did not involve hydrolysis or enzymic degradation it is clear that the fibrils released were not linked to each other within a fiber by stable covalent bonds. The failure of this procedure to solubilize the entire tissue does suggest, however, that some interfibrillar covalent linkages are present in the fibers. The normal electron microscopic appearance of the fibrils, and the difficulty of preparing SLS segments from them indicate that the monomers are linked together in their native staggered array <u>within</u> the filaments. The chromatographic and disc electrophoretic data support the conclusion of extensive cross-linking. Thus, these data support the concept of the limiting microfibril arrangement within the collagen fibers and indicate that one important cross-linking network is within and restricted to the limiting fibrils.

ACKNOWLEDGEMENT

A report of work done under contract No. 12-14-100-8933(73) with the U.S. Department of Agriculture and authorized by the Research and Marketing Act of 1946. The contract is being supervised by the Eastern Utilization Research and Development Division of the Agricultural Research Service.

REFERENCES

Bailey, A.J. (1968). Biochim. Biophys. Acta 160, 447.

Bailey, A.J., Fowler, L.J. and Peach, C.M. (1969). Biochem. Biophys. Res. Comm. 35, 663.

Bailey, A.J. and Lister, D. (1968). Nature 220, 280.

Bornstein, P. and Piez, K.A. (1964). J. Clin. Invest. 43, 1813.

Clark, C.C. and Veis, A. (1968). Biochim. Biophys. Acta 154, 175.

Drake, M.P., Davison, P.F., Bump, S. and Schmitt, F.O. (1966). Biochemistry 5, 301.

Hodge, A.J. and Petruska, J.A. (1963). In Aspects of Protein Structure, p. 289. Ed. by Ramachandran, G.N. Academic Press, New York.

Stevens, F.S. (1964). Ann. Rheum. Dis. 23, 300.

Stevens, F.S. (1967). Biochim. Biophys. Acta 140, 522.

Smith, J.W. (1968). Nature 219, 157.

Veis, A. and Anesey, J. (1965). J. Biol. Chem. 240, 3899.

Veis, A., Anesey, J. and Cohen, J. (1960). J. Amer. Leather Assoc. 55, 548.

Veis, A., Anesey, J. and Mussell, S. (1967). Nature 215, 931.

Veis, A. and Cohen, J. (1956). J. Amer. Chem. Soc. 78, 6238.

Veis, A. and Cohen, J. (1958). J. Phys. Chem. 62, 459.

ISOLATION AND PARTIAL CHARACTERIZATION OF INTERMOLECULAR CROSSLINKS FROM RECONSTITUTED COLLAGEN FIBRILS

Marvin L. Tanzer

Knowledge about the details of collagen crosslinking has particular relevance with respect to interactions in self-ordering systems, and may bear upon time-dependent biologic phenomena such as aging.

One model system which has proven useful in the study of fibril self-assembly is the phase transition of collagen solutions into native-type fibrils (Gross and Kirk, 1958). An interesting feature of this system is the progressive development of fibril insolubility, apparently due to the formation of intermolecular bonds between adjacent collagen molecules (Gross, 1964). One class of covalent intermolecular crosslinks which rapidly and spontaneously form in the reconstituted fibrils seem to be Schiff bases, which can be converted into stable secondary amines by reduction with sodium borohydride (Tanzer, 1967). The borohydride treated fibrils become quite insoluble and physicochemical studies show that a covalently linked fibrillar network accounts for their insolubility (Tanzer, 1968). The studies reported below concern the isolation and partial characterization of the borohydride-reduced crosslinks from these fibrils.

Native-type fibrils were reconstituted from solutions of calf skin collagen and the protein suspension treated with sodium borotritide as previously described (Tanzer and Mechanic, 1968).

The lyophylized fibrils were hydrolyzed at 108°C in 3 N HCl for 24 hr and the hydrolysate dried in a rotary evaporator. These conditions of hydrolysis were chosen

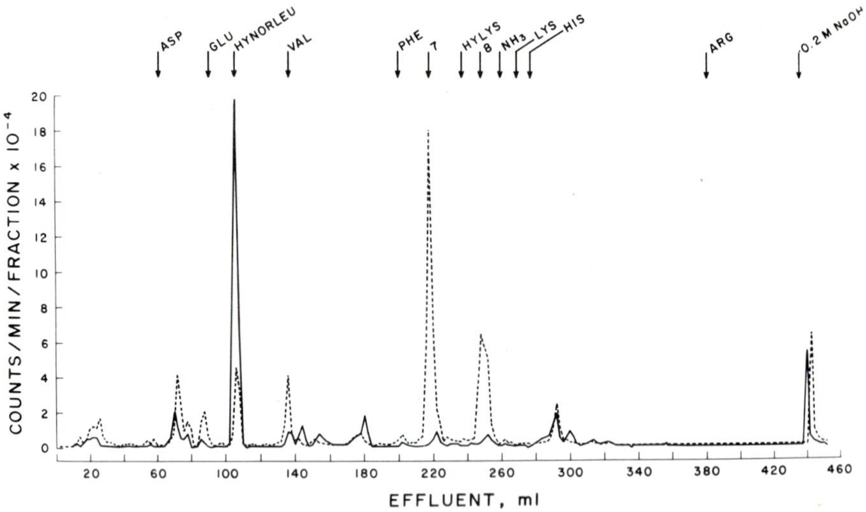

Fig. 1. Chromatographic fractionation of hydrolysates of borotritide treated collagen fibrils and collagen solutions. 300 mg of each hydrolysate (found to have similar specific activities) were applied to a 0.9 x 60-cm column of Beckman resin UR-30 at 50°C and the chromatogram developed with citrate buffers and a 9-chambered Varigrad. Two-milliliter fractions were collected and a small portion of each fraction was measured for radioactivity by liquid scintillation spectrometry using Bray's solution (Bray, 1961) containing 5% cab-o-sil. The position of the reference compounds was determined by using the analytical section of a Beckman 116 amino acid analyzer.
Collagen solution (—); collagen fibrils (----).

because control studies showed that: 1) the conversion of hydroxynorleucine to chloronorleucine occured to the extent of less than 10%; 2) the amino acid composition of collagen hydrolysates from 3 N HCl and 6 N HCl (at the same temperature and duration of hydrolysis) were very similar; 3) comparison of the release of all the radioactive components into the 3 N HCl and 6 N HCl hydrolysates as a function of time (temperature being constant) showed no significant differences. Thus, hydrolysis of collagen for 24 hr in 3 N HCl at 108°C was routinely adopted in these studies.

Two methods of initial fractionation of the radioactive components were carried out, as illustrated in Figs. 1 and 2. In both methods, the radioactive components were found to be contaminated with nonradioactive amino acids and further purification was accomplished by gel filtration,

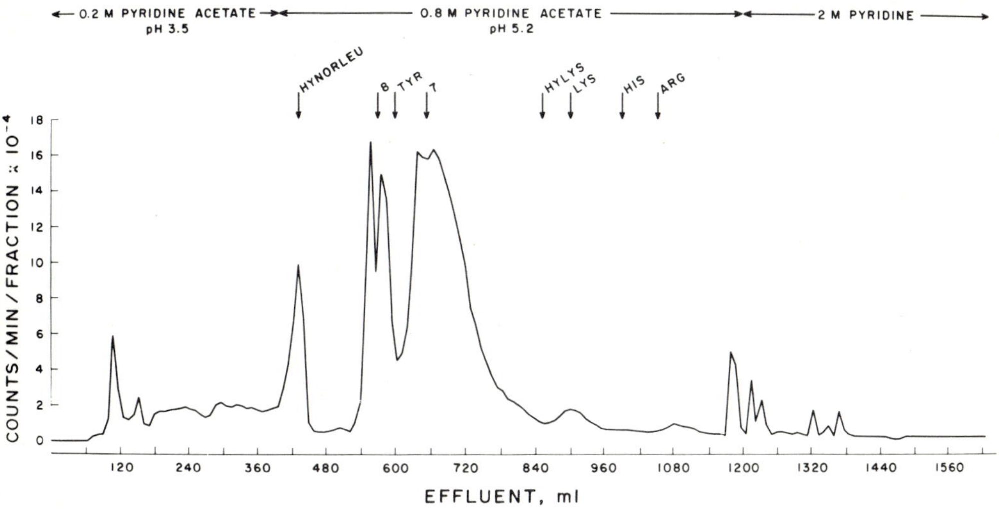

Fig. 2. Chromatographic fractionation of a hydrolysate of borotritide treated collagen fibrils. Two grams of hydrolysate in 0.01 N HCl were applied to a 4 x 52-cm column of BioRad AG-50W-X8, 200-400 mesh, which had been equilibrated with 0.2 M pyridine-acetate, pH 3.50. The column was eluted stepwise with the solvents shown and 2.5-ml fractions were collected. A small portion of each fraction was measured for radioactivity by liquid scintillation spectrometry using Bray's solution (Bray, 1961). The position of the reference compounds was determined by using the ninhydrin reaction. The relative location of compounds 7 and 8 on this chromatogram was established by chromatographing a portion of each of them by the procedure outlined in Fig. 1.

ion-exchange chromatography, and paper chromatography. The fractionations procedure outlined in Fig. 2 was more useful than that of Fig. 1 because larger amounts of hydrolysate could be processed and no desalting was required prior to the next purification step. As shown, the compounds labelled 7 and 8 in Figs. 1 and 2 represented a considerable proportion of the radioactivity of the hydrolyzed crosslinked fibrils. In contrast, hydroxynorleucine (the reduction product of α amino adipic semialdehyde) is the major radioactive component (Fig. 1) of collagen which was reduced in solution, and which does not become crosslinked. The most likely explanation for these results is that α amino adipic semialdehyde contributes a portion of the

TABLE I

Electrophoretic and Chromatographic Properties of the Presumptive Crosslinks

Compound	Electrophoretic migration		Chromatographic migration	
	Solvent A	Solvent B	Solvent C	Solvent D
	(CM from origin)		(Rf)	
7	11.7	1.4	.42	.21
8	8.5	1.1*	.12,.04	.03
Lysine	21.0	5.0	.65	.49
Hydroxylysine	19.0	3.8	.54	.38
Lysinonorleucine	----	----	.54	---

The location of the radioactive compounds was determined with a strip scanner and the reference compounds were located after reaction with ninhydrin.

Solvents and conditions: Whatman 3MM Paper was used throughout.

A) Pyridine-acetate, pH 6.4, 45 V/cm, 60 min.
B) Ammonium-acetate, pH 9.0, 20 V/cm, 60 min.
C) Methanol:water:10 N HCl:pyridine, 80:17:2.5:10.
D) Chloroform:methanol:15% NH_4OH, 40:40:15.

*Migrated towards the anode at this pH. All other distances recorded are for migration towards the cathode.

structure of compounds 7 and 8, which are the presumptive crosslinks. Interestingly, under several different conditions of ion-exchange chromatography or paper chromatography, compound 8 was found to partially fractionate into 2 components (Fig. 2), perhaps representing isomers. When highly purified, both moieties of compound 8 were found to be quite unstable, particularly at acid pH. Comparison of Figs. 1 and 2 also illustrates that the relative elution positions of compounds 7 and 8 will vary with the solvent employed, although similar types of cation exchange resins were used in both instances. The behaviour of these compounds upon electrophoresis and chromatography is shown in Table 1, comparing them with lysine and hydroxylysine. The electrophoretic studies indicate that compound 8 has a lower isoelectric point than compound 7, which would be consistent with its elution position in Fig. 2 but not

Fig. 1. Another unusual feature of compound 8 is its slow migration on paper chromatography in solvents in which lysine, hydroxylysine, lysinonorleucine and compound 7 all migrate well. Both compounds 7 and 8 react with ninhydrin to yield a colored complex which absorbs well at 570 mμ; sufficient material has not been obtained to quantitatively determine the molar color yield after reaction with ninhydrin.

Preliminary mass spectroscopic studies have been carried out on several derivatives of these compounds but their full structure has not been elucidated to date. It has been determined, however, that part of the structure of compounds 7 and 8 is consistent with their genesis via reduction of a Schiff base of α amino adipic semialdehyde.

An important aspect of these investigations concerns the quantitative distribution of the radioactivity. As previously shown, under the conditions of borohydride reduction employed, approximately 1 mole of tritium is incorporated per mole of collagen. We find that virtually all of the radioactivity in the hydrolysates applied to the ion-exchange columns is eluted by the buffer systems used. Consequently, the results in Figs. 1 and 2 demonstrate that in the crosslinked protein, about 75% of the total radioactivity can be accounted for by compounds 7 and 8. Thus, most of the α amino adipic semialdehyde in the reconstituted fibrils becomes involved in intermolecular crosslinking.

ACKNOWLEDGEMENTS

This work was carried out during the tenure of an Established Investigatorship from the American Heart Association and was supported in part by National Science Foundation Grant #GB-7903 and by USPHS Grant #AM-12683.

REFERENCES

Bray, G. (1961). Anal. Biochem. 1, 279.

Gross, J. (1964). Science 143, 960.

Gross, J. and Kirk, D. (1958). J. Biol. Chem. 233, 355.

Tanzer, M. L. (1967). Biochem. Biophys. Acta 133, 584.

Tanzer, M. L. (1968). J. Biol. Chem. 243, 4045.

Tanzer, M. L. and Mechanic, G. (1968). Biochem. Biophys. Res. Commun. 32, 885.

INTERMOLECULAR CROSS-LINKS IN RAT-SKIN AND RAT-TAIL TENDON COLLAGENS

M. Rojkind, A. Hamabata, E. González and G. Rendón

Collagen from different animal species has been shown to contain both intramolecular and intermolecular cross-links. The intramolecular cross-links have been located near the amino terminal end of the protein (Rojkind, Blumenfeld and Gallop, 1964, 1966; Bornstein and Piez, 1966; Kang, Bornstein and Piez, 1967) and are formed via aldol condensation of two α-amino adipic δ-semi-aldehydes from adjacent chains (Bornstein and Piez, 1966; Rojkind, Rhi and Aguirre, (1968). This aldol product has been recently identified as the actual cross-link in rat-skin collagen (Rojkind, Gutierrez, Zeichner and Lent, 1969) and chick-skin collagen (Kang, Faris and Franzblau, 1969).

The existence of intermolecular cross-links in collagen has been established by the presence of β22 dimers (Bornstein and Piez, 1964) and γ components made of three α1 or three α2 chains (Veis and Anesey, 1965). The exact location of the intermolecular bonds remains to be determined, but it has been suggested that the B end of the molecule plays an important role in the formation of such bonds (Drake and Davison, 1968).

It has been also shown (Tanzer, 1968) that native collagen fibrils can be reduced with NaB^3H_4 to yield large molecular weight aggregates. These aggregates are not obtained when the reduction is performed with "segment-long-spacing" fragments (SLS) or with native collagen in solution (Tanzer, 1968), thus suggesting that the ordered arrangement of the fibrils (one-quarter staggering) is a prior step to cross-linking. Borohydride reduction is also accompanied by a decrease of the aldehydes normally present in collagen and new radioactive components are formed (Tanzer and Mechanic, 1968; Bailey, 1968; Bailey and Lister, 1968). With this information, it has been suggested that the intermolecular cross-link is an aldimine bond between the aldehydes present in collagen and the ε-amino group of a reactive lysyl or hydroxylysyl residue. Accordingly, the formation of such bonds should be inhibited by blocking either the aldehydes or the free ε-amino groups of the protein. It has been already demonstrated that lathyritic collagen which is aldehyde deficient (Bornstein and Piez, 1966; Rojkind and Juarez, 1966; Page and Benditt, 1968) does not form aggregates when reduced with NaB^3H_4 (Tanzer, 1968). Furthermore, amidinated collagen has a similar behavior to lathyritic collagen (Tanzer and Mechanic, 1968) and is unable to form intermolecular cross-links "in vitro" (Deshmukh and Nimni, 1969).

Recently, a new cross-linking amino acid has been obtained from native rat-tail tendon collagen reduced with NaB^3H_4, and its structure determined (Bailey and Peach, 1968). The compound thus obtained, is the reduced Schiff's base of α-amino adipic δ-semialdehyde and the ε-amino group of a hydroxylysyl residue.

We have been studying the reactivity of the ε-amino groups in native rat-skin collagen, and attempting to determine the location of the reactive groups involved in intermolecular cross-linking. In this communication we shall summarize the results obtained in our laboratory for the past 12 months.

I EXPERIMENTAL APPROACH

A. LOCATION OF THE INTERMOLECULAR CROSS-LINKS IN RAT-TAIL TENDON COLLAGEN

To study the location of the intermolecular cross-links, native rat-tail tendon collagen was reduced in suspension with calibrated NaB^3H_4 (Blumenfeld and Gallop, 1966; Gallop, Blumenfeld, Henson and Schneider, 1968) and treated with CNBr under conditions known to cleave a single peptide containing 14 or 15 amino acid residues from the amino terminal end (limited cleavage) Bornstein, Kang and Piez, 1966). Duplicate samples of rat-tail tendon collagen were first cleaved with CNBr and later reduced with calibrated NaB^3H_4 and used as a control. Both control and experimental samples were heat denatured and chromatographed on CM-cellulose columns as previously described (Piez, Eigner and Lewis, 1963). The results obtained are shown in Fig. 1 and 2.

As can be seen, the control sample (Fig. 1) showed 4 fractions, three of them (A,B,C) were eluted with the normal gradient and the last fraction (U) was eluted with 6 M urea containing 2 N NaCl. Fractions A and B contained over 90% of the total counts (see Table I) and the specific activity of fraction A was 7.3 x 10^4 dpm/mg of protein. When fraction B was subjected to further digestion with CNBr (Bornstein and Piez, 1965) over 30% of the counts were recovered in peptides similar to the peptides of fraction A, thus suggesting that most of the counts were present in the aldehyde containing peptides (α1-CB1, β11-CB1 and β12-CB1) normally found in the latter fraction.

TABLE I

Recovery of Protein and Radioactivity in the Control and Experimental Samples Cleaved With CNBr, and Chromatographed on CM-Cellulose

	Control		Experimental	
Fraction	Protein %	Counts %	Protein %	Counts %
A	4.9	55.0	4.8	27.2
A'	-	-	19.0	29.7
B	59.0	37.0	39.3	15.0
C	32.5	6.0	30.1	20.6
U	3.6	0.4	6.8	7.3

In contrast to the control, the experimental sample showed 5 fractions (see Fig. 2). Four of these fractions (A,B,C,U) were similar to the control but contained a

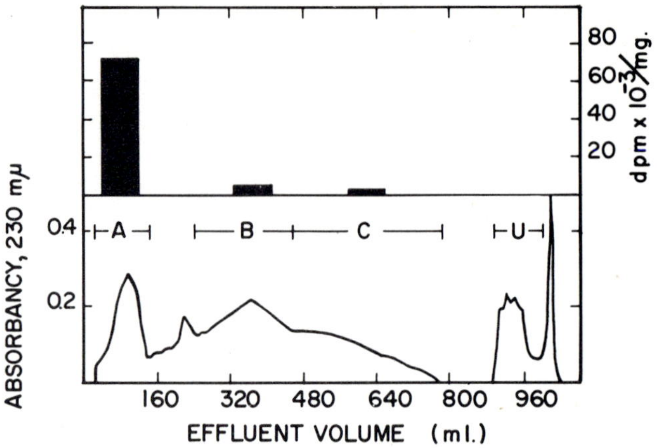

Fig. 1. Chromatographic separation on CM-cellulose (2.5 x 18 cm) of 50 mg of rat-tail tendon collagen cleaved with CNBr and reduced with NaB^3H_4. Elution was achieved in 0.06 M acetate buffer, pH 4.8, using a linear gradient of NaCl from 0.0 to 0.1 M. The total volume of the gradient was 800 ml. At the end of the gradient the column was washed with 6 M urea in 2 N NaCl.

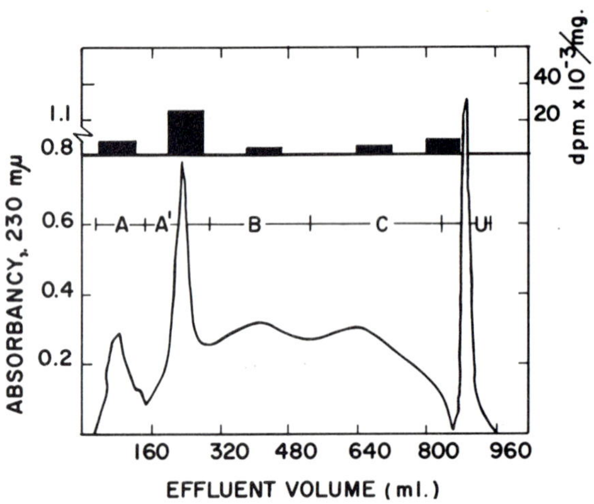

Fig. 2. Chromatographic separation on CM-cellulose (2.5 x 18 cm) of 100 mg of rat-tail tendon collagen reduced with NaB^3H_4 and cleaved with CNBr. Elution was achieved in 0.06 M acetate buffer, pH 4.8, using a linear gradient of NaCl from 0.0 to 0.1 M. The total volume of the gradient was 800 ml. At the end of the gradient the column was washed with 6 M urea in 2 N NaCl.

different proportion of counts (Table I). Fractions A and B only contained 43% of the total radioactivity (Table I) and the specific activity of fraction A was 7.4×10^3 dpm/mg.

The missing counts were distributed among fraction A' (27%), fraction C (20.6%) and in the peak eluted with urea (7.3%). These results clearly suggest that borohydride reduction produced large molecular weight aggregates and that the aldehyde-containing peptides known to be involved in intramolecular cross-links also participate in interchain cross-links. Furthermore, the presence of a new polypeptide after "limited cleavage" of the tail-tendons with CNBr, suggests that the new bond formed is at either end of the molecule. Although we have been unable to completely purify fraction A', some of the amino acids present in this fraction indicate that this particular bond may be located near the C-terminal end of the protein. Fraction A' contains equal amounts of 3-hydroxyproline and histidine, and these amino acids have been found together only in the C-terminal peptides obtained after CNBr cleavage of purified α chains from rat-skin and chick-bone collagens (Butler, Piez and Bornstein, 1967; Miller, Lane and Piez, 1969; Lane and Miller, 1969).

B. LOCATION OF THE REACTIVE ε-AMINO GROUPS IN RAT-SKIN COLLAGEN.

The reactivity of the free amino groups in collagen has already been investigated. It has been shown that two hydroxylysyl residues and one lysyl residue in native collagen react with pyridoxal phosphate and the Schiff's base formed can be stabilized by the addition of $NaBH_4$ (Page, Benditt and Kirkwood, 1968). However, even with the denatured protein only a small number of groups react. Using other reagents such as KCNO and 2,4,6-trinitrobenzene-1-sulfonic acid (TNBS) we have been able to show that close to 100% of the free amino groups in the denatured protein react, but only 2 to 3 groups are available in the native protein (Gonzalez, Hamabata and Rojkind, unpublished data). Collagen containing 3 trinitrophenyl groups (TNP-groups) per α chain has the same intrinsic viscosity as the control, suggesting that no major conformational change has occured during the reaction. Collagen containing larger proportion of TNP-groups showed an intrinsic viscosity similar to the parent gelatin, indicating that the protein was already denatured.

Native collagen incubated for 1 hr at 25°C with increasing ratios of TNBS (assuming 30 free amino groups per α chain) showed two different reaction rates. When the concentration of reagent was increased from 0.25 to 1 mole/mole of free amino groups the reaction was linear and showed proportionality between the concentration of reagent and the number of groups blocked. With higher concentrations of reagent, the reaction was also linear but the slope was less steep (Fig. 3).

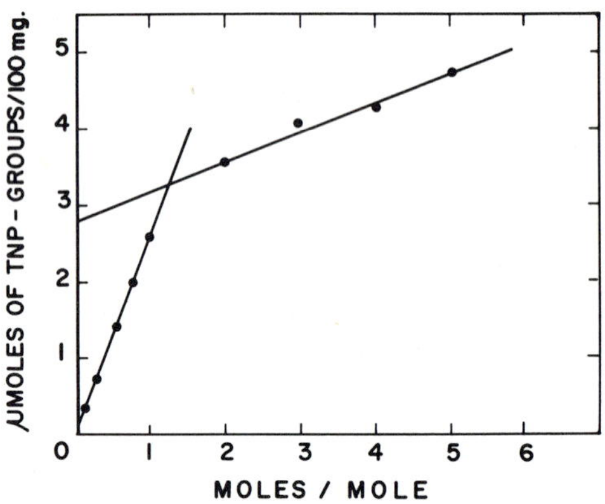

Fig. 3. Effect of reagent concentration (TNBS) on the number of ε-TNP-groups formed. A 0.3% solution of native collagen in 0.1 M phosphate buffer at pH 8.0 was incubated for 1 hr at 25°C with different concentration of TNBS. The reaction was stopped by lowering the pH to 3.0.

Three different collagen preparations incubated with 1 molar excess of TNBS at pH 8.0 and 25°C showed a similar amount of TNP-groups, and the values obtained ranged from 2.3 to 2.6 μmoles per 100 mg of protein. In order to study the exact location of the reactive groups, purified α1 and β11 fractions from TNBS-treated collagen were cleaved with CNBr as already described (Bornstein and Piez, 1965) and the fragments separated on CM-cellulose columns (Butler, et al., 1967). Over 40% of the 340 mμ absorbing material was recovered in four peaks (Fig. 4). The last peak (α1-CB8) was further purified by gel filtration chromatography on Bio-Gel P-100 column and its amino acid composition determined after acid hydrolysis in 6 N HCl. As can be seen (Table II)

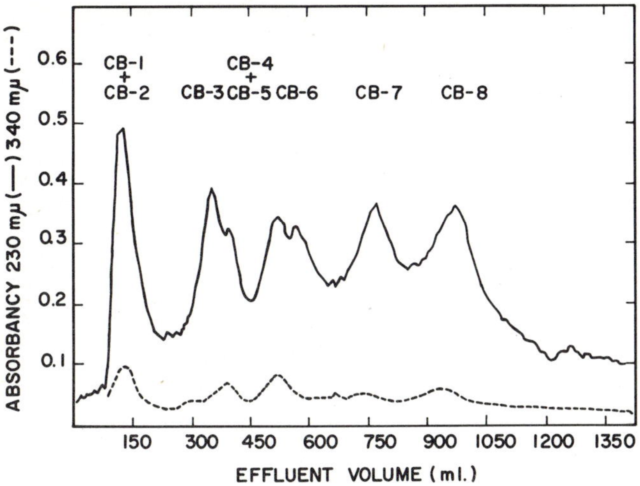

Fig. 4. CM-cellulose elution pattern of the CNBr peptides derived from α1-β11 chains of neutral-salt extractable rat-skin collagen treated with TNBS. Elution was achieved in 0.02 M citrate, pH 3.6,using a linear gradient of NaCl from 0.04 to 0.14 M. The total volume of the gradinet was 1600 ml.

two different preparations of α1-CB8 have very similar amino acid composition and in both cases 0.3 residues of hydroxylysine were missing. From the absorption at 340 mμ, and using an extinction coefficient of 16 x 10^3 (Kakade and Liener, 1969) it was calculated that the sample placed on the amino acid analyzer contained 0.3 residues of a TNP-derivative. A duplicate sample of α1-CB8 was hydrolyzed for 1 hr in 6 N HCl and after thin layer chromatography in butanol:acetic acid (9:1) it was shown to contain a single yellow spot corresponding to ε-TNP-hydroxylysine.

II GENERAL DISCUSSION

Although we hve been unable to establish the exact location of the intermolecular cross-links, the results presented in this communication suggest the involvement of at least two different regions of the protein; the α1-CB8 which has been shown to be located between the first and second quarter of the molecule, and α1-CB6 which is the C-terminal end of the protein (Piez et al., 1968; Miller et al., 1969).

Although we used two different types of collagen and a

different experimental approach in each case, we arrived at the same conclusions. The reactive ε-amino groups which may be involved in interchain cross-links are hydroxylysyl residues and are present in both α1CB6 and α1CB8. The exact location of the reactive groups in each peptide remains to be elucidated, but it may well correspond to a single and specific residue. The reproducible results obtained with 3 different collagen preparations strongly support this suggestion. However, one has to bear in mind that partial hydroxylation of lysyl residues occurs in collagen (Butler, 1968). Accordingly, different lysyl residues of different molecules may be partially hydroxylated. The reproducible and constant value of 0.3 residues of TNP-hydroxylysine obtained in this work suggests, that at least certain lysyl residues along the tropocollagen molecule are always hydroxylated with the same efficiency. It is also possible that these hydroxylysyl residues are exposed and available for cross-linking.

TABLE II

Composition of α1-CB8 from TNBS Treated Collagen

	Prep I	Prep II	Control*
Hydroxyproline	25.0	25.0	27.0
Asparatic acid	10.0	10.0	10.0
Threonine†	5.0	4.0	5.0
Serine†	9.0	8.0	10.0
Proline	29.0	33.0	31.0
Glutamic acid	19.0	17.0	19.0
Glycine	89.0	87.0	87.0
Alanine	32.0	28.0	36.0
Valine	4.0	4.0	5.0
Isoleucine	1.0	1.0	1.0
Leucine	4.0	4.0	4.0
Phenylalanine	2.0	3.0	3.0
Hydroxylysine	0.7	0.7	1.0
Lysine	9.0	9.0	9.0
Arginine	14.0	14.0	14.0
TNP-ε-Hydroxylysine	0.3‡	0.3‡	-
Homoserine+			
Homoserine Lactone	1.0	present	1.0

*Taken from Butler et al., 1967.
+ Uncorrected for loses after acid hydrolysis.
‡ Calculated using a molar extinction coefficient of 16 x 10^3 at 340 mμ.

The NaB^3H_4 experiments were performed to stabilize the Schiff's base between the aldehyde (s) and the ε-amino groups of hydroxylysine (s) and to determine if the reactive residues are the ones involved in these cross-links.

After reduction of native tail-tendon fibrils with NaB^3H_4 and limited cleavage with CNBr, we isolated a fraction containing radioactivity and an amino acid composition similar to the composition reported for the C-terminal end of α1 chains in rat-skin and chick-skin collagens (Butler et al., 1967; Miller et al., 1969). The modified α chains contained a large proportion of the total counts, indicating that areas other than α1-CB6 are involved in these cross-links. Furthermore, the peak containing the α1-CB1 and β11-CB1 peptides showed 50% of the radioactivity present in the controls, thus suggesting the participation of the aldehyde-containing peptides in the interchain cross-links.

The presence of intermolecular cross-links between the aldehydes of collagen (α1-CB1 or β11-CB1) and the ε-amino groups of hydroxylysyl residues in α1-CB8 (between the first and second quarter of the molecule) and α1-CB6 (C-terminal end) would support the earlier model for collagen in which the A end of one tropocollagen molecule is one quarter staggered with respect to a second molecule and at the same time may be close to the B end of a third tropocollagen molecule (Gross, Highberger and Schmitt, 1954; Hodge and Petruska, 1963).

ACKNOWLEDGEMENTS

This work was supported by Grant R01-AM11045 from the National Institute of Health, USPHS.

REFERENCES

Bailey, A.J. (1968). Biochim. Biophys. Acta 160, 447.

Bailey, A.J. and Lister, D. (1968). Nature 220, 280.

Bailey, A.J. and Peach, C.M. (1968). Biochem. Biophys. Res. Communs. 33, 812.

Blumenfeld, O.O. and Gallop, P.M. (1966). Proc. Nat. Acad. Sci. (Wash.) 56, 1260.

Bornstein, P. and Piez, K.A. (1964). J. Clin Invest. 43, 1813.

Bornstein, P. and Piez, K.A. (1965). Science 148, 1353.

Bornstein, P. and Piez, K.A. (1966). Biochemistry 5, 3460.

Bornstein, P., Kang, A.H. and Piez, K.A. (1966). Biochemistry 5, 3803.

Butler, W.T., Piez, K.A. and Bornstein, P. (1967). Biochemistry 6, 3771.

Butler, W.T. (1968). Science 161, 796.

Deshmukh, K. and Nimni, M.E. (1969). J. Biol. Chem. 244, 1787.

Drake, M.P. and Davison, P.F. (1968). J. Biol. Chem. 243, 2890.

Gallop, P.M., Blumenfeld, O.O., Henson, E. and Schneider, A.L. (1968). Bichemistry 7, 2409.

Gross, J., Highberger, J.H. and Schmitt, F.O. (1954). Proc. Nat. Acad. Sci. (Wash.) 40, 679.

Hodge, A.J. and Petruska, J.A. (1963). In Aspects of Protein Structure, p. 289. Ed. by Ramachandran, G.N. Academic Press, New York.

Kakade, M.L. and Liener, I.E. (1969). Anal. Biochem. 27, 273.

Kang, A.H., Bornstein, P. and Piez, K.A. (1967). Biochemistry 6, 788.

Kang, A., Faris, B. and Franzblau, C. (1969). Biochem. Biophys. Res. Communs. 36, 345.

Lane, J.M. and Miller, E.J. (1969). Biochemistry 8, 2134.

Miller, E.J., Lane, J.M. and Piez, K.A. (1969). Biochemistry 8, 30.

Page, R.C. and Benditt, E.P. (1968). Lab. Invest. 18, 124.

Page, R.C., Benditt, E.P. and Kirkwood, C.R. (1968). Biochem. Biophys. Res. Communs. 33, 752.

Piez, K.A., Bladen, H.A., Bornstein, P., Butler, W.T., Kang, A.H., Lane, J.M. and Miller, E.J. (1968). Brookhaven Symp. Biol. 21, 345.

Piez, K.A., Eigner, E.A. and Lewis, M.S. (1963). Biochemistry 2, 58.

Rojkind, M., Blumenfeld, O.O. and Gallop, P.M. (1964). Biochem. Biophys. Res. Communs. 17, 320.

Rojkind, M., Blumenfeld, O.O. and Gallop, P.M. (1966). J. Biol. Chem. 241, 1530.

Rojkind, M., Gutierrez, A.M., Zeichner, M. and Lent. R.W. (1969). Biochem. Biophys. Res. Communs. 36, 350.

Rojkind, M. and Juarez, H. (1966). Biochem. Biophys. Res. Communs. 25, 481.

Rojkind, M., Rhi, L. and Aguirre, M. (1968). J. Biol. Chem. 243, 2266.

Tanzer, M.L. (1968). J. Biol. Chem. 243, 4045.

Tanzer, M.L. and Mechanic, G. (1968). Biochem. Biophys. Res. Communs. 32, 885.

Veis, A. and Anesey, J. (1965). J. Biol. Chem. 240, 3899.

STABLE INTERMOLECULAR CROSSLINKS IN COLLAGEN AFTER REDUCTION

Gerald Mechanic

The formation of stable intermolecular crosslinks in biological macromolecules correlates intimately with growth and development. Many of these processes involve formation, maturation and ageing of the fibrous structural proteins.

The system which is ideal for study is that involving collagen where spontaneous formation of intermolucular crosslinks occur. The body contains soluble collagen (tropocollagen) and insoluble collagen. A small portion of the soluble collagen is newly formed and extractable with salt solutions. As the collagen maturates more powerful solvents are needed to extract it from skin. The collagen left behind after extensive extraction with salt and dilute acids is termed by definition insoluble collagen. The formation of insoluble collagen may well coincide with the artificial stabilization of soluble collagen fibrils by reduction with sodium borohydride (Tanzer, 1967). It was indicated at the time that the compounds so stabilized were Schiff bases reduced to secondary amines forming a collagen which was relatively insoluble (Tanzer, 1968). This study extends the work of Tanzer and Mechanic (1968) and presents some exploratory experiments as to the type of intermolecular crosslink formed in collagen fibrils upon mild reduction.

Soluble collagen as tropocollagen and reconstituted collagen fibrils of the native-type from calf skin were treated with sodium borotritiide as previously described (Tanzer and Mechanic, 1968).

The collagens after lyophilization were hydrolyzed at 105°C with 6 N HCl and 2 N NaOH in evacuated sealed tubes for 24 hr and 18 hr, respectively. Aliquots of the acid hydrolyzed products were treated with metaperiodate according to Bohak (1964). The alkaline hydrolyzates were acidified and desalted on a Dowex-50 column in the H+ form.

Portions of each hydrolyzate representing 10 mg of collagen were chromatographed on a rapid single-column amino acid analyzer using a variable gradient. Two-mililiter fractions were collected and 0.2 ml from each was pipetted into a scintillation vial containing 10 ml of Bray's solution (Bray, 1961), which was 5% with respect to Cabosil. Approximately the same amount of radioactivity was contained in each aliquot chromatographed.

The results of this series of experiments are shown in Figures 1-6. Figure 1 contains the radioactive elution profile of collagen treated with sodium borotritiide while in solution as tropocollagen. Peaks 4 and 7 are 2-amino-6-hydroxyhexanoic acid (Hydroxynorleucine) and 2-amino-6-chlorohexanoic acid (chlorornorleucine) respectively. These were identified by cochromatography with synthetic samples. The conversion of the hydroxyl function to the chloro derivative under the conditions of hydrolysis was shown previously (Paz et al. 1969). The 2-amino-6-hydroxyhexanoic acid results from the reduction of 5-amino-5 carboxypentanal (α-aminoadipic semialdehyde). Fibrils first reduced, hydrolyzed and chromatographed in the identical manner as above resulted in the pattern observed in Fig. 2. Note here that peaks 4 and 7 are considerably reduced which seems to indicate that 5-amino-5-carboxypentanal is partaking in cross-link formation spontaneously upon fibrogenesis. Peaks 5 and 6 also contain much less radioactivity. We now see appearing F_1, F_2 and F_3 which are new to the radioactive elution profile. Figure 3 represents alkali hydrolyzed collagen that was reduced in solution. Peak 4 is very much enhanced since there can be no conversion of the hydroxy compound to the chloro derivative under these conditions. Instead we observe another peak 7 which eluted in the same area as the aldol condensation product of 5-amino-5carboxypentanal as shown by Paz et al. (1969).

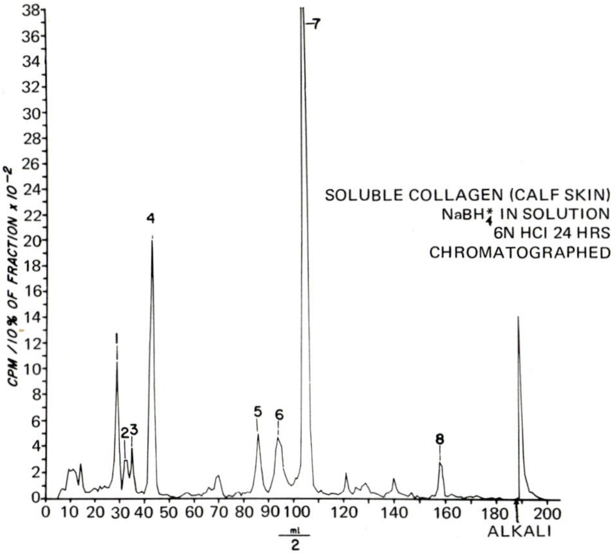

Fig. 1. Ten mg of collagen reduced while in solution. Hydrolyzed with acid and chromatographed. 2-ml Fractions collected from a 58-cm single column eluted with a 9-chambered varigrad. Position of natural amino acids depicted in Fig. 5.

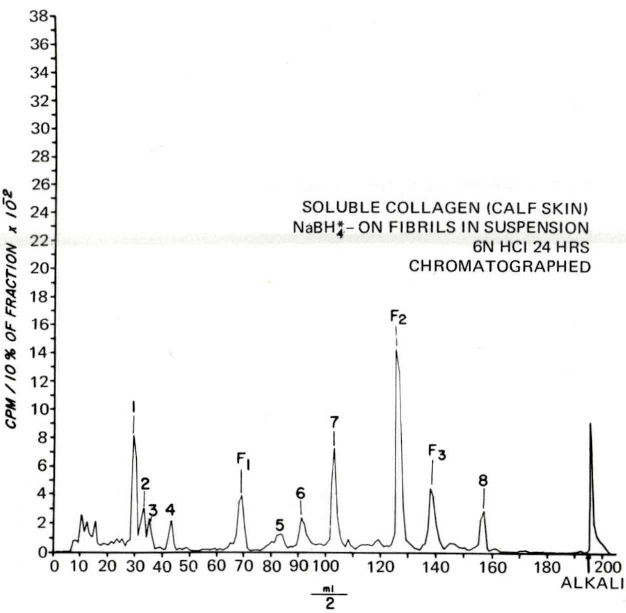

Fig. 2. Ten mg of collagen reduced as fibrils and hydrolyzed with acid.

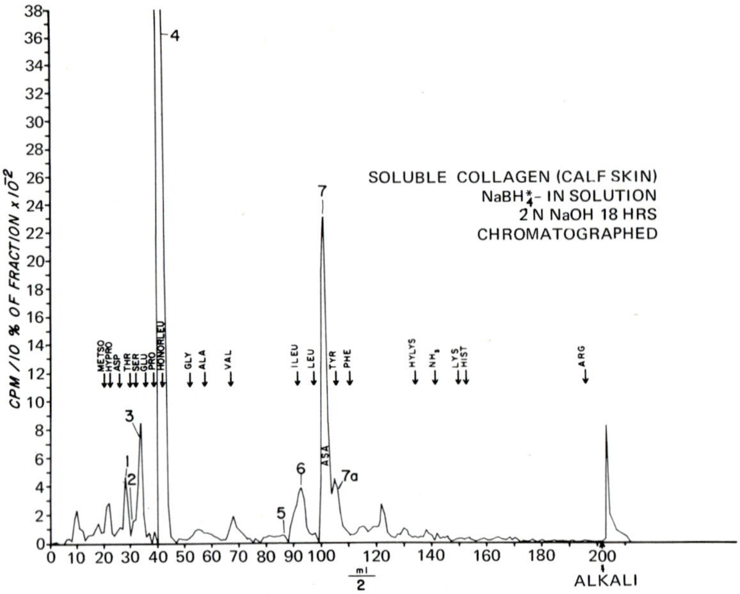

Fig. 3. Ten mg of collagen reduced while in solution hydrolized with 2 N NaOH.

This compound is then presumed to be the reduced dehydrated aldol 2-(4-amino-4-carboxybutyl)-5-amino-5-carboxy-2-hexenol or the reduced aldol product 2-(4-amino-4-carboxybutyl)-2-hydroxy-5 amino-5-carboxyhexanol. In each case the aldehyde would be the precursor product. Appearing also is another peak labeled 7a in Fig. 3. Peaks 5 and 8 which are absent and may be labile to alkaline hydrolysis or artifacts of acid hydrolysis as peak 7 is in Fig. 1. When the reduced fibrils were hydrolyzed with 2 N NaOH and chromatographed, the elution profile obtained is that shown in Fig. 4. Here a marked decrease in peaks 4,7 and a disappearance of 7a is noted. F_1, F_2 and F_3 are readily apparent although F_2 and F_3 are markedly reduced. This elution pattern confirms the observation noted previously that 5-amino-5 carboxypentanal forms intermolecular crosslinks in collagen fibrils. From this data it may also be presumed that the self aldol condensation product of 5-amino-5-carboxypentanal, 2-(4-amino-4-carboxy-butyl)-2-hydroxy-5-amino-5-carboxyhexanal also forms an intermolecular crosslink along with the unknown peak 7a.

The acid hydrolyzates of reduced tropocollagen and

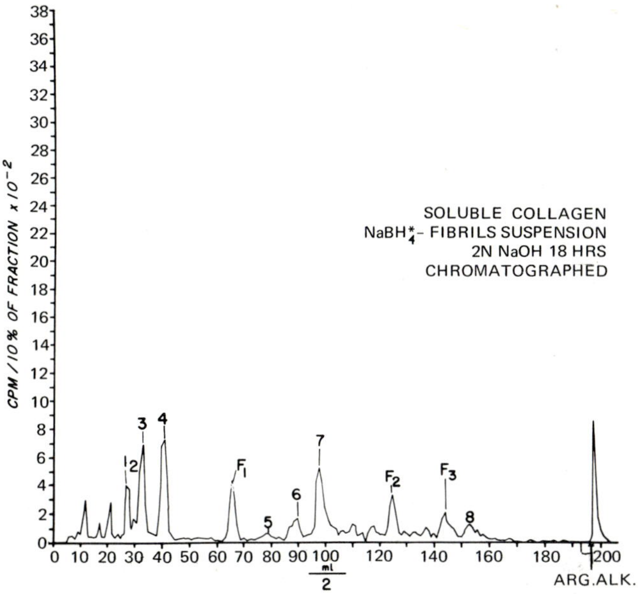

Fig. 4. Ten mg of collagen reduced as fibrils and hydrolyzed with alkali.

collagen fibrils treated with periodate were chromatographed and resulted in the elution profiles seen in Figs. 5 and 6 respectively. It can be seen that Fig. 5 is virtually identical to Fig. 1 except for a reduction of peak 1. When comparing Fig. 6 with Fig. 2 we note the same reduction of peak 1. Since this peak occurs in Figs. 1 and 2 it is presumed that it does not partake in crosslink formation. Significantly F_2 has virtually disappeared from the chromatograph. It was thought that prior to periodate oxidation this was the compound hydroxylysine norleucine (Bailey and Peach, 1968). According to Bohak (1963) periodate oxidation of this radioactive compound as produced by the reduction of 7,8-didehydro-Nε-(5-amino-4-carboxypentanyl)hydroxylysine (Bailey and Peach, 1968) would result in the production of radioactive lysine which was not found in any chromatogram. Therefore, it is probable that F_2 is not hydroxylysine norleucine but another type of periodate labile compound. Further investigations in the isolation of F_1, F_2 and F_3 and their subsequent identification is in progress. Their structure should go far in elucidating the intermolecular covalent crosslinks.

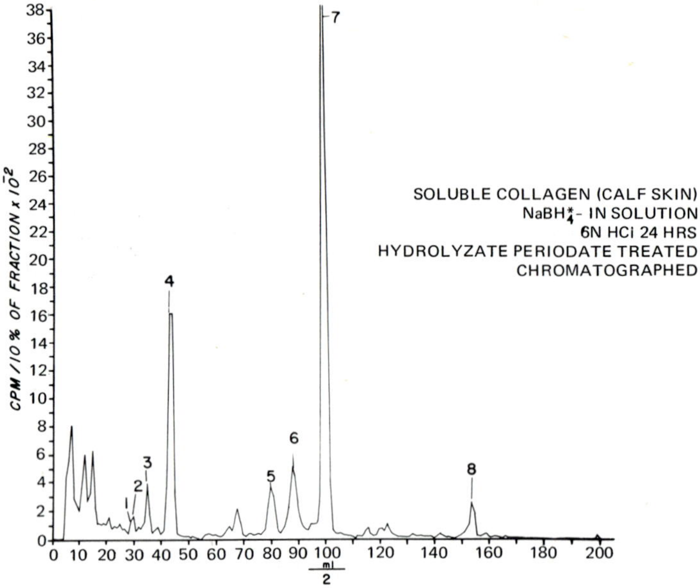

Fig. 5. Ten mg of hydrolyzed, reduced solution collagen treated with periodate.

present in collagen.

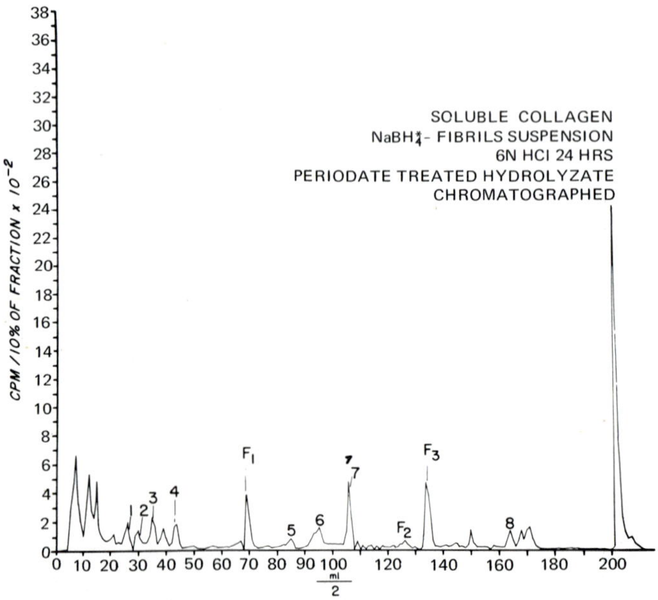

Fig. 6. Ten mg of hydrolyzed, reduced fibril collagen treated with periodate

ACKNOWLEDGEMENTS

This work was supported in part by USPHS Grant No. DE-02668-03.

REFERENCES

Bailey, A.J. and Peach, C.M. (1968). Biochem. Biophys. Res. Communs. 33, 812.

Bohak, Z. (1964). J. Biol. Chem. 239, 2878.

Bray, G. (1961). Anal. Biochem. 1, 279.

Paz, M.A., Lent, R.W., Faris, B., Franzblau, C., Blumenfeld, O.O., and Gallop, P.M. (1969). Biochem. Biophys. Res. Communs. 34, 221.

Tanzer, M.L. (1967). Biochem, Biophys. Acta 133, 584.

Tanzer, M.L. (1968). J. Biol. Chem. 243, 4045.

Tanzer, M.L. and Mechanic, G. (1968). Biochem. Biophys. Res. Communs. 32, 885.

SWELLING AND TRANSPORT PROPERTIES OF COLLAGEN FILMS

A. Gliozzi, R. Morchio and A. Ciferri

When immersed in a salt solution, a collagen membrane interacts with the solution and its degree of swelling and its structure change with salt type and concentration. At certain critical values of concentration, the collagen undergoes melting, or helix-coil transformation, with macroscopic changes in the dimensions of the membrane. Thus, this system offers an opportunity for investigating the transport properties both when the membrane is undergoing alterations in swelling (in the crystalline as well as in the amorphous state) and when it is undergoing a conformational transition. Determination of the transport properties of collagen films may also be a useful tool for elucidating fine details of the swollen structure which are not revealed by the swelling behavior. In addition, Tasaki (1959) has suggested that the permeability change during the excitation of biological membranes may be related to a conformational transition. Therefore collagen films may be a useful model for assessing the role of a phase transition on transport properties.

I EXPERIMENTAL TECHNIQUES

The membranes chosen are crosslinked collagen films near the isoelectric point. Collagen films, 25 μ thick, were kindly supplied by Dr. J. Nichols of Ethicon, Inc. (Somerville, New Jersey, U.S.A.).

The films were prepared by casting a dispersion of fibrils obtained from steer tendons. Electron micrographs of the membranes revealed the occurrence of the typical tropocollagen unit with the 700 Å-spacing (Veis, 1964). Although the films were not subject to any deliberate orientation, during the drying process the fibrils spontaneously arranged themselves in layers forming oriented bundles. Figure 1 shows the film surface as it appears at the scanning microscope at two different magnifications. Figure 2 shows the swelling as a function of concentration in three different salt solutions at 26°C (Ciferri, Rajagh and Puett, 1965).

Our present experiments consisted in measuring the volume flow through the membrane clamped between two aqueous solutions when a hydrostatic pressure difference was applied. The salt concentration was the same on both sides of the membrane and the temperature was kept constant at 26 ± 0.1°C (Fig. 3a). We measured the volume flow at a fixed pressure gradient by following the movement of the meniscus in the horizontal capillary as a function of time. A typical plot is given in the lower part of Fig. 3. Since the concentration of salt was found to remain the same on the two sides of the membrane, the filtration coefficient L_p was simply obtained by the slope of the line (J_v = volume flux per unit time and area) divided by ΔP.

II RESULTS AND DISCUSSION

The values of L_p obtained for KSCN are reported in Fig. 4b as a function of salt concentration C_s. One can observe a strong dependence of the filtration coefficient on salt concentration. The discontinuity of L_p corresponds to the occurrence of a phase transition which was also observed independently by means of optical techniques. Thus, the full line refers to the crystalline state and the broken line to the amorphous state.

In order to explain the effects, the filtration data

Fig. 1. Scanning micrographs of the membrane surface at two different magnifications (2200 X and 6300 X) (courtesy of Prof. P. Graziadei, Florida State University, Fla.).

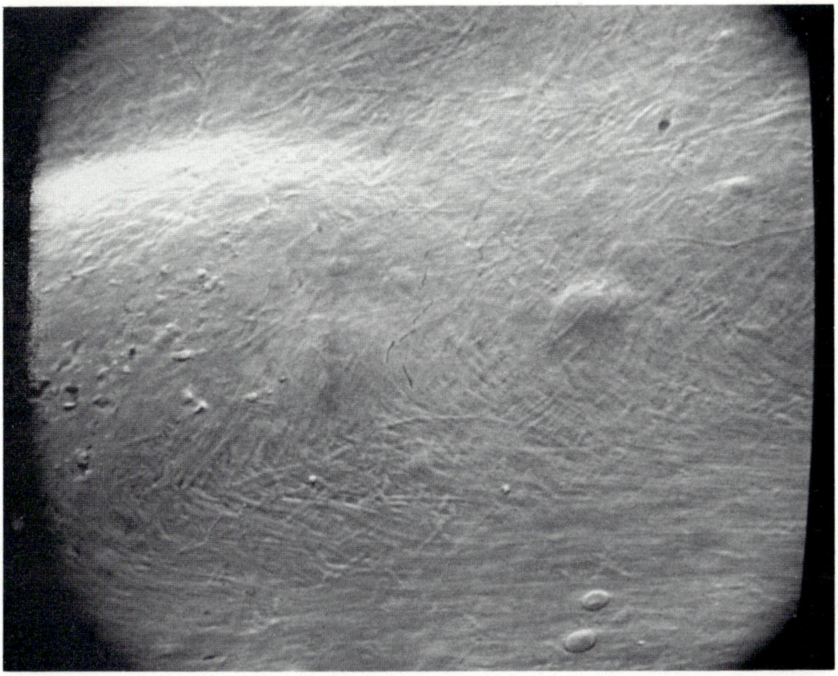

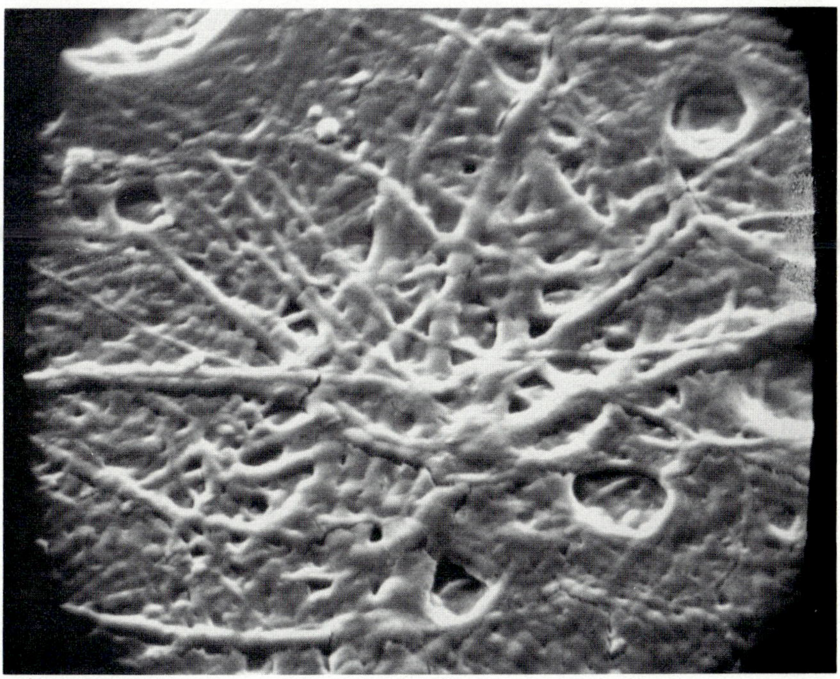

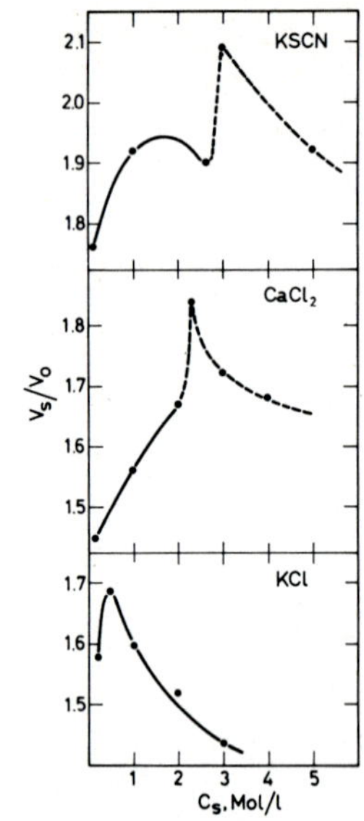

Fig. 2. Ratio of swollen volume V_s to dry volume V_o for collagen films as a function of concentration in various salt solutions.

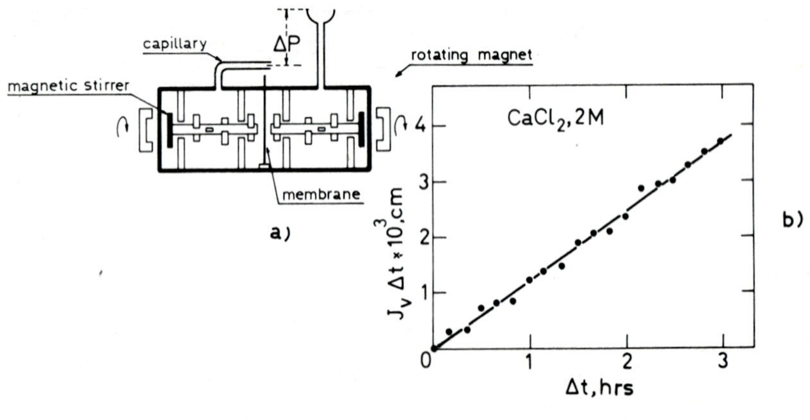

Fig. 3. a) The experimental apparatus; b) volume displacements (cm^3/cm^2) versus time in a typical experimental run.

have been related to the swelling behavior. Fig. 4a shows the changes in the thickness Δx due to swelling in KSCN solutions. As in the case with the volume swelling presented in Fig. 2, the cross-sectional swelling Δx

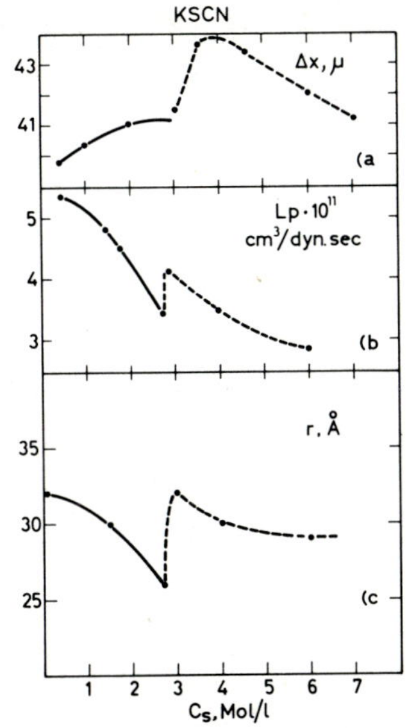

Fig. 4. a) Thickness Δx; b) filtration coefficient L_p; and c) equivalent pore radius r, plotted against KSCN concentration.

increases with increasing salt concentration in the crystalline state, rises suddenly at the transition to the amorphous state, and then starts to decrease.

Since L_p and Δx vary in a similar way with the concentration in the amorphous state and oppositely in the crystalline state, it is clear that the macroscopic swelling is inadequate to explain the overall permeability behavior so that other factors must be taken into consideration. To this end we have performed diffusion measurements with tritiated water under no pressure gradient. The tritium permeability ω_T was obtained by the Fick relation $J_t = RT\omega_T \Delta c_T$ where Δc_T is the difference in tritiated water content in the two half cells. According to irreversible thermodynamics treatment (Thau, Block and Kedem, 1966) the ratio $g = L_p/\overline{V}_w\omega T$ (where $\overline{V}_w$ is the partial molar volume of the solvent) is a measure of the relative importance of solvent-solvent versus solvent-polymer interaction inside the membrane. In particular, if we consider the solvent transport as a viscous flow through the pores of the membrane, g is a measure of the size of the pores. According to this approximation, we have (Paganelli and Solomon, 1957):

$$r = \frac{8\eta D \bar{V}_w g}{RT}$$

(where D and η are the diffusion coefficient and the viscosity of the solution through the pores, respectively). This relationship may be used for the evaluation of the "equivalent pore radius", as seen in Fig. 4c. We find that $\underline{r}$ decreases with C_s in the crystalline as well as in the amorphous state, while it increases abruptly during the transition. The trend is similar to that of L_p and in contrast to the variations of Δx.

Thus, at least qualitatively, the variation of L_p seems to be controlled by the effect of the solvent on pore size. However, this raises the problem of the relationship between macroscopic swelling and porosity. It is interesting to observe that in the crystalline state an increase of swelling (which indicates a favorable collagen-KSCN solution interaction; Ciferri et al., 1965) corresponds to a decrease of porosity, while in the amorphous state a decrease of porosity corresponds to a decrease of swelling. We interpret this effect in the following way. In the amorphous state one has to distinguish between bound salt and water and relatively more mobile solvents. In line with previous work (Orofino, Ciferri and Hermans, 1967), the affinity of the latter towards the protein is reduced in the salting-out region which occurs when $C_s > 3$ $\underline{M}$ KSCN. The resulting de-swelling (cf. Figs. 2, 4) causes a reduction of pore size since the amorphous network does not possess a rigid structure: the situation may be similar to that occurring in a sponge where the pore size increases by swelling and decreases by de-swelling.

A different situation occurs, however, in the crystalline state where, among interfibrillar spaces, there are large pores which are relatively rigid owing to the rigidity of the overall structure. Water and salt which are admitted within the crystalline structure and bound to the protein walls of the pore, may then effectively close up the pores, or reduce porosity. An additional contribution to the closing up of the pores may arise from an expansion of regions surrounding the pore (note, however, the X-ray evidence (Puett, Ciferri and Rajagh, 1967) indicates no alteration of the lattice spacings upon swelling). At the melting point, the disorganisation of the structure and the sudden increase of swelling generate new pores and a consequent increase of L_p.

In order to test the generality of the above effects, other data for $CaCl_2$ are reported in Fig. 5. The same general features observed in the case of KSCN are shown. In particular, the slopes $\delta L_p/\delta C_s$ and $\delta \Delta x/\delta C_s$ have the same sign in the amorphous state and different sign in the crystalline state and there is a sudden increase of L_p at the transition. The case of KCl reported in Fig. 6, is apparently different from the situation observed for KSCN and $CaCl_2$ but, in effect, adds support to our proposed interpretation. The interaction between collagen and KCl solutions has been described previously (Ciferri et al., 1965). The salting out character of this salt is shown by the lack of a chemical melting at room temperature and by the de-swelling of the crystalline membrane (cf. Figs. 2,6) on increasing C_s. To the observed de-swelling corresponds an increase of L_p, in contrast to the cases of KSCN and $CaCl_2$ when swelling increases with C_s in the crystalline state, and L_p decreases with C_s. The pore size (cf. Fig. 6) increases with C_s in the crystalline state, again in contrast with the observation made for KSCN and $CaCl_2$. We think this is coherent with our model for the crystalline membrane. If there are large rigid pores which can be closed by absorption of solvent in the case of KSCN and $CaCl_2$, it is only natural that they should be opened by desorption of solvent in the case of KCl thus leading to observed increase of L_p.

Finally, we report in Fig. 7 the results of the variation of L_p with pH at low ionic strength. In this case the phase transition occurs because of the electrostatic repulsion of the charges on the ε-amino groups. As

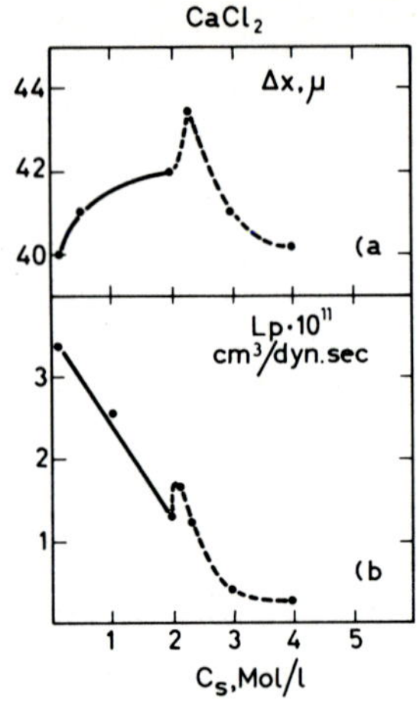

Fig. 5. a) Thickness Δx; and b) filtration coefficient L_p plotted against $CaCl_2$ concentration.

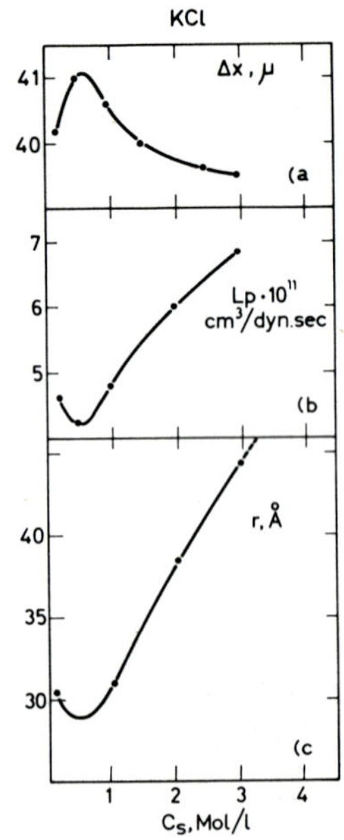

Fig. 6. a) Thickness Δx; b) filtration coefficient L_p; and c) equivalent pore radius plotted against KCl concentration.

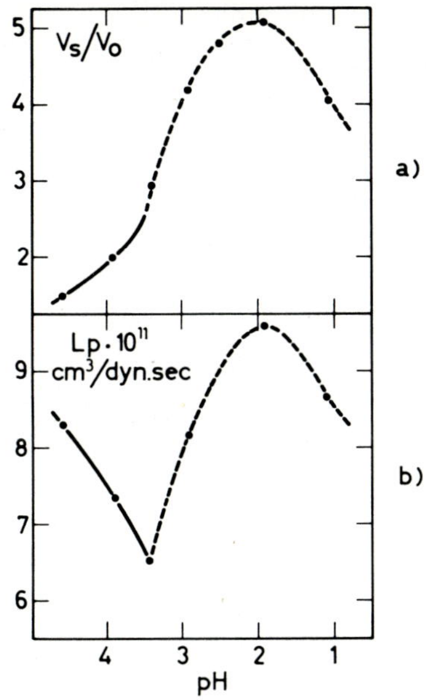

Fig. 7. a) Ratio of swollen volume V_s to dry volume V_o at different pH in KCl 10^{-2}M; b) the filtration coefficient L_p as a function of pH in KCl 10^{-2}M.

in the previous cases, the increase of swelling in the crystalline state (which is here particularly large due to Donnan effect) is accompanied by a decrease of L_p with decreasing pH. L_p increases at the transition and decreases in the amorphous state when the charge on the polymer has reached a constant value and further addition of acid causes a de-swelling.

ACKNOWLEDGEMENTS

The authors are indebted to Dr. V. Vittoria for the determination of permeability data at low pH and to Dr. R. Pierantoni (Florida State University) for the scanning electronmicrographs of the membrane surface.

REFERENCES

Ciferri, A., Rajagh, L. and Puett, D. (1965). Biopolymers 3, 461.

Orofino, T.A., Ciferri, A. and Hermans, J.J. (1967). Biopolymers 5, 773.

Paganelli, C.V. and Solomon, A.K. (1957). J. Gen. Physiol. 41, 259.

Puett, D., Ciferri, A. and Rajagh, C. (1967). Biopolymers 5, 439.

Tasaki, I. (1959). J. Physiol. 148, 306.

Thau, G., Block, R. and Kedem, O. (1966). Desalination 1, 129.

Veis, A. (1964). The Macromolecular Chemistry of Gelatin. Academic Press, New York.

AN INVESTIGATION OF THE THERMAL SHRINKAGE OF BOVINE ACHILLES TENDON

D.R. Gee, T.P. Melia, R.E. Morgan and G.O. Phillips

Heat capacity measurements on polymers over a temperature range extending down to the absolute zero are of considerable current interest (Melia, 1964; Dole, 1960). In the first place they represent a fundamental approach to the problem of understanding the structure and internal motion of a polymer. Secondly, they can be used to evaluate the entropy, enthalpy and free energy functions as well as the changes in these functions associated with crystallisation, melting, glass transitions and denaturation. Thirdly, they can be used to test the validity of various theoretical treatments of the heat capacity of chain polymer crystals (Melia, 1964) and in the verification of the Third Law of thermodynamics (Westrum and McCullough, 1963). Fourthly, they provide a means whereby such features as the temperature and temperature range of reversible and irreversible transitions, the influence of chain orientation and its effect on total crystallinity, and the change in thermal properties resulting from a change in molecular configuration can be studied (Westrum and McCullough, 1963).

A comprehensive investigation of the thermal properties of the relatively simple synthetic polymers which form the basis of the plastics industry has been carried out by Melia (1964) and other workers (Dainton, Evans, Hoare and Melia, 1962b,c; Melia and Tyson, 1967; Clegg, Gee, Melia and Tyson, 1968; Melia, Clegg and Tyson, 1968; Gee and Melia, 1968; Clegg, Gee and Melia, 1968). However, such data about biopolymers are meagre. This prompted the present research programme which has as its initial object the provision of thermal data for biopolymers and, as its ultimate aim, application of the method in the characterisation and deduction of the detailed molecular structures of biologically important macromolecules.

Achilles Tendon collagen was chosen as the material for this preliminary investigation. Recently considerable effort (Ramachandran, 1967a,b) has been directed towards the elucidation of its molecular structure and to ascertaining the nature of the transformation which occurs when collagen is heated whilst immersed in a swelling agent such as water. X-ray diffraction (Cowan, North and Randall, 1955), calorimetric (Kuntzel and Doehner, 1939), volume dilatometric (Flory and Garrett, 1958), spectroscopic (Wetlaufer, 1962) and optical rotation techniques (Harrington and Von Hippel, 1961) have been used to study this transformation. From the results of such studies Flory and Garrett (1958) conclude that the transformation is a first-order phase transition involving the melting of crystalline regions in the collagen molecule. So far most physicochemical studies of this transition have been carried out in the presence of diluent (Ramachandran, 1967a). In the present investigation this transition has been investigated in the solid state using differential scanning calorimetry.

I EXPERIMENTAL TECHNIQUES

A. CALORIMETRY

The differential scanning calorimeter used in the present investigation has been described previously (Clegg et al., 1958). The weights of collagen used varied between 20 and 30 mg. Heating rates of 4°K per min were employed. The overall precision of the measurements is better than ±2%.

B. MATERIALS

Sample 1 is bovine achilles tendon, freshly excised from adult cows. This was subsequently extracted according

TABLE I

Amino Acid Analysis of the Collagen Samples (Results Expressed in Residues of Amino Acid Per 1000 Total Residues)

	Sample 1	Sample 2	Sample 3	Sample 4	Sample 5	Sample 6
Lysine	22.4	24.3	24.2	24.3	22.9	24.3
Histidine	4.50	5.00	4.55	4.32	6.37	5.89
Arginine	49.7	49.6	50.6	52.4	49.4	52.1
3-Hydroxyproline	1.86	0.34	0.34	0.33	0.31	0.25
4-Hydroxyproline	92.7	85.5	90.3	91.0	89.3	92.5
Aspartic acid	48.5	45.0	45.7	47.0	47.4	48.0
Threonine	18.6	17.8	18.3	17.2	19.3	18.4
Serine	36.8	36.5	36.5	36.5	37.7	37.0
Glutamic acid	77.6	70.1	71.9	74.4	75.3	76.1
Proline	120.0	122.8	119.8	105.1	112.1	123.7
Glycine	330.8	347.1	342.0	342.2	339.4	314.8
Alanine	116.0	112.1	110.2	113.2	110.9	111.8
Valine	24.0	22.3	21.6	23.8	21.9	22.6
Methionine	4.50	4.86	2.73	4.27	3.56	5.31
Iso-leucine	12.3	11.6	11.8	12.8	11.9	11.3
Leucine	26.9	25.5	26.0	27.0	27.4	27.0
Tyrosine	5.00	3.79	5.41	5.55	4.94	4.82
Phenylalanine	13.5	11.7	11.4	14.4	12.7	13.9
Hydroxylysine	8.9	8.89	9.39	8.98	10.6	10.3

to the method of Einbinder and Schubert (1951) with 3% Na_2HPO_4, 25% KCl and water and air dried without prior ethanol treatment (sample 2). Sample 3 was the residue obtained after treating sample 2 with ether at 4°C for 24 hr; sample 4 was the residue remaining after extracting sample 2 with acetone at 4°C for 24 hr; sample 5 was the residue obtained after extraction of sample 2 with ethanol at 4°C for 24 hr. Sample 6 is sample 2 after ether, acetone and ethanol extraction. These treatments do not grossly influence distribution of amino acids in the proteins of the individual achilles tendon samples (Table I).

II RESULTS

The heat capacity of sample 2 was measured over the temperature range 200 to 430°K. Typical results are presented in Fig. 1. Samples 1 and 3-6 were investigated over the temperature range 310-430°K. The results are presented in Table II.

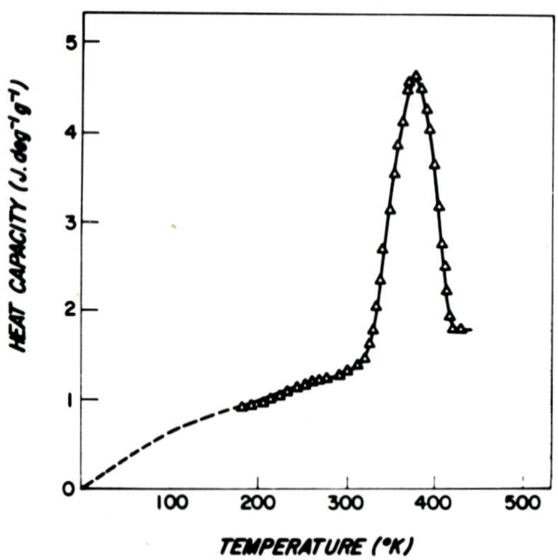

Fig. 1. Observed heat capacities of tendon (sample 2). (Heating rate 4°K min^{-1}).

TABLE II

Observed Values of the Denaturation Transition in Tendon

Sample No.	w^* (%)	Transition energy $J.g^{-1}$	$w\Delta H_v$ $J.g^{-1}$	ΔH_d $J.g^{-1}$
1	6.4	196±4	144±4	52±8
2	7.3	219±4	165±4	54±8
3	6.0	195±4	137±4	58±8
4	6.2	200±4	141±4	59±8
5	6.1	209±4	138±4	71±8
6	5.7	212±4	127±4	85±8

*w = observed weight loss during experiment

For sample 2 heat capacity data below 200°K were obtained using the Kelley, Parks and Huffmann (1929) extrapolation procedure. Polyethylene, for which heat capacity data are available (Dainton, Evans, Hoare and Melia, 1962a; Tucker and Reese, 1967) down to 2.5°K, was chosen as the standard substance for this extrapolation. Derived values of the entropy and enthalpy of sample 2 are presented in Figs. 2 and 3, respectively. Again these plots emphasize the diffuse nature of the transition which occurs in the temperature range 310 to 430°K. The entropy and enthalpy were obtained by evaluating the thermodynamic relations

$$S^o_T - S^o_T = \int_0^T \frac{C}{T}\,dT \qquad (1)$$

$$H^o_T - H^o_0 = \int_0^T C\,dT \qquad (2)$$

where $(S^o_T - S^o_0)$ and $(H^o_T - H^o_0)$ are the entropy and enthalpy relative to absolute zero.

The most significant feature of the heat capacity versus

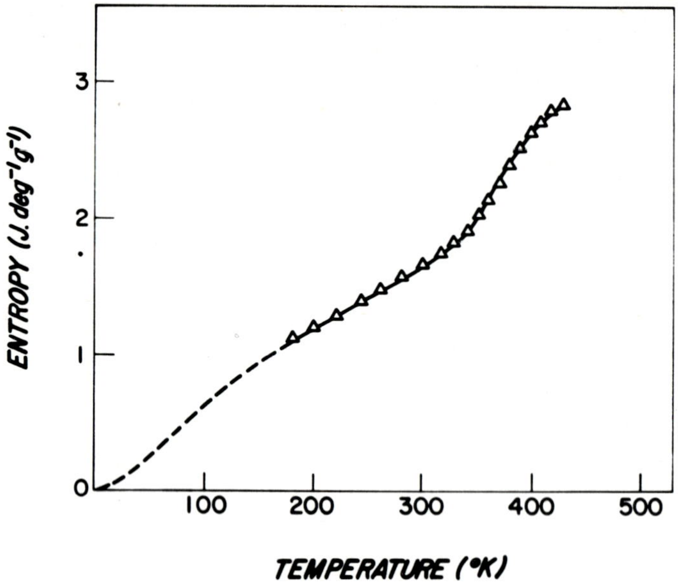

Fig. 2. Entropy-temperature plot for tendon (sample 2).

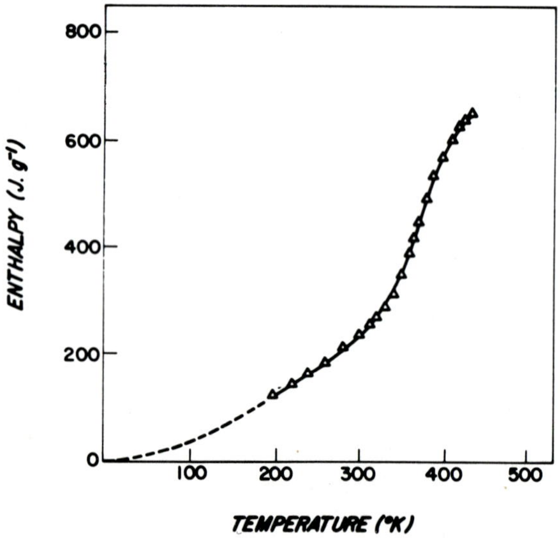

Fig. 3. Enthalpy-temperature plot for tendon (sample 2).

temperature plot in Fig. 1 is the diffuse transition observed over the temperature range 310 to 430°K. This diffuse, endothermic peak has a maximum at 373°K. During the experiments a pronounced weight loss of between 5 and 7% was observed with all samples. Thermogravimetric analysis indicates that this weight change is associated with the loss of water.

III DISCUSSION

The diffuse endothermic peak observed in all the collagen samples studied is probably a composite of several endothermic processes of which dehydration and denaturation are the principals. Denaturation in collagen is associated with the heat induced collagen → gelatin transition, which at the molecular level involves the conversion of the rigid, three-chain collagen molecule to random-coil gelatin. This transition is known to proceed extremely slowly (Von Hippel and Wong, 1963). Consequently, because of the short time scale of the differnetial scanning calorimetry experiments, the transition appears diffuse.

The total energy involved in this transition is shown in Table II. To assess the energy associated with denaturation (ΔH_d) the total energy must be corrected for the contribution from the dehydration process. Using the value 2260 ± 1 $J.g^{-1}$ for the heat of vaporisation of water (ΔH_v) and the observed weight loss (w) during the experiment, the values of $w\Delta H_v$ given in column 4 of Table II are obtained. These values were subtracted from the total transition energy to obtain ΔH_d.

The untreated tendon shows the lowest value for ΔH_d (52 ± 8). Despite the fact that this sample is predominantly collagen, it also contains cells, extracellular proteins and proteoglycans, and small metabolites. The treatments with Na_2HPO_4, KCl and water (sample 2), ether (sample 3) and acetone (sample 4) only lead to a relatively small increase in ΔH_d. The large increase obtained for samples 5 and 6, both of which had been ethanol extracted, indicates that this treatment is the most critical.

In interpreting these data it is not possible at this stage to decide unequivocally whether the molecular structure of collagen is influenced by the ethanol treatments or whether some other components of the tendon are removed or denatured.

Flory and Garrett (1958) studied the thermal shrinkage of a collagen sample similar to sample 6, in the presence of ethylene glycol, over the temperature range 323 to 373°K using volume dilatometry. They also observed a diffuse first-order transition and calculated the values 100 ± 20 $J.g^{-1}$ and 418°K for the transition enthalpy and the temperature at which the transition is complete in "pure" collagen, respectively. This compares with the value of 85 ± 8 $J.g^{-1}$ and 419°K, respectively, obtained in this work.

Flory and Garrett (1958) studied the thermal shrinkage of a collagen sample similar to sample 6, in the presence of ethylene glycol, over the temperature range 323 to 373°K using volume dilatometry. They also observed a diffuse first-order transition and calculated the values 100 ± 20 $J.g^{-1}$ and 418°K for the transition enthalpy and the temperature at which the transition is complete in "pure" collagen, respectively. This compares with the value of 85 ± 8 $J.g^{-1}$ and 419°K, respectively, obtained in this work.

It is current practice in the purification of "insoluble collagen" to utilise solvent treatment procedures such as we have adopted here, despite the fact that no evaluation is possible of their overall effects on the nature of the "insoluble collagen" samples. The present work indicates that ΔH_d could be a reasonable parameter for the identification and characterisation of individual collagen samples.

REFERENCES

Clegg, G.A., Gee, D.R. and Melia, T.P. (1968). Makromolekulare Chem. 116, 130.

Clegg, G.A., Gee, D.R., Melia, T.P. and Tyson, A. (1968). Polymer (London) 9, 501.

Cowan, P.M., North, A.C.T. and Randall, J.T. (1955). Symp. Soc. Exp. Biol. 9, 115.

Dainton, F.S., Evans, D.M., Hoare, F.E. and Melia, T.P. (1962a). Polymer (London) 3, 277.

Dainton, F.S., Evans, D.M., Hoare, F.E. and Melia, T.P. (1962b). Polymer (London) 3, 286.

Dainton, F.S., Evans, D.M., Hoare, F.E. and Melia, T.P. (1962c). Polymer (London) 3, 297.

Dole, M. (1960). Fortschr. Hochpolymeren-Forsch 2, 221.

Einbinder, J. and Schubert, M. (1951). J. Biol. Chem. 188, 335.

Flory, P.J. and Garrett, R.R. (1958). J. Am. Chem. Soc. 80, 4836.

Gee, D.R. and Melia, T.P. (1968). Makromolekulare Chem. 116, 122.

Harrington, W.F. and Von Hippel, P.H. (1961). Adv. Protein Chem. 16, 1.

Kelley, K.K., Parks, G.S. and Huffmann, H.M. (1929). J. Phys. Chem. 33, 1802.

Kuntzel, A. and Doehner, K. (1939). Angew. Chem. 52, 175.

Melia, T.P. (1964). J. Appl. Chem. 14, 461.

Melia, T.P., Clegg, G.A. and Tyson, A. (1968). Makromolekulare Chem. 112, 84.

Melia, T.P. and Tyson, A. (1967). Makromolekulare Chem. 109, 87.

Ramachandran, G.N. (1967a). Treatise on Collagen, vol. 1. Academic Press, New York.

Ramachandran, G.N. (1967b). Conformation of Biopolymers, vol. 2. Academic Press, New York.

Tucker, J.E. and Reese, W. (1967). J. Chem. Phys. 46,1388.

Von Hippel, P.H. and Wong, K.Y. (1963). Biochemistry 2, 1387.

Westrum, E.F. and McCullough, J.P. (1963). Physics and Chemistry of the Organic Solid State. Interscience, New York.

Wetlaufer, D.B. (1962). Adv. Protein Chem. 17, 304.

Chapter II

Metabolism of Collagen

INTRACELLULAR BIOSYNTHESIS OF COLLAGEN AND INTERACTIONS OF PROTOCOLLAGEN PROLINE HYDROXYLASE WITH LARGE POLYPEPTIDES

Darwin J. Prockop

I GENERAL SCHEME FOR THE INTRACELLULAR BIOSYNTHESIS OF COLLAGEN

Work from a number of laboratories over the past several years has demonstrated that the intracellular biosynthesis of collagen involves a pathway which has several unusual features (for recent reviews, see Gould, 1968; Chvapil, 1968; Rosenbloom and Prockop, 1969a). One of the most striking features of this pathway is that several critical enzymatic steps occur after the first macromolecular intermediate is synthesized and after all the information available in messenger-RNA is translated. The general steps of the pathway are: (a) assembly on ribosomal complexes of a proline-rich and lysine-rich polypeptide we have called "protocollagen"; (b) hydroxylation of appropriate prolyl and lysyl residues, in protocollagen to hydroxyproline and hydroxylysine; (c) glycosylation of some of the hydroxylysyl residues to galactosylhydroxylysine and glucosylgalactosylhydroxylysine before the completed collagen molecule is extruded (Fig. 1). Data primarily from our own laboratory suggested that these enzymatic steps occur as discrete processes so that one step does not begin until the previous reaction is largely complete and that the whole pathway operates like an assembly-line process (Rosenbloom and Prockop, 1969a; Blumenkrantz, Rosenbloom and Prockop, 1969). Most of the published evidence on the intracellular biosynthesis of collagen has been summarized in recent reviews (see above), and, therefore, the present discussion will be limited to several points which are either still uncertain or controversial.

One of the unsettled questions about the intracellular biosynthesis of collagen concerns the stage at which the two

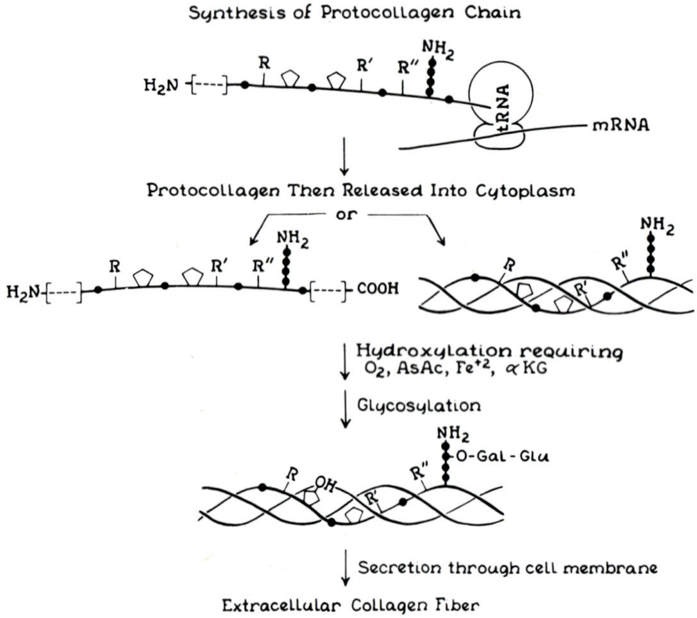

Fig. 1. General scheme for the intracellular biosynthesis of collagen. As indicated, the cofactors or cosubstrates for the hydroxylation of proline and lysine in protocollagen are O_2, ferrous iron, α-ketoglutarate, and probably ascorbate. Initial observations (Hutton, Tappel and Udenfriend, 1967; Kivirikko and Prockop, 1967c) suggested that ascorbic acid was a cosubstrate for the hydroxylation of proline, but the requirement for ascorbic acid is not highly specific, and a recent report (Lindbald, Lindstedt, Tofft and Lindstedt, 1969) suggests that α-ketoglutarate is the principal reducing factor for hydroxylases which utilize α-ketoglutarate. The latter results raise the possibility that additional reducing agents such as ascorbate serve only to keep the ferrous iron in the protocollagen hydroxylase from being oxidized through side reactions. Recent results suggest that two separate enzymatic sites and perhaps two separate enzymes are involved in the hydroxylations (Weinstein, Blumenkrantz and Prockop, 1970). The glycosylation of the hydroxylysine (Butler and Cunningham, 1966) involves two UDP-transferases (Bosmann and Eylar, 1968; Spiro and Spiro, 1968) which are probably present in the plasma membrane (Hagopian et al., 1968). Reproduced by permission (Rosenbloom and Prockop, 1969a).

α1 and one α2 chains come together to form the triple helical structure found in tropocollagen (Fig. 1). Three laboratories reported that protocollagen proline hydroxylase will hydroxylate native and denatured protocollagen at about the same rate (Kivirikko and Prockop, 1967b; Hutton, Tappel and Udenfriend, 1967; Kivirikko, Bright and Prockop, 1968; Nordwig and Pfab, 1968), and at the moment it is not clear whether the helical structure is formed before or after protocollagen is hydroxylated.

One of the most controversial points concerning the intracellular biosynthesis of collagen is the question of whether the hydroxylations of proline and lysine can occur while protocollagen is still being assembled on ribosomal complexes, or whether the hydroxylations only occur after the protocollagen polypeptides are released from ribosomes (Gould, 1968; Rosenbloom and Prockop, 1969a). The experimental evidence clearly indicated that under some experimental conditions the hydroxylations occur after protocollagen is released from ribosomal complexes. The only point which still seems debatable is whether the hydroxylations always occur after protocollagen is released from ribosomes or whether under some conditions the hydroxylations occur at an earlier stage.

Evidence that protocollagen can be hydroxylated intracellularly after it is released from ribosomes came from experiments in which the hydroxylases were intermittently inhibited by incubating embryonic cartilage without oxygen (Juva, Prockop, Cooper and Lash, 1966) or with an iron chelator (Hurych and Chvapil, 1965). When the hydroxylases were inhibited, protocollagen synthesis continued at 40-90% of the control rate for several hours (Juva et al., 1966; Bhatnagar and Prockop, 1966). This observation indicated that hydroxylation is not essential for protocollagen to be released from ribosomes, since if it were essential, inhibition of the hydroxylases would quickly fill all the active ribosomes in the cell with protocollagen molecules, and protein synthesis would be completely inhibited in a matter of minutes. In the same series of experiments (Juva et al.,

1966) it was found that if the hydroxylases were inhibited for several hours and then inhibition of the hydroxylases was reversed by exposing the tissue to oxygen or iron, the protocollagen which had accumulated during the period of inhibition was hydroxylated to the same extent as the protocollagen in control tissues. Studies with a metal chelator which does not enter cells (Hurych and Nordwig, 1967) and experiments with puromycin (Bhatnagar, Kivirikko, Rosenbloom and Prockop, 1967a) demonstrated that protocollagen proline hydroxylase is an intracellular enzyme. Accordingly, the fact that protocollagen can by hydroxylated in the tissue up to 2 hr after it is synthesized indicated that it remains intracellular, and that under the conditions of this experiment it can be hydroxylated long after it is released from ribosomal complexes. Autoradiographs of the tissue supported these conclusions (Juva et al., 1966; Cooper and Prockop, 1968).

Several different types of experimental evidence have been cited as indicating that the hydroxylation of proline can occur before complete assembly of the polypeptides of collagen. One type of observation in favor of this possibility was the isolation of small peptides which contained high specific activity hydroxyproline from connective tissues incubated with radioactive active proline (Chvapil, Holecková, Cmuchalová, Kobrle and Hurych 1962; Woessner and Boucek, 1961; Bekhor, Mohseni and Bavetta, 1966). However, a number of investigators have emphasized the technical problems in obtaining reliable data from such experiments, because of the difficulty of accurately measuring the specific activity of hydroxyproline in small molecular weight fractions of systems synthesizing collagen, and because of the possibility that the small peptides might come from the degradation of newly-synthesized collagen (Kivirikko, 1963; Lukens, 1965, 1966). In fact, an attempt to repeat the experiments of Chvapil et al. (1962) indicated that the original interpretations of the data were in error (Chvapil and Jackson, 1964).

A second type of observation supporting hydroxylation of proline at an early stage was found in two reports (Manner and Gould, 1963; Manning and Meister, 1966) indicating that puromycin did not inhibit the synthesis of [^{14}C]hydroxyproline as much as it inhibited the incorporation of [^{14}C]proline, and therefore the ratio of [^{14}C]hydroxyproline to total [^{14}C] increased. Since puromycin inhibits polypeptide synthesis after the assembly of new chains is begun but before it is completed (Yarmolinsky and de la Haba, 1959), the results suggested that the hydroxylation of proline occurs before the assembly of protocollagen polypeptides is completed. The data in these two reports, however, have not been confirmed by other laboratories. Manner and Gould (1963) found the increase in the ratio of [^{14}C]hydroxyproline to total ^{14}C only when they compared free [^{14}C]-hydroxyproline to total ^{14}C in protein. Manning and Meister (1966) and especially Lukens (1965) examined this question in considerable detail, but they found no significant synthesis of free [^{14}C]hydroxyproline with or without the addition of puromycin to their systems. Manning and Meister (1966), on the other hand, found the increase in the ratio of [^{14}C]-hydroxyproline to total ^{14}C only in the fraction of their system (minces of carrageenin granulomas) which was soluble in cold trichloroacetic acid (TCA). At about the same time, however, Lukens (1965) reported that he did not find any change in the ratio of [^{14}C]hydroxyproline to total ^{14}C in the cold TCA soluble fraction of chick embryo minces, and he documented the fact that this fraction of his system contained a significant amount of radioactivity in compounds with chromatographic properties very similar to hydroxyproline. In addition, we have found that if one examines the total non-dialyzable fraction of embryonic cartilage (i.e. the fraction which contains most of the incorporated ^{14}C), puromycin decreases rather than increases the ratio of [^{14}C]hydroxyproline to total ^{14}C. In fact, such fractions are sufficiently deficient in [^{14}C]hydroxyproline that we have been able to use them as substrates for protocollagen hydroxylase. The data of Manner and Gould (1962) on the collagen fractions from their system indicate the same effect of of puromycin as we obtained (Juva and Prockop, 1966; Bhatnagar, Kivirikko, Rosenbloom and Prockop, 1967a). Manning and Meister (1966) also reported that if they reduced the microsomal fraction from their system with $LiBH_4$, they obtained a small amount of [^{14}C]hydroxyprolinol. Since $LiBH_4$ reduction should give the alcohol derivative only if the hydroxyproline was in an ester linkage, they interpreted their results as indicating the presence of peptidyl-[^{14}C]hydroxyprolyl-tRNA in the microsomal fraction. Although the data support this conclusion, it would be important to have experiments of this type confirmed by other laboratories, since the yields of [^{14}C]hydroxyprolinol were small, and since recent results in other situations have indicated that reduction of collagen with borohydride may give unexpected products (Gallop, 1969).

Much of the current evidence that protocollagen can be hydroxylated on ribosomal complexes consists of experiments in which tissues were labeled with [^{3}H] or [^{14}C]proline and then polyribosomal complexes were isolated which contained peptide-bound [^{14}C] or [^{3}H]hydroxyproline (Lowther, Green and Chapman, 1961; Malt and Speakman, 1964 and 1965; Kretsinger, Manner, Gould and Rich, 1964; Manner, Kretsinger, Gould and Rich, 1967; Fernández-Madrid, 1967; Goldberg and Green, 1967). These reports clearly demonstrate that it is possible to isolate subcellular fractions which have many of the sedimentational properties of polyribosomes, and which contain both ribosomes and peptide-bound hydroxyproline. The principal difficulty with these reports is that relatively long labeling periods with radioactive proline were used and the results do not convincingly prove that the labeled-hydroxyproline in the isolated complexes was in fact in nascent polypeptides. In particular, the experimental controls provided do not completely rule out the possibility that the isolated fractions contained labeled hydroxyproline simply because the polyribosomal complexes were contaminated by collagen of high specific activity which had already been released from ribosomal complexes into other cellular compartments or into the extracellular matrix.

One of the first attempts at experiments of this type was the report of Lowther et al. (1961) in which they isolated microsomal fractions from carregeenan granulomas and they showed that these fractions contained [^{14}C]hydroxyproline of high specific activity. The labeling period they used, however, was 45 min, and therefore a large part of the protein-bound [^{14}C]hydroxyproline in the microsomal fractions could have represented already completed collagen molecules (see below). Lowther et al. (1961) also reported that collagen fibrils were not seen in electron micrographs of their microsomal fractions, even though Eastoe (1961) extracted quantitative amounts of salt soluble collagen from the same fractions. The failure to demonstrate fibrils suggested that the collagen in the microsomal fractions was in a newly-synthesized, nonhelical, form, but Lowther et al. (1961) pointed out that "as the total collagen present was only 0.5 to 1 per cent of dry weight, the significance of such negative findings is uncertain."

One type of control provided is several subsequent reports consisted of treating the ribosomal complexes with ribonuclease. However, the large polyribosomal fractions isolated by Manner et al. (1967), Fernández-Madrid (1967), and Goldberg and Green (1967) were relatively resistant to ribonuclease. The smaller polyribosomal fractions were disrupted by ribonuclease (Manner et al. 1967; Goldberg and Green, 1967). Although this observation indicated that the smaller fractions contained polyribosomes, it does not necessarily prove that the peptide-bound hydroxyproline in the fractions represented nascent ribosomal polypeptides. The same result might be expected if the fractions contained collagen which had nonspecifically aggregated with polyribosomes. Since the polyribosomes themselves were presumably linked by messenger-RNA, digestion of the messenger-RNA with ribonuclease could greatly reduce the sedimentation rate of the RNA and the peptide-bound hydroxyproline in the fractions whether the peptide-bound hydroxyproline was in nascent polypeptides or it was in contaminating collagen from other cell fractions.

In a second type of control for these experiments, Manner et al. (1967) showed that their polyribosomal complexes did not absorb radioactive proteins when they were mixed with labeled soluble proteins from their system. This control is also not convincing, since if the polyribosomal complexes form nonspecific agregate with collagen, the complexes Manner et al. (1967) isolated were probably saturated with collagen before they were mixed with the labeled soluble proteins. Also, the main source of contamination in such experiments would come from particulate fractions.

Goldberg and Green (1967) attempted to carry out a more direct type of control by pulse-labeling and chasing the peptide-bound hydroxyproline in the polyribosomal fractions from their system. However, the 3-min pulse and 90-min chase periods they employed were far too long to be conclusive proof that the labeled hydroxyproline was in nascent polypeptides, since in most biological systems the time required to synthesize complete polypeptides on ribosomes is one minute or less (Winslow and Ingram, 1966; Rosenblom, Bhatnagar and Prockop, 1967).

We ourselves have tried to examine this question by applying a number of different experimental techniques to isolated embryonic cartilage, a convenient tissue which synthesizes collagen at a rapid rate in vitro. The two most convincing observations are: (1) the time required to synthesize a protocollagen molecule de novo is about 1 min, but the time required to hydroxylate the proline (Rosenblom et al., 1967) and lysine (Fig. 2) in a newly-synthesized protocollagen molecule is considerably longer.

Earlier data by Manner and Gould (1962, 1963) clearly indicated that the hydroxylation of proline lagged behind the incorporation of proline by 6-10 min. We ourselves were initially unable to demonstrate the effect (Juva and Prockop, 1966), but we subsequently learned that this was because we terminated the pulse-labeling period by freezing the tissues. The effect was easily demonstrated when more vigorous precautions were taken to stop all enzymatic activity (Rosenbloom et al., 1967). The same effect is apparent in the data published by several other laboratories (See Goldberg and Green, 1967; and in particular Fessler, 1969). Our results (Rosenbloom et al., 1967) simply emphasized that if polypeptide

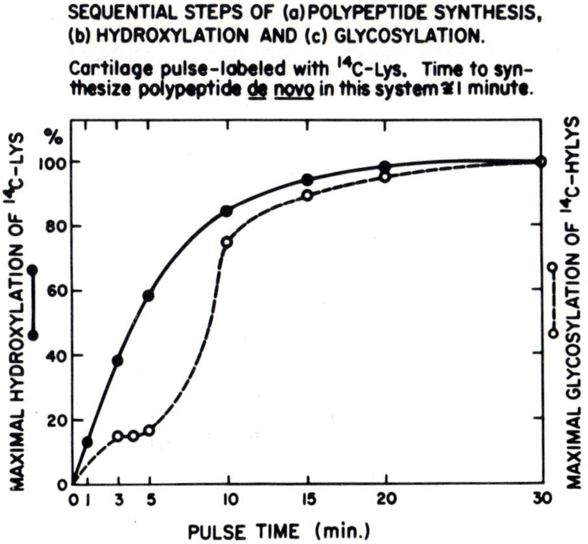

Fig. 2. Time course for the hydroxylation of lysine and glycosylation of hydroxylysine in isolated cartilage from chick embryos. Values reflect ratio of [^{14}C]hydroxylysine/ total ^{14}C incorporated into protein, and ratio of glycosylated[^{14}C]hydroxylysine to total [^{14}C]hydroxylysine. Figure is adapted from the data of Blumenkrantz et al. (1969).

synthesis is occurring at a reasonable rate, a delay of 5 min or more in the hydroxylation is too long to be consistent with the assumption that the hydroxylation occurs before the polypeptides are released from ribosomal complexes. After the tissue is treated with either of two inhibitors which prevent completion of nascent polypeptide chains, protocollagen-like molecules which have molecular weights considerably greater than 10,000 and which contain little or no hydroxyproline (Juva and Prockop, 1966; Bhatnagar, Rosenbloom, Kivirikko and Prockop, 1967) or hydroxylysine (Table I) can be isolated from the tissue. In reviewing these experiments we have been aware that our data do not conclusively exclude the possibility that a small amount of the proline and lysine near the H_2N-terminal end of the nearly complete polypeptide is hydroxylated while the HOOC-terminal end is still attached to ribosomes (Rosenblom and Prockop, 1969a). Also the results do not exclude the possibility that the hydroxylations may occur at an earlier stage in biological systems which differ significantly from the system we have studied, e.g. cells with more limited amounts of endoplasmic reticulum and therefore with less separation between active ribosomal complexes and other cellular compartments. The data do establish, however, that in the biological system we have examined most of the protocollagen polypeptide is assembled before any significant hydroxylation occurs.

Another point about the intracellular biosynthesis of collagen (Fig. 1) which has recently been debated is the question of whether protocollagen can be released from cells without being hydroxylated. Gribble, Comstock and Udenfriend (1969) indicated that protocollagen-like polypeptides can be recovered from the medium of tissue culture cells at early stages of the culture growth. Chvapil and Hurych (1966) reported that protocollagen-like polypeptides can be isolated in fractions from carregeenan granulomas which contain most of the insoluble collagen of this tissue. Although these two reports have not excluded the possibility that the extracellular polypeptides are degradative products of protocollagen it should be noted that most of the published observations indicating that protocollagen is not extruded have been based on relatively short-term observations of 4 hr or less (Rosenbloom and Prockop, 1969a). If the consequences of these observations are extrapolated for longer periods of time, it is clear that cells cannot indefinitely continue to synthesize protocollagen at the initial rate without some further change in the system. Eventually one of two changes must occur: One possibility is that the synthesis of protocollagen stops as a result of some type of delayed repression, feed-back inhibition, or simply cell death. The other possibility is that after the intracellular pool of protocollagen has increased sufficiently, protocollagen is extruded from the cells at a rate comparable to its rate of synthesis.

Another incompletely resolved point concerning the intracellular biosynthesis of collagen is the question of which cellular compartments are involved in various stages of the

TABLE I

Synthesis of Non-dialyzable Polypeptides Deficient in Hydroxylysine Under Conditions Where the Protocollagen Hydroxylases are not Inhibited

	Total ^{14}C incorp.* (dpm x 10^{-5}	$[^{14}C]$Hylys synth.+ (dpm x 10^{-4}	100 x $\frac{[^{14}C]\text{Hylys}}{\text{total }^{14}C}$ (%)
Control	104	95.0	9.13
Puromycin (50 μg/ml)	4.3	.69	1.6
Cycloheximide (100 μg/ml)	1.5	.08	<.5

*Total ^{14}C incorporated as $[^{14}C]$lysine and $[^{14}C]$hydroxylysine into nondialyzable protein of the tissue.

+Total $[^{14}C]$hydroxylysine recovered from dialyzed homogenates of the tissue.

Chick embryo cartilage was incubated with $[^{14}C]$lysine and the amounts of puromycin and cycloheximide indicated. Values are taken from the data of Blumenkrantz et al. (1969). Control experiments indicated that puromycin and cycloheximide did not inhibit protocollagen proline hydroxylase (Bhatnagar et al., 1967a,b) or protocollagen lysine hydroxylase (Blumenkrantz et al., 1969) in the tissue.

process. Although it was originally suggested that collagen was extruded via the Golgi vacuoles (Revel and Hay, 1963), recent reports appear to exclude this possibility (Ross and Benditt, 1965; Saltpeter, 1968; Cooper and Prockop, 1968). The two other possibilities which have been considered are (1) collagen is synthesized in the cisternae of the endoplasmic reticulum, it passes into the ground cytoplasm, and then it is extruded, or (2) collagen is synthesized in the cisternae and then it is extruded directly from the cisternae either through the plasma membrane or through openings between the cisternae and the extracellular space. Ross and Benditt (1965) presented results tending to support the latter possibility, but our results (Cooper and Prockop, 1968) favor extrusion from the ground cytoplasm. The question has not been competely resolved in part because it is difficult to obtain clean subcellular fractions from cells synthesizing collagen (see above). Most of the evidence is based on autoradiographic techniques in which it is difficult to distinquish radioactivity in collagen from radioactivity in other proteins, and in which the limits of resolution of the techniques make it difficult to localize radioactivity in small compartments such as the cisternae of the endoplasmic reticulum. The approaches we used in cartilage had several advantages over earlier observations in that the tissue was highly labeled, 50-65% of the radioactivity in the tissue was in collagen or related polypeptides, and it was possible to correlate changes in the distribution of grains with chemical assays of labeled protocollagen and collagen (Cooper and Prockop, 1968). When the tissue was incubated without 0_2 so that protocollagen labeled with [^{3}H]proline accumulated, the autoradiographs indicated an increased concentration of radioactivity over the ground cytoplasm. When the tissue was subsequently exposed to 0_2 so that the accumulated [^{3}H]protocollagen was converted to [^{3}H]collagen, there was a marked decrease in concentration of radioactivity over the ground cytoplasm and an increase over the matrix. Statistical evaluation of the data indicated that there was no significant change in the concentration of radioactivity over any other cellular compartment. The results suggested therefore that when the protocollagen hydroxylases are inhibited, protocollagen accumulates in the ground cytoplasm, and that when the inhibition is reversed, the molecules are extruded directly through the plasma membrane. The results did not necessarily prove that protocollagen passes into the ground cytoplasm when the hydroxylases are not inhibited, but the results strongly supported this scheme. Two independent observations with protocollagen proline hydroxylase also supported this scheme. Experiments with homogenates of cartilage which had been incubated with [^{14}C]proline and cycloheximide indicated that nascent ribosomal polypeptides are in a compartment (presumably the cisternae) which prevents their hydroxylation by either endogenous or added protocollagen hydroxylase (Bhatnagar et al. 1967). Fractionation of chick embryo homogenates indicated that protocollagen proline hydroxylase is recovered in the soluble protein fraction (Kivirikko and Prockop, 1967a), and therefore it presumably is found in the ground cytoplasm. We initially (Prockop and Juva, 1965a; 1965b) detected protocollagen proline hydroxylase in particulate fractions of embryonic cartilage, but subsequent work demonstrated that only a small part of the total enzyme was recovered in such fractions (Kivirikko and Prockop, 1967a) and that the enzyme detected in these early experiments was probably in the form of enzyme-substrate complexes (Juva and Prockop, 1969).

Saltpeter (1968) independently reported autoradiographic results suggesting that collagen is extruded directly from the ground cytoplasm through the plasma membrane in salamander limb buds. Hagopian, Bosmann and Eylar (1968) presented results suggested that the UDP-transferases which glycosylate the hydroxylysine in collagen are present in plasma membrane fractions, but this observation is of course consistent with extrusion through the plasma membrane from either the cisternae or the ground cytoplasm.

II INHIBITION OF PROTOCOLLAGEN PROLINE HYDROXYLASE BY POLYMERS OF POLYPROLINE OF VARYING SIZE

Since hydroxylysine and hydroxyproline can be synthesized after the assembly of protocollagen (above), it is clear that the protocollagen hydroxylases can act on macromolecular substrates. Extensive studies with protocollagen proline hydroxylase have in fact demonstrated that the enzyme will not hydroxylate free proline or proline in tripeptides such as Gly-Pro-Pro, and that large polypeptides with the appropriate amino acid sequences are generally more effective substrates than shorter polypeptides with the same repeating sequences (Table II) (Kivirikko and Prockop, 1967c; Hutton, Tappel and Udenfriend, 1967; Kivirikko et al., 1968; Hutton et al., 1968;

Kivirikko, Prockop, Lorenzi and Blout, 1969; Prockop and Kivirikko, 1969). There have, however, been several technical difficulties in using the available substrates to examine in detail the effect of polypeptides size on the interaction with the enzyme (Prockop and Kivirikko, 1969). We have recently (Prockop and Kivirikko, 1969) examined the effect of polypeptide size on interaction with protocollagen proline hydroxylase by using different molecular weight fractions of polyproline as inhibitors for the enzyme. The use of polyproline for this purpose had several advantages: large molecular weight polymers can be synthesized, the polymers are water-soluble in the form II conformation, and the polymers have a relatively rigid helical structure which is independent of size over a broad range (Carver and Blout, 1968).

The synthetic polymer $(Pro\text{-}Gly\text{-}Pro)_n$ was used as a substrate for protocollagen proline hydroxylase, and different molecular weight fractions of polyproline II were used as inhibitors. With 6.3 μg per milliliter of each of the polyproline fractions, the percent inhibition of the reaction increased with the size of the inhibitor polypeptide (Fig. 3). Double reciprocal plots of initial velocity and substrate concentration indicated that polyproline was a competitive inhibitor, and that the K_i values decreased with size of polymer with fractions ranging in molecular weight from 1,600 to 15,000 or 20,000 (Figs. 4 and 5). Of special interest was the observation that the K_i values decreased even when the values were expressed in molar concentration of prolyl residues (upper curve in Fig. 5), indicating that the binding of the enzyme per prolyl residues was greater with the larger molecular weight fractions than in the small ones.

Polyproline II polymers in the range of sizes used in these experiments can be regarded as having a rigid, helical structure in solution without any signicant interaction between individual chains and without any size-dependent differences in structure (for review, see Carver and Blout, 1968). Accordingly, the decrease in K_i values with size suggests that the interaction between the enzyme and the polymer has some unusual size-dependent feature. The data can be explained by any one of three possible schemes for the interaction: (A) separate short segments of the large polymers might bind several enzyme molecules; (B) the inhibitor site on the enzyme might be an extensive one, and the large polymers might have lower K_i values because they occupy more of the site; and (C) the enzyme might move laterally along the polypeptide substrates or inhibitors, and the larger polyproline fractions might be better inhibitors because on the average the enzyme spends more time in contact with them.

Scheme (A) is unlikely for several reasons. If the reaction involved non-cooperative binding of several enzyme molecules, the K_i values should be the same for large and small fractions of polyproline when the values are expressed on the basis of molar concentration of prolyl residues. As indicated (Fig. 5), K_i values expressed on this basis decreased with the size of the polymer. If there were cooperative binding to the inhibitor, it is unlikely that double reciprocal plots of initial velocity and substrate concentration would be linear, or that they would indicate a purely competitive type of inhibition. Also, the K_i values observed with cooperative binding should vary with enzyme or inhibitor concentration, but such effects could not be demonstrated (Prockop Kivirikko, 1969).

The available data do not distinguish between the other two schemes (Fig. 6). Recent physical measures on pure protocollagen proline hydroxylase by Kivirikko (1969) suggest that the enzyme is not large enough to accommodate scheme B (upper model in Fig. 6), but this scheme has not been completely excluded.

III FORMATION OF ENZYME-SUBSTRATE COMPLEXES WITH PROTOCOLLAGEN PROLINE HYDROXYLASE AND LARGE POLYPEPTIDE SUBSTRATES

As indicated above, kinetic studies with various substrates indicated that large polypeptides were better substrates for protocollagen proline hydroxylase than short poly-

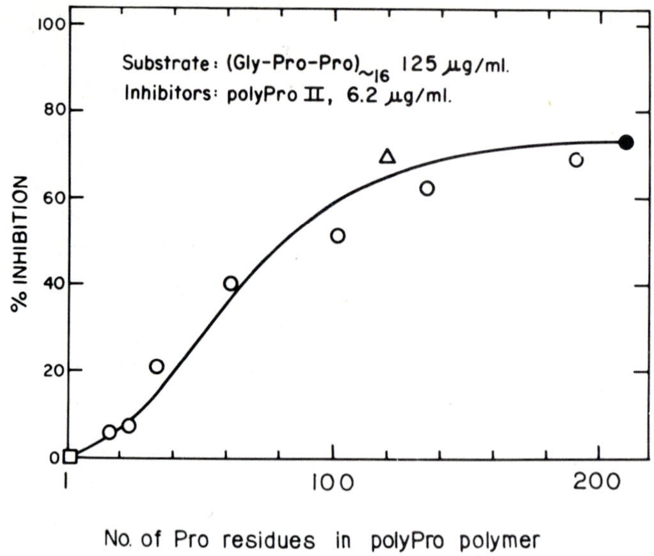

Fig. 3. Inhibition of protocollagen proline hydroxylase with polyproline (polyPro) polymers of varying sizes. The enzyme was incubated with 125 μg per ml $(Pro-Gly-Pro)_n$ as substrate and with 25 μg per ml of L-proline or 6.2 μg per ml of the polyproline polymers indicated. Symbols: L-Proline (open squares); fractions of polyproline separated by gel filtration (open circles); unfractionated polyproline with an average molecular weight of about 21,000 (filled circles). Reproduced by permission from Prockop and Kivirikko (1969).

peptides. The K_m values observed with some of the larger substrates were as low as 10^{-7} or 10^{-8} M polypeptide (Table II), indicating that the enzyme had an unusually high affinity for these polypeptides. In order to examine further the high affinity of the enzyme for large polypeptides, we prepared a protocollagen-like substrate of high specific activity, and we examined the binding of the substrate to enzyme by gel filtration (Juva and Prockop, 1969).

The substrate for these experiments was prepared by incubating cartilage from chick embryos with [^{14}C]proline and puromycin, and then extracting the non-dialyzable polypeptides which were labeled with [^{14}C]proline (Table III). Substrate prepared in this matter was heterogeneous but it was of high specific activity, its average molecular weight was greater than that of the available synthetic polypeptides,

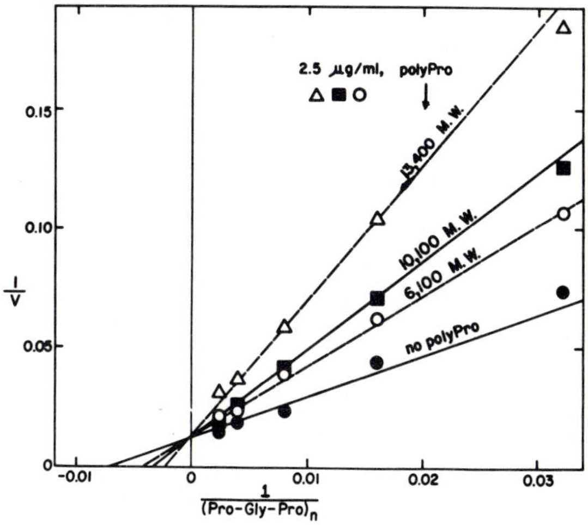

Fig. 4. Inhibition of protocollagen proline hydroxylase with polyproline fractions of varying size. The preparation of most of the polyproline polymers used in these experiments was kindly carried out for us by Dr. Volker Ganser in the laboratory of Dr. Jürgen Engel, The Max-Planck-Institut für Eiweiss-und Lederforschung, Munich, Germany. Dr. Ganzer also carried out most of the fractionations and molecular weight measurements on the polymers. Symbols: no addition of polyproline (filled circles); 2.5 μg per ml of fractionated polyproline with an average molecular weight of 6,100 (open circles); 2.5 μg per ml of fractionated polyproline with an average molecular weight of 10,100 (filled squares) and 2.5 μg per ml of fractionated polyproline with an average molecular weight of 13,400 (open triangles). Reproduced from Prockop and Kivirikko (1969).

and it could be examined readily by gel filtration.

The ^{14}C-labeled substrate was eluted in a broad peak near the middle of the total eluted volume of a Bio-Gel P-300 or Sephadex G-200 column (Fig. 7). Most of the protein and all of the enzymatic activity in partially purified preparations of protocollagen proline hydroxylase appeared near the exclusion volume of the column. When the substrate was mixed with enzyme and the mixture was chromatographed, a significant fraction of the substrate appeared with the enzyme in the exclusion volume. Rechromatography of the fractions recovered in the exclusion volume gave a single peak in the second gel column (Fig. 7). Incubation of the fractions recovered in the exclusion volume with the cofactors

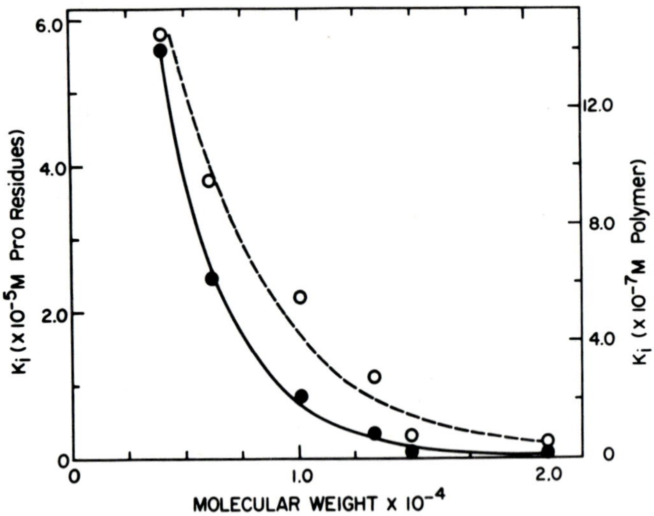

Fig. 5. Plot of K_i values against molecular weight of polyproline polymers. The preparation of most of the polyproline polymers used in these experiments was kindly carried out for us by Dr. Volker Ganser in the laboratory of Dr. Jürgen Engel, The Max-Planck-Institut für Eiweiss-und Lederforschung, Munich, Germany. Dr. Ganser also carried out most of the fractionations and molecular weight measures on the polymers. Symbols: K_i values expressed as molar concentration of prolyl (Pro) residues (open circles); and K_i values expressed as molar concentration of polyproline polymer (filled circles). Reproduced from Prockop and Kivirikko (1969).

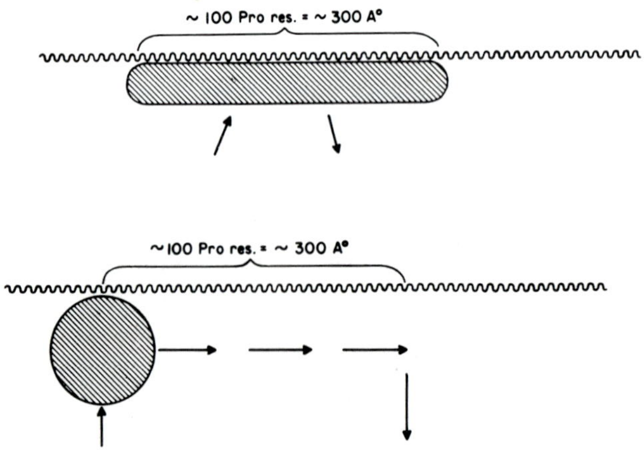

Fig. 6. Two possible schemes for the interaction between protocollagen proline hydroxylase and polyproline polymers. Brackets indicate that at least 100 prolyl residues (Pro res.) are involved in the interaction. Physical measurements on polyproline II indicate that polymers of the size used here (Figs. 3-5) are relatively rigid helices with three residues per turn and an axial spacing of about 3Å between successive residues.

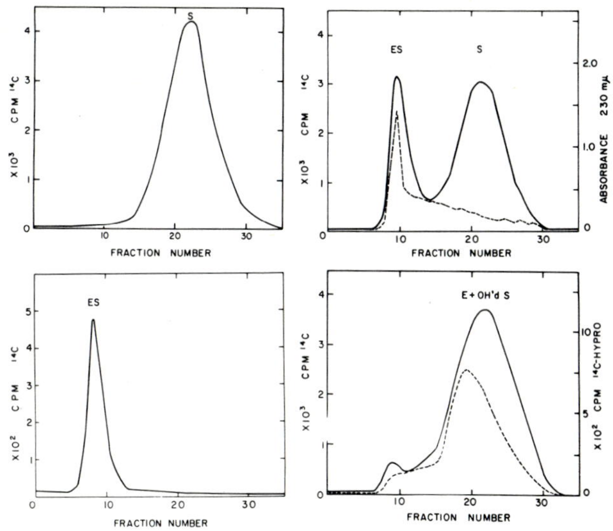

Fig. 7. Gel filtration of protocollagen proline hydroxlase and [^{14}C]proline-labeled substrate. The substrate was prepared by incubating chick embryo cartilage with [^{14}C]proline and puromycin as described in Table II.

Upper left: About 600,000 dpm of [^{14}C]proline-labeled puromycinpeptides in a volume of 0.9 ml were chromatographed on a P-300 polyacrylamide column at 4°C.

Upper right: Protocollagen proline hydroxylase, 9.4 Units, was mixed with 600,000 dpm ^{14}C-labeled puromycin-peptides, and the mixture in a final volume of 0.9 ml was chromatographed under the same conditions used in upper left figure. Symbols: (_____) ^{14}C; (-----) absorbance at 230 mμ.

Lower left: The first peak from a chromatograph similar to that shown in the upper right figure was re-chromatographed under identical conditions on a second column of P-300 Polyacrylamide.

Lower right: Gel filtration of puromycine-peptides after complete hydroxylation with protocollagen proline hydroxylase. [^{14}C]Proline-labeled puromycin-peptides, 1.2. x 10^6 dpm, were incubated at 36°C for 1 hr with 28 Units of protocollagen proline hydroxylase and the standard concentrations of the required cofactors. About 5.4 x 10^5 dpm of the reactions mixture was then chromatographed under the same conditions used in upper right figure. Symbols: (_____) ^{14}C in fraction; (-----) [^{14}]hydroxyproline in fractions. Reproduced by permission from Java and Prockop (1969).

of the reaction resulted in the synthesis of [^{14}C]hydroxyproline (Fig. 8). When the substrate was maximally hydroxylated by prior incubation with enzyme and cofactors, it was no longer bound to enzyme in the gel filtration column (Fig. 7). These results suggested that the fractions re-

TABLE II

Substrates and Inhibitors

Protocollagen Proline Hydroxylase[1]

Oligopeptide or polymer	Number of tripeptide Units[2] (n)	Conc. of tripeptide units[3] ($\times 10^{-6}$ M)	Conc. of polypeptide[3] ($\times 10^{-8}$ M)
SUBSTRATES:			
$(Ala\text{-}Pro\text{-}Gly)_n$	2		
	4	>>2,000	>>100,000
		1,600	40,000
$(Pro\text{-}Pro\text{-}Gly)_n$[4]	5	500	10,000
	10	200	2,000
	20	(80)[5]	(400)[5]
Ascaris cuticle			
Collagen (denatured)	∿200	40	20
Vertebrate protocollagen	∿330	3	1
INHIBITORS:			
$(Gly\text{-}Pro\text{-}Gly)_n$	4	120	3,000
$(Pro\text{-}Pro\text{-}Pro)_n$	4	>200	>5,000
	∿21	130	60
	∿71	7	1

[1]For experimental conditions and sources of data see Kivirikko et al. (1969).

[2]The number of tripeptide units for the Ascaris cuticle collagen, vertebrate protocollagen, and the polyproline polymers were estimated from their average molecular weights.

[3]K_m and K_i values are presented both in molar concentration of tripeptide units and in molar concentration of polypeptide. Neither method of expressing the values is entirely satisfactory on a theoretical basis, since a single encounter between enzyme and polypeptide probably involves more than one tripeptide unit but less than the complete length of a large polypeptide (see text).

[4]Values shown were obtained with polytripeptides prepared by Drs. Y. Kishida and S. Sakakibara, The Peptide Center,

Osaka University, Osaka, Japan, with a new modification of a Merrified-type procedure. The polytripeptides have physical properties (Sakakibara, Kishida, Kikuchi, Sakai and Kakiuchi, 1968) closer to those of collagen than polymers of the same sequence prepared by the tetraethyl pyrophosphite procedure (Engel, Kurtz, Katchalski and Bergen, 1966). The K_m values shown are lower than those previously obtained with $(Pro\text{-}Gly\text{-}Pro)_n$ of about the same molecular weight synthesized by polymerization techniques (Kivirikko and Prockop, 1967c; Hutton et al., 1968; Kivirikko et al., 1969).

[5]K_m values too low for accurate measurement.

---

covered in the exclusion volume contained enzyme-substrates complexes, and further study of the systems confirmed this conclusion (Juva and Prockop, 1969).

The formation of E-S complexes in the system was independent of the flow-rate of the column, and it did not require addition of ascorbate, α-ketoglutarate, or ferrous iron to dialyzed preparations of the enzyme. Accordingly, freely dissociable forms of these cofactors and cosubstrates were not essentially for the binding step.

Under the conditions employed (Fig. 7) the enzyme in the isolated complexes was readily saturated with substrate (Juva and Prockop, 1969). It was difficult, however, to saturate the substrate with enzyme. With high concentrations of enzyme relative to substrate, the initial velocity for the reaction was greater than the initial velocity observed with the isolated E-S complexes (Fig. 8), and the results suggested therefore that one molecule of polypeptide substrate could bind more than one molecule of enzyme.

The E-S complexes were in relatively rapid equilibrium with free enzyme and substrate, since addition of a competing polypeptide produced a dissociation of the initial complexes in the gel filtration column (not shown), and a rapid inhibition of the hydroxylation of the substrate (Fig. 9). Most of the substrate was still recovered in the E-S complexes under conditions where the over-all concentration of substrate was about 2×10^{-10} M polypeptide (Juva and Prockop, 1969). The enzyme was saturated with substrate under these conditions, and the mean concentration of free substrate was less than 25% of the total, or less than 0.5×10^{-10} M poly-

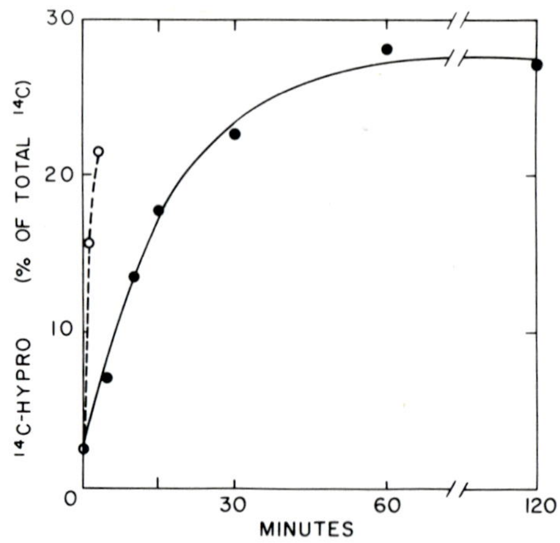

Fig. 8. Synthesis of [^{14}C]hydroxyproline with isolated enzymesubstrate complexes. In one experiment fractions containing E-S complexes from a chromatograph similar to that shown in Fig. 7 (upper right) were pooled and divided into seven equal fractions each containing 19,000 dpm ^{14}C. The fractions were than incubated at 37°C with 2 mM ascorbic acid, 0.5 mM α-ketoglutarate, and 0.04 mM $FeSO_4$ for the times indicated. In a second experiment 31,000 dpm of unfractionated substrate was incubated under the same conditions with a large excess (117 Units) of protocollagen proline hydroxylase. Symbols: (0.___0) [^{14}C]hydroxyproline synthesized with isolated E-S complexes; (0----0) [^{14}C]hydroxyproline synthesized when the ratio of enzyme: substrate was much greater than in the isolated E-S complexes. Reproduced with permission from Juva and Prockop (1969).

peptide. On the assumption that the concentrations of both free enzyme and free substrate were 0.5×10^{-10} M or less, the results suggested that the dissociation constant expressed on the basis of the <u>molar concentration of substrate polypeptide</u> was no greater than $(0.5 \times 10^{-10})^2/(1.5 \times 10^{-10})$, or about 2×10^{-11}M.

Although the affinity of the enzyme for the initial substrate was high enough to permit demonstration of E-S complexes by gel filtration, the affinity decreased markedly after partial hydroxylation of the substrate. After one-sixth of the available [^{14}C]proline in the substrate was converted to [^{14}C]hydroxyproline, it was no longer possible to demonstrate E-S complexes in the gel filtration column (Fig. 10).

The results of these experiments allow us to add several features (Fig. 11) to the two schemes suggested for the inter-

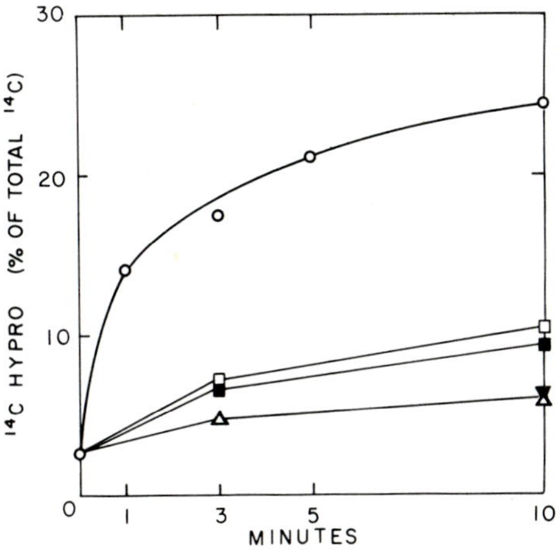

Fig. 9. Effect of polyproline and denatured Ascaris collagen on the synthesis of [^{14}C]hydroxyproline after the formation of the initial E-S complexes. Each sample contained 39 Units of protocollagen proline hydroxylase in 7.1 ml buffer with 2 mM ascorbic acid and 0.0 mM $FeSO_4$. The samples were equilibrated at 37°C, and then 34,00 dpm of puromycin-peptides in 0.1 ml buffer was added. After 60 seconds, the reaction was initiated by the addition of 0.8 ml of 4 mM α-ketoglutarate. Symbole: (open circles) synthesis of [^{14}C] hydroxyproline under control conditions; (filled squares) 200 g per ml polyproline with an average molecular weight of about 12,000 added to the enzyme 30 seconds before the substrate peptides were added; (open squares) 200 g per ml of polyproline were added 30 seconds after the substrate was added; (filled triangles), 200 g per ml of denatured and carboxymethylated collagen from Ascaris cuticle were added to the enzyme 30 seconds before the substrate peptides were added; (open triangles) 200 g per ml of denatured and carboxymethylated collagen from Ascaris cuticle added 30 seconds after the substrate. Reproduced with permission from Juva and Prockop (1969).

action between the enzyme and large polypeptides (Fig. 6). Although the interaction involves a large segment of the polypeptide, a single encounter between enzyme and a large substrate does not result in the complete hydroxylation of the substrate, and multiple encounters are required to complete reaction. This is true even though recently completed experiments (Juva and Prockop, (1969) in dicate that a single encounter between enzyme and a large substrate usually results in the hydroxylation of several prolyl residues. Since the initial velocity of the reaction increases when the ratio of

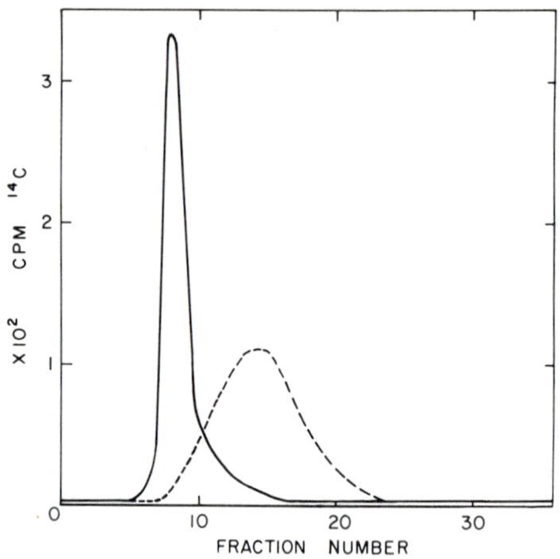

Fig. 10. Re-chromatography after partial hydroxylation of the substrate in the enzyme-substrate complexes. A mixture of 3.6 x 10^5 dpm puromycin-peptides and 12 units of protocollagen proline hydroxylase were chromatographed under the same conditions as were used in Fig. 7 (upper right). The E-S fractions were pooled, and one-third of the sample was incubated at 37°C for 1 hr with 2 mM ascorbic acid, 0.04 mM $FeSO_4$; and no α-ketoglutarate. Another third of the sample was incubated at 37°C for 1 hr with 2 mM ascorbic acid; 0.04 mM $FeSO_4$; and 0.001 mM α-ketoglutarate so that about one-sixth the available substrate [^{14}C]proline was converted to [^{14}C]hydroxyproline. Symbols: (___) sample incubated without α-ketoglutarate; (---) sample incubated with limiting amount of α-ketoglutarate. Reproduced with permission from Juva and Prockop (1969

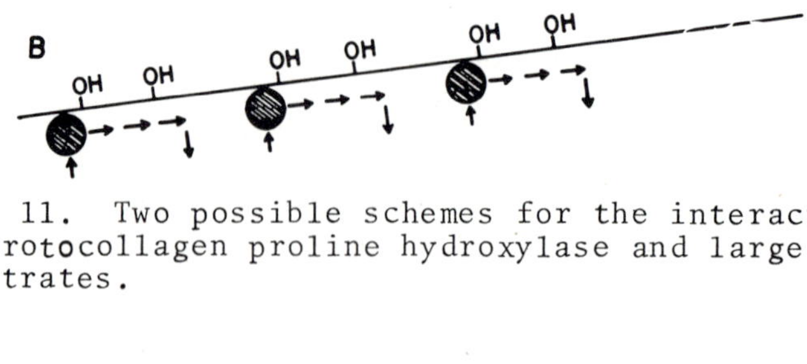

Fig. 11. Two possible schemes for the interaction between protocollagen proline hydroxylase and large polypeptide substrates.

TABLE III

PREPARATION OF SUBSTRATE FOR ISOLATION

OF ENZYME-SUBSTRATE COMPLEXES BY GEL FILTRATION

	100 x [^{14}C]Hypro/total ^{14}C
Initial value	2-3%
After maximum hydroxylation with protocollagen hydroxylase	20-24%

Cartilage from 10-day-old chick embryos was incubated with [^{14}C]proline and 40 μg per ml puromycin for 4 hr. The tissues were homogenized in distilled water, and the homogenates were exhaustively dialyzed. The dialyzed sample was boiled for 5 min, and centrifuged at 100,000 x g for 60 min. The 100,000 x g supernate was used as a substrate for the synthesis of [^{14}C]hydroxyproline. The molecular weights of labeled polypeptides inthe preparation ranged from about 10,000 to almost 100,000. From 50 to 60% of the total ^{14}C was [^{14}C]proline in protocollagen-like polypeptides (Juva and Prockop, 1969).

enzyme to substrate is greater than 1:1 (Fig. 8), a large substrate polypeptide can simultaneously accommodate more than one enzyme molecule.

IV INCORPORATION OF PROLINE ANALOGUES INTO PROTOCOLLAGEN AND THE HYDROXYLATION OF THE ANALOGUE-CONTAINING PROTOCOLLAGEN

A number of proline analogues are now available and several of these have been shown to be incorporated into protein in place of proline (Fowden and Fichmond, 1963; Fowden, Neale and Tristram, 1963). We have been particularly interested in examining the effects of three proline analogues on collagen synthesis: L-azetidine-2-carboxylic acid, *cis*-4-flouroproline, and 3,4-dehydroproline (Fig. 12).

When incubated with embryonic cartilage, all three of the analogues were incorporated into protocollagen and collagen in place of proline. In the case of L-azetidine-2-carboxylic acid and 3,4-dehydroproline, incorporation of the analogues was demonstrated by using ^{14}C-labeled preparations of the analogues, and recovering [^{14}C]azetidine carboxylic acid (Takeuchi and Prockop, 1969), and [^{14}C]3,4-dehydroproline (Rosenbloom and Prockop, 1968b) from protein fractions of the tissue. Although an earlier report (Gottlieb, Fujita, Udenfriend and Witkop, 1965) indicated that both _trans_- and _cis_-isomers of 4-flouroproline were incorporated into collagen, our results suggested that only _cis_-4-flouroproline was incorporated by our system (Takeuchi and Prockop, 1969), and it clearly had more dramatic effects than _trans_-4-flouroproline (see below).

Incorporation of any of the three analogues by cartilage had a number of effects on the cellular system and on the nature of the collagen which was synthesized. One interesting effect was that the altered collagen containing the analogues was not extruded from the cells at a normal rate. Autoradiographs prepared from embryonic cartilage incubated with [^{3}H] proline indicated that after 2 hr a large fraction of the collagen containing _L_-azetidine carboxylic acid or _cis_-fluoroproline remained intracellular, whereas most of the normal collagen synthesized by control tissues was in the extracellular matrix (Fig. 13). Similar results were obtained with 3,4-dehydroproline (Rosenbloom and Prockop, 1969b). Control experiments indicated that the analogues themselves did not affect the rate of extrusion of normal collagen by the cells (Takeuchi, Rosenbloom and Prockop, 1969).

Another feature of the collagen synthesized in the presence of these three analogues was that the proline and lysine in the molecule were under-hydroxylated and under-glycosylated compared to normal collagen synthesized by the same tissue (Table IV). The analogues themselves did not inhibit the protocollagen hydroxylases, and gel filtration indicated that the altered collagen synthesized in the presence of the analogues was of the same size as normal collagen from the same tissue (Rosenbloom and Prockop, 1969b). Further observations indicated that the under-hydroxylation of the collagen was explained by the fact that the analogue residues in the procollagen adversely affected the interaction between the polypeptide and the protocollagen hydroxylases. Kinetic studies

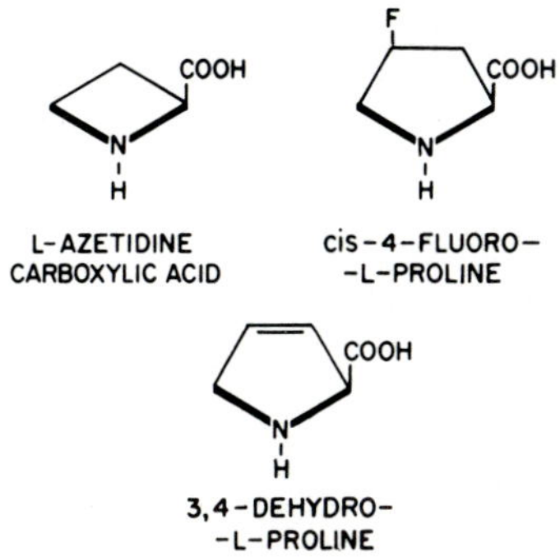

Fig. 12. Three proline analogues which are incorporated into protocollagen and collagen (see text).

with purified protocollagen proline hydroxylase indicated a significant difference between the ratio of $K_m:V_{max}$ for normal protocollagen and for protocollagen containing either L-azetidine carboxylic acid or cis-fluoroproline (Takeuchi and Prockop, 1969). 3,4-Dehydroproline had a more marked effect than the other two analogues on the extent of hydroxylation and glycosylation of the collagen (Table IV).

Incubation of the collagen containing, 3,4-dehydroproline with excess protocollagen proline hydroxylase and the required cofactors indicated that two-thirds of the normally available prolyl sites in protocollagen are totally inaccessible to the enzyme (Rosenbloom and Prockop, 1969b). Related to this finding was the observation that substrate containing, 3,4-dehydroproline formed ES-complexes with protocollagen proline hydroxylase even after the substrate was maximally hydroxylated with the enzyme (Fig. 14). Accordingly, the presence of 3,4-dehydroproline in the substrate molecule greatly increased the affinity of the enzyme for the polypeptide.

V CONSEQUENCES OF THE PROPERTIES OF THE PROTOCOLLAGEN HYDROXYLASES

The studies to date on protocollagen proline hydroxylase have indicated that it belongs to a new and interesting class of hydroxylases requiring O_2, ferrous iron, and α-ketoglutarate (Lindbald, Lindstedt, Tofft, M. and Lindstadt, 1969). In addition, the work has demonstrated that it belongs to the limited group of enzymes which function with macromolecular

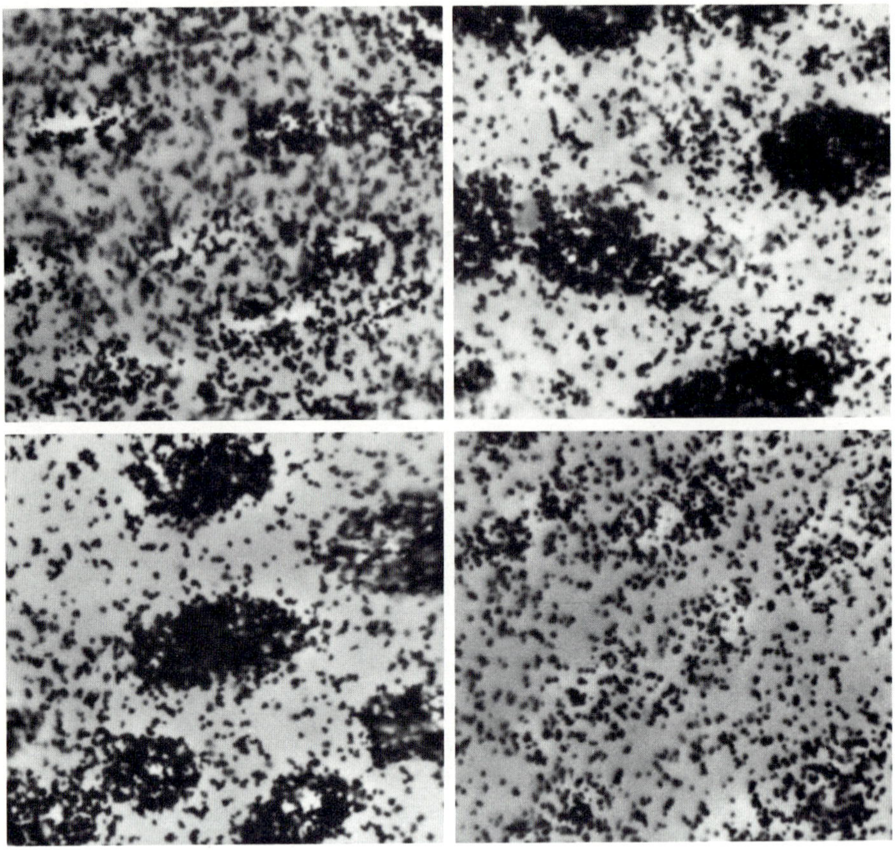

Fig. 13. Autoradiographs prepared after incubating embryonic cartilage with [^{3}H] proline for 2 hr. For conditions, see Takeuchi et al. (1969).

Upper left: Control tissue with grains fairly evenly distributed over cells and extracellular matrix.

Upper right: Tissue incubated with 200 μg per ml L-azetidine carboxylic acid. A major part of the grains are still over the cells.

Lower left: Tissue incubated with 200 μg per ml cis-4-fluoro-L-proline. A major part of the grains are still over the cells.

Lower right: Tissue incubated with 200 μg per ml trans-4-fluoro-L-proline. Distribution of grains is indistinguishable from control tissue, and chemical data suggest trans-isomer is not incorporated into protein (Takeuchi & Prockop, 1969). Reproduced by permission (Takeuchi et al, 1969).

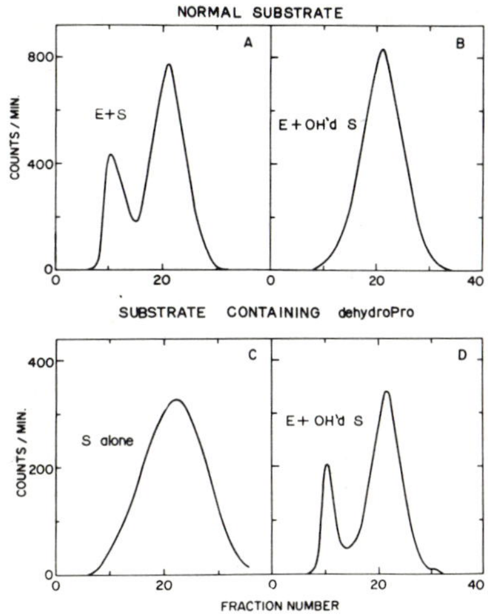

Fig. 14. Formation of E-S complexes with substrate containing 3,4-dehydroproline (dehydroPro). A: Control showing formation of E-S complexes as in Fig. 7.above. B: Dissociation of the E-S complexes after hydroxylation of the normal substrate. C: Gel filtration of substrate containing 3,4-dehydroproline. Substrate was prepared as described in Table II except that incubation medium contained 200 μg per ml 3,4-dehydro-DL-proline in addition to puromycin and [^{14}C] proline. D: Gel filtration of enzyme and substrate after substrate containing 3,4-dehydroproline was maximally hydroxylated by incubation with excess protocollagen proline hydroxylase and the required cofactors.

substrates. One of the consequences of the unusual properties of the enzyme is that conditions which do not affect other cellular processes may have profound effects on the amount and kind of collagen synthesized. For example, limiting the concentration of O_2 or ferrous iron clearly reduces the amount of hydroxyproline and hydroxylysine introduced into the molecule in short-term experiments with isolated tissues (above). Introduction of any of three proline analogues into protocollagen had similar effects. The presence of the analogue resulted in the synthesis of an altered collagen, but within the time periods studied there was no marked effect on other cellular processes, such as the rate of protein synthesis or the rate of the extrusion of normal collagen (Takeuchi and Prockop, 1969; Takeuchi et al., 1969).

A further consequence of the unusual properties of protocollagen proline hydroxylase is that even under what might be considered optimal conditions, it is difficult for the enzyme to synthesize homogeneous molecular products. Multiple collisions between enzyme and substrate are required to complete the hydroxylation of a large polypeptide substrate, but the affinity of the enzyme for the substrate markedly decreases after partial hydroxylation of the substrate (Fig. 10). The hydroxylation of any given substrate molecule, therefore, becomes less and less favorable as the reaction proceeds. It is apparent that very high concentrations of enzyme, or long reaction times would be necessary to give complete hydroxylation of all the available prolyl residues in large substrates. From the point of view of the reaction mechanism, it is not surprising that the hydroxylation of specific prolyl residues is variable and incomplete (Bornstein, 1967; Piez, 1969; Butler, 1969, Rhoads, Udenfriend and Bornstein, 1969). In fact, from this viewpoint an interesting question is why the hydroxylation is usually completed to about the same high level in most vertebrate collagens? The answer to this question is probably that most cells synthesizing collagen contain relatively large concentrations of the enzyme compared to substrate concentrations, and that the protocollagen substrate spends a relatively long time in the same compartment as the enzyme (Fig. 2). Even with these favorable conditions, the hydroxylated polypeptides produced by the reactions are highly heterogeneous (Bornstein, 1967; Miller, Lane and Piez, 1969; Piez, 1969; Butler, 1969). Although a separate enzyme is probably involved (Weinstein, Blumenkrantz and Prockop, 1970), the enzymatic reaction for the hydroxylation of lysine in protocollagen probably involves mechanisms similar to the hydroxylation of proline, and it also gives a heterogeneous product (Miller et al., 1969; Butler 1969). Since the glycosylating reactions depend on the presence of hydroxylysine in the molecule, heterogeneity introduced at the level of the lysine hydroxylase is probably compounded during the glycosylating reactions. These considerations as well as other features of the biosynthetic pathway (Fig. 1) suggest that the amount and specific kind of collagen

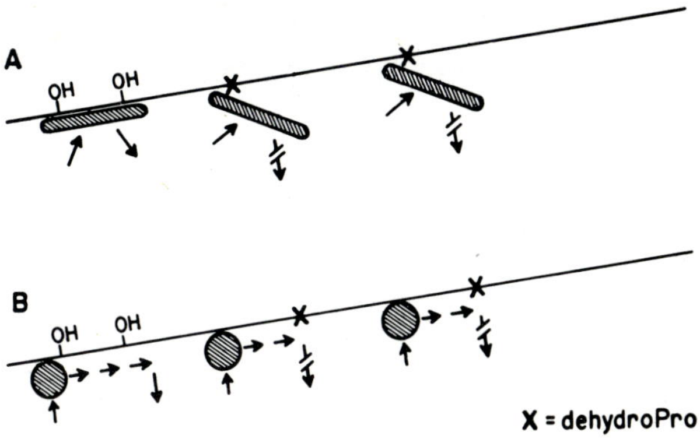

Fig. 15. Two possible schemes for the interaction between protocollagen proline hydroxylase and a large polypeptide substrate containing 3,4-dehydroproline.

synthesized by a cell is affected by an unexpectedly large number of factors. It seems probable that the kind of collagen synthesized would be affected by variations in the rate of protocollagen synthesis, the intercellular levels of the hydroxylating enzymes, the levels of the glycosylating enzymes, and the nature of the membrane barrier which apparently limits the rate of extrusion until the molecule has reached a given level of "completeness". Other factors such as the intracellular concentrations of O_2, iron, α-ketoglutarate, UDP-galactose, and UDP-glucose may be rate limiting under some conditions, and, therefore, they might also affect the extent to which collagen is hydroxylated and glycosylated before it is extruded.

ACKNOWLEDGEMENTS

Recent work from our own laboratory reported in this paper was carried out in collaboration with Drs. Joel Rosenbloom, Kari Kivirikko, Nelly Blumenkrantz, Kale Juva, and Mrs. Elsa Weinstein. The work was supported in part by N.I.H. research grants HD-107, AM-5459, GM-14583, and FR-107 from the U.S. Public Health Service.

TABLE IV

SYNTHESIS OF ALTERED COLLAGENS CONTAINING PROLINE ANALOGUES

Analogue added	100 x [^{14}C]Hypro/ total ^{14}C*	100 x [^{14}C]Hylys/ total ^{14}C$^+$	100 x Glyc. [^{14}C]Hylys/ total ^{14}C$^+$
None	19-20	12-14	6.4-8.4
Azetidine carboxylic acid	13.4	6.3	2.1
cis-Fluoro-proline	12.3	8.4	4.4
3,4-Dehydro-proline	7.5	3.5	1.0

*Results obtained when [^{14}C]proline was used. Values are based on [^{14}C] hydroxyproline (Hypro) and total ^{14}C in dialyzed homogenates of the tissue. Essentially all of total ^{14}C was accounted for by [^{14}C]proline and [^{14}C]hydroxyproline.

$^+$Results obtained when [^{14}C]lysine was used. Values are based on total [^{14}C]hydroxylysine (Hylys), glycosylated [^{14}C]hydroxylysine (Glyc. Hylys), and total ^{14}C in dialyzed homogenates of the tissue. Essentially all the total ^{14}C was accounted for by total [^{14}C]hydroxylysine and [^{14}C]lysine.

REFERENCES

Bekhor, I., Mohseni, A. and Bavetta, L.A. (1966). _Fed. Proc._ 25, 715.

Bhatnagar, R.S. and Prockop, D.J. (1966). _Biochim. Biophys. Acta_ _130_, 383.

Bhatnagar, R.S. Kivirikko, K.I., Rosenbloom, J. and Prockop, D.J. (1967a). _Proc. Nat. Acad. Sci., Wash._ _58_, 248.

Bhatnagar, R.S., Rosenbloom, J., Kivirikko, K.I., and Prockop, D.J. (1967b). _Biochim. Biophys. Acta_ _149_, 273

Blumenkrantz, N., Rosenbloom, J. and Prockop, D.J. (1969). _Biochim. Biophys. Acta_ (In press.)

Bornstein, P. (1967). _Biochemistry_ _6_, 3082.

Bosmann, H.B. and Eylar, E.H. (1968). _Biochem. Biophys. Res. Commun._ _30_, 89.

Butler, W.T. (1969). This book, p. 149.

Butler, W.T. and Cunningham, L.W. (1966). J. Biol. Chem. 241, 3882.

Carver, J. and Blout, J.R. (1968). In Treatise on Collagen vol. 1, p. 441. Ed. by Ramachandrandran, G.N. Academic Press, London and New York.

Chvapil, M. (1968). In International Review of Connective Tissue Research, vol. 4, p. 67. Ed. by Hall, D.A. Academic Press, London and New York.

Chvapil, M. and Jackson, D.S. (1964). In Fourth National Collagen Symposium, Hluboka, Czechoslovakia; Collagen Curr. 5, 161.

Chvapil, M., Holecková, E., Cmuchalová, B., Kobrle, V. and Hurych, J. (1962). Exptl. Cell Res. 26, 1.

Cooper, G. and Prockop, D. J. (1968). J. Cell Biol. 38, 523.

Eastoe, J.E. (1961). Biochem. J. 79, 648.

Engel. J., Kurtz, J., Katchalski, E. and Berger, A. (1966). J. Mol. Biol. 17, 255.

Fernandez-Madrid, F. (1967). J. Cell Biol. 33, 27.

Fessler, J.H. (1969). This book, p. 457.

Fowden, L. Richmond, M.H. (1963). Biochim. Biophys. Acta 71, 459.

Fowden, L., Neale, S. Tristram, H. (1963). Nature 199, 35.

Gallop, P. (1969). This book, p. 179.

Goldberg, B., Green, H. (1967). J. Mol. Biol. 26, 1.

Gottlieb, A.A., Fujita, Y., Udenfriend, S. Witkop, B. (1965). Biochemistry 4, 2507.

Gould, B.S. (1968). In Treatise on Collagen, vol. 2, p. 139. Ed. by Ramachandran and Gould, B.S. Academic Press, London and New York.

Gould, B.S. and Manner, G. (1962). In Collagen, Central Leather Research Institute Symp. p. 311. (1960, Madras, India) Interscience, New York.

Gribble, T.J., Comstock, J.P. and Udenfriend, S. (1969). Arch. Biochem. Biophys. 129, 308.

Hagopian, A., Bosmann, H.B. and Eylar, E.H. (1968). Arch Biochem. Biophys. 128, 387.

Hurych, J. and Chvapil, M. (1965). Biochim. Biophys. Acta 97, 361.

Hurych, J. and Nordwig, A. (1967). Biochim. Biophys. Acta 140, 168.

Hutton, J.J., Marglin, A., Witkop, B., Kurtz, J., Berger, A. and Udenfriend, S. (1968). Arch. Biochem. Biophys. 125, 779.

Hutton, J.J., Tappel, A.L. and Udenfriend, S. (1967). Arch Biochem. Biophys. 118, 231.

Juva, K. and Prockop, D.J. (1966). J. Biol. Chem. 241, 4419.

Juva, K. and Prockop, D.J. (1969). J. Biol. Chem. (In press)

Juva, K., Prockop, D.J., Cooper, G. and Lash, J.W. (1966). Science 152, 92.

Kivirikko, K.I. (1963). Acta Physiol. Scand. 60, Suppl. 219, 1.

Kivirikko, K.I. (1969). This book, p. 411.

Kivirikko, K.I. and Prockop, D.J. (1967a). Arch. Biochem. Biophys. 118, 611.

Kivirikko, K.I. and Prockop, D.J. (1967b). Biochem. J. 102, 432.

Kivirikko, K.I. and Prockop, D.J. (1967c). J. Biol. Chem. 242, 4007.

Kivirikko, K.I., Bright, H.J. and Prockop, D.J. (1968). Biochim. Biophys. Acta 151, 558

Kivirikko, K.I., Prockop, D.J., Lorenzi, G.P. and Blout, E.R. (1969). J. Biol. Chem. 244, 2755.

Kretsinger, R.H., Manner, G., Gould, B.S. and Rich, A. (1964). Nature, Lond. 202, 438.

Lindbald, B., Lindstedt, G., Tofft, M. and Lindstedt, S. (1969). J. Am. Chem. Soc. 91, 16.

Lowther, D.A., Green, N.M. and Chapman, J.A. (1961). J. Biophys. Biochem. Cytol. 10, 373.

Lukens, L.N. (1965). J. Biol. Chem. 240, 1661.

Lukens, L.N. (1966). Proc. Nat. Acad. Sci., Wash. 55, 1235.

Malt, R.A. and Speakman, P.T. (1964). Life Sci. 3, 81

Malt, R.A. and Speakman, R.T. (1965). Surgery 58, 248

Manner, G. and Gould, B.S. (1963). Biochim. Biophys. Acta 72, 243.

Manner, G., Kretsinger, R.H., Gould, B.S. and Rich, A. (1967). Biochim. Biophys. Acta 134, 411.

Manning, J.M. and Meister, A. (1966). Biochemistry 5, 1154

Miller, E.J., Lane, J.M. and Piez, K.A. (1969). Biochemistry 8, 30.

Nordwig, A. and Pfab, F.K. (1968). Biochim. Biophys. Acta 154, 603.

Prockop, D.J. and Juva, K. (1965a). Biochem. Biophys. Res. Comm. 18, 54.

Prockop, D.J. and Juva, K. (1965b). Proc. Nat. Acad. Sci., Wash. 53, 661.

Prockop, D.J. and Kivirikko, K.I. (1969). J. Biol. Chem. (In press)

Piez, K. (1969). This book, p. 117.

Revel, J.P. and Hay, E.D. (1963). Z. Zellforsch. Mikroskop. Anat. 61, 110.

Rhoads, R., Udenfriend, S. and Bornstein, P. (1969). Federation Proc. 28, 408.

Rosenbloom, J. and Prockop, D.J. (1960a). In Repair and Regeneration, The Scientific Basis of Surgical Practice, p. 117. Ed. by Dunphy, J.E. and Van Winkle, Jr., W. McGraw-Hill Book Company, New York.

Rosenbloom, J. and Prockop, D.J. (1969b). Federation Proc. 28, 408.

Rosenbloom, J., Bhatnagar, R.S. and Prockop, D.J. (1967). Biochim. Biophys. Acta 149, 259.

Ross, R. and Benditt, F.P. (1965). J. Cell Biol. 27, 83.

Takeuchi, T. and Prockop, D.J. (1969). Biochim. Biophys. Acta 175, 142.

Takeuchi, T., Rosenbloom, J. and Prockop, D.J. (1969). Biochim. Biophys. Acta 175, 156.

Sakakibara, S., Kish da, Y., Kikuchi , Y., Sakai, R. and Kakuchi, K. (1968). Bull. Chem. Soc. Japan 41, 1273.

Saltpepter, M.M. (1968). J. Morph. 124, 387.

Spiro, R.G. and Spiro, M.J. (1968). Federation Proc. 27, 245.

Weinstein, E., Blumenkrantz, N. and Prockop, D.J. (1970). Biochim. Biophys. Acta (In press)

Winslow, R.M. and Ingram, V.M. (1966). J. Biol. Chem. 241, 1144.

Woessner, J.F., Jr. and Boucek, R.J. (1961). Arch. Biochem. Biophys. 93, 85.

Yarmolinsky, M.D. and de la Haba, G.L. (1959). Proc. Nat. Acad. Sci. Wash. 45, 1721.

BIOSYNTHESIS OF HYDROXYPROLINE IN COLLAGEN

Sidney Udenfriend

The unique presence of hydroxyproline in collagen, where it represents a substantial proportion of the protein, has attracted the attention of many investigators for some time. Today, although we have learned a great deal about the mechanisms involved in the biosynthesis of hydroxyproline, we have yet to determine what function is served by this imino acid. Unlike hydroxylysine, hydroxyproline does not serve as a site for covalent linkage to other substituents. Furthermore, the unique physical properties of the tropocollagen molecule seem to be adequately explained by its total imino acid content, the ring hydroxyl making no apparent contribution to the various models which have been proposed Ramachandran (1967). Nevertheless, one must conclude that hydroxyproline formation serves some important function in the biosynthesis of collagen because of the widespread occurrence of a unique and elaborate catalytic system for proline hydroxylation in all collagen forming tissues.

It has been established that in animals hydroxylation of proline to hydroxyproline occurs after the proline has been incorporated into peptide linkage (Udenfriend, 1966). There have been several reports of hydroxylation of t-RNA proline, but Urivetsky, Frei and Meilman (1966) showed that the apparent t-RNA-hydroxyproline is not incorporated into collagen. Present studies are concerned with the nature of the hydroxylating enzyme, the mechanism of hydroxylation, and substrates for hydroxylation, natural and synthetic. The development of sensitive and rapid methods for measuring enzyme activity has been a most important factor in these studies.

I COLLAGEN PROLINE HYDROXYLASE

Before the enzyme had been detected in homogenates, it had already been established with the aid of [$^{18}O_2$] that it was an oxygenase (Fujimoto and Tamiya, 1962; Prockop, Kaplan and Udenfriend, 1962). At the homogenate level, requirements for Fe^{++} and ascorbic acid were shown (Peterkofsky and Udenfriend, 1965; Prockop and Juva, 1965). The Fe^{++} chelating agent α,α-dipyridyl is a potent inhibitor of the hydroxylase (Hurych and Chvapil, 1965) and a reagent for preparing "unhydroxylated collagen". As purification of the enzyme proceeded, another dialyzable factor became limiting. This turned out to be a α-ketoglutarate (Hutton, Tappel, and Udenfriend, 1967). Further purifications of the enzyme have been carried out in the presence of optimal amounts of Fe^{++}, ascorbic acid, and α-ketoglutarate.

Collagen proline hydroxylase is found in essentially all animal tissues. Initial attempts at purification were carried out with chick embryos. More recently, we have been using fetal rat skin because homogenates are richer in the enzyme and contain less interfering substances. Robert Rhoads in our laboratory has purified the fetal rat skin enzyme to where it shows essentially one component on disc-gel electrophoresis and shows only a minor component on sedimentation in the ultracentrifuge. The latter studies yielded an $S_{20,w}$ value of 7S, suggesting a molecular weight of about 150,000 for a symmetrical molecule. The ultraviolet and visible absorption spectra of the purified enzyme show only the bands characteristic of protein thereby ruling out a flavin cofactor.

The purified enzyme shows almost a total dependence on Fe^{++}, ascorbic acid and α-ketoglutarate. The requirements for Fe^{++} is a specific one. Studies with various iron chelators suggest that the iron binds at a hydrophobic site on the enzyme. The role of ascorbic acid in the overall mechanism must be reconsidered now that the enzyme has been purified. Even in crude preparations it was obvious that the requirement was not specific and ascorbic acid analogues and tetrahydropteridines were shown to be fairly effective (Peterkofsky and Udenfriend, 1965). As the enzyme was purified, additional factors were required for maximal activity. Low concentrations of dithiothreotol and certain proteins, particularly bovine serum albumin (BSA), were found to stimulate activity markedly when added during incubation (Rhoads, Hutton and Udenfriend, 1967). These findings point to a sulfhydryl involvement near the active site. More direct evidence for this was recently reported by Popenoe, Aronson and Vas Slyke (1969) With appropriate amounts of Fe^{++}, α-ketoglutarate, bovine serum albumin and dithiothreotol, ascorbic acid can be omitted and most of the activity retained. Thus, ascorbic acid is not an obligatory requirement of collagen proline hydroxylase as are Fe^{++} and α-ketoglutarate. It remains to be determined whether ascorbic acid or some other reducing agent is utilized for proline hydroxylation in vivo. Hydroxyproline formation is diminished in scorbutic guinea pigs. However, it has been shown that protein synthesis is markedly diminished in scorbutic guinea pigs and that their tissues contain less proline hydroxylase. The enzyme deficiency can account for the diminution in hydroxyproline formation.

The finding that α-ketoglutarate is an obligatory requirement for proline hydroxylation revealed an entirely new class of oxygenases. The initial report concerning its role in proline hydroxylation (Hutton, Tappel and Udenfriend, 1967) led other investigators to look into its possible role in other hydroxylation reactions. α-Ketoglutarate has now been shown to be an obligatory requirement for several enzymes involved in the oxidative demethylation of thymine to uracil (Abbott, Schandl, Lee, Parker and Midgett, 1967) and in the hydroxylation of γ-butyrobetaine to carnitine (Lindstedt, Lindstedt, Midtwedt and Tofft, 1967). These enzymes also show a requirement for Fe^{++} and ascorbic acid.

With the purified fetal rat skin enzyme it was possible to show that α-ketoglutarate is stoichiometrically consumed during the hydroxylation and that succinate and CO_2 are formed in amounts equivalent to the newly formed hydroxyproline (Rhoads and Udenfriend, 1968). Lindstedt, Lindstedt, Olander and Tofft, 1968) reported similar findings with the γ-butyrobetaine hydroxylase. It appears, therefore, that we are dealing with a new class of enzymes in which α-ketoglutarate decarboxylation is coupled to hydroxylation of an aliphatic substrate. The purified proline hydroxylase does not, however, resemble α-ketoglutarate dehydrogenase in its spectral or physical properties. It will be interesting to see just how this coupling does occur. Recently Holme, Lindstedt, Lindstedt and Tofft (1968) ruled out succinic semi-aldehyde as an intermediate in γ-butyrobetaine hydroxylation.

II SUBSTRATES OF THE ENZYME

In the earliest studies proline hydroxylase activity was detected by conversion of [^{14}C] proline residues to [^{14}C] hydroxyproline residues in "unhydroxylated collagen" in microsomes (Peterkofsky and Udenfriend, 1965). Subsequently it was shown that labelled unhydroxylated collagen, prepared by incubating chick embryo with radioactive proline in the presence of an iron-chelator, could be gelatinized and used as a soluble substrate (Prockop and Juva, 1965). Such solubilized unhydroxylated collagen was shown to contain Gly-Pro-Pro sequences which could be hydroxylated stoichiometrically to Gly-Pro-Hyp sequences (Hutton, Kaplan and Udenfriend, 1967). Synthetic peptide polymers of the type (Gly-Pro-Pro)$_n$ prepared by condensation of the tripeptide were first shown to be substrates of collagen proline hydroxylase by Kivirikko and Prockop (1970). This was soon verified in our laboratories (Hutton et al., 1968). With synthetic peptides ranging in size from about 1200 to 8000 (obtained by fractionation of the polymer) it was shown that the enzyme affinity (apparent Km) increased

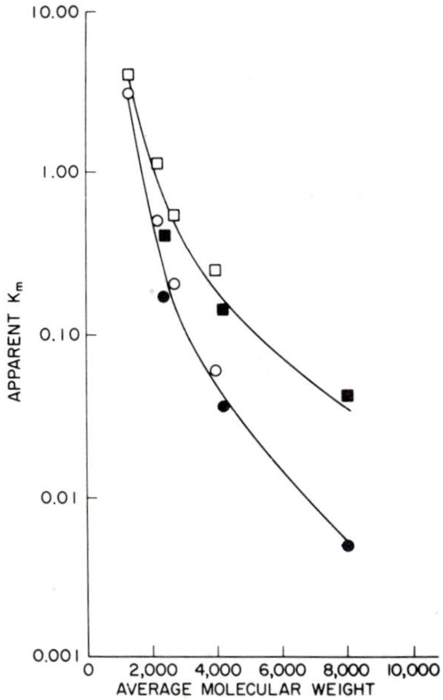

Fig. 1. Plot of apparent Km as a function of weight-average molecular weight of fractions of (3,4-H-Pro-Gly-Pro)n. The Km is plotted on a log scale; molecular weight on a linear scale. Circles indicate Km in mM; squares indicate Km in mg/ml. The open symbols represent an experiment using the first batch of polymer and a rather crude enzyme preparation; the filled symbols represent another experiment using a second batch of polymer and more highly purified enzyme (Hutton et al., 1968).

markedly with size, Fig. 1. Free proline and the tripeptide, Gly-Pro-Pro, are not substrates. Activity can just be detected with the hexapeptide and becomes meaningful at the nonapeptide stage. Arnold Marglin (Hutton et al., 1968) synthesized such sequences by the solid state procedure to make certain that the observed activity obtained with the smaller peptides isolated by fractionation of the polymerized tripeptide was not due to contamination with small amounts of high molecular weight material. In these studies it became evident that with increasing size of peptides, the V_{max} remains constant as the apparent Km decreases.

Rat skin collagen and tail-tendon collagen have been shown to contain sequences which are incompletely hydroxyl-

TABLE I

Comparative Hydroxylation of α_1-CB_2 Peptide from Tendon and Skin

	Tendon peptide (11.7 nmoles)		(Skin peptide (11.0 nmoles)	
Enzyme (ng)	New hydroxyproline (nmoles)	Theoretical maximum (%)	New hydroxyproline (nmoles)	Theoretical maximum (%)
0	0	50	0	82
115	12.1	--	0.9	--
585	19.4	--	2.8	--
1150	21.9	81	4.4	88

ated at the hydroxyproline residues (Bornstein, 1967). One of the cyanogen bromide peptides (α_1CB_2) varies considerably in the degree of hydroxylation at a number of residues which appear susceptible of hydroxylation. When samples of the same cyanogen bromide derived sequence (α_1CB_2) from rat skin and rat tail collagen were treated with purified fetal rat skin hydroxylase, they were both hydroxylated to almost the same limiting value (Rhoads, Udenfriend and Bornstein, 1969) (Table I). It is evident, therefore, that factors other than primary sequence limit the degree of hydroxylation of these residues in the two collagens in vivo and limit them to different extents.

Ascaris cuticle collagen contains very little hydroxyproline and consequently unusually large amounts of proline. For some reason little hydroxylation of susceptible proline residues occurs in Ascaris cuticle in vivo. It is not surprising that Ascaris cuticle collagen (denatured) serves as an excellent substrate of collagen proline hydroxylase (Rhoads and Udenfriend, 1968; Fujimoto and Prockop, 1968). In recent studies in our laboratory we have found that all samples of isolated collagen can be further hydroxylated following denaturation. As shown in Table II, some colla-

TABLE II

Increased Hydroxylation of Collagen from Various Sources*

Experiment	Source	New Hydroxylation (nmoles/50 μg protein)	% Increases (based on Hyp)
1	Rat tail tendon	8.7	18.7
	Calf skin	8.3	15.5
2	Rat tail tendon	5.4	11.6
	Rat skin	4.5	9.5
	Carp swim bladder	4.8	12.3
	Dogfish skin	2.9	9.4
	Rabbit skin	3.0	6.1
	Chick skin	2.9	5.3
	Guinea pig skin	2.2	4.6

*Rhoads, R.E. for Ph.D. thesis preparation

gens can be hydroxylated an additional 15%.

Elastin, which seems to contain small amounts of hydroxyproline, is very rich in glycine and proline. We have shown that proline residues in oxalate extracted elastin[1] can be hydroxylated by rat skin proline hydroxylase (Rhoads and Udenfriend, 1969).

A most interesting observation was that the vasoactive peptide bradykinin can serve as a substrate o proline hydroxylase (Rhoads and Udenfriend, 1969). In this peptide whose structure is H-Arg^1-Pro^2-Pro^3-Gly^4-Phe^5-Ser^6-Pro^7-Phe^8-Arg^9-OH only the proline at position 3 is hydroxylated by the enzyme. Thus, a -Gly-X-Pro*-sequence is not apparently the recognition sequence for hydroxylation. It may be that the glycine subsequent to the susceptible proline (the one at position 4) may serve the key role in en-

*The sample of oxalate extracted elastin was kindly supplied by Dr. Jerome Gross, Harvard Medical School.

zyme recognition (-X-Pro*-Gly). Thus far, all susceptible sites for proline hydroxylation have been of the sequence A-X-Pro-Gly- where A has generally been glycine but can be replaced by arginine in bradykinin. The residue at X is not critical, and hydroxylation has been shown to occur in sequences where X is proline, alanine, leucine, or methionine. Since hundreds of bradykinin analogues have been prepared, this series of peptides should prove useful in elucidating the recognition site for the enzyme.

III REGULATION OF PROLINE HYDROXYLATION

Several approaches to the problem of regulation have been made. Mussini et al. (1967) showed that the hydroxylase is widely distributed in all animal tissues and is present in much higher concentration in tissues of younger animals. This corroborates data obtained by measuring urinary excretion of hydroxyproline (Lindstedt and Prockop, 1961). In scorbutic guinea pigs, it was shown that the proline hydroxylase activity was diminished consistent with the previously observed decline in hydroxyproline content. However, the diminished enzyme activity was shown to be due largely to diminished synthesis of the hydroxylase rather than to the ascorbic acid deficiency (Mussini et al., 1967). These findings, together with the previously discussed non-specificity of ascorbic acid as reductant with purified enzyme, suggest that the observed diminution in collagen hydroxyproline in scurvy is most likely related to a disturbance in protein synthesis.

Another observation made by Mussini et al.,(1967) is that following a lag period, proline hydroxylase activity increases markedly at the site of a wound. The enzyme is highly localized to the wound site and remains elevated until the healing process is over. The factors involved in increasing and decreasing proline hydroxylase and the other enzymes related to collagen production at the site of a wound are undoubtedly related to fibroblasts. This led to an investigation of fibroblasts in tissue culture.

With cultured L-929 cells, it was shown that the appearance of proline hydroxylase activity lags behind cell growth and protein synthesis. In fact, hydroxylase activity does not appear until the end of the log-phase of growth. In the early log-phase before hydroxylase activity appears, "unhydroxylated collagen" is formed and is secreted into the medium. Towards the end of the log-phase, proline hydroxylase activity appears and the cells now contain hydroxylated collagen. A most interesting finding is that the appearance of hydroxylase in the late log-phase is not due to new protein synthesis but involves activation of an inactive form of the enzyme to an active form. The activation was shown to be related to cell crowding and may be related to some metabolites which accumulate in the medium with increased cell density.

Another important point concerns the normal site of hydroxylation within cells. Complete unhydroxylated chains or molecules (protocollagen) have been postulated as obligatory intermediates in collagen biosynthesis (Kivirikko and Prockop, 1967). It has been suggested that protocollagen must be released from the polysomes before hydroxylation occurs. Hydroxylation has also been suggested to be a requirement before collagen chains can be released from cells (Kivirikko and Prockop, 1968). All these points must be questioned. Totally unhydroxylated collagen can appear experimentally (anaerobically, in the presence of Fe^{++} chelators, tissue culture) or normally as in Ascaris cuticle. However, evidence has been presented by Meister and Manning (1966) and Bavetta (1967) that hydroxylation occurs on nascent chains. R. Miller in our laboratory has shown that [^{14}C] hydroxyproline appears on nascent chains when guinea pig granuloma minces are incubated with [^{14}C] proline corroborating the findings of Meister and Manning (1966). Ronald Miller has recently shown that the [^{14}C]hydroxyproline is associated with polysomes in a form which can be released by puromycin and activating enzymes.

Hydroxylation appears to be a process independent of collagen chain formation. Under normal circumstances both occur concurrently. It appears, however, that even under normal conditions many proline residues in primary sequences which should be susceptible to hydroxylation are not hydroxylated. In the case of Ascaris cuticle collagen or L-929 cells in the early log-phase of tissue culture, chains are completed essentially unhydroxylated. All of the above forms of collagen, hydroxylated fully, partially, or not at all can be secreted by the cells.

IV PROCEDURES FOR ASSAY OF COLLAGEN PROLINE HYDROXYLASE

Finally, and most important, are the methods which have been developed to assay proline hydroxylase (Udenfriend, Rhoads and Roberts, in press). The first method developed in our laboratory involved incorporation of [^{14}C] proline into an unhydroxylated collagen (Peterkofsky and Udenfriend, 1965). The latter was then used as a substrate and the activity determined by the appearance of [^{14}C] hydroxyproline measured by the method of Peterkofsky and Prockop (1962). Modifications of this procedure have been used in many other laboratories. However, the procedure is lengthy since it involves protein hydrolysis and separation of hydroxyproline from proline.

When 3,4[^{3}H]proline became available, it suggested the possibility of following hydroxylation of the 4-position of proline by release of tritium and its appearance as tritium water (THO). Attempts in this laboratory to use proline-3,4 [^{3}H] to follow the overall formation of hydroxyproline in collagen of intact chick embryos were not successful because considerable amounts of tritium water were formed as a result of other routes of proline metabolism. However, Stone and Meister (1962) were successful in using proline-3,4[^{3}H] to study the overall process (chain formation plus hydroxylation) in intact guinea pig granuloma cells. This was possible because in granuloma cells, degradative metabolism of proline is low compared to its utilization in collagen synthesis. In cell-free systems, the measurement of THO released from 3,4[^{3}H]proline became meaningless since it resulted from more than one enzyme reaction. Only when 3,4[^{3}H] proline was incorporated into a protein substrate of proline hydroxylase could it be used to assay the enzyme. Hutton et al. (1966) labelled unhydroxylated chick embryo collagen with 3,4[^{3}H]proline and showed that the THO released with purified hydroxylase was equivalent to the appearance of 3[^{3}H]hydroxyproline. The tritium assay is rapid since the tritium water can be rapidly distilled from all other radioactive materials. Although the tritium release assay made possible many advances in our laboratory, it has certain limitations which are due to the necessity for preparation of a labelled substrate. One can use synthetic substances (Gly-Pro-Pro*)n with the Pro* being 3,4,[^{3}H]proline. However, this is a costly and exacting procedure and does not generally lead to very active peptide substrates because their weight is seldom above 8000. Alternatively, one can incubate collagen forming tissues (intact cells) with 3,4[^{3}H]proline in the presence of α,α dipyridyl and extract the unhydroxylated collagen (Hutton, Tappel and Udenfriend, 1966) as was done by Hutton et al. (1967). Highly active substrates can be prepared in this manner; however, there is variability in the activity from preparation to preparation. The important limitation is that the 3,4[^{3}H]proline is diluted to a large and unknown extent during the preparation and the substrate extract is composed of trace amounts of newlyformed, labelled collagen extracted along with large amounts of unlabelled old collagen. It is apparent, therefore, that labelled "substrate" prepared in this manner either with [^{14}C] or tritium can be used only to determine relative activity in terms of c.p.m. They cannot be used stoichiometrically.

The demonstration that α-ketoglutarate is stoichiometrically converted to succinate and CO_2 during the hydroxylation of peptidyl proline to hydroxyproline (Rhoads and Udenfriend, 1968) has made it possible to devise a simple and stoichiometric procedure for assaying collagen proline hydrosylase. The specific activity of 1[^{14}C]α-ketoglutarate (commercially available) is established and then any unlabelled substrate can be utilized in the assay. We have found that oxidized and denatured Ascaris cuticle collagen is an excellent substrate; only microgram quantities are needed per assay. It should soon be possible to obtain this material from commercial sources.

Following incubation, the resulting [$^{14}CO_2$] is trapped on base impregnated filter paper in the incubation vessel and transferred to a vial containing an appropriate scintillation cocktail. Under these conditions [$^{14}CO_2$] evolution is a direct measure of the moles of hydroxyproline formed. This is the simplest and most direct assay which has been developed for proline hydroxylase. It too, has limitations. In intact cells and whole homogenates there will obviously be substantial liberation of [$^{14}CO_2$] by other pathways of α-ketoglutarate metabolism. In partially purified preparations of fetal rat skin, this extraneous [$^{14}CO_2$]evaluation has been of a magnitude which can be corrected for in controls. As enzyme purification proceeds, the only interference will be from similar α-ketoglutarate requiring hydroxylases. In collagen forming tissues there are three such hydroxylations which are known to occur: proline-4-hydroxylase, lysine-5-hydroxylase, and proline-3-hydroxylase. The significance of the latter is not yet known and the amount formed in vivo is small. The most purified preparations of the fetal rat skin peptidyl proline hydroxylase prepared in this laboratory do not hydroxylate lysine (Rhoads and Udenfriend, 1969).

ACKNOWLEDGEMENT

This is mainly a summary of work in the author's laboratory. The data represent studies that have been carried out over the last few years with several collaborators. These include: John J. Hutton, Arnold Marglin, Robert E. Rhoads, John T. Gribble, John P. Comstock, Ronald Miller, and Nelson Roberts.

REFERENCES

Abbott, M.T., Schandl, E.K., Lee, R.F., Parker, T.S. and Midgett, R.J. (1967). Biochem. Biophys. Acta 132, 525.

Bekhor, I. and Bavetta, L.A. (1967). P.N.A.S. 58, 2351.

Bornstein, P. (1967). Biochemistry 6, 3082.

Fujimoto, D. and Prockop, D.J. (1968). J. Biol. Chem. 243, 4138.

Fujimoto, D. and Tamiya, N. (1962). Biochem. J. 84, 333.

Holme, E., Lindstedt, G., Lindstedt, J. and Tofft, M. (1968). Febs Letters 2, 29.

Hurych, J. and Chvapil, M. (1965). Biochem. Biophys. Acta 97, 361.

Hutton, J.J., Kaplan, A. and Udenfriend, S. (1967). Arch. Biochem. Biophys. 121, 384.

Hutton, J.J., Marglin, A., Witkop, B., Kurtz, J., Berger, A. and Udenfriend, S. (1968). Arch. Biochem. Biophys. 125, 779.

Hutton, J.J., Tappel, A.L. and Udenfriend, S. (1966). Anal. Biochem. 16, 384.

Hutton, J.J., Tappel, A.L. and Udenfriend, S. (1967). Arch. Biochem. Biophys. 118, 231.

Kivirikko, K.I. and Prockop, D.J. (1967a). J. Biol. Chem. 242, 4007.

Kivirikko, K.I. and Prockop, D.J. (1967b.) Biochem. J. 102, 432.

Lindstedt, G., Lindstedt, S., Midtwedt, T. and Tofft, T. (1967). Biochem. J. 103, 19P.

Lindstedt, G., Lindstedt, S., Olander, B. and Tofft, M. (1968). Biochem. Biophys. Acta 158, 503.

Lindstedt, S. and Prockop, D.J. (1961). J. Biol. Chem. 236, 1399.

Manning, J.M. and Meister, A. (1966). Biochem. J. 5, 1154.

Mussini, E., Hutton, J.J. and Udenfriend, S. (1967). Science 157, 927.

Peterkofsky, B. and Prockop, D.J. (1962). Anal. Biochem. 4, 400.

Peterkofsky, G. and Udenfriend, S. (1965). Proc. Nat'l. Acad. Sci., U.S. 53, 335.

Popenoe, E.A., Aronson, R.B. and Vas Slyke, D.D. (1969). Arch. Biochem. Biophys. (133, 286).

Prockop, D.J. and Juva, K. (1965). Proc. Nat'l. Acad. Sci., U.S. 53, 661.

Prockop, D., Kaplan, A. and Udenfriend, S. (1962). Biochem. Biophys. Res. Commun. 9, 162.

Ramachandran, G.N. (1967). In Treatise on Collagen, Vol. I., p. 103. Ed. by Ramachandran, G.M. Academic Press, New York.

Rhoads, R.E., Hutton, J.J. and Udenfriend, S. (1967). Arch. Biochem. Biophys. 122, 805.

Rhoads, R.E. and Udenfriend, S. (1968). Proc. Nat'l. Acad. Sci., U.S. 60, 1473.

Rhoads, R.E. and Udenfriend, S. (1969). Arch. Biochem. Biophys. 133, 108.

Rhoads, R.E., Udenfriend, S. and Bornstein, P. (1969). Fed. Proc. 28, 408.

Stone, N. and Meister, A. (1962). Nature 194, 555.

Udenfriend, S. (1966). Science 15,

Udenfriend, S., Rhoads, R.E. and Roberts, Methods in Enzymology (in press).

Urivetzky, M., Frei, J.M. and Meilman, E. (1966). Arch. Biochem. Biophys. 117, 224.

THE BIOSYNTHESIS OF INTERMOLECULAR CROSSLINKS IN COLLAGEN

A.J. Bailey, Catherine M. Peach and L. J. Fowler

The unique properties that allow collagenous tissue to act as the major supporting tissue of the body are largely dependent on the high tensile strength of the collagen fibers. It is generally accepted that this property is dependent on the biosynthesis of a system of covalent crosslinks between the tropocollagen molecules making up the fibres (for reviews see Bailey, 1968a; Ramachandran, 1967). The need for these crosslinks can be demonstrated very dramatically in experimental lathyrism, when injection of β-amino propionitrile (βAPN) into animals results in tissues that have no mechanical strength yet the collagen aggregates normally and appears to be chemically identical (Levene and Gross, 1959). Examination of the denatured forms, however, revealed the absence of the stabilizing interchain crosslinking system (Martin, Lewis and Piez, 1963). In contrast, native collagen is highly crosslinked, resulting in a protein that is virtually insoluble without denaturation, thus increasing the difficulties involved in the study of the chemistry of such a protein. Despite these difficulties a great deal has been learned of the nature of these crosslinks. The present paper considers the evidence available on the various crosslinks and presents some recent studies on the nature of the crosslinks stabilizing the collagen fibre.

I THE NATURE OF THE INTRAMOLECULAR CROSSLINKS

The simplest collagen system to work with is the small proportion extractable as tropocollagen by the use of acid buffers. The three peptide chains of tropocollagen may be crosslinked intramolecularly by covalent bonds to give β components (2 α chains) and ∂ components (3 α chains). From a comprehensive study of these solutions, largely due to Piez (1968) and his colleagues (Bornstein and Piez, 1960; Piez et al., 1968), considerable information is now available on the biosynthesis of the intramolecular crosslinks.

Although the actual crosslink has not yet been isolated and characterised, substantial indirect evidence indicated that both the β11 and β12 crosslinks were derived from two lysine aldehydes, i.e. α amino adipic δ - semialdehyde, by an aldol condensation (Bornstein and Piez, 1960). The crosslink was shown to be present in the N-terminal telopeptide region of the tropocollagen molecule. Further studies also established the presence of the biosynthetic precursor of the crosslink, the lysine aldehyde (allysine), in the telopeptide region. Examination of lathyritic collagen clearly demonstrated that injection of βAPN inhibits the conversion of this telopeptide lysine to allysine. Sequence analyses of the N-terminal peptide from lathyritic collagen from rat skin showed that the lysine residue occurs at position 9 from the N-terminal pyrrolidone carboxylic acid on the α1 chain and at position 6 on the α2 chain (Piez et al., 1968).

An alternative intramolecular crosslink has been proposed by Gallop and his coworkers (Blumenfeld and Gallop, 1966). The crosslink di-enosaline was isolated from reduced gelatin and identified from the fragmentation pattern in the mass spectrometer. No molecular mass ion by high resolution mass spectrometry was reported. The relationship of the compound to lathyrism, and indeed its involvement as a crosslink was not demonstrated.

Despite the absence of conclusive evidence the most satisfactory explanation is that the biosynthesis of the intramolecular crosslinks is mediated through the enzymic oxidation of the ε-NH_2 group of a specific lysine in the telopeptide region. The reaction of two of these lysines to give an aldol then constitutes the crosslink. The aldol may dehydrate spontaneously or exist in vivo as the aldol and dehydrate under the acid conditions used to isolate the peptide contain-

Aldol Crosslink (Bornstein and Piez, 1960)

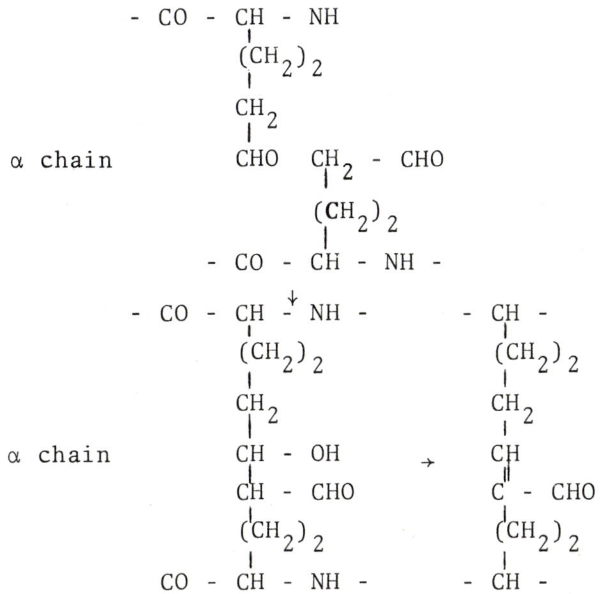

Di-enosaline Crosslink (Blumenfeld and Gallop, 1966)

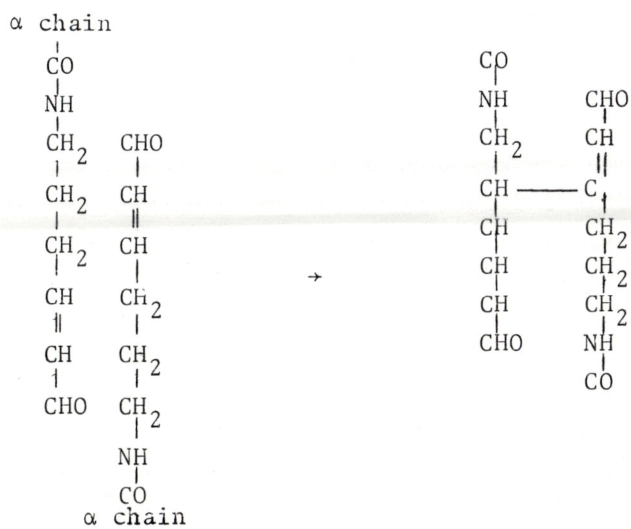

ing the crosslink.

II THE NATURE OF THE INTERMOLECULAR CROSSLINKS

From a functional point of view it is unlikely that this intramolecular crosslink contributes to the stability of the larger structural units of the fibril since it must be the bond between molecules that prevents slippage of adjacent molecules (Fig. 1). In fact, the function of the intramolecular crosslink has not been established although it may be an intermediate, the aldehyde function reacting further to give an intermolecular crosslink. Unfortunately, the study of these intermolecular crosslinks is more difficult since their presence results in an insoluble collagen. Although there is convincing evidence on the chemical nature of the intramolecular crosslink, there is little known of the chemistry of the intermolecular crosslinks. The ability of lathyrogens to render tissue fragile and inhibit the synthesis of all crosslinks strongly suggest a common biosynthetic route for both the intra- and intermolecular crosslinks involving the lysine derived aldehydes.

The existence of covalent intermolecular crosslinks has been demonstrated by Veis and his colleagues (Veis and Ansey, 1965) by examination of the denatured collagen derived from the more insoluble bovine collagens. The presence of double and triple chain components was observed and these were identified as $\beta 22$ and $\gamma 222$. These components could not have arisen intramolecularly from tropocollagen molecules containing two $\alpha 1$ chains and one $\alpha 2$ chain. Furthermore, a series of components of higher molecular weight than γ were present, thus confirming the existence of intermolecular covalent crosslinks. Our recent studies have been concerned with at attempt to study the nature of the intermolecular bonds and subsequently isolate and identify them.

We initially employed a different approach to the question of crosslinks by studying the stability of the intact fibres to gain an insight into the nature and stability of the intermolecular bond, on the assumption that changes in the tensile strength must reflect changes in the intermolec-

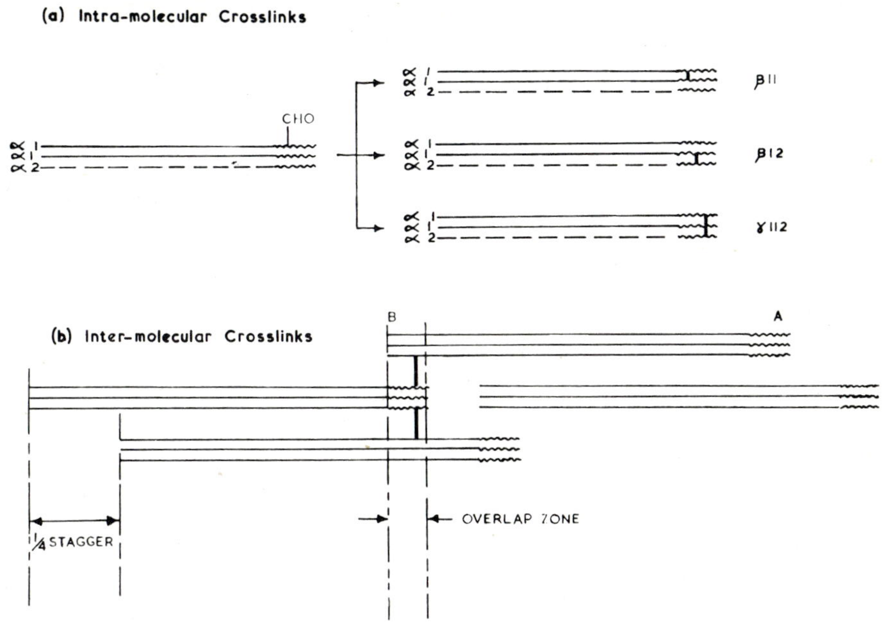

Fig. 1. Diagrammatic representation of the location of (a) the intra-molecular crosslinks; and (b) the possible location of the crosslinks along adjacent tropocollagen molecules arranged within a fibril in the quarter-stagger alignment.

ular bond.

Following the studies of Harkness and Harkness (1966) on the effect of various chemical reagents on the mechanical strength of skin, the increased solubility of rat skin in amino β thiols demonstrated by Nimni (1966), and the studies on the cleavage of β bonds with the lathyritic agent βAPN (Fessler and Bailey, 1966), we studied the effect of different reagents on the strength of intact collagen fibres. We used rat-rail tendon as a reasonably pure form of collagen rather than the complex tissue skin used by the other workers. EDTA and mercaptoethanol affected little change in the fibre strength suggesting that crosslinks involving metals, or disulphide bonds, do not play a major role in the stability of the fibre. The most effective compounds were those shown by Harkness and his colleagues to have a dramatic effect on the more complex tissue skin. However, the most significant observation was that reduction of the fibres with sodium borohydride completely inhibited their susceptibility to these reagents. Since it is unlikely that borohydride would introduce crosslinks the effect of reduction must be to stabilize labile bonds already present. Given the presence of lysine-derived aldehydes in the telopeptide region of the tropocollagen molecule a possible reaction of these aldehydes is with the εNH_2 of a lysine residue to form an aldimine bond or Schiff base. From the observations on the stability of the bond in the intact fibre particularly the ready cleavage by acids, bases and α-amino β thiols, the reversible nature of the bonds and the ability to be stabilized by reduction, it was proposed that the predominant intermolecular bonds in rat tail tendon collagen involved an aldimine bond (Bailey, 1967). During the course of this work, Tanzer (1967) similarly concluded that reprecipitated collagen fibrils were stabilized by a Schiff base. However, we have confined ourselves to intact fibres since the small proportion of tropocollagen extracted is hardly representative of the crosslinking systems in vivo.

III ISOLATION AND CHARACTERISATION OF THE LABILE INTERMOLECULAR CROSSLINKS

Confirmation of the proposed aldimine bond must lie in the isolation and identification of the crosslink.

To distinguish the crosslink from other amino acids reduction was carried out with tritiated sodium borohydride prior to acid hydrolysis and separation of the amino acids subsequently carried out with a Technicon automatic amino acid analyzer. Compounds such as aldehydes and aldimine bonds should then be readily detectable from the tritium activity. About six radioactive peaks were obtained (Bailey, 1968b). Before attempting the formidable task of isolating and identifying the radioactive components under the peaks it was considered necessary to demonstrate their involvement in the crosslinking system and their relationship to the intermolecular bonds cleaved by α-amino β thiols and dilute acids.

Reduction before and after treatment with D-penicillamine established that Peaks B and C (Fig. 2) were absent in the latter case demonstrating that these components were involved in the cleavage of intermolecular crosslinks by α-amino β thiols (Bailey and Lister, 1968). Similarly, reduction of tropocollagen, i.e. in the absence of intermolecular crosslink again demonstrated the absence of Peaks B and C and suggested that the peaks eluting near tyrosine were involved in the intramolecular crosslink. These results confirmed that peaks B and C were related to the labile intermolecular bonds. Reduction of thermally denatured fibres demonstrated that the bonds were also thermally labile (Bailey and Lister, 1968). Reduction of highly purified reprecipitated collagen fibres produced a basically similar pattern, although more complex and the peaks B and C were less dominant, presumably due to rupture of the native labile bonds during dissolution and the less precise orientation of the fibrils. The importance of the alignment of the molecules in the fibre and their ability to be rendered insoluble by borohydride reduction has been very neatly demonstrated by Tanzer (1968).

The relationship of these peaks to lysine was established by injection of [^{14}C]lysine into rats and subsequent reduction of the collagen fibres with nonradioactive borohydride. All the major reducible peaks were again radioactive confirming that they were derived from lysine.

Fraction B was, therefore, isolated and its identity established by mass spectrometry. The tetra-trifluoracetyl methyl ester of the isolated compound was prepared, and exact mass measurement by peak matching against perfluorokerosene gave a mass ion of 703.44. Comparison of its electrophoretic mobility with lysine, lysinonorleucine and merodesmosine indicated that the material was slightly less basic than lysinonorleucine. These results identified the compound as Nε-(5-amino 5 carboxy pentanyl)-hydroxylysine or, using the trivial nonmenclature, hydroxylysinonorleucine (Bailey and Peach, 1968).

Confirmation of the structure was achieved by chemical synthesis of the compound from dihydropyran (Bailey and Peach, 1968). δ-Bromobutylhydantoin was first synthesised from

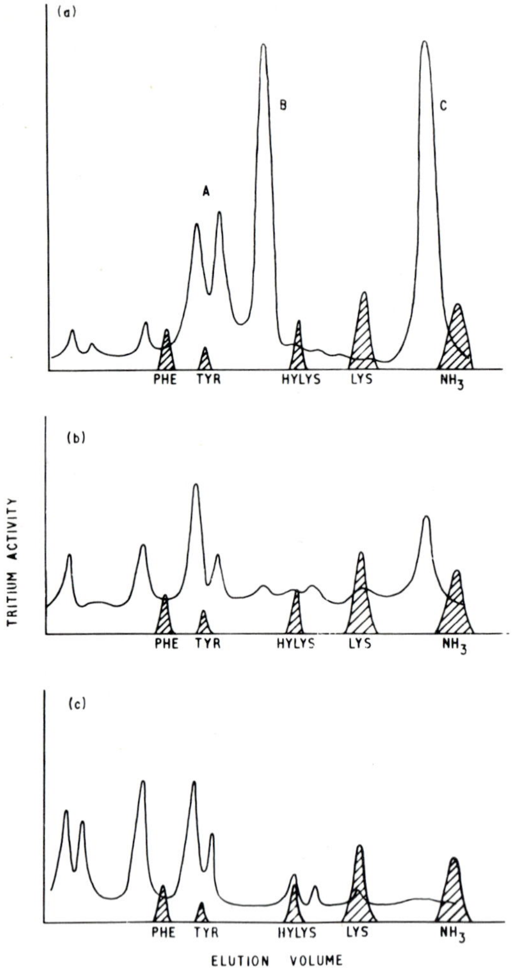

Fig. 2. Elution patterns of acid hydrolysates of rat tail tendon collagen reduced with tritiated sodium borohydride. (a) Native collagen fibres: (b) fibres reduced after treatment with D-penicillamine (0.01 M); and (c) reduced tropocollagen solution.

dihydropyran and then reacted with hydroxylysine α-N-trifluoroacetate. The product was hydrolysed with 2 N NaOH and purified by fractionation on the amino acid analyzer. The properties of the purified compound were identical to the material isolated from reduced collagen. The material eluted as a twin peak in the Beckman amino acid analyzer (Fig. 3). The presence of isomers is to be expected since the molecule can undergo epimerisation at C-2 during acid hydrolysis analogous to hydroxylysine.

Since the compound appears in the acid hydrolysis products only after reduction it must be concluded that it exists in the collagen fibre in the labile aldimine bond form, i.e. Δ 6, 7-dehydro hydroxylysinonorleucine. The

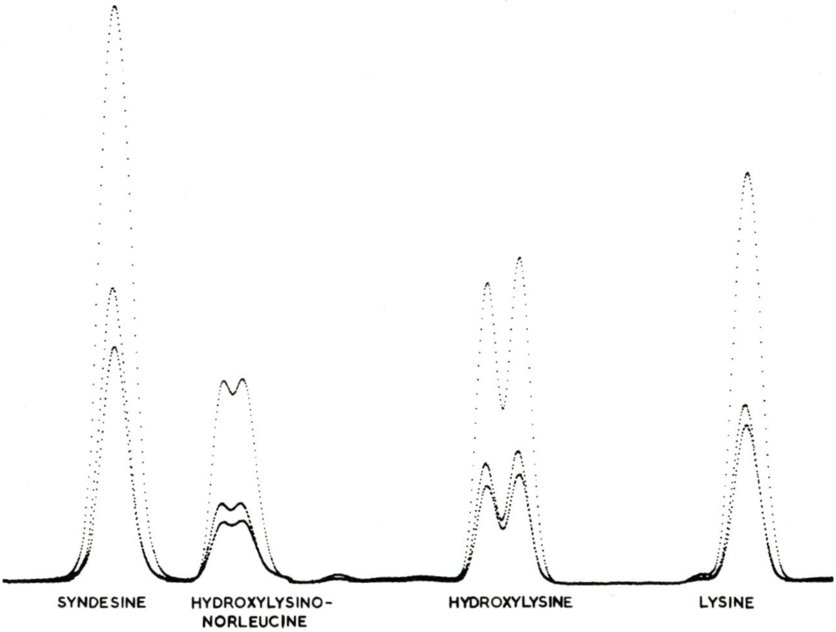

Fig. 3. Elution pattern depicting the position, on an extended basic column of the Beckman autoanalyzer, of the reduced forms of the two isolated crosslinks.

compound could be formed biosynthetically through the condensation of the carbonyl function of the allysine, with the ε-NH_2 group of hydroxylysine.

The precursor, allysine, was also isolated and identified in its reduced form, hydroxynorleucine, from the telopeptides cleaved from the tropocollagen molecule by digestion with chymotrypsin or pepsin. Since amino acid sequence determinations have demonstrated the absence of hydroxylysine in the telopeptide region of rat skin and tendon collagen (Piez et al., 1968), it may be concluded that the isolated crosslink exists as an intermolecular bond between the telopeptide region of one molecule and the body of a second adjacent molecule. This would be consistent with the generally accepted "quarter stagger" of the molecules in the native fibres. However, the actual location of the crosslink remains to be elucidated.

The identification of the second labile intermolecular crosslink peak C (Fig.22) remains to be completed, preliminary studies suggest that it is more complex than hydroxylysinonorleucine and may crosslink several molecules together.

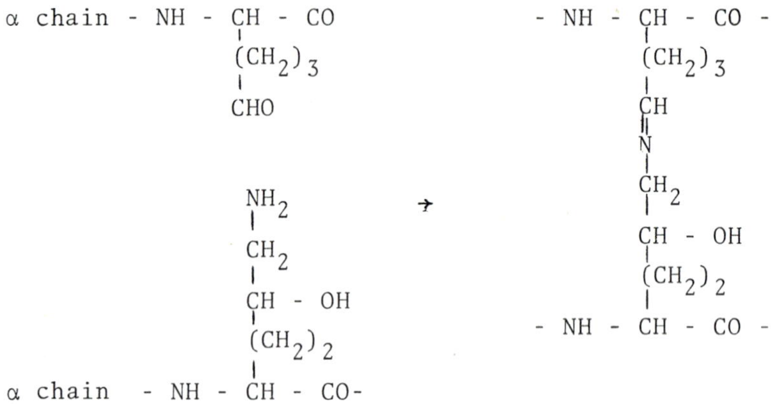

IV ISOLATION AND PARTIAL CHARACTERISATION OF A STABLE INTERMOLECULAR CROSSLINK

Both crosslinks (components B and C, Fig. 2) were shown to be labile to dilute acids and thermal denaturation of the collagen, thus, although they confer stability on the fibre in the physiological state and account for the ready solubility of rat tail and rat skin collagen in weak acids and α-amino β thiols they do not account for the insolubility, or the presence of crosslinked components after gelatinization, of the majority of other fibres. Additional crosslinks may be present in the more insoluble collagens, or these labile aldimine bonds may undergo further reaction to stabilize themselves. The isolated crosslinks can be considered as intermediate in the biosynthetic processes of the crosslinking system. Further studies have suggested that both these proposals are probably true.

A. EFFECT OF AGE

Reduction of fibres isolated from tissues of increasing age show a marked decrease in the proportion of reducible component (fig. 4) and this is concomitant with the decrease in solubility (Bailey, 1969). Similarly the in vitro incubation of rat tail tendons at 38°C shows a decrease in the reducible components together with a rapid decrease in the solubility. The routes by which these intermediate bonds are stabilized remain to be elucidated.

The most obvious mode of stabilization would be in vivo reduction of the aldimine bond. This type of reduction has a precedent in the reduction of a similar bond in elastin to produce lysinonorleucine. However, we have been unable to demonstrate the presence of the reduced form of the crosslink, hydroxylysinonorleucine, in aged but non-reduced collagen.

B. ADDITIONAL CROSSLINKS

The second proposal that additional stable bonds may be present was confirmed by analysis of the reduction products obtained from the less soluble collagens. For these studies we turned to similar but less soluble tissues, e.g. the achilles tendon. Reduction of rat achilles tendon indicated the presence of another important component and this was confirmed by reduction of the even less soluble bovine achilles tendon when the new component was found to be present in the same proportion as hydroxylysinonorleucine (Fig. 5b). Further confirmation was achieved by reduction of the completely insoluble bone and dentine collagens. For these collagens the new component was by far the major reducible component (Fig. 5a). In contrast to the aldimine bond this component was stable to D-penicillamine and thermal denaturation. The stability of the crosslink to the former reagent accounts for the decreased ability of α-amino β thiols to solubilize collagenous tissue other than rat tendon and rat skin. Studies were, therefore, again carried out to establish whether this component played a role in the crosslinking process.

Reduction of lathyritic chick bones showed a steady decrease in the amount of the reduced component with increasing doses of βAPN indicating involvement of the component

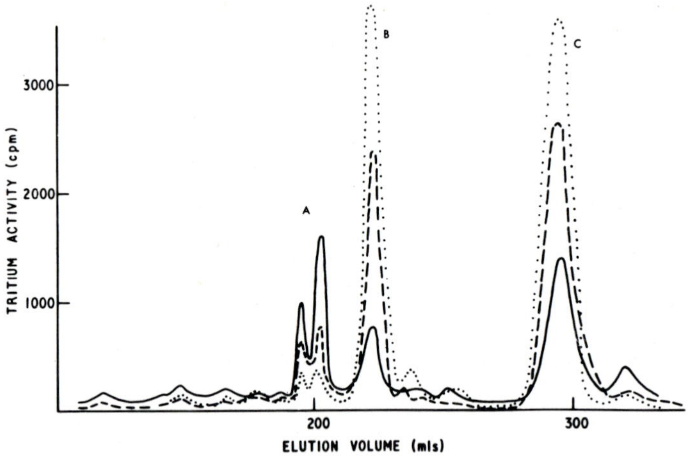

Fig. 4. Effect of age on the elution pattern of acid hydrolysates from sodium borotritide reduced rat tail tendon. ...., 3-month-old rat; ----, 9-month-old rat; ——, 2-year-old rat.

in the biosynthesis of the crosslinks. Injection of [^{3}H] lysine into the embryonic chicks and reduction of the bones and leg tendons with nonradioactive borohydride again produced radioactive peaks confirming that the component was derived from lysine or hydroxylysine.

These facts confirmed that the two major reducible peaks were involved in the crosslinking process. This type of study is essential to avoid the tedious isolation of components not involved in the biosynthesis of crosslinks, and is particularly important in the case of collagen where one is expecting to isolate less than one residue in a 1,000.

The reduced component under the peak was, therefore, isolated and analysed by mass spectrometry. The trifluoroacetyl methyl ester gave a mass ion of $^{m}/e$ 816. Peak matching against pfk. gave an exact mass measurement of 816.10. The ethyl ester has a mass ion of 844 the difference of 28 between this mass and the mass of the methyl ester confirmed the presence of two carboxyl groups.

From the exact mass ion, the presence of two amino acid residues, its derivation from lysine and its nitrogen content it was concluded that the compound was a reduced aldol derived from the δ-semialdehydes of lysine and hydroxylysine (Bailey,

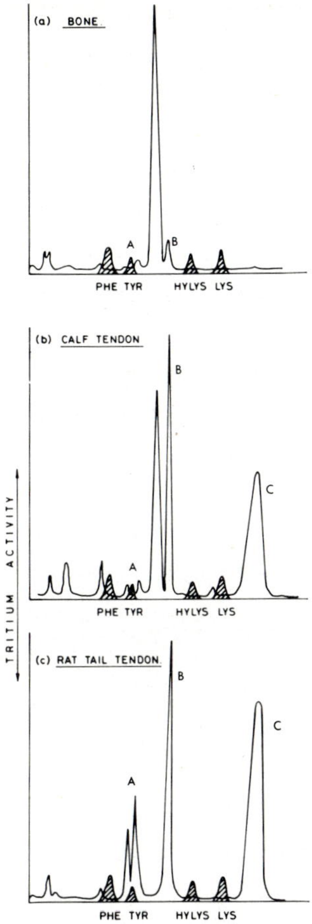

Fig. 5. Distribution of radioactivity of acid hydrolysates of collagen reduced with tritiated sodium borohydride.
(a) Decalcified bone
(b) calf achilles tendon;
(c) rat tail tendon.

Fowler and Peach, 1969). We intend to refer to the crosslink as "syndesine" and the reduced form isolated in these experiments as "syndesinol."

The configuration of two of the possible isomers may be written

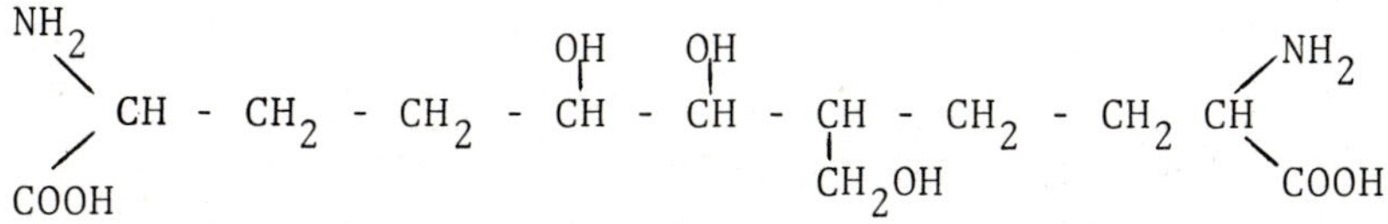

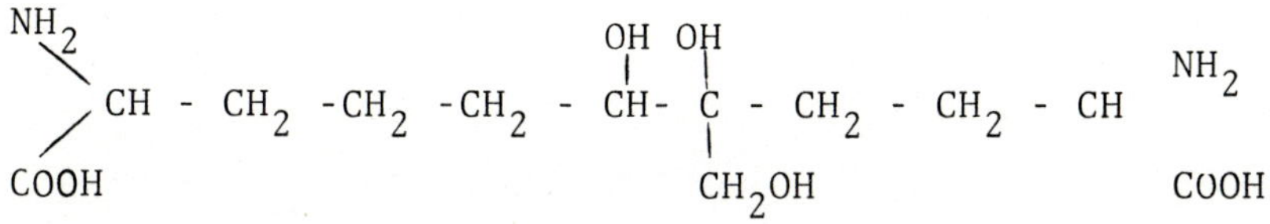

Unfortunately, knowledge of the stereochemistry of the aldol condensation is limited, the reaction generally leading to a mixture of the isomers but very often one predominates. From the limited number of examples available it appears that the aldol results from attack by the aldehyde with the lesser number of α substituents on the α carbon atom of the aldehyde having the greater number of α substituents (Nielsen and Houlihan, 1968) (Lieben's rule). However, increased substitution of groups in the β position favours the reversal of this rule. Chemical studies, e.g. periodate oxidations are now being carried out to confirm the proposed structure, and establish whether both isomers are present.

The nature of the non-reduced form of the crosslink readily accounts for the previously observed ability of periodate to solubilize dentine (Veis and Schlueter, 1964) and the involvement of hydroxylysine may also account for the decrease in hydroxylysine content of bone with increase in age of the tissue (Miller, Martin, Piez and Powers, 1967).

Studies with embryonic chicks previously injected with [^{3}H]lysine demonstrated that one aldol bond was present per tropocollagen molecule, and it must, therefore, be a major factor in stabilizing the structure. Although the aldol crosslink was found to be stable during denaturation and resists weak acids and penicillamine further studies should establish whether with increase in age these bonds remain as aldols or that they are intermediate bonds that undergo further reaction with other active groups.

However, it is significant that even embryonic chick bone collagen is virtually insoluble and the "syndesine" peak is the only major component involving a lysine derivative, which suggests that in the case of bone there is a need for the rapid production of stable crosslinks and further modification is unnecessary. The rapid reaction may be due to the reactive nature of the δ-semialdehyde of hydroxylysine.

V LOCATION OF THE CROSSLINK

Miller, Lane and Piez (1969) have recently demonstrated the presence of hydroxylysine in the telopeptide region of lathyritic bone. More specifically they demonstrated that the lysine found at position 9 in all the different collagens so far studied, is 50% hydroxylated in bone collagen. Thus, both lysine and hydroxylysine are present in a region accessible to enzymes for conversion to δ-semialdehyde. On reduction of tropocollagen extracted from calf tendon and that from embryonic bone the aldol was not present indicating that the compond constituted an intermolecular crosslink. However, if the aldehydes only occur in the N-terminal telopeptide region this would entail a side to side aggregation of the tropocollagen molecules with their N-terminal ends in register. On the quarter stagger hypothesis only a small proportion would have their ends aligned in this manner. Alternatively, assuming the quarter stagger hypothesis to be correct it is necessary to postulate that the lysine aldehydes also occur along the body of the molecule, in addition to the telopeptide ends. Detailed studies on the peptide chains have only been carried out on rat skin, which does not possess the aldol crosslink. Further sequence studies on bovine tendon might reveal additional aldehydes along the body of the molecule. The recent studies of Kuhn and his colleagues (1966) are of interest since they suggest that side to side crosslinks occur in bovine tendon but not in rat tail or rat skin collagen. It is possible that syndesine may be related to the side to side crosslink.

VI ENZYMIC BIOSYNTHESIS OF THE INTERMOLECULAR CROSSLINKS

Although it is generally accepted that an amine oxidase is involved in the oxidative deamination of the lysine to give allysine the actual enzyme has not been isolated. A number of workers have postulated that certain amine oxidases, e.g. benzylamine oxidases are involved. However, the most con-

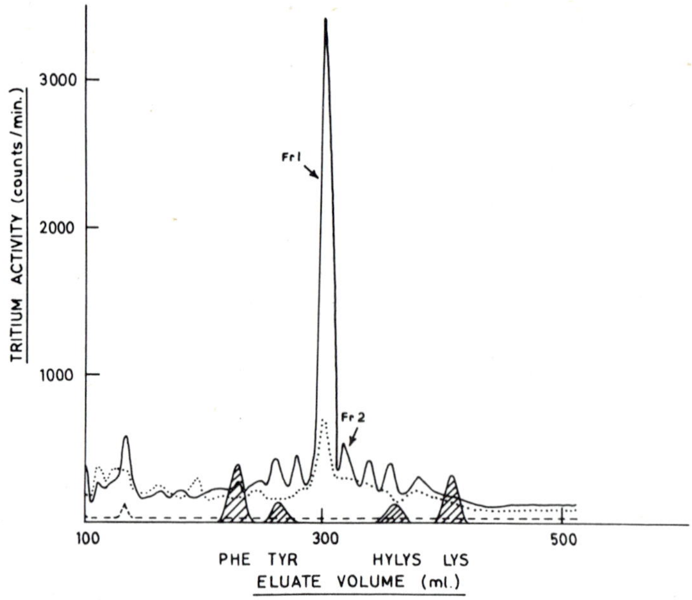

Fig. 6. Elution pattern of reducible components obtained from an acid hydrolysate of enzyme treated lathyritic chick bone collagen reduced with tritiated sodium borohydride. ——, $NaBT_4$ reduced lathyritic bones; ····, $NaBT_4$ reduced enzyme extract. Fr. 1 denotes "syndesine" peak and Fr 2 hydroxylysinonorleucine.

convincing study is that of Pinnell and Martin (1968) who demonstrated the presence of an enzyme system capable of converting lysine in peptide linkage to allysine using elastin as a substrate.

Using the same procedure as these workers we extracted the enzyme system from embryonic chick bones. However, rather than incubate the extracts with highly crosslinked collagen we incubated the enzyme extract with lathyritic bone, since the lysine and hydroxylysines that are normally involved in further oxidation to aldehydes are still available. In addition, this procedure should provide a low background of reducible crosslinks, thus permitting the detection of small amounts of new reducible crosslinks synthesized by the enzyme system. On reduction of the lathyritic bone after incubation with the enzyme extract both crosslinks, syndesine and hydroxylysinonorleucine previously observed in the reduced form in normal and reduced bone (Bailey and Fowler, 1969) were again present, whilst they were barely detectable in the lathyritic control (Fig. 6). Incubation of tendon with the enzyme digest similarly resulted in the formation of the intermolecular crosslinks. These studies also provided further evidence for the involvement of these components in the crosslinking process. The presence of the reduced form of allysine had been demonstrated previously but reduction of the bone after enzymic incubation revealed the presence of an additional peak eluting prior to hydroxynorleucine. Preliminary studies indicate that this component is the reduced form of the aldehyde derived from hydroxylysine.

VII CONCLUDING REMARKS

The chemistry of the primary structure of collagens of different tissues appear to be virtually identical. The differentiation of the various tissues probably depends on the extent and nature of changes collagen undergoes after synthesis (Piez et al., 1968). Hydroxylation of the prolines and lysines occurs, addition of carbohydrates also occurs and finally oxidative deamination of the lysines and hydroxylysines occurs to produce crosslinks and to form a mechanically stable, insoluble supporting tissue. The involvement of hydroxylysine in the crosslinks suggests that this could be a controlling factor in the extend of the crosslinking. The greater the proportion of the specific lysine hydroxylated, probably the telopeptide lysine, the more hydroxylysine available for enzymic conversion to the aldehyde and subsequent crosslink formation. If indeed this is the case future investigations should reveal a smaller proportion of the telopeptide lysines converted to hydroxylysine in calf tendon collagen, (compared to the 50% in bone collagen). This would be consistent with the smaller proportion of aldol crosslinks in calf tendon and their absence from rat tail tendon and rat skin collagen.

The other role reported for this unique amino acid is its ability to attach mono and disaccharide units of galactose and glucose (Butler and Cunningham, 1966; Spiro, 1967).

The relationship, if any, of this to crosslinking is not at present clear although the possibility of the Gal-Glu, disaccharide unit sterically hindering the involvement of this specific hydroxylysine from crosslink formation cannot be overlooked, particularly in view of its position on the molecule, i.e. at the end of the overlap region.

Based on the present studies the biosynthesis of the intermolecular crosslinks of collagen appears to be based on a system of crosslinks mediated through the δ-semialdehyde derived from lysine and hydroxylysine by enzymic oxidation. Presumably the oxidative deamination takes place extracellularly on the surface of the fibril although this point requires clarification.

Fibre formation by aggregation of the tropocollagen molecules extruded from the fibroblast most probably occurs by charge interactions of the amino acid side chains along the length of the molecule. These interactions would in the case of collagen locate the molecule precisely on the collagen fibril. This precise location is essential to provide the correct juxtaposition of the reactive aldehyde groups, thus increasing their effective concentration many fold to permit spontaneous reaction of the aldehydes in an environment which might be inaccessible to enzymes.

From the studies to date it is clear that the fibres contain both labile and stable intermolecular crosslinks. The labile crosslinks are aldimine bonds whilst the stable crosslinks appear to be aldols. Rat tail tendon and rat skin collagen are different from most other mammalian collagen in not possessing the stable syndesine crosslink. The proportion of syndesine, at least within the ranges of collagens examined, appears to be greatest in the more insoluble collagen. With increase in age of a particular tissue there is a marked decrease in solubility and an increase in the extent of crosslinking. At the same time there is a decrease in the identified reducible crosslinks suggesting that further stabilization of these crosslinks occurs to produce a non-reducible crosslink.

Although there is some evidence for other functions of collagen (Stuart and Moscona, 1967) its major function is mechanical, and for this reason the most important current aspect of the biochemistry of collagen is the elucidation of the nature and biosynthesis of the stabilizing crosslinks.

Even though some progress in the elucidation of the chemistry of the crosslinks is now being made, considerable effort is still required for a complete picture of the biosynthesis of the collagen crosslinking system. The site of enzymic oxiaative deamination has not been established, nor whether an enzyme is involved in the reaction of the aldehydes. Further studies are required to establish the role of the carbohydrate linked to hydroxylysine, the actual location of the different crosslinks, and their relationship to tissue function. Finally, at a morphological level the factors controlling the fibre size and fibre orientation required elucidation.

ACKNOWLEDGEMENTS

This work was supported in part by a grant from the Nuffield Foundation. We are grateful to Mr. A.H. Whiting for technical assistance and to Mrs. J. James for carrying out the mass spectra. Thanks are also due to Dr. S.M. Partridge for continued interest and encouragement.

REFERENCES

Bailey, A.J. (1967). Biochem. J. 105, 34 P.

Bailey, A.J.(1968a). In Comprehensive Biochemistry, vo. 260B, p. 297. Elsevier, New York.

Bailey, A.J. (1968b). Biochim. Biophys. Acta., 160, 447.

Bailey, A.J. (1969). Gerontologia, 15, 65.

Bailey, A.J. and Fowler, L.J. (1969). Biochem. Biophys. Res. Communs. 35, 672.

Bailey, A.J., Fowler, L.J. and Peach, C.M. (1969). Biochem. Biophys. Res. Communs. 35, 663.

Bailey, A.J. and Lister, D. (1968). Nature 220, 280.

Bailey, A.J. and Peach, C.M. (1968). Biochem. Biophys. Res. Communs. 33, 812.

Blumenfeld, O.O. and Gallop, P. (1966). Proc. Natl. Acad. Sci. 56, 1260.

Bornstein, P. and Piez, K.A. (1960). Biochemistry 5, 3460.

Butler, W.T. and Cunningham, L.W. (1966). J. Biol. Chem. 241, 3882.

Fessler, J.N. and Bailey, A.J. (1966). Biochim. Biophys. Acta. 117, 368.

Harkness, M.L.R. and Harkness, R.D. (1966). Nature 211, 496.

Kühn, K., Fietzek, P. and Kühn, J. (1966). Biochem Z. 344, 418.

Levene, C.I. and Gross, J. (1959). J. Exptl. Med. 110, 771.

Martin, S.R., Lewis, M.A. and Piez, K.A. (1963). Biochim. Biophys. Acta. 69, 471.

Miller, E.J., Lane, J.M. and Piez, K.A. (1969). Biochemistry, 8, 30.

Miller, E.J., Martin, G.R., Piez, K.A. and Powers, M.J. (1967). J. Biol. Chem. 242, 5481.

Nielsen, A.T. and Houlihan, W.J. (1968). Organic Reactions, vol. 16, p. 1.

Nimni, M. (1966). Biochem. Biophys. Res. Communs. 25, 434.

Piez, K.A. (1968). Ann. Rev. Biochem. 37, 547.

Piez, K.A., Bladen, H.A., Lane, J.M., Miller, E.J., Bornstein, P., Butler, W.T. and Kang, A. H. (1968). Brookhaven Symposium.

Pinnell, S.R.and Martin, G.R. (1968). Proc. Natl. Acad. Sci. (U.S.) 708.

Ramachandran, G.N. (1967). Treatise on Collagen, vol. I. Academic Press, New York.

Spiro. R.G. (1967). J. Biol. Chem. 242, 4813.

Stuart, E.S. and Moscona, A.A. (1967). Science 157, 947.

Tanzer, M.L. (1967). Biochim. Biophys. Acta. 133, 584.

Tanzer, M.L. (1968). J. Biol. Chem. 243, 4045.

Veis, A. and Anesey, J. (1965). J. Biol. Chem. 240, 3899.

Veis, A. and Schlueter, R.J. (1964). Biochemistry 3, 1650.

LYSYL OXIDASE: THE ENZYMATIC STEP IN COLLAGEN AND ELASTIN CROSSLINKING

George R. Martin, Sheldon R. Pinnell, Robert C. Siegel and Elliot R. Goldstein

I BIOGENESIS OF CROSSLINKS

Current evidence, although not complete in all details, clearly indicates that collagen and elastin are crosslinked in a similar series of reactions. Certain lysines in these proteins are oxidatively deaminated to form an aldehyde, α-aminoadipic-δ-semialdehyde, (allysine*), and these lysine derived aldehydes are used to form the actual crosslinks (Piez, 1968). The oxidative deamination of these lysines is enzymatic (Pinnell and Martin, 1968), whereas the subsequent formation of the crosslinks is probably spontaneous (Schiffmann and Martin, 1969).

Working primarily with chick embryos, we have detected an enzyme in extracts of several tissues that converts peptide-bound lysine to peptide bound allysine (Pinnell and Martin, 1968). Lysyl oxidase would seem a suitable name for this enzyme. Detection of lysyl oxidase was dependent upon the development of senstive assays for measuring the lysyl-allysyl conversion. Two such assays were developed. The tritium release assay detects the tritium released from collagen or elastin labeled biosynthetically [3H]6-lysine as lysyl groups are oxidatively deaminated (Fig. 1). The tritium released from the protein is isolated by distillation and measured by standard counting techniques. This assay

* We have given α-amino adipic-δ- semialdehyde the trivial name allysine in order to indicate that it is an aldehyde derived from lysine.

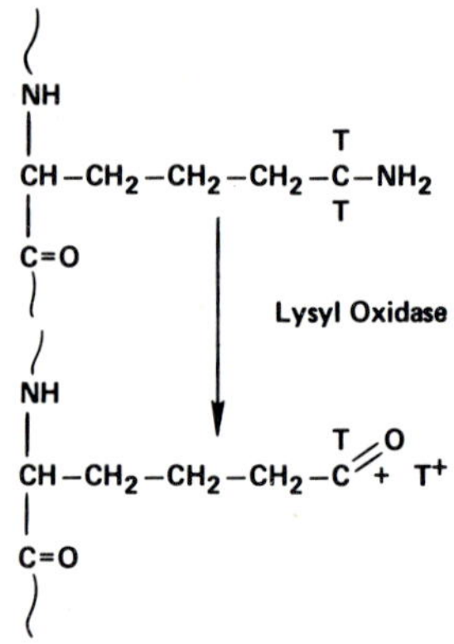

Fig. 1. Basis of the tritium release assay. Concomitant with the enzymatic synthesis of peptide-bound allysine from lysyl residues in collagen or elastin labeled with [3H]6-lysine is the releasr of tritium. Enzyme activity is followed by isolating and assaying the tritium released from the protein.

is sensitive and rapid. In the $[^{14}C]\alpha$-aminoadipic acid assay, collagen or elastin is labeled biosynthetically with $[^{14}C]$U-lysine. The $[^{14}C]$U-lysine labeled collagen or elastin is purified and used as a substrate for the enzyme. After incubation with enzyme, the reaction mixture is oxidized with performic acid in order to convert allysine to α-aminoadipic acid. Following hydrolysis the amino acids are separated on an automatic amino acid analyzer and the radioactivity in α-aminoadipic acid is measured by passing the effluent through a liquid scintillation counter equipped for flow counting. This assay though cumbersome measures allysine production directly.

II LYSYL OXIDASE

In our initial studies on lysyl oxidase we have used elastin as a substrate rather than collagen, since many more lysines in this protein are converted to allysine during crosslinking. When elastin prepared from embryonic chick aorta, biosynthetically labeled with $[^{3}H]$6-lysine in tissue culture, is incubated with a 10^{5}xg supernatant of an extract of chick cartilage, tritium is released at a linear rate for several hours (Fig. 2). Addition of the lathyrogen, β-

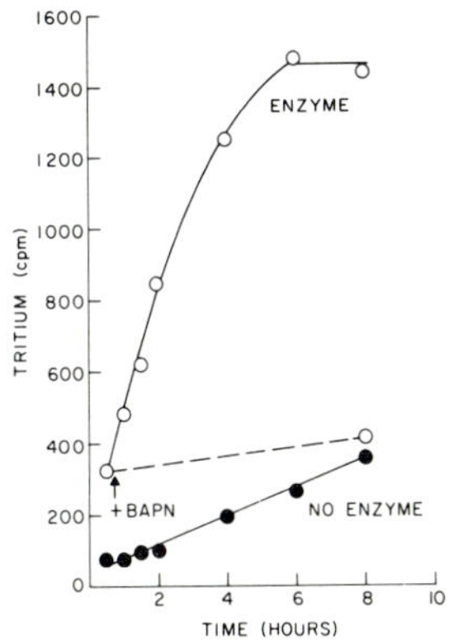

Fig. 2. Release of tritium from [^{3}H]6-lysine-labeled substrate. β-Aminopropionitrile (50 μg/ml) was added to one of the tubes containing substrate and enzyme 30 min after the start of the reaction, in order to demonstrate that the lathyrogen inactivates lysyl oxidase.

aminopropionitrile (βAPN) after 30 min of incubation largely abolishes further enzyme action. Previous work has established that βAPN prevents the crosslinking of both elastin and collagen by inhibiting the oxidative deamination of lysines in these proteins. Using the [^{14}C]α-amino-adipic acid assay we have determined in other studies (Pinnell and Martin, 1968) that, allysine formation is proportional to tritium release. Some tritium is released from the substrate in the absence of added enzyme but this represents only a small fraction of that observed with enzyme.

The tritium release assay can be used to measure quantitatively the amount of enzyme present in an extract. When varying amounts of enzyme are incubated with a constant amount of [^{3}H]6-lysine-labeled substrate, tritium release is proportional to the amount of enzyme added (Fig. 3). Using such an assay, we have measured the enzyme content of cartilage in chicks of different ages. These studies have shown that the enzyme is highest in cartilage from chick embryos 17 days of age and that the amount of enzyme decreases rapidly after hatching. Quantitative enzyme assays carried out on copper-deficient and copper-supplemented chickens indicate that lysyl oxidase is missing from the copper deficient chicks 8 days after being placed on the diet. These obser-

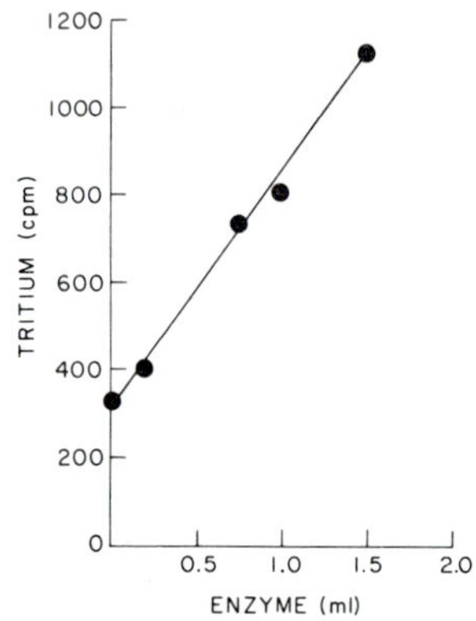

Fig. 3. Relationship between tritium released and amount of enzyme added.

vations are in accord with earlier studies that indicated that the crosslinking of collagen and of elastin is impaired in copper-deficient animals.

The enzyme is precipitated from the 105,000 G extract of cartilage by $(NH_4)_2SO_4$ (20-60% cut). When concentrated in this fashion and examined on a molecular sieve, the enzyme activity elutes in a single peak with a mobility expected from a globular protein of relatively high molecular weight (greater than 70,000)(Fig. 4).

Because far fewer lysines in collagen than elastin are converted to aldehydes, it has proven more difficult to study collagen as a substrate for the enzyme. However, by growing embryonic chick bone in culture with the appropriate isotope and βAPN to block crosslinking, we have been able to isolate and purify collagen which is suitable for study as substrate. When this collagen labeled with $[^3H]$6-lysine is incubated with our extracts containing lysyl oxidase, tritium is released and this activity is blocked by βAPN (Table I). In addition, some of the lysine in collagen labeled with $[^{14}C]$-lysine was converted to $[^{14}C]$-allysine. As expected, βAPN inhibited this conversion. More recently, we have isolated the α chains of collagen following incubation with lysyl oxidase and found that they indeed contain the allysine generated by the enzyme.

In order to determine if the tertiary structure of collagen is required by the enzyme, we have studied both native

TABLE I

Comparison of Tritium Release and [^{14}C]Allysine Formation using Biosynthetically Labeled Chick Tibia Collagen.

	TRITIUM RELEASE (cpm)	[^{14}C]αAMINOADIPIC ACID (cpm)
Collagen + Buffer	703	200
Collagen + Enzyme	1869	652
Collagen + Enzyme + BAPN	575	182

and denatured collagen as substrates for lysyl oxidase. Indeed, denatured collagen was found to be a substrate for lysyl oxidase when tested by both the tritium release and [^{14}C]allysine production assays. The extent of reaction was similar in both native and denatured collagen. This result may be fortuitous since our current enzyme preparations contain a significant amount of protease activity which might degrade these substrates to inactive fragments. Further work is necessary in order to define the specificity of the enzyme.

Other investigators have called attention to the possible role of monoamine oxidase in crosslinking. Both allysine formation and amine oxidation would appear to involve

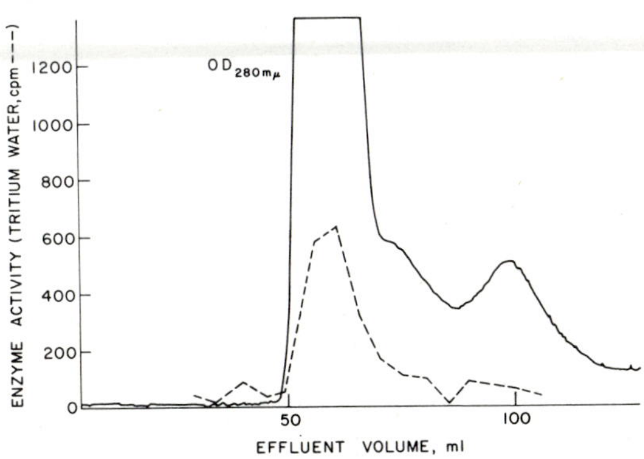

Fig. 4. Molecular sieve chromatogram (10% agarose, 180 ml column) of lysyl oxidase.

an oxidative deamination. Both activities require copper and are inhibited by βAPN. However, the enzyme catalyzing lysine oxidation is inactivated by 5×10^{-6} M βAPN whereas βAPN is metabolized by monoamine oxidase and concentrations of 10^{-3}M are required to demonstrate competitive inhibition. In addition, it has been reported that monoamine oxidase levels are normal in animals given βAPN, whereas lysyl oxidase activity is not detected in cartilage from chicks injected with βAPN. Current evidence, therefore, indicates that the two are separate and distinct enzymes.

REFERENCES

Piez, K.A. (1968). In Annual Review of Biochemistry. Ed. by Boyer, P.D., Palo Alto.

Pinnell, S.R. and Martin, G.R. (1968). Proc. Acad. Sci. 61, 708.

Schiffmann, E. and Martin, G.R. (1969). Fed. Proc. 28, 407.

ISOLATION OF HIGHLY PURIFIED PROTOCOLLAGEN PROLINE HYDROXYLASE

Kari I. Kivirikko, Jouko Halme and Kai Simons

The enzyme protocollagen proline hydroxylase synthesizes hydroxyproline by hydroxylation of proline in protocollagen, the large proline-rich and lysine-rich polypeptide precursor of collagen (for review see Udenfriend, 1966; Prockop and Kivirikko, 1967). The enzyme has previously been partially purified and characterized from chick embryo extracts (Kivirikko and Prockop, 1967a,b; Hutton, Tappel and Udenfriend, 1967) and foetal rat skin (Rhoads and Udenfriend, 1968), and the synthesis of hydroxyproline by partially purified preparations of the enzyme has been shown to require molecular oxygen, ascorbate, α-ketoglutarate and ferrous iron (Kivirikko and Prockop, 1967a, Hutton et al., 1967). Initial attempts to further purify the enzyme from chick embryo extracts were unsuccessful, because the enzyme rapidly lost its activity during the purification process. A recent study indicated that protocollagen proline hydroxylase is relatively stable in buffers containing free glycine and having a pH value around 8 (Halme and Kivirikko, 1968). This has enabled us to produce highly purified preparations of protocollagen proline hydroxylase.

I EXPERIMENTAL METHODS

The protocollagen proline hydroxylase was prepared from extracts of 13-day-old chick embryos (200 embryos per batch). For the purification all buffers contained glycine. Their pH was 7.8 except for those used in DEAE-cellulose chromatography. Ammonium sulphate fractionation of the chick embryo extract and the calcium phosphate gel step were performed as described previously (Halme and Kivirikko, 1968; Kivirikko, Bright and Prockop, 1968). A 5x35-cm column was used for DEAE-cellulose chromatography. It was equilibrated with a solution containing 0.2 M NaCl, 0.2 M glycine and 0.01 M Tris-HCl buffer, pH 7.0 at 4°C, and eluted in steps with solutions containing 0.20 M, 0.25 M, 0.30 M and 0.40 M NaCl and glycine, and 0.01 M Tris-HCl buffer pH 7.0. Twelve milliliter fractions were collected in tubes containing 3.0 ml 0.2 M glycine-NaCl buffer, pH 8.7. Fractions containing the enzyme were pooled and concentrated by ultrafiltration to a final volume of 3 ml. This enzyme preparation was applied to a 2.5x90-cm column of Bio-Gel A-1 5 m, which was equilibrated and eluted with 0.2 M NaCl, 0.2 M glycine and 0.01 M Tris-HCl buffer, pH 7.8. The void volume (174 ml) was determined with blue dextran. The same agarose column was calibrated with ceruloplasmin, serum albumin and cytochrome C, which had elution volumes of 290 ml, 340 ml and 430 ml, respectively. The peak enzyme activity had an elution volume of about 245 ml, and the specific activity of the enzyme in the fractions eluted between 210 and 250 ml differed by less than 10%. These fractions were pooled, and constituted the purified enzyme preparation.

The activity of the enzyme was assayed in a final volume of 4 ml containing 10-200 μg/ml enzyme protein; 125 μg/ml $(Pro\text{-}Gly\text{-}Pro)_n$, M.W. 6600 (Miles-Yeda); 0.08 mM $FeSO_4$; 0.5 mM α-ketoglutarate; 2 mM ascorbic acid; 0.2 mg/ml catalase (Kivirikko and Prockop, 1967c); 0.1 mM dithiothreitol; 2 mg/ml bovine serum albumin (Rhoads, Hutton and Udenfriend, 1967), and 0.05 M Tris-HCl buffer, adjusted to pH 7.8 at 25°C. The samples were incubated at 37°C for 1 hr. as described earlier (Kivirikko and Prockop, 1967c), and, after hydrolysis, the amount of hydroxyproline was measured (Kivirikko, Laitinen and Prockop, 1967). The protein content of the enzyme preparations was determined by absorbance at 225 nm, and by ninhydrin assays of acid hydrolysates. The sedimentation coefficient of the enzyme preparation was measured using a Spinco Model E analytical ultracentrifuge with a rotor speed of 42,040 rpm at 23°C. Disc electrophoresis was carried out in a 6.5% polyacrylamide gel with Tris-glycine buffer, pH 9 (Jovin, Chrambach, and Naugton, 1964), and the amino acid analysis of the enzyme preparation was performed on a Beckman Model 120-C amino acid analyzer [^{14}C]Lysine-labelled protocollagen was hydroxylated and the [^{14}C]hydroxylysine formed was measured as described previously (Kivirikko and Prockop, 1967b).

II RESULTS AND DISCUSSION

The procedure for the purification of protocollagen proline hydroxylase consisted of fractionations with ammonium sulphate and calcium phosphate gel, and chromatography on DEAE-cellulose and Bio-Gel A-1.5 m (Table I). The final purified enzyme preparations synthesized about 300 μg hydroxyproline per milligram protein per hour with 125 μg/ml of the synthetic polytripeptide substrate; and about 600 μg hydroxyproline per milligram protein per hour with a saturating concentration of the substrate. The starting material, which was the 15,000 x g supernatant of the embryo homogenates, contained inhibitory substances (Kivirikko and Prockop, 1967c), making the exact degree of purification difficult to express. However, purification increased the specific activity of the enzyme several thousand times (Table I).

The purified enzyme preparation only gave one component in the analytical ultracentrifuge. The sedimentation coefficient was 6.7 S. This suggests a molecular weight of about 150,000 if the enzyme is a fairly symmetric globular protein with a normal amount of hydration. However, the elution pattern in gel filtration suggests a molecular weight of about 350,000, and it thus seems that the enzyme is a relatively asymmetric molecule.

Disc electrophoresis showed one major band and one minor band (Fig. 1). When the fractions eluted from the Bio-Gel A-1.5 m column behind the enzyme peak were analyzed by disc electrophoresis the minor band was much stronger than in Fig. 1. The minor band, therefore, is probably a contaminant,

TABLE I

Purification of Protocollagen Proline Hydroxylase*

Enzyme fraction	Total protein (mg)	Specific activity (units/mg)+
15,000xg supernatant	84,700	(0.03-0.1)‡
Ammonium sulphate	23,700	1.0
Calcium phosphate gel	910	15
DEAE-cellulose	46	91
Bio-Gel A-1.5 m	8	290

*The starting material was 1.4 kg of 13-day-old chick embryos.

+One unit of enzymatic activity was defined as the amount of enzyme required to synthesize 1 μg hydroxyproline in 1 hr. with 125 μg/ml of $(Pro\text{-}Gly\text{-}Pro)_n$ as substrate.

‡According to Prockop, Juva and Engel, 1967.

and the major band the enzyme. Densitometry suggested that only about 5% of the total protein in the enzyme preparation is contaminant if both proteins stain in a similar way with amido black. It thus seems that the enzyme preparation is relatively pure.

Preliminary amino acid analysis of the purified enzyme preparation indicated relatively large amounts of acidic amino acids: about 90 residues of aspartic acid and 180 residues of glutamic acid per 1000 residues. This agrees with the relatively strong binding of the enzyme to DEAE-cellulose. We also found relatively high amounts of serine, glycine and lysine.

Earlier studies (Kivirikko and Prockop, 1967b) indicated that partially purified preparations of protocollagen proline hydroxylase hydroxylate lysine as well as proline residues in protocollagen. Both hydroxylations required molecular oxygen, ascorbate, α-ketoglutarate and ferrous iron. Our highly purified enzyme preparation did not hydroxylate lysine residues in protocollagen (Table II). Thus, it seems that two separate enzymes, protocollagen proline hydroxylase and protocollagen lysine hydroxylase, are involved in the hydro-

TABLE II

Hydroxylation of [^{14}C]Lysine in Protocollagen with Different Preparations of Protocollagen Proline Hydroxylase

Enzyme preparation	Units of enzyme added	[^{14}C]Hydroxylysine formed (dpm)
Ammonium sulphate	30	9120
Calcium phosphate gel	30	9410
Bio-Gel A-1.5 m	60	220

Values indicate dpm [^{14}C]hydroxylysine synthesized with 300,000 dpm [^{14}C]lysine-labelled protocollagen as substrate.

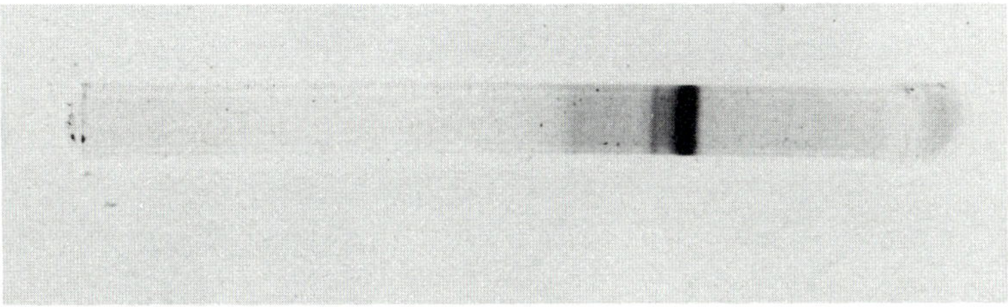

Fig. 1. Disc electrophoresis of the purified enzyme preparation.

xylation of proline and lysine in protocollagen.

ACKNOWLEDGEMENTS

This study was supported by a grant from the National Research Council for Medical Sciences, Finland.

REFERENCES

Halme, J. and Kivirikko, K.I. (1968). FEBS Letters 1, 223.

Hutton, J.J., Tappel, A.L. and Udenfriend, S. (1967). Arch. Biochem, Biophys. 118, 231.

Jovin, T., Chrambach, A. and Naughton, M.A. (1964). Biochemistry 9, 351.

Kivirikko, K.I., Bright, H.J. and Prockop, D.J. (1968). Biochim. Biophys. Acta 151, 558.

Kivirikko, K.I., Laitinen, O. and Prockop, D.J. (1967). Anal. Biochem. 19, 249.

Kivirikko, K.I. and Prockop, D.J. (1967a). Arch. Biochem. Biophys. 118, 611

Kivirikko, K.I. and Prockop, D.J. (1967b). Proc. Natl. Acad. Sci. (U.S.) 57, 782.

Kivirikko, K.I. and Prockop, D.J. (1967c). J. Biol. Chem. 242, 4007

Prockop, D.J., Juva, K. and Engel, J. (1967). Z. Physiol. Chem. 348, 553.

Prockop, D.J. and Kivirikko, K.I.(1967). Ann. Internal Med. 66, 1243.

Rhoads, R.E., Hutton, J.J. and Udenfriend, S. (1967). Arch. Biochem. Biophys. 122, 805.

Rhoads, R.E. and Udenfriend, S. (1968). Proc. Natl. Acad. Sci. (U.S.) 60, 1473.

Udenfriend, S. (1966). Science 152, 1335.

MECHANISM OF INHIBITION OF COLLAGEN CROSSLINKING AND DEPOLYMERIZATION OF AN INCOMPLETELY CROSSLINKED FORM OF INSOLUBLE COLLAGEN CAUSED BY D-PENICILLAMINE

Marcel E. Nimni, Kalindi Deshmukh and Arvind Deshmukh

The involvement of collagen in the pathogenesis of lathyrism was first demonstrated by Levene and Gross (1959). The neutral salt soluble collagen which accumulates in the tissues of animals treated with β-aminopropionitrile (βAPN) and other lathyrogens has proven of great value in beginning to understand the nature of the covalent crosslinks which stabilize the collagen fiber. A few years ago, it was reported from our laboratory (Nimni and Bavetta, 1965; Nimni, 1965) that the administration of D-penicillamine, (ββ-dimethyl cysteine) was able to produce an accumulation of neutral salt soluble collagen in soft tissues, in a fashion which resembled the changes seen in lathyrism. In addition to preventing the formation of crosslinks between newly synthesized tropocollagen subunits, the administration of penicillamine was shown to cause a degradation of a certain fraction of insoluble collagen, presumably that which had not attained the completion of stable intermolecular crosslinks (Nimni, 1968). This depolymerizing effect of penicillamine could also be observed in vitro, since this compound and various analogues with α-aminothiol structures were able to solubilize significant amounts of rat skin insoluble collagen at neutral pH and at 4°C (Nimni, 1966). The collagenous material obtained from normal animals which can be solubilized in vitro under these conditions contains 30-50% of β-components, depending on the age of the tissue. On the other hand, however, the neutral salt soluble collagen extracted from rats treated with penicillamine yields mostly α-components upon denaturation. This seems to indicate that in vivo the blockage in the crosslinking process accounts for a major part of the soluble material which accumulates in soft tissues, and the degradation of insoluble collagen yielding subunits with stable intramolecular crosslinks contributes to a lesser extent to this soluble pool. In spite of apparent similarities in the effects of penicillamine and lathyrogens (Martin, Gross, Piez and Lewis, 1961), some major discrepancies became evident, which proved to be of value in our further attempt to elucidate the mechanism underlying the change induced by penicillamine.

I FIBER FORMATION

In contrast to the lathyritic collagen, which even after extensive purification fails to form stable fibers in vitro (Gross, 1963), the collagen isolated from the animals treated with penicillamine will form stable crosslinked fibers which will not redissolve upon cooling. Figure 1 summarizes these observations. Collagen from normal and penicillamine-treated animals aggregated very rapidly and reached a maximum optical density within 10 min. of incubation at 37°C. Collagen from lathyritic animals showed a retarded capacity to gel, but eventually reached the same maximum optical density. After incubation at 37°C for 7 days and subsequent cooling at 2°C, the gels from the control and penicillamine collagen did not show significant redissolution, while the optical density of the β-aminoproprionitrile collagen dropped rapidly, with complete liquefaction of the gel structure. As a matter of fact, in several experiments, the penicillamine collagen showed an enhanced capacity to gel at 37°C as well as a greater stability than the controls when subsequently cooled at 2°C.

The amino acid composition, specific optical rotation and melting temperature of the various soluble collagens isolated from normal, βAPN and penicillamine-treated animals, failed to reveal any differences (Deshmukh and Nimni, 1969a).

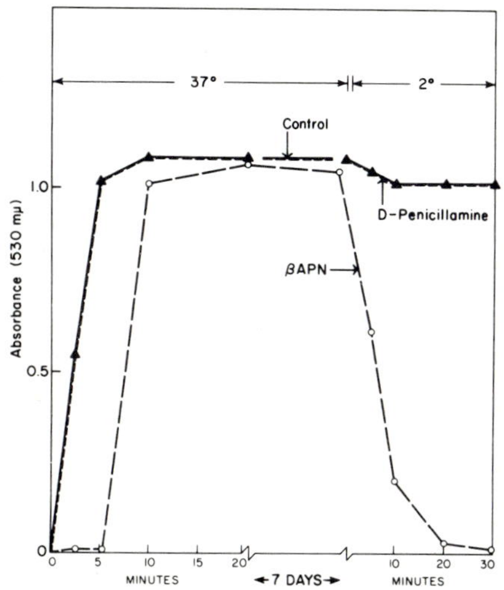

Fig. 1. Solutions of neutral salt-soluble collagen from normal, β-aminoproprionitrile (βAPN) and penicillamine-treated rats in 0.45 M NaCl, pH 7.0, were incubated at 37°C for 7 days and cooled at 2°C. The rate of thermal aggregation and redissolution of gels was measured by changes in absorbance.

II ALDEHYDES IN TROPOCOLLAGEN

A. ESTIMATION

The aldehyde residues, which are implied to be involved in the formation of crosslinks, are known to be reduced in quantity in the collagen obtained from the lathyritic rats (Rojkind and Juarez, 1966; Bornstein and Piez, 1966). Since the incapacity of this type of collagen to crosslink in vitro as well as in vivo could be attributed to such a deficiency, it seemed of interest to look at the aldehyde content of the collagen isolated from the penicillamine-treated rats.

The aldehyde contents of different neutral salt soluble collagen preparations are given in Table I. Our findings confirm those of previous investigators, in that, the collagen from lathyritic animals is deficient in aldehydes. On the other hand, collagen from penicillamine-treated rats has significantly more aldehydes than normal. This observation reflects a major difference between the modes of action of

TABLE I

Aldehyde Content of Neutral Salt-soluble Collagen from Skin of Normal, Lathyritic, and Penicillamine-treated Rats

Collagen sample	Aldehyde content (μmoles acetaldehyde eq/100mg collagen)
Normal	0.87
βAPN*-treated	0.49
Penicillamine-treated	1.60

*β-Aminopropionitrile

βAPN and penicillamine.

B. BLOCKING MECHANISM

It has been previously reported (Nimni, 1968) that addition of D-penicillamine to normal salt-soluble collagen affects its behavior during thermal aggregation. At a high concentration, such as 0.2 M, it causes a complete blockage of the polymerization process, while at lower concentrations, it does not significantly affect the rate of aggregation. but causes redissolution to occur after cooling at 4°C. Along with D-penicillamine, other compounds such as β-aminopropionitrile, N-acetylpenicillamine, and sodium bisulfite were tested. Figure 2 shows that at 10^{-2} M concentration none of these compounds inhibit the thermal aggregation of neutral salt-soluble collagen from normal animals. Upon storage for 4 days at 37°C with subsequent cooling at 4°C, the presence of penicillamine in the media caused complete liquefaction of the gel structure, whereas, N-acetylpenicillamine or βAPN had no such effect. Sodium bisulfite caused the gel to dissolve completely at 4°C. This compound was found to be effective at concentrations of 10^{-3} or 10^{-4} M. Such action of sodium bisulfite can be attributed to its capacity to form addition products with aldehydes and low molecular weight ketones. Modification of the collagen molecule, such as by

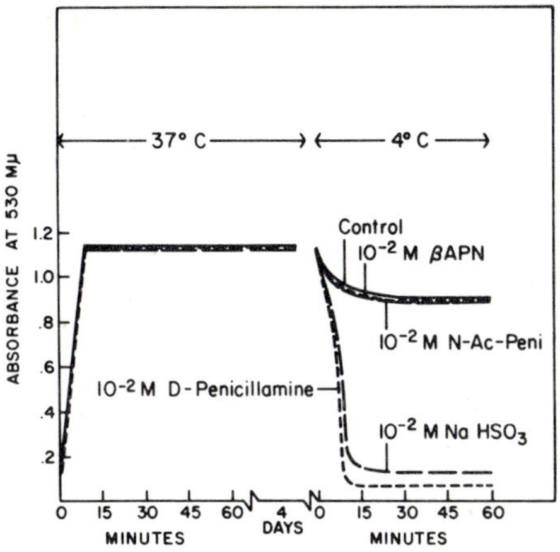

Fig. 2. The effects of the addition of β-aminopropionitrile (βAPN), D-penicillamine, N-acetyl-D-penicillamine (N-Ac-Peni), and sodium bisulfite to neutral salt-soluble collagen were monitored by studying the rate of thermal aggregation at 37°C and redissolution at 4°C. All of the gels were stored at 37°C for 4 days prior to cooling.

reducing the aldehydes with $NaBH_4$ under nondenaturing conditions, or blockage of the ε-amino groups of lysine with ethyl acetimidate also inhibited the formation of stable crosslinks (Deshmukh and Nimni, 1969).

C. BINDING STUDIES

The interactions of penicillamine and other thiol-amine compounds with tropocollagen or parent gelatin was next investigated. Preliminary experiments using film dialysis gave evidence of such an interaction. When mixtures of collagen or the parent gelatin and labeled thiol-amines were placed in a dialysis sack, and dialyzed against excess solvent, the rate of removal of the labeled ligand from the dialysis bag was inversely proportional to the number of aldehyde residues on the collagen molecule. Collagen reduced with $NaBH_4$ showed the minimum degree of interaction.

It seemed likely that cysteine and its analogues were binding to the collagen molecule by weak forces and that the nature of the collagen-mercaptoethylamine interaction involved an unstable binding which could be dissociated by exhaustive dialysis. Therefore, the method of equilibrium dialysis as used by Klotz, Walker, and Pivan (1946), to study binding of organic ions to protein molecules and developed further by Hunter and Commerford (1955), for interactions of amino acids with proteins was applied to this system. In addition to the collagen and gelatin samples used in the film dialysis experiment, periodate oxidized gelatin served as a material rich in aldehydes. Commercial gelatin (Knox) was oxidized with sodium periodate in alkaline media or with periodic acid. The amount of aldehydes increased after oxidation and the hydroxylysine to lysine ratio changed from the normal range of 0.2 to a value of 0.04. Data in Table II indicates that when equilibrium was reached, the binding of cysteine to collagen (or gelatin) was directly proportional to the amount of aldehydes on the molecule. The reversibility of the changes induced in vivo by D-penicillamine can be explained quite readily on the basis of its unstable interaction with potential crosslinking groups present in collagen. The fact that neutral salt soluble collagen from rats treated with D-penicillamine cannot crosslink in vivo when the carbonyl groups are blocked, but will form stable fibers in vitro once these groups have been exposed during purification agrees with the postulate of a dissociable interaction.

III FORMATION OF NEW INTRAMOLECULAR CROSSLINKS

If this was the case, that is, that the potential crosslinking groups are being exposed during the removal of the bound penicillamine, new intramolecular and intermolecular crosslinks should become evident. A demonstration of such an effect could be seen when acid soluble collagen from D-penicillamine treated rats (which has a preponderance of α-components) was chromatographed on carboxymethyl cellulose or separated by acrylamide disc electrophoresis before and after incubation at 37°C (Deshmukh and Nimni, 1969). The formation of these new intramolecular crosslinks was time dependent and no significant amount of

TABLE II

Binding of [^{14}C]cysteine to Collagen or Gelatin Studied by Equilibrium Dialysis

Collagen specimen	Observed binding ratio*	Molar binding ratio (cysteine to tropocollagen)	Residues of acetaldehyde/ tropocollagen+
None (control)	0.998	0	
Neutral salt-soluble-reduced	1.017	1.0	0
Lathyritic (βAPN‡)	1.043	2.5	1.5
Geletin (Knox)	1.062	3.6	1.8
Neutral salt-soluble	1.076	4.47	2.6
Cysteamine-soluble	1.240	14.1	8.0
Alkali-oxidized gelatin	1.300	17.6	14.1
Acid-oxidized gelatin	1.385	22.6	17.2

* Moles of labeled cysteine inside dialysis bag (free and bound to protein) per moles outside dialysis bag.

\+ Assuming a molecular weight of tropocollagen to be 300,000; aldehydes estimated by the method of Paz et. al. (1965). In the case of gelatin results are expressed assuming a tropocollagen equivalent molecular weight.

‡ β-Aminopropionitrile.

crosslinks formed prior to 16 hr of incubation; also, as was to be expected, the presence of carbonyl trapping agents (such as penicillamine) in the media prevented this reaction.

Figures 3 and 4 summarized our observations in this connection. Figure 3 shows the elution patterns from carboxymethyl cellulose (Piez, Eigner and Lewis, 1963) after incubation at 37°C, at pH 7.0, in the absence or presence of 0.01 M penicillamine. Because of the high tendency of this collagen to polymerize (probably related to its high aldehyde content), the yields were not quantitative and decreased with increasing time of incubation at 37°C. The higher molecular

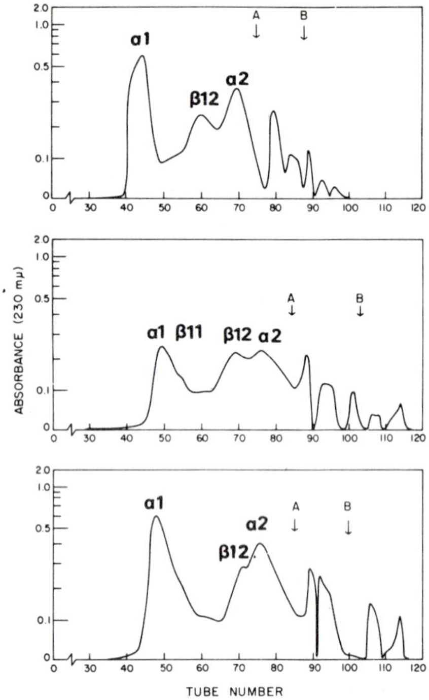

Fig. 3. Carboxymethylcellulose chromatograms of denatured skin collagen extracted from penicillamine-treated rats with 0.5 M acetic acid. Conditions were: 50 mg collagen; 40°C; column size, 2 x 18 cm; flow rate, 150 ml/hr; buffer, sodium acetate, pH 4.8; Γ/2 = 0.06; linear gradient to 0.1 M NaCl. Arrow A and B indicate elution with starting buffer containing 0.44 M NaCl and 6.0 M urea plus 1.0 M NaCl, respectively. (Untreated sample-top; sample incubated for 96 hr - middle; and sample incubated in presence of 0.01 M penicillamine - bottom)

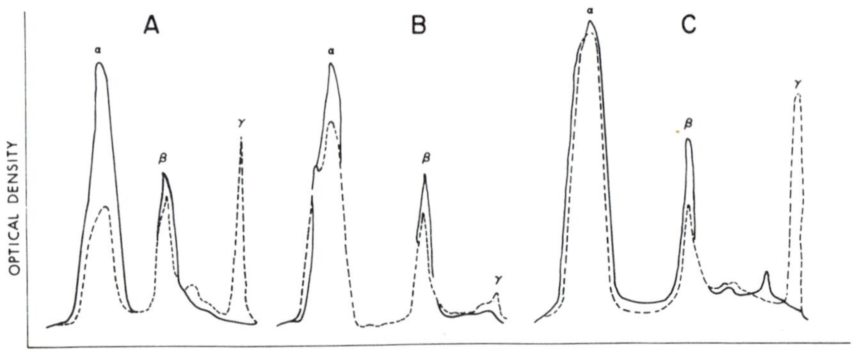

Fig. 4. Densitometric tracings corresponding to heat denatured acid soluble collagen from penicillamine and βAPN treated rats. Solid line refers to the subunits present in the initial collagen specimen; dotted line to that same sample incubated at 37°C at neutral pH for 72 hr. (A) Acid-soluble collagen from penicillamine-treated rats. (B) Same, but incubated in the presence of 0.01 M penicillamine. (C) Acid-soluble collagen from βAPN-treated rats.

weight polymeric material could not be eluted from these columns even at higher ionic strengths or by addition of 6 M urea (Veis and Anesey, 1965). Figure 4 represents the densitometric tracing of acrylamide gels, stained with Amido Black and scanned with a Gilford Spectrophotometer. The full line corresponds to the subunits present in the original acid soluble collagen; the dotted line to the same sample incubated at 37°C at neutral pH for 72 hr. Acid-soluble collagens from penicillamine-treated rats (in the absence A, or in the presence of .01 M D-penicillamine B) and from βAPN treated rats was examined. It is of interest that incubation at 37°C of all sources of acid soluble collagen gave rise to higher molecular weight aggregates which could now be visualized and that they barely penetrated the gel (γ's or greater). These polymeric forms did not form in the presence of 0.01 M penicillamine.

IV DEPOLYMERIZATION OF INSOLUBLE COLLAGEN

After rat skin has been exhaustively extracted with 0.45 M NaCl, an additional amount of collagen can be dispersed by either dilute organic acids (citric, acetic) or by compounds such as cystemine or penicillamine (0.01 to 0.2 M at 4°C, in 0.45 M NaCl at pH 7.0). In rats younger than 60 days, practically all the skin collagen can be dispersed by thiol-amines to yield a collagen soluble in 0.45 M NaCl pH 7.0, with an intrinsic viscosity of 25 dl/g, which reflects a mixture of tropocollagen with polymeric aggregates. This material will withstand centrifugation at forces greater than 100,000 x g for several hours without appreciable precipitation.

The solubilizing effect of thiol-amines on this form of collagen which cannot be dissolved by neutral salt solutions decreases as the age of the tissue increases (Nimni, Deshmukh, and Bavetta, 1967). We can assume, therefore, that the material dispersed under these conditions, as well as, that fraction of "insoluble collagen" which can be depolymerized in vivo by penicillamine, is a form of incompletely cross-linked insoluble collagen. These incomplete crosslinks may well be of the Schiff base type recently described by Lent and Franzblau (1967) in elastin, and by Bailey and Peach in collagen (1968). Additional evidence supporting this type of crosslinking entity comes from the previously discussed requirement of free aldehyde and ε-amino groups on adjacent polypeptide chains for stable crosslink formation. More recent studies using model Schiff base compounds using γ-amino butyric acid and pyridoxal phosphate clearly showed the acid and thiol-amine catalized cleavage of such Schiff bases (Deshmukh, Rojkind and Nimni, unpublished data). It is of interest that reagents that tend to disperse the fibrous collagen aggregates (e.g. dilute acetic acid, acid citrate buffers, cysteamine at neutral pH), provide environments where synthetic Schiff bases are rapidly cleaved. On the other hand, however, neutral or slightly basic pH's, where a Schiff base shows maximum stability in aqueous media, coincides with conditions which are most unfavorable for the depolymerization of collagen aggregates.

V CONCLUSIONS

Figure 5 shows in a schematic form some of the fundamental steps involved in the polymerization of tropocollagen and indicates the most likely sites of action of βAPN and penicillamine. After the tropocollagen molecule has been extruded by the cell, some specific ε-amino groups of lysine are converted to aldehydes. Although lathyritic collagen has most of the physical and chemical characteristics of normal collagen, it is defective in aldehydes. The enzyme involved, which is heat-labile and inhibited by physiological levels of βAPN, has been detected in the 100,000 x g supernatant of extracts prepared from bone, aorta, and skin (Pinnell and Martin, 1968). Consequently, if the formation of aldehydes is inhibited, the subsequent condensation step and formation of stable crosslinks cannot occur.

On the other hand, the administration of penicillamine to animals does not affect the rate or nature of the tropocollagen synthesized; but nevertheless, it interferes with

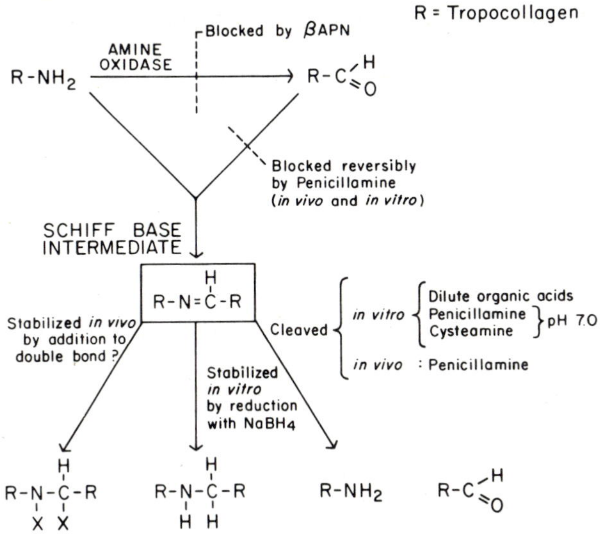

Fig. 5.

the crosslinking, presumably by reacting with aldehyde groups on the macromolecule. Compounds with neighboring thiol and amino groups, such as cysteine and penicillamine, will readily form condensation products with aldehydes (Schubert, 1936). The nature of the ring substituents, the composition and pH of media and many cations will shift the equilibrium of this reaction (Cook and Heilbron, 1949). Blockage or absence of either the amino or sulfhydryl groups gives rise to highly dissociable Schiff's bases or hemimercaptals, but when both functional groups are present on the same addend in a suitable proximity, the product is a relatively stable complex containing a thiazolidine ring (Buell and Hanson, 1960). Studying the kinetics of the reaction of pyridoxal 5'-phosphate with thiol-amino acids, Mackay obtained evidence that this involved the formation of a Schiff's base intermediate rather than a hemimercaptal prior to cyclization to a thiazolidine derivative (Mackay, 1962). Under the appropriate conditions, the thiazolidine structure postulated for this interaction can dissociate to regenerate normal collagen with reactive aldehydes and the metabolic inhibitor. This mechanism agrees with the observation that the inhibition of crosslinking will reverse in vivo once the drug is discontinued, as well as by dialysis, which removes the interacting penicillamine. It also explains the effects in vitro of penicillamine, since concentrations as low as $4x10^{-4}$ M penicillamine, or its analogues will prevent the crosslinking of normal collagen, and blocking the amino group by acetylation or the sulfhydryl group by alkylation will render the compound inactive in vivo and in vitro.

Once the Schiff base intermediate has formed, it must become stabilized. This can be done in vitro exposing polymerized tropocollagen to $NaBH_4$ and reducing the C:N double bond. Under physiological conditions this does not seem to be the most likely mechanism for stabilization since the resulting product, lysinonorleucine is only present in small amounts after reduction indicating that it may result from the stabilization of an intermediate. More so, this compound is present in even smaller amounts if older collagen is used as a substrate for the $NaBH_4$.

The solubilizing effect that the thiol-amines exhibit in vivo and in vitro on an "intermediately crosslinked" form of insoluble collagen can also be explained on the basis of the information available. At the stage of a Schiff base intermediate, this link could be easily split by dilute acids, thus explaining the high dispersing effect of these agents on collagen fibers. In addition, Schiff bases could be sensitive to nucleophilic attack by the mercapto group of penicillamine or could participate in an exchange reaction with an activated amino group, such as that encountered in the amino-thiols. We have observed that, whereas recently aggregated tropocollagen can be almost completely solubilized by 0.2 M penicillamine, this effect can be prevented if the collagen aggregate is reduced with $NaBH_4$. This stabilization had previously been evidenced by decreased solubility (Tanzer, 1968), changes in mechanical properties (Harkness and Harkness, 1968) and decreased sensitivity to pH changes

(Bailey, 1968). In the situation in vivo this could occur by reduction, but more likely by other means such as the formation of addition compounds across the double bond, an event which could then represent the final step in the synthesis of a covalent crosslink.

REFERENCES

Bailey, A.J. (1968). Biochim. Biophys. Acta 160, 447.

Bailey, A.J. and Peach, C.M. (1968). Biochem. Biophys. Res. Commun. 33, 812.

Bornstein, P. and Piez, K.A. (1966). Biochemistry 5, 3460.

Buell, M.V. and Hanson, R.E. (1960). J. Amer. Chem. Soc. 82, 6042

Cook, A.H. and Heilbron, I.M., (1960). In The Chemistry of Penicillin, p. 92. Ed. by Clark, H.T., Johnson, J.R. and Robinson, R. Princeton University Press, Princeton.

Deshmukh, A. and Nimni, M.E. (1969). Biochim. Biophys. Res. Commun. 35, 845.

Deshmukh, K. and Nimni, M.E. (1969). J. Biological Chem. 244, 1787.

Gross, J. (1963). Biochim. Biophys. Acta. 71, 250.

Harkness, M.L.R. and Harkness, R.D. (1968). Biochim. Biophys. Acta. 154, 553.

Hunter, M.J. and Commerford, S.L. (1955). J. Amer. Chem. Soc. 77, 4857.

Klotz, I.M., Walker, F.M., and Pivan, R.B. (1946). J. Amer. Chem. Soc. 68, 1486.

Lent, R. and Franzblau, C. (1967). Biochem. Biophys. Res. Commun. 26, 43.

Levene, C.I. and Gross, J. (1959) J. Exp. Med. 110, 771.

Mackay, D. (1962). Arch. Biochem. Biophys. 99, 93.

Martin, G.R., Gross, J., Piez, K.A. and Lewis, M.S. (1961) Biochim. Biophys. Acta. 53, 599.

Nimni, M.E. (1965) Biochim. Biophys. Acta. 111, 576.

Nimni, M.E. (1966). Biochim. Biophys. Res. Commun. 25, 434.

Nimni, M.E. (1968). J. Biological Chem. 243, 1457.

Nimni, M.E. and Bavetta, L.A. (1965). Science 150, 905

Nimni, M.E., Deshmukh, K., and Bavetta, L.A. (1967). Arch. Biochem. Biophys. 122, 292.

Paz, M.A., Blumenfeld, O.O., Rojkind, M., Henson, E., Furfine, C. and Gallop, P.M. (1965). Arch. Biochem. Biophys. 109, 548.

Piez, K.A., Eigner, E.A. and Lewis, M.S. (1963). Biochemistry, 2, 58.

Pinnell, S.R. and Martin, G.R. (1968). Proc. Nat. Acad. Sci. (U.S.) 61, 708.

Rojkind, M. and Juarez, H. (1966). Biochim. Biophys. Res. Commun. 25, 481.

Schubert, M.P. (1936). J. Biol. Chem., 144, 341.

Tanzer, M.L. (1968). J. Biol. Chem. 243, 4045.

Veis, A. and Anesey, J. (1965). J. Biol. Chem. 240, 3499.

POSSIBLE FOLATE-ASCORBATE INTERACTION IN COLLAGEN FORMATION

Bernard S. Gould

It has been generally assumed that ascorbic acid is an essential requirement for collagen biosynthesis. However, chick lung fibroblasts cultured on presumably ascorbic acid-free media (Woessner and Gould, 1957) were found to produce small but definite amounts of collagen. On this basis Woessner and Gould postulated that there might exist both ascorbic acid-dependent and ascorbic acid-independent collagen formation. This hypothesis was tested (Gould, 1961) by showing that young guinea pigs deprived of ascorbic acid lost most of the ability to produce collagen in repair long before they failed to form collagen in growth. These observations, among others, raise the question whether other factors may not be effective in replacing ascorbic acid entirely or potentiate low levels of ascorbic acid in some collagen formation.

It is quite clear that one of the central aspects of collagen biosynthesis involves the hydroxylation of proline and lysine. Many aspects of this mechanism have been elucidated (Prockop, 1967; Udenfriend, 1966; Chvapil, 1968) and it is generally accepted that the hydroxylase involved belongs to the "mixed function" oxidases which catalyze a reaction of the type

$$RH + O_2 + XH_2 \text{ ---- } ROH + H_2O + X$$

At least three different kinds of electron donors (XH_2) have been found to function as co-enzymes or co-reactants in different hydroxylating systems: (1) ascorbate (2) tetrahydropteridines and (3) NADPH. In collagen formation the essential factors appear to be ascorbate, Fe^{2+}, α-ketoglutarate and O_2.

In several hydroxylating systems tetrahydropteridines have been shown to be co-enzymes (Kaufman, 1959; Nair and Vining, 1965); Vaughan and Butt, 1967; and Nakamura, 1965) but the mechanism by which they act is not known. Particularly interesting is the fact that certain of these can replace ascorbate in certain hydroxylating systems. More specifically, 2-amino-4-hydroxy-tetrahydropteridine could in large part replace ascorbate in collagen proline hydroxylation and NADPH was about half as effective as ascorbate (Peterkofsky and Udenfriend, 1965; Hutton, Tappel and Udenfriend, 1967). Udenfriend reported at this meeting that for hydroxylation in vitro ascorbic acid is not essential and can be replaced by other suitable reducing compounds that can maintain the iron in the reduced state.

A possible potentiation between ascorbate and tetrahydropteridines has been suggested by Priest and Bublitz (1967) from their studies on cultured cells. In addition, there are some reports (Calnan and Davies, 1965) which have shown that wound healing is impaired when a folate antagonist is administered to rats; that bone repair is impaired (Mangioni and Taverna, 1964) as is liver regeneration under similar conditions (Song, 1966).

Presented here are preliminary results of experiments designed to test further the hypothesis that some collagen formation in vivo may in fact not involve ascorbic acid. The experiments involve a study of collagen formation in folic acid deficiency in rats induced by antagonists and in young guinea pigs which have been maintained on a folic acid deficient diet with and without added ascorbate.

I EXPERIMENTAL PROCEDURES

A. ANIMALS

Young guinea pigs (ca. 200 g each) were used. These have a dietary requirement for both ascorbate and folate. Until ready for study they were kept on a commercial laboratory diet. The diet used to induce folic acid deficiency was that of Reid, Martin and Briggs (1956) with ascorbic acid omitted. 10 milligrams ascorbic acid was administered daily by mouth except when indicated. Calcium folinate, made up freshly just before use, was injected intraperitoneally when desired.

Guinea pigs were desaturated of ascorbic acid by maintaining them on the diet for 4-6 days and of folic acid after 14 days on the diet.

Rats weighing about 150 g were of the Wistar Strain and were maintained on a commercial pellet diet. Methotrexate (4-amino-$\underline{N}^{10}$-methylpteroylglutamate) was administered intraperitoneally daily to induce a folic acid deficiency.

B. METHODS

Collagen formation was studied in subcutaneously implanted polyvinyl sponges. Total collagen, and in certain instances salt-soluble collagen, were determined on the basis of the hydroxyproline content of hydrolyzates of the autoclaved extracts of the sponges. The methods are essentially those described previously (Gould, 1958).

II RESULTS AND DISCUSSION

A. COLLAGEN FORMATION IN SUBCUTANEOUSLY-IMPLANTED POLYVINYL SPONGES IN METHOTREXATE-TREATED RATS

Sponges were implanted in the usual way into a number of 150-g rats maintained on a commercial laboratory diet. Groups of 3-6 animals were maintained as controls or were injected intraperiteally daily with either 0.075 mg or 0.150 mg of methotrexate for 8 days, a suitably long period for the accumulation of substantial amounts of collagen in the control sponges. The results shown in Table I indicate that chemical determination of collagen formation in implants parallels the observations of Calnan and Davies (1965) who studied the effects of folate deficiency induced by methotrexate on wound healing as measured by tensile strength. The lower concentration (0.075 mg/day) affects the level of salt-soluble and insoluble collagen equally;

TABLE I

Collagen Formation in Subcutaneous Polyvinyl (Ivalon) Sponge Implants in Methotrexate-treated Rats

	Untreated	Methotrexate-treated (mg/day) 0.075	0.150
	(μg collagen/sponge)		
0.45 M NaCl-soluble collagen	160	64.2	28.5
Insoluble collagen	2990	1300	62.3

Implants were removed and analyzed after 8 days.

Methotrexate treatment was begun immediately after implanting.

at the higher level of antagonist the effect on insoluble collagen formation is much more pronounced than on the accumulation of salt-soluble collagen. It is amply clear that methotrexate inhibits collagen formation; the mechanism by which it does so is not clear. It may be through inhibition at the molecular level or through cytoxic effects of the drug.

B. THE EFFECT ON COLLAGEN FORMATION OF FOLIC ACID DEPLETION AND THE EFFECT OF THE ADMINISTRATION OF FOLIC ACID AND OF ASCORBIC ACID TO DEPLETED GUINEA PIGS

Groups of 15-30 guinea pigs (200 g each) were subdivided into groups of 5 for the following studies. Preliminary experiments involving the withdrawal of folic acid for varying periods of time before implanting the sponges indicated that a preparation period of 11-14 days was necessary to deplete the animals of folic acid--as determined by their inability to form substantial amounts of collagen. A 7-day period on the folic acid deficiency diet before implantation resulted in a 30% impairment of collagen formation. In these experiments all animals were depleted of folic acid by maintaining them on the deficient diet for 11-14 days. They were depleted of ascorbic acid by withdrawing the latter from the diet 4-6 days before implantation.

TABLE II

The Effects of Folinic Acid and of Ascorbic Acid on Collagen Formation in Folic Acid-Depleted Guinea Pigs

Treatment (days)	Ascorbic acid-depleted + Ascorbic acid	Folic acid-depleted + Folinic acid + Ascorbic acid (a)	Folic acid-depleted + Folinic acid + Ascorbic acid (b)	Folic acid-depleted ascorbic acid-depleted + Folinic acid (a)	Folic acid-depleted ascorbic acid-depleted + Folinic acid (b)
	(Collagen, μg/sponge)				
5	130	62.3		58	
8	600	232.		106	
12	975	875	345 (14 d)	372 (15 d)	101 (14 d)

Sponges were implanted after 11 days on the folic acid-deficient diet and ascorbic acid was withdrawn 4 days prior to implantation.

(a) Treatment with folinic acid (calcium salt) 0.5 mg/day commenced immediately after implantation

(b) Treatment with folinic acid (calcium salt) 0.5mg/day commenced 5 days after implantation

Sponges in animals continued on the folic acid-free diet with added ascorbate (10 mg/day) after implantation contained 313 μg collagen after 12 days.

Table II summarizes the results of a number of preliminary experiments. It is clear that folic acid deficiency even when the animal is saturated with ascorbic acid results in markedly impaired collagen formation. Folic acid depleted animals continued on the deficiency diet after implantation and supplemented with ascorbic acid accumulated a small amount (313 μg/sponge) of collagen. This amount is somewhat greater than that (175 μg/sponge) produced by ascorbic acid depleted animals maintained on a scorbutigenic diet after implantation.

When folic acid-depleted animals were treated with 0.5 mg folinic acid and 10 mg. ascorbic acid daily immediately post-implantation collagen formation was restored but at a slower rate compared to that by ascorbic acid-depleted guinea pigs in response to ascorbic acid. Within 12 days however similar levels are attained. This may involve the time to attain adequate levels in the tissues or for the conversion to the proper folate compound. It is quite evident that folinic acid cannot replace ascorbic acid since the administration of the former without the latter resulted in what appears to be the formation of a relatively small amount of collagen. Further experiments will determine the significance of this increase.

It is notable that when folinic acid was withheld for 5 days post-implantation, after which it was administered for 14 days, collagen formation was markedly impaired in the ascorbic acid-supplemented as well as in the unsupplemented animals.

These preliminary data suggest that in the absence of either folic acid or of ascorbic acid, guinea pigs are unable to accumulate substantial amounts of collagen in polyvinyl sponge implants. Neither can substitute entirely for the other in vivo.

Folic acid deficiency in the rat induced by methotrexate, a folic acid antagonist, results in markedly impaired collagen formation.

REFERENCES

Calnan, J. and Davies, A. (1965). Br. J. Cancer 19, 502.

Chvapil, M. (1968). Int. Rev. Conn. Tissue Res. 4, 68.

Gould, B.S. (1958). J. Biol. Chem. 232, 637.

Gould, B.S. (1961). Ann. N.Y. Acad. Sci. 92, 168.

Hutton, J.J., Tappel, A.L. and Udenfriend, S. (1967). Arch. Biochem. Biophys. 118, 231.

Kaufman, S. (1959). J. Biol. Chem. 234, 267.

Mangioni, F. and Taverna, L. (1964). Bull. Soc. Ital. Biol. Sper. 40, 711.

Nair, P.M. and Vining, L.C. (1965). Phytochemistry 4, 161.

Nakamura, S., Ichiyama, A. and Hayaishi, O. (1965). Fed. Proc. 24, 604.

Peterkofsky, B. and Udenfriend, S. (1965). Proc. Nat. Acad. Sci. 53, 335.

Priest, R.E. and Bublitz, C. (1967). Lab. Invest. 17, 371.

Prockop, D.J. (1967). Ann. Intern. Med. 66, 1243.

Reid, M.E., Martin, M.G. and Briggs, G.M. (1956). J. Nutr. 59, 103.

Song, K.J. (1966). Chungang Vihak 11, 701.

Udenfriend, S. (1966). Science 152, 1335.

Vaughan, P.F.T. and Butt, V.S. (1967). Biochem. J. 104, 658.

Woessner, J.F. and Gould, B.S. (1957). J. Biophys. Biochem. Cytol. 3, 685.

MECHANISM OF ACTION OF ASCORBIC ACID IN THE BIOSYNTHESIS OF COLLAGEN

F. Fernández-Madrid and J. Pita, Jr.

This work describes an effect of ascorbic acid different than the direct enhancement of the hydroxylation of collagen proline. Several years ago electron miscroscopic studies of skin wounds and tendon regeneration in the scorbutic guinea pig respectively (Peach, 1962; Ross and Benditt, 1964), showed that the rough surfaced endoplasmic reticulum (ER) of the scorbutic fibroblasts was considerably reduced in extent and differed in form, from the rough-surfaced ER of fibroblasts from animals receiving ascorbic acid. The ribosomes of the fibroblasts from nondeficient animals were highly organized in the form of paralled rows of particles, curved or linear. This characteristic geometry of the ribosomes of the ER was lost in scorbutic fibroblasts and began to reappear early after ascorbic acid administration, when extracellular collagen fibrils also began to reappear. It was suggested that there may be a relationship between the aggregation of the ribosomes of the ER of the fibroblast and the aggregation of tropocollagen leading to the deposition of fibrous collagen (Ross and Benditt, 1964).

Collagen has been shown to be synthesized on large polyribosomes in several systems (Kretsinger, Manner, Gould and Rich, 1964; Malt and Speakman, 1965; Fernández-Madrid, 1967), though collagen synthesis in fibroblasts in tissue culture seems to occur on small polyribosomes (Goldberg and Green, 1967). If the orderly arrangement of the ribosomes of fibroblasts described by electron microscopic studies corresponds to the polyribosomes synthesizing collagen, it could be expected that changes in the particle size distribution of the collagen-synthesizing polyribosomes may occur in scurvy.

The system used in this work was the guinea pig carrageenan granuloma. All male guinea pigs were placed on a scorbutigenic diet supplemented with vitamins A and D. Pair-feeding method was used (Friberg, 1958), and all animals were supplemented with a casein hydrolysate and dextrose administered daily by a thin polyethylene tube. Pair-fed guinea pigs were given 50 mg ascorbic acid daily per os. Carrageenan granulomas were produced in the guinea pig (Robertson and Schwartz, 1953) 10-14 days after beginning the scorbutigenic diet. The animals were killed after 16-20 days on the ascorbic acid deficient diet by decapitation. The molars and incisors were examined for evidence of the scorbutic state. There was also a striking difference in the macroscopic appearance and in the total collagen content of granulomas from scorbutic and pair-fed animals. In addition to scorbutic and pair-fed animals, the effect of a systemic injection of 100 mg ascorbic acid given to scorbutic animals 18-24 hr prior to the experiment was studied (recovery animals). Non-growing animals at the time of the experiment were discarded.

Slices of granuloma tissue from pair-fed guinea pigs were incubated in vitro with [^{14}C]proline for 45 min, the tissue was homogenized in Tris 0.01 M, KCl 0.01 M, $MgCl_2$ 0.0015 M, pH 7.4, and subjected to cell fractionation. The 105,000xg pellet was gently resuspended in the same buffer and centrifuged at 4000xg for 5 min. The supernatant, labeled resuspended ribosomes, was then layered on 15-60% linear sucrose gradients and centrifuged in the SW25.1 head of the Spinco ultracentrifuge. The absorbancy at 260 mμ was monitored and the ^{14}C total radioactivity determined in sucrose gradient fractions. Thereafter, the fractions were hydrolysed in 6 N HCl and proline was separated from hydroxyproline by paper chromatography in two different solvent systems (Fernández-Madrid, 1967). It is seen in Fig. 1 that the guinea pig carrageenan granuloma polyribosomes are large

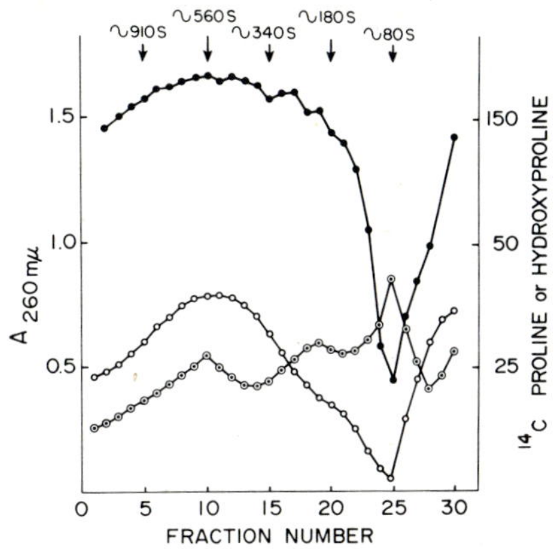

Fig. 1. Particle size, [^{14}C]proline and [^{14}C]hydroxyproline distribution in pair-fed guinea pig carrageenan granuloma polyribosomes. Sedimentation values at the top are approximate, in reference to T_2 bacteriophage marker. A_{260} mμ, dotted circles; [^{14}C]proline, filled circles; [^{14}C]hydroxyproline, open circles.

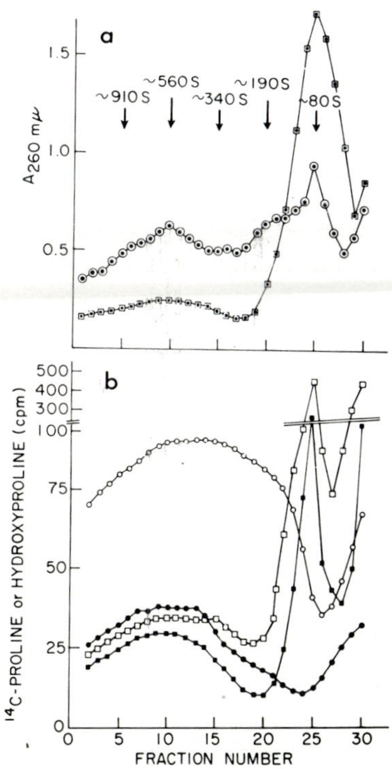

Fig. 2. Effect of ribonuclease on pair-fed guinea pig carrageenan granuloma polyribosomes. Experimental conditions as in Fig. 1. (a) control, dotted circles; RNase, dotted squares; (b) [^{14}C]proline control, open circles; [^{14}C] proline RNase, open squares; [^{14}C]hydroxyproline control, closed circles; [^{14}C]hydroxyproline RNase, closed squares.

and polydisperse with sedimentation constants ranging from 200 S to more than 1000 S. It is seen that the largest [^{14}C]hydroxyproline content was on the large aggregates (>400 S) and that the [^{14}C]pro/[^{14}C]hydroxyproline ratio in that region was about 2.5, indicating that in this area there is a mixture of collagen-synthesizing polyribosomes and aggregates engaged in non-collagenous protein synthesis. As usual the single ribosomes had the least amount of radioactivity.

Figure 2 shows the effect of 50 μg pancreatic RNase at 4°C during 30 min on this polyribosome distribution. It is seen that RNase removes 50-60% of the ultraviolet-absorbing material on the large polyribosome area, which now accumulates in the single ribosomal region (a). The radioactivity is removed by RNase following a similar pattern (b), but [^{14}C]proline is removed preferentially by the enzyme; the [^{14}C]proline to [^{14}C]hydroxyproline ratio being slightly above unity in the material not susceptible to RNase attack. This experiment, in agreement with previous reports (Kretsinger et al., 1964; Malt and Speakman, 1965; Goldberg and Green, 1967; Fernández-Madrid, 1967) indicates that the material which is resistant to RNase contains a large proportion of collagen-synthesizing polyribosomes and that the enzyme removes preferentially aggregates involved in the synthesis of non-collagenous protein. This material resistant to RNase was completely degraded by ethylenediaminetetraacetic acid (EDTA) in low Mg^{2+} buffer to 50 S and 30 S ribosomal subunits and was therefore formed chiefly by ribosomes. Thus, this preparation isolated by conventional techniques to prepare polyribosomes incorporates rapidly radioactive amino acids, and though it is only partially sensitive to RNase, it may be completely degraded by EDTA to ribosomal subunits.

Figure 3 shows the effect of the scorbutigenic diet on the particle size distribution of these polyribosomes. It is seen that the large polyribosomes (>400 S), are reduced in the scorbutic tissue, there being an increased proportion of single ribosomes and small polyribosomes.

Figure 4 shows the polyribosome size distribution (a)

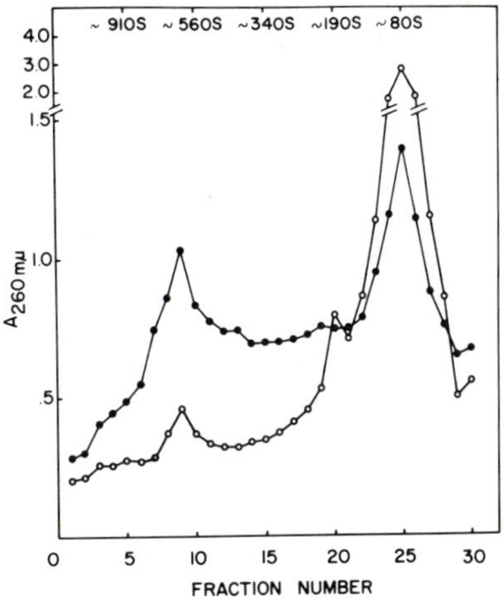

Fig. 3. Particle size distribution of polyribosomes from pair-fed and scorbutic guinea pig carageenan granulomas. Pair-fed, closed circles; scorbutic, open circles.

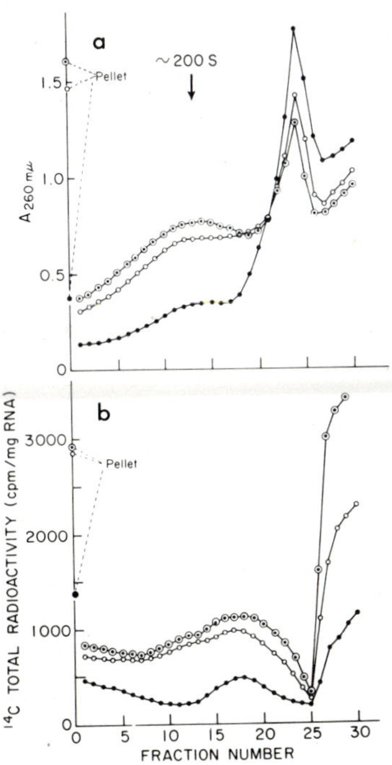

Fig. 4. Particle size distribution (a) and aminoacid incorporating activity (b) of scorbutic, pair-fed and recovery guinea pig carrageenan granuloma polyribosomes. Fifteen to thirty per cent linear sucrose gradient. Centrifugation time 2 hr. Other experimental conditions as in Fig. 1. Pair-fed, dotted circles; recovery, open circles; scorbutic, closed circles.

and amino acid incorporating ability (b) of scorbutic, pair-fed and recovery guinea pig carrageenan granuloma polyribosomes. The absorbancy profile shows the large difference in the proportion of large polyribosomes between the pair-fed and the scorbutic tissue. The recovery animals showed an increased proportion of aggregates of large size approaching the concentration found in pair-fed animals. In (b) it is seen that there is a severe reduction of the ^{14}C-radioactivity precipitable with cold trichloroacetic acid (TCA) in the individual sucrose gradient fractions. In the scorbutic polyribosomes [^{14}C]hydroxyproline was present, but so much decreased that no consistent [^{14}C]proline to [^{14}C]hydroxyproline ratios could be obtained. The recovery animals presented a content of [^{14}C]hydroxyproline quite similar to that of the pair-fed animals.

Since it has been shown that the effect of ascorbic is local rather than systemic (Gould, 1958; Robertson, Hewitt and Herman, 1959) the same type of experiment was performed in vitro. Granuloma slices from scorbutic animals were incubated in vitro in Krebs-Ringer phosphate solution, pH 7.5, for 1 hr with [^{14}C]proline, in the presence or absence of 50 μg/ml of ascorbic acid. After cell fractionation and isolation of the ribosomes, aliquots of both preparations were incubated with highly purified bacterial collagenase (0.3 mg/ml) at 25°C for 30 min, prior to zone centrifugation through sucrose gradients. It is seen (Fig. 5a) that ascorbic acid also stimulates the formation of large polyribosomes, in vitro. In addition, collagenase completely obliterated the action of ascorbic acid suggesting that this stimulation was probably due to enhancement of aggregation of nascent collagen chains on the polyribosomes. Figure 5b shows the effect of collagenase on the ^{14}C-radioactivity incorporated by scorbutic polyribosomes. It is seen that collagenase removes very little radioactivity from polyribosomes of all sizes indicating that some, but very reduced synthesis of peptides susceptible to collagenase is occurring. Figure 5c shows the effect of collagenase on the radioactivity incorporated into scorbutic polyribosomes stimulated by ascorbic acid in vitro.

The large surge of radioactivity found in the large polyribosomes stimulated by ascorbic acid is removed by digestion with collagenase; radioactive material now accumulated in areas of the gradient corresponding to smaller particles. These experiments describe an effect of ascorbic acid influencing the assembly of large polyribosomes

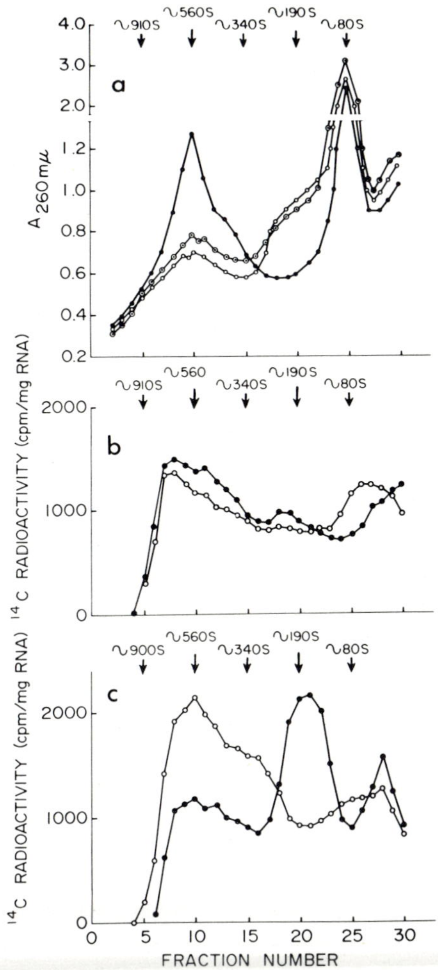

Fig. 5. (a) Effect of ascorbic acid on scorbic acid on scorbutic polyribosomes in vitro (cells intact); scorbutic, dotted circles; ascorbic acid added; closed circles; ascorbic acid and collagenase added, open circles. (b) Effect of collagenase on the ^{14}C-radioactivity incorporated by scorbutic polyribosomes after incubating the tissue with [^{14}C] proline in vitro; scorbutic, filled circles; scorbutic treated with collagenase, open circles. (c) Effect of collagenase on the ^{14}C-radioactivity incorporated by scorbutic polyribosomes stimulated by ascorbic acid in vitro; scorbutic, ascorbic acid added, open circles; scorbutic, ascorbic acid and collagenase added, closed circles.

(350-1000 S) which are severely reduced in scurvy; these large aggregates stimulated by ascorbic acid incorporate more radioactivity per ribosome than scorbutic polyribosomes and contain as much labeled hydroxyproline as polyribosomes from pair-fed animals.

The influence of inanition was eliminated by using careful pair-feeding controls, by the use of recovery animals which were not allowed to eat after the injection of ascorbic acid and finally by the effect observed in vitro. The stimulation of collagen-synthesizing polyribosomes by ascorbic acid in vitro is in agreement with a direct, local action of this vitamin.

It has been suggested that ascorbic acid might produce its effect on the aggregation of the ribosomes by inducing the synthesis or availability of mRNA for collagen (Ross and Benditt, 1964). However, tritiated uridine incorporation was not stimulated by ascorbic acid, in vivo or in vitro, though the usual effect on the collagen-synthesizing polyribosomes was observed. This is in agreement with reports of increased hydroxyproline content in ascorbic acid deficient chick embryo tibias that had been incubated with actinomycin D and therefore presumably in the absence of mRNA synthesis, though these results were attributed to the action of ascorbic acid on the hydroxylation of proline (Jeffrey and Martin, 1966).

If the action of ascorbic acid is local on the polyribosomes, it should be possible to detect incorporation of labeled ascorbic acid into the polyribosomes. Figure 6 shows the incorporation of [^{14}C]ascorbic acid into scorbutic guinea pig carrageenan granuloma polyribosomes.

It is seen that the label precipitated in sucrose gradient fractions by cold TCA is preferentially incorporated into the large (>400 S) polyribosomes, which have the highest [^{14}C]hydroxyproline content. Also it is seen that there is no incorporation of labeled ascorbic acid at 0°C. Since ascorbic acid increases very rapidly the content of [^{14}C]hydroxyproline of the large polyribosomes, it could be argued that the effect on aggregation is secondary to the effect on hydroxylation. This does not appear to be the case since

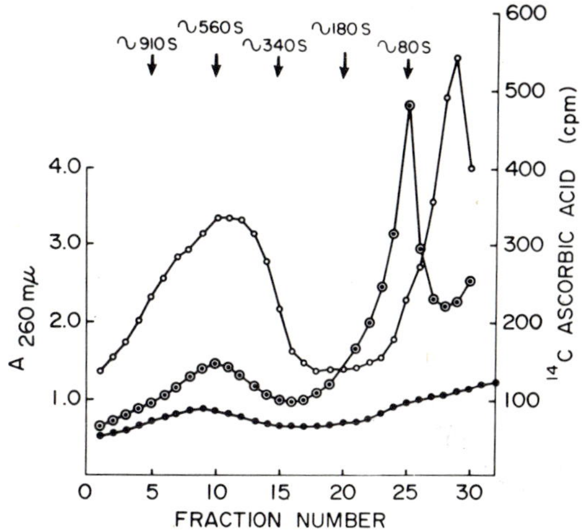

Fig. 6. Incorporation of [^{14}C]ascorbic acid into TCA-precipitable material from scorbutic guinea pig carrageenan granuloma polyribosomes. Except for incubation of the granuloma slices with 10 μC [^{14}C]ascorbic acid at 37°C or at 0°C for 1 hr the experimental conditions were as in Fig. 1; A_{260} mμ, 0° and 37°C incubation, dotted circles; [^{14}C] ascorbic acid 37°C, open circles; [^{14}C]ascorbic acid, 0°C, closed circles.

blocking the hydroxylation reaction with the alpha-alpha'-dipyrididyl does not modify the sedimentation properties of these polyribosomes. The influence of ascorbic acid on the assembly of the large polyribosomes and the rapid enhancement of collagen synthesis revealed by the increase of [^{14}C] hydroxyproline content suggests a relationship between aggregation of ribosomes and aggregation of collagen. The effect of collagenase probably indicates, that the shift of polyribosome size toward the bottom of the gradient upon stimulation with ascorbic acid, is due to interaction of collagen peptides leading to the formation of poly-polyribosomes. It is suggested that the enhancement of collagen synthesis by ascorbic acid may be largely due to its influence on the polyribosomes and the formation of the large collagen-synthesizing polyribosomes leading to rapid collagen fibrillogenesis.

ACKNOWLEDGEMENTS

This work was supported by PHS Program Project Grant No. 5 P01 HE-11035 from the National Heart Institute and by Grant No. AM 12571 from the National Institute of Arthritis and Metabolic Diseases.

REFERENCES

Fernández-Madrid, F. (1967). J. Cell Biol. 33, 27.

Friberg, U. (1958). Arkiv. Kemi. 12, 501.

Goldberg, B. and Green, H. (1967). J. Mol. Biol. 26, 1.

Gould, B.S. (1958). J. Biol. Chem. 232, 637.

Jeffrey, J.J. and Martin, G.R. (1966). Biochem. Biophys. Acta 121, 281.

Kretsinger, R.H., Manner, G., Gould, B.S. and Rich, A. (1964). Nature 202, 438.

Malt, R.A. and Speakman, P.T. (1965). Sugery 58, 248.

Peach, R. (1962). J. Ultrastructure Res. 6, 679.

Robertson, W. van B., Hewitt, J. and Herman, C. (1959). J. Biol. Chem. 234, 105.

Robertson, W. van B. and Schwartz, B. (1953). J. Biol. Chem. 201, 689.

Ross, R. and Benditt, E.P. (1964). J. Cell Biol. 22, 365.

THE PROPERTIES OF COLLAGEN IN TISSUES OF PENICILLAMINE TREATED RATS

Suzanne Bazin and Albert Delaunay

Some papers previously issued from our laboratory have described the accumulation and the resorption of collagen in granulation tissue of several types of experimentally produced inflammation (Bazin and Delaunay, 1964, 1966a,b, 1967). A special collagenolytic cathepsin appeared as an effective agent in the degradation of the collagen synthesized in the granulation tissue (Bazin and Delaunay, 1966b, 1968), such an enzyme being active presumably in the phagocytic vacuoles of inflammatory cells. In vitro, this cathepsin degraded acid-soluble collagen more rapidly than insoluble collagen, suggesting that in vivo collagen might be removed more or less easily according to its cross-linkage.

The present paper describes the first group of experiments we have carried out to investigate how a more or less cross-linked collagen can be degraded in vivo by the collagenolytic cathepsin we have isolated and characterized (Bazin and Delaunay, 1969). Growing rats, bearing the granulation tissue of a subacute inflammation, were treated by penicillamine, a substance known as able to break some weak cross-links of collagen fibres in vitro and in vivo and also to prevent the formation of bonds in the newly formed collagen.

In the penicillamine treated animals, were studied first the amount and the cross-linkage of collagen, then the enzymatic activity of collagenolytic cathepsin.

I MATERIAL AND METHODS

A. GRANULATION TISSUE AND NORMAL SKIN

Forty young 150-g rats had two pieces of plastic sponge implanted under the dorsal skin by our usual method (Bazin and Delaunay, 1964). Five days after implantation, 20 of the animals received 30 mg penicillamine daily, per os, dissolved in 0.5 ml isotonic saline (containing 0.10 mg pyridoxine to avoid B_6 avitaminosis).

The other 20 were used as controls and received 0.5 ml isotonic saline daily. After 16 days treatment, the animals were sacrificed and the sponge implants of all the animals were removed, minced and pooled. The ventral skin of the same animals was taken off, carefully shaved, and freed from subcutaneous fat, minced and pooled.

The pooled granulation tissues and skins were divided into three fractions: one was used to extract the collagenolytic cathepsin, as previously described (Bazin and Delaunay, 1966b, 1969); another was dehydrated, defatted and used to extract the total collagen by hot 5% trichloacetic acid (Fitch, Harkness and Harkness, 1955); the third one was used to extract the non and weakly cross-linked collagen, as indicated below.

B. EXTRACTIONS OF COLLAGEN FRACTIONS

The pooled tissues were first homogenized twice in phosphate buffer 0.066 M, pH 7.8, then centrifuged at 30,000xg and 10% NaCl was added to the supernatant. The precipitate formed contained the neutral soluble collagen which was collected by centrifugation and purified by dissolution in N/100 acetic acid and reprecipitation with NaCl.

The residue was then homogenized twice in citrate buffer 0.1 M pH 3.6 and centrifuged. The supernatant contained the acid soluble collagen which was purified as for the neutral soluble collagen. All these operations were carried out at 0 + 4°C.

The residue was homogenized in 0.2 M phosphate buffer

pH 6.4, containing 0.25 M NaCl and maintained for 1 hr at 60°C with constant stirring, centrifuged and the supernatant collected. This supernatant, containing the 60°C labile collagen, was dialyzed and then lyophilized.

The residue of the last homogenate was treated by hot trichloracetic acid (Fitch et al., 1955) to extract the insoluble collagen. A sample of each fraction was hydrolysed in 6 N HCL and the hydroxyproline content determined by Stegemann's method (1958).

C. COLLAGENOLYTIC CATHEPSIN

The "free" collagenolytic cathepsin was extracted from homogenate of granulation tissue and from normal skin as previously described (Bazin and Delaunay, 1966a). The "bound" collagenolytic cathepsin was freed from the particulate phase of the tissue homogenates by saponin. Both extracts were partly purified before testing their collagenolytic activity on purified acid soluble collagen from rat tail tendon by our usual methods (Bazin and Delaunay, 1966a, 1969).

D. FREE ALDEHYDES OF COLLAGEN

Aldehydes were determined in acid soluble and 60°C-labile collagen fractions without previous hydrolysis, by the method of Paz et al. (1955). Aldehydes were not determined in neutral salt soluble collagen because the amount collected was not sufficient for analysis. The determination of free aldehydes was also impossible in the insoluble collagen because solubilization by hydrolysis would lead to structural modification.

II RESULTS

The total collagen and the proportions of its soluble and 60°C-labile fractions, in neutral skin and in sponge granulation tissue of normal and of penicillamine treated rats, are given in Fig. 1. The activity of the collageno-

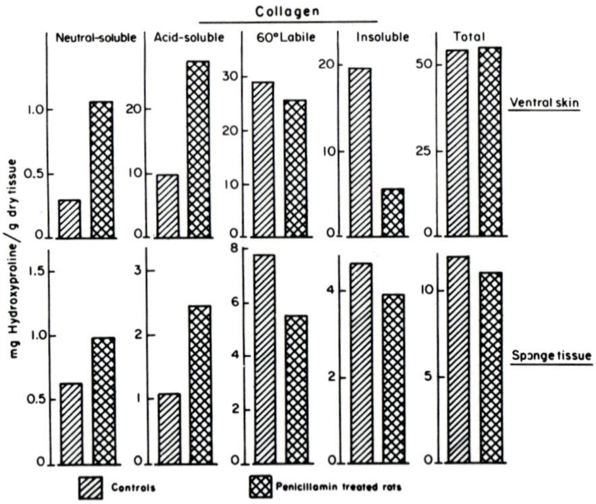

Fig. 1. Total collagen and its neutral soluble, acid-soluble, 60°C labile and insoluble fractions in normal skin and in sponge granulation tissue of normal or penicillamine treated rats.

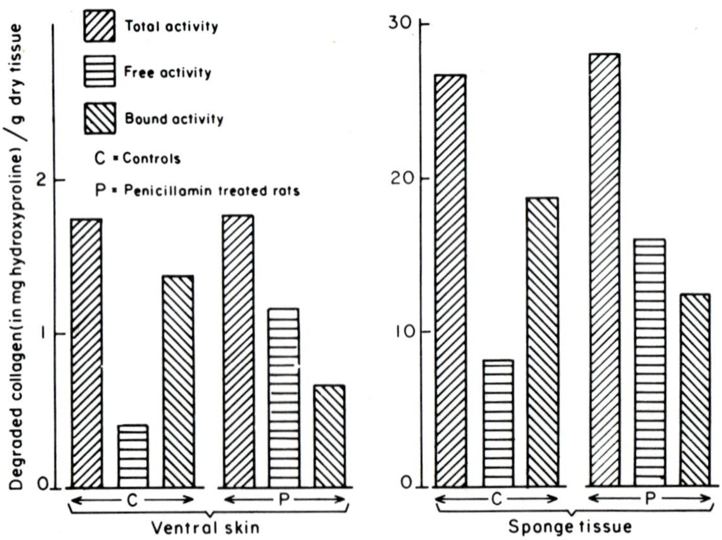

Fig. 2. Activity of collagenolytic cathepsin and its distribution into "free" and "bound" activities in normal skin and in sponge granulation tissue of normal or penicillamine treated rats.

TABLE I

Free Aldehydes (in μM acetaldehyde equivalents/100 mg Collagen) in Collagen Fractions of Normal and Penicillamine Treated Rats

	Ventral skin		Sponge tissue	
	C(1)	P(2)	C(1)	P(2)
Citrate-soluble collagen	1.58	2.13	1.62	2.58
60°C-labile collagen	3	4.20	1.03	2.05

(1) C = Control group
(2) P = Penicillamine treated group

lytic cathepsin in the tissues of the same groups of rats, are given in Fig. 2.

The free aldehyde groups of citrate soluble and 60°C-labile collagen fractions are given in Table 1.

III DISCUSSION

The collagen of the studied tissues was fractionated into four fractions: neutral soluble, acid soluble, 60°C-labile and insoluble collagen. These fractions, solubilized under successive, more and more drastic treatments, correspond to more and more cross-linked collagen.

As shown in Fig. 1, the penicillamine treatment of rats increased the proportion of neutral soluble and acid soluble collagen fractions, without significantly modifying the total collagen of skin and of sponge granulation tissue. Consequently the 60°C-labile and the insoluble fractions are decreased in both tissues. However, the insoluble collagen is proportionately more decreased in skin (73% less) than in granulation tissue (25% less).

Our results are in agreement with those obtained by Nimni and Bavetta (1965); Youssef, Grever and Levenson (1966); and Chvapil, Hurych and Ehrlichova (1968) who observed that penicillamine treatment increases the salt soluble and citrate soluble collagens in the skin of growing rats and in granulation tissues of sponge implants, skin wounds and silica induced fibrosis of the liver. All these observations have shown that, in vivo, penicillamine is able to prevent the formation of cross-links in the newly synthesized collagen and to cleave some weak bonds in the collagen formed before the treatment and not yet completely matured. Thus in a tissue where the biosynthesis of collagen is very active, such as a granulation tissue, the prevention of cross-linkage is predominant. In a tissue where the biosynthesis is less active, such as the skin, bonds are prevented in newly formed collagen and other bonds can be cleaved in the more recently deposited fibres. Such differences in the effect of penicillamine treatment according to the characteristics of collagen in a tissue is evidenced in our results showing a larger decrease of insoluble collagen in skin than in granuloma. Similar differences were also noted by Nimni (1968) who observed that the highly cross-linked, slowly turning over collagen of old animals is only slightly sensitive to penicillamine treatment.

The bonds affected by penicillamine can be detected through the determination of the free aldehyde groups. We have observed that penicillamine treatment has increased the proportion of aldehyde groups in acid soluble collagen and in 60°C-labile collagen (see Table I). This result is in agreement with the work of Deshmukh and Nimni (1968), showing that the collagen, extracted from rat skin, soaked in vitro in a cysteamine solution, is richer in aldehyde groups than the collagen extracted from untreated skin.

It can be seen in Table I that, in normal animals, the citrate soluble collagen from ventral skin and of granulation tissue contains approximately the same number of aldehyde groups. The 60°C-labile collagen, on the contrary, appears richer in aldehydes in the ventral skin than in the granulation tissue. In penicillamine treated rats the increase of the number of aldehyde groups is higher in collagen fractions of granulation tissue (60-99%) than in the similar fractions of ventral skin (35-40%). These observations show that the aldehyde-mediated cross-links, fewer in the young immature collagen of a granulation tissue than in the more mature collagen of the skin, are,however, more sensitive to penicillamine.

In the tissues of the penicillamine treated rats, the total activity of the collagenolytic cathepsins is not significantly modified. But in both ventral skin and sponge granulation tissue, the proportion of "free" cathepsin has increased (Fig. 2). This result indicates that under penicillamine treatment, the enzyme has been freed from the lysosomes into the phagocytic vacuoles of cells or into the extracellular spaces. As it is now well known that collagen fibres are easily degraded in cytoplasmic vacuoles (Grillo, Lapiere, Dresden and Gross, 1968; Parakkal, 1969), our results suggest that penicillamine has increased the degradation of collagen fibres inside the phagocytic cells. Since the level of total collagen has not significantly changed in the tissues of penicillamine treated rats, an increased turnover might then be postulated. Such an hypothesis is supported by Nimni's results (1968) showing that in young rats treated with penicillamine and injected with labeled proline the collagen turnover is accelerated.

A similar acceleration had been already observed in lathyrism (Kühn et al., 1964; Tanzer and Gross, 1964), it is interesting to note that an increase of cathepsin activity had also been observed in the serum of lathyric animals (Holzmann, Korting and Mosches, 1965).

REFERENCES

Bazin, S. and Delaunay, A. (1964). Ann. Inst. Pasteur 107, 163.

Bazin, S. and Delaunay, A. (1966a). Ann. Inst. Pasteur 110, 192.

Bazin, S. and Delaunay, A. (1966b). Ann. Inst. Pasteur. 110, 347.

Bazin, S. and Delaunay, A. (1967). Ann. Inst. Pasteur 112, 316

Bazin, S. and Delaunay, A. (1968). C.R. Acad. Sci. 266, 973.

Bazin, S. and Delaunay, A. This book, p. 1727.

Chvapil, M., Hurych, J. and Ehrlichova, E. (1968). Hoppe Seyler's Z. Physiol. Chem. 349, 218.

Deshmukh, K. and Nimni, M. (1968). Bioch. Bioph. Acta 154, 258.

Fitch, S.M., Harkness, M.L. and Harkness, R.D. (1955). Nature 176, 163.

Grillo, H.C., Lapiere, C.M., Dresden, C.M. and Gross, J. (1968). Develop. Biol. 17, 571.

Holzmann, H., Korting, G.W. and Mosches, B. (1965). Naturwiss. 52, 308.

Kühn, K., Kurutti, M., Iwangoff, P., Hammerstein, F., Stecker, K., Holzmann, H. and Korting, W. (1964). Hoppe Seyler's Z. Physiol. Chem. 336, 4.

Nimni, E. (1968). J. Biol. Chem. 243, 1457.

Nimni, E. and Bavetta, L.A. (1965). Science 150, 905.

Parakkal, P.F. (1969). J. Cell Biol. 41, 345.

Paz, M.A., Blumenfeld, O.O., Rojkind, M., Henson, E., Furfine, C. and Gallop, P.M. (1965). Arch. Bioch. Biophys. 109, 548.

Stegemann, H. (1958). Hoppe Seyler's Z. Physiol. Chem. 311, 41.

Tanzer, M.L. and Gross, J. (1964). J. Exp. Med. 119, 275.

Youssef, S.A., Grever, E.F. and Levenson, S.M. (1966). Surgical Forum 17, 89.

COLLAGEN SYNTHESIS BY CELLS IN CULTURE

J. H. Fessler and Lona A. Smith

This paper reports on how much time is available within a cell for the assembly and hydroxylation of collagen molecules, and their secretion from the cell. This was made possible by studying cells in culture, which release a collagen-like material into the culture medium. They were given [14C] proline and for 3 hr the production of radioactive, protein-bound hydroxyproline and proline were followed both in the medium and in the cells plus medium. These materials accumulated linearly with time, after initial lag times characteristic for each material (Figs 1a, b and 2). Protein-bound proline appeared within the cells 13 min after administering proline to the cells, cellular protein-bound hydroxyproline appeared after 23 min and protein-bound hydroxyproline was released into the medium after 61 min, while proline bound to protein other than collagen appeared earlier in the medium, after 41 min. As these times were obtained as intercepts of the linear plots of accumulation with the time axis, they represent time intervals for radioactive materials flowing through cells in a steady state.

I EXPERIMENTAL

Chick cells were secondary cultures derived 3-5 weeks earlier from trypsinised, 9-day-old eviscerated and decapitated embryos, grown in modified Dulbecco-Vogt medium (Smith, Freeman, Vogt and Dulbecco 1960) containing 5% or 10% calf serum, 0.5% lactalbumin hydrolysate, ascorbic acid 10 ug/ml, penicillin G 1,000 units/ml and strepto-

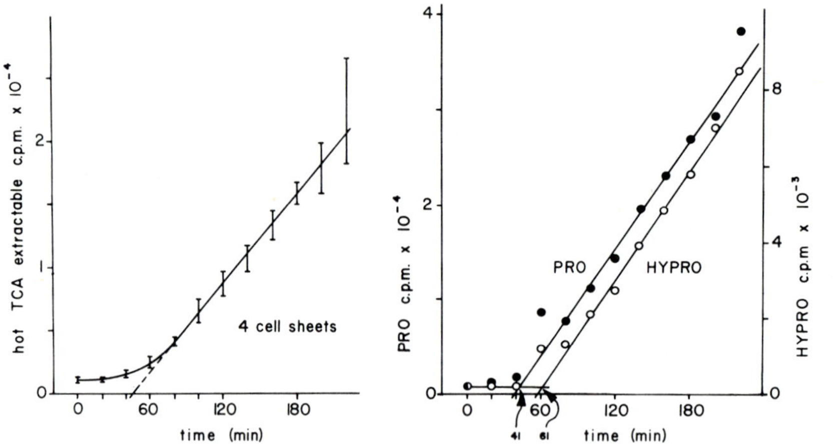

1a 1b

Fig 1a and 1b. Appearance in medium of radioactivity in protein soluble in 5% TCA at 90°C measured (1a) on individual cultures and (1b) after separation into proline and hydroxyproline contributions. Bars join maximum and minimum values.

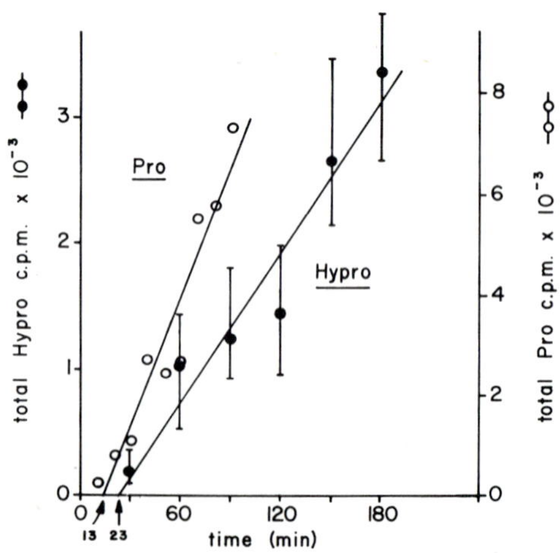

Fig 2. Incorporation of total proline and total hydroxyproline into proteins of the cultures (cells plus medium). Bars join maximum and minimum values.

mycin 2.5 mg/ml, under 5% CO_2 at 38°C. Glass Petri dishes (10 cm diameter) were seeded with 3 x 10^6 cells and used when grown to 2-5 x 10^7 cells per dish.

Uniformly labelled [14C]L-proline (specific activity 250 mC/mM, 2 or 4 μC per dish) was added and either the contents of the whole plate analysed after the specified time, or 1-ml samples of medium were withdrawn at intervals and replaced with 1 ml of fresh medium containing radioactive proline at the original concentration. At 0°C cells were homogenized and proteins precipitated with trichloroacetic acid (TCA), final concentration 15%. The precipitate was washed 3 times with 15% TCA, 3 ml. Collagen-like materials were solubilized in 1.5 ml hot 5% TCA (90°C, 1 hr). Radioactivity of an aliquot sample of supernatant was measured. One micromole each of proline and hydroxyproline was added as carrier and TCA was removed from the supernatant by 3 extractions with 3 ml diethyl ether. After hydrolysis (6NHCl, 140°C/3 hr) and removal of HCl, hydroxyproline and proline were quantitatively isolated on a Beckman amino acid analyser (Model 120B) and radioactivity measured (statistical error $\pm$ 5% or better, Beckman LS-150 scintillation system, 1.5 ml Biosolve 3, Beckman, per 15 ml toluene scintillation solution). Some TCA precipitates of washed cells only were hydrolysed without prior removal of TCA.

II RESULTS

Figure 1a shows the appearance of total hot TCA soluble protein-bound radioactivity and Fig 1b of protein-bound hydroxyproline and proline in the medium. The hydroxyproline was assumed to represent collagen, as will be discussed later, and correspondingly the proline data was corrected to represent, as plotted, proline bound to noncollagenous proteins. Best straight lines and their intercepts were calculated by the method of least squares for the data obtained at 90-200 min. Intercepts were also obtained for lines differing from the best straight line by plus or minus one standard deviation of the slope of the best straight line. The values were for hydroxyproline 61 min (64 min, 59 min) and for proline 41 min (45 min, 39 min). These data were obtained by the method of repetitive sampling of medium and are presented as total production of a given material up to that time by the whole cell sheet in a Petri dish. Bars join the highest and lowest values obtained from four plates seeded from one suspension of cells. Similar results were obtained in other experiments. Samples from the four dishes were pooled for proline and hydroxyproline isolation.

Figure 2 shows the appearance of total protein-bound proline and hydroxyproline in the system. Contents of individual Petri dishes were analysed and variation from dish to dish introduced scatter into the data which was greater than when the medium of a given dish was sampled repetitively. Bars join the maximum and minimum values and dots indicate the mean. The scatter of the data was not significantly decreased by correction for the number of cells in individual dishes, which were members of sets of dishes seeded from one cell suspension. Best straight lines were calculated as described previously and the intercepts on the time axis were for proline 13 min (16 min, 9 min) and for hydroxyproline 23 min (32 min, 11 min). Small variations of synthetic ability and timing between individual plates of cells would cause a disproportionate scatter of results in this method and current improvement in technique should allow us to delineate these times better. Repeated measurements on these and other cells show, however, that while proline incorporation occurs rapidly after addition of the amino acid, very little, if any, hydroxyproline is found within the first half hour.

III DISCUSSION

The time intervals found are interpreted as average times which are required for radioactive imino acid to traverse biochemical pools of chick cells in a steady state, independently of the initial time taken for equilibration of the pools. The only exception to this is the 13-min interval for protein-bound proline to appear; it is measured from an arbitrary zero time and includes the initial times required for addition of proline and its uptake by cells. Small variations of these processes between plates will, however, cause scatter in the results. Proline attached to transfer RNA will have been measured as cell protein-bound proline, but this cell pool should have been equilibrated rapidly and is unlikely to have affected substantially the results obtained over a prolonged period.

The delay between the incorporation of proline into protein and the appearance of hydroxyproline fits in well with the current views of hydroxylation of proline after peptide synthesis, reviewed by Prockop, and by Udenfriend elsewhere in this symposium. Other interpretations are possible, such as a separate, additional pool of imino acid for hydroxylation causing an additional delay, but this is most unlikely.

The time required for the synthesis of an α strand of collagen is not known. By analogy with reticulocyte hemoglobin synthesis (Attardi, 1967) 2 1/2-8 min may be expected; the time will also vary with physiological conditions. A cell-free bacterial system completes de novo synthesis of enzymatically active lysozyme in less than 1 min (Salser 1969), corresponding to less than 6 min for the collagen α-strand. We found an interval of approximately 10 min between two intercepts: one for protein-bound proline, the other for protein-bound hydroxyproline. Each intercept represents an average: thus proline residues near the beginning of a peptide chain would give rise to an intercept earlier than 13 min while terminal residues would give rise to a later one; the 13-min intercept represents an average for all the prolines incorporated into the various proteins which the cells synthesize. On this basis one would expect collagen α strand synthesis to be completed within the first few minutes of the approximately 10-min interval. It seems unlikely that there would be a pause prior to hydroxylation, though transport to a neighboring part of the cytoplasm may be necessary. A likely explanation is that hydroxylation is a protracted process: some hydroxyl groups being introduced soon after peptide synthesis, others a good deal later than the average 10-min interval.

The 20-min delay ((48 min-28 min) after synthesis) in the time of release of hydroxyproline containing protein into the media as compared with other proline containing proteins suggests that either collagen is transported through the cell more slowly than the average protein, or that it is released from the cell more slowly, or both. Although heterogeneity of the cell population cannot be excluded, it is unlikely to be the cause of this difference because similar results were obtained with a line of mouse fibroblasts (PR 105) derived by Dr. R. E. Priest and kindly donated by him (Fessler and Smith, 1969). This difference of time of passage through the cell for collagen and for other proline containing proteins suggests caution in using autoradiographic techniques for such studies.

According to our results about 48 min elapse between initiation of synthesis of collagen and release from the fibroblast. It is assumed that the hydroxyproline containing ing material is collagen. Preliminary gel filtration and acrylamide gel electrophoresis experiments, after denaturation, showed materials with the behavior of collagen α chains, and of higher apparent molecular size.

The reasons for the release, into the medium, of such material is not known. Cell sheets cultured for a prolonged time had collagen associated with them, as shown by chemical determination of hydroxyproline after hydrolysis. It is unlikely that collagenolytic action occurred because the culture medium contained serum, which inhibits such enzymes; furthermore the conclusions would not be affected by any degradation of collagen subsequent to release from the cell. The release of incomplete collagen molecules or α-chains is, however, not excluded.

ACKNOWLEDGEMENTS

We thank Mrs. June Baumer, Mrs. Jeanene Cooper and Mrs. Ann Bradley for assistance with imino acid analyses and gratefully acknowledge financial support from the Arthritis Foundation (Southern California Chapter); U.S.

Public Health Service, Grant 5-R01-AM 11546 and Cancer Research Committee, University of California.

REFERENCES

Attardi, G., (1967) Ann. Rev. Microbiol 21, 283.

Fessler, J. H., and Smith, L. A., this symposium. P. 465.

Salser, W. (1969) personal communication.

Smith, J. W., Freeman, G., Vogt, M., and Dulbecco, R., (1960) Virology 12, 185, 1960.

ASCORBIC ACID STIMULATION OF A MOUSE FIBROBLAST CELL LINE

J. H. Fessler and Lona A. Smith

The stimulating effect of ascorbic acid on collagen synthesis is well known (reviewed by Gould, 1968), and has been linked particularly with hydroxylation mechanisms. The report by Udenfriend in this book (see page 363) that α-ketogluterate and not ascorbic acid is the substance directly participating in hydroxylation of proline, again opens the question of the function of ascorbic acid. From the study which we report here we conclude that a cell-line of mouse fibroblasts responds in at least three ways to ascorbic acid added to the culture medium (1) total synthesis of protein-bound hydroxyproline is increased (2) release of this material into the culture medium is stimulated and (3) non-collagen protein synthesis is also increased.

The mouse fibroblast cell-line PR 105 was obtained from R. E. Priest (Davies, Priest and Priest, 1968). Experimental conditions and methods were as described in another paper in this book (see page 457, Fessler and Smith, 1969), except that ascorbic acid was omitted from the medium in which the cells were grown. Cells were subcultured at approximately 10-day intervals.

Ascorbic acid was added to the media of cell cultures (final concentration 0, 1, 5, 10, 25 μg/ml) and 1 hr later each culture received 2 μC L-proline. Aliquots were taken from each culture medium at 0, 1/2, 1, 2, 4, 22 hr and the radioactivity measured of the total material which was solubilized by hot 5% TCA (90°C/1 hr) from a washed 15% TCA precipitate. This radioactivity increased linearly after an initial lag period, closely similar to the findings with chick cells described elsewhere (see page 458, Fessler and Smith, 1969, page 457). The stimulatory effect of ascorbic acid was clearly evident in the 2-hr and later data (i.e. 3 hr after addition of ascorbic acid) and increased progressively with ascorbic acid concentration up to 10 μg/ml.

After 22 hr media and cell sheets were analysed for protein-bound proline and hydroxyproline. Assuming the hydroxyproline to represent collagen of usual composition, and the imino acids of this newly formed collagen to have the same specific activity, a proportional amount of the proline radioactivity was denoted as non-collagen protein. The results are shown in Figs 1, 2 and 3. The stimulation of collagen production by ascorbic acid is evident in Fig 1, and is appreciably more for the material released into the medium than that in the cell sheet. The apparently linear relationships of Figs 2 and 3 indicate that ascorbic acid also, proportionately, stimulates the formation of proteins other than collagen. Should these relationships hold at low rates of synthesis, then they would indicate that a basal synthesis of non-collagenous proteins occurs even when collagen synthesis is absent, which is reasonable.

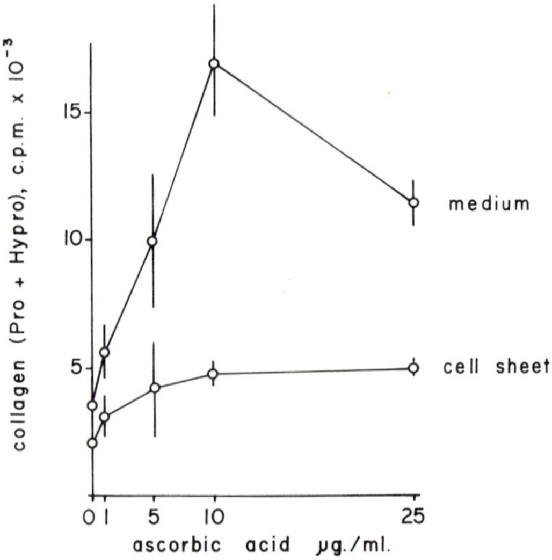

Fig 1. Effect of ascorbic acid on collagen formation after 22 hr incubation; cells and culture media analysed separately; bars indicate maximum and minimum values.

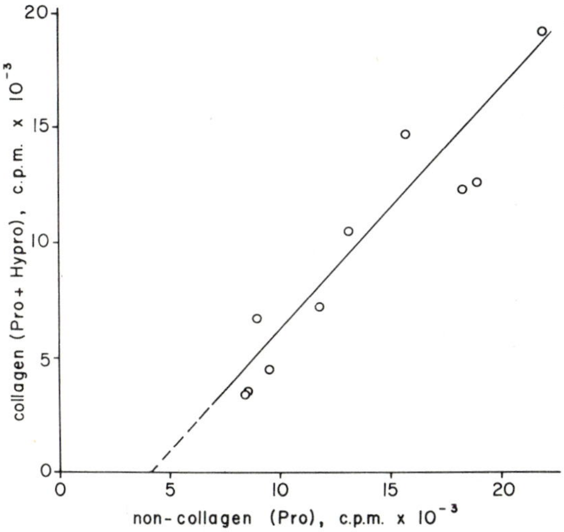

Fig 2. Radioactivity of proteins soluble in hot TCA and found in the medium after 22 hr incubation at different ascorbic acid concentrations. See text for definitions of collagen and non-collagen proteins.

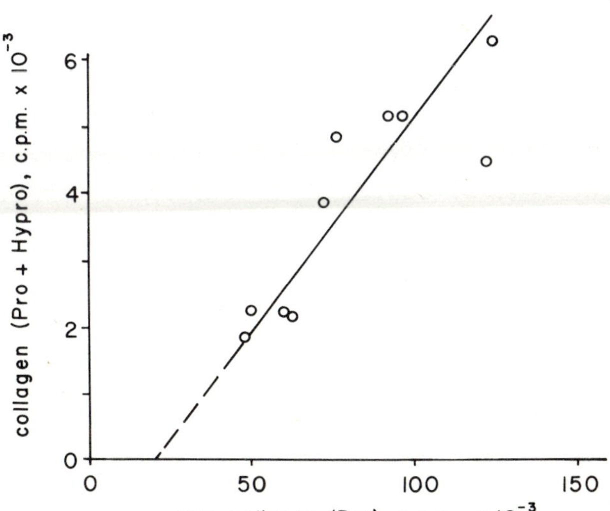

Fig 3. Radioactivity of proteins found in the cell sheets after 22 hr incubation at different ascorbic acid concentrations. See text for definitions of collagen and non-collagen proteins.

These results show that (1) ascorbic acid stimulates total protein synthesis of these cells within 3 hr after addition, that (2) collagen and non-collagen syntheses are stimulated proportionally, and (3) that the production of extracellular materials, both collagenous and non-collagenous proteins, is stimulated more than the formation of cellular and associated materials.

ACKNOWLEDGEMENTS

We are grateful to Dr. R. E. Priest for a gift of PR 105 cells, to Mrs. Jeanene Cooper and Mrs. June Baumer for imino acid analyses, and for financial support from the Arthritis Foundation (Southern California Chapter); U. S. Public Health Service, Grant 5-R01-AM11546, and Cancer Research Committee, University of California.

REFERENCES

Davies, L. M., Priest, J. H., and Priest, R. E. (1968). Science 159, 91.

Fessler, J. H., and Smith, L. A. (1969) (elsewhere in this Symposium).

Gould, B. S. (1968) In Treatise on Collagen, vol. 2A, ch. 8, p. 323. Ed. by Gould, B. S. Academic Press, New York.

Chapter III

Chemistry and Structure of Basal Lamina

EPITHELIAL BASEMENT MEMBRANE: ORIGIN, DEVELOPMENT AND ROLE IN DISEASE

G. Barry Pierce

Basement membranes have been recognized by histologists as thin eosinophilic hyaline membranes which separate certain cells from their environment. For the purpose of this discussion, emphasis will be placed on epithelial basement membranes, but basement membranes are also associated with endothelial cells, nerve sheath and muscle cells. With the electron microscope, epithelial basement membranes are described as being amorphous or finely fibrillar, depending upon the methods of fixation. They lie at the epithelial stromal junction in juxtaposition to the cell membrane or separated from it by a narrow electron lucent space, and they are so intimately associated with collagen fibrils as to be inseparable from them with the usual means of tissue fractionation (Figs. 1 and 2).

The origin of basement membrane has been controversial. Because of the anatomical relationship to collagen and intracellular ground substance, it is not surprising that epithelial basement membrane was considered to be a component of the connective tissues, presumably formed by polymerization of ground substance (Gersh and Catchpole, 1960). This idea was questioned by Kurtz (1958), Farquhar, Wissig and Palade (1961), and Andres, Morgan, Hsu, Rifkind and Seegal (1962), who obtained indirect evidence compatible with the idea that some basement membranes might be synthesized by epithelial cells.

Many ideas have been offered concerning the possible function of basement membrane. Because it is conspicuously located in the capillary loops of the glomerulus, where it

Fig. 1. This drawing illustrates the relationship of epithelial basement membrane to the epithelial cells of the glandular acinus (right), and endothelial basement membrane to the capillary (left). Note the intimate relationship of collagen fibrils to the basement membrane.

Fig. 2. Basement membranes of renal glomerulus, tubule, and arteriole are illustrated. The basement membrane of the glomerular tuft (A) has a trilaminar appearance. that of Bowman's capsule (B) is homogenous and blends with the basement membrane of the tubule (C). The muscle (M) of the arteriole is invested by a thin basement membrane which blends with that of the endothelial cell (E) at X. (X14,000). (Pierce et al., 1963).

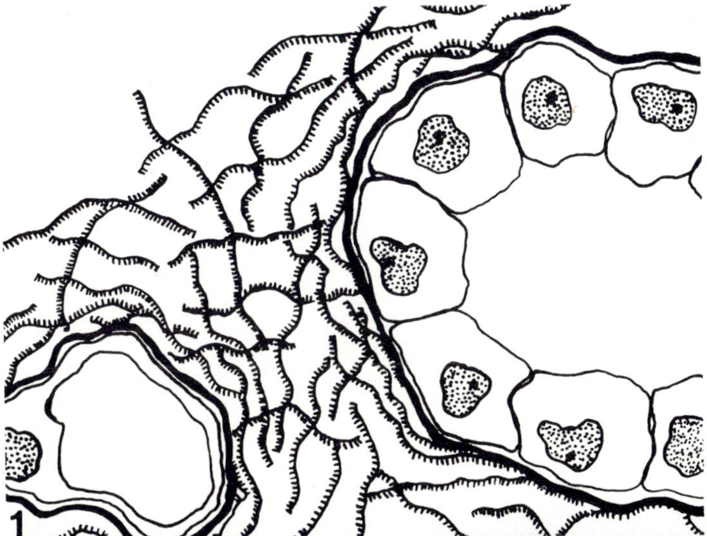

1

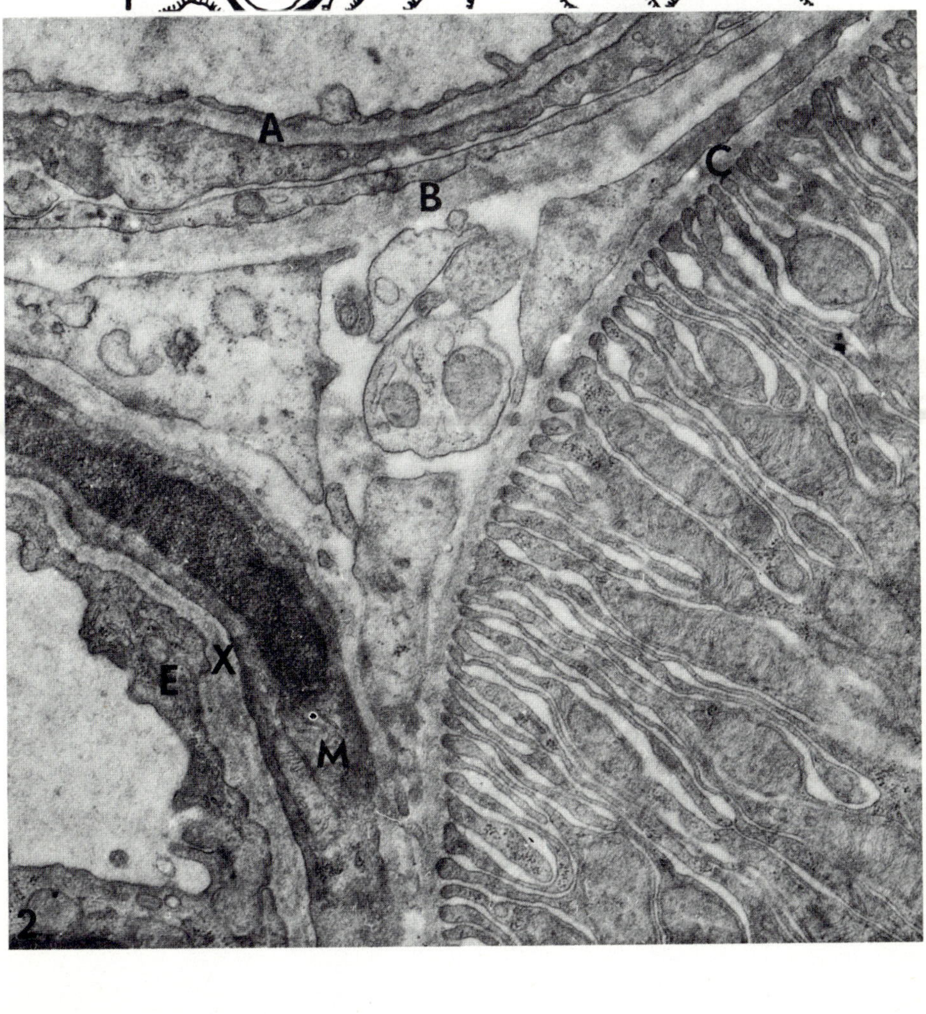

2

Fig. 3. The anatomic relationships of Reichert's membrane (arrow) may be seen in relationship to the trophoblastic giant cells of the placenta (bottom) and to the small, darkly stained parietal yolk sac epithelium which secretes the membrane. (S192). (Pierce et.al., 1964).

Fig. 4. The neoplastic basement membrane (NBM) separates clumps and cords of parietal yolk sac carcinoma cells. Capillaries and mesenchymal cells (arrows) of the stroma are embedded in the NBM. (X300). (Pierce et al.,1964).

Fig. 5. a. Monolayer of parietal yolk sac carcinoma cells, maintained in vitro for 4 months and stained with hematoxylin and eosin to illustrate the appearance of the cells. b. Similar monolayer stained with fluorescein-labeled anti-epithelial basement membrane. The brightly fluorescent epithelial basement membrane antigen may be seen at the arrow. (X385). c. Control monolayer, to indicate immunological specificity, was stained with fluorescein-labeled anti-epithelial basement membrane that had been absorbed with this antigen prior to staining. This section is negative. (X385).

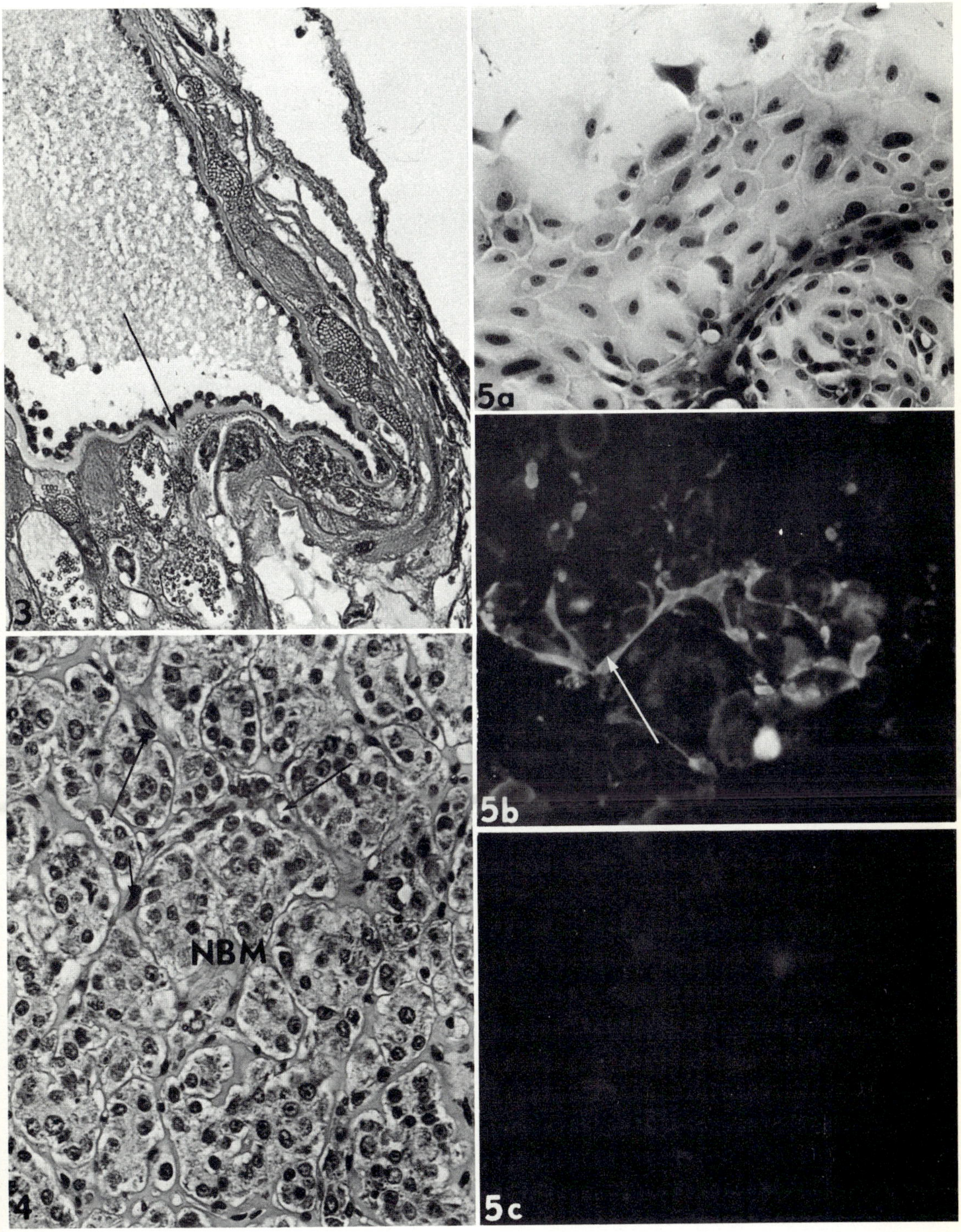
3
4
NBM
5a
5b
5c

forms a continuous membrane, it is believed by many to be the renal filter (Robbins, 1968). Obviously, fluid traverses the glomerular basement membrane. It also is clear that nutritional elements for the glandular acinus illustrated in Fig. 1 must cross the capillary basement membrane and the basement membrane of the acinus. While it is not disputed that material flows across basement membrane, there is no direct evidence to the effect that basement membrane serves as a filter. If it is a mechanical filter, it should have a pore size in physiologic range, and come equipped with a mechanism for self cleansing. Techniques are available to determine whether or not it filters on the basis of molecular sieving or ion exchange, but these experiments have not been done.

Basement membranes are involved in a number of important disease processes, including nephrosis, glomerulonephritis, and asthma. Each of these diseases is characterized by abnormal thickening of basement membranes, but the role played by the thickened basement membrane in the disease processes is not known.

Factual knowledge of epithelial basement membrane, as it existed recently, could be summarized by stating that it is an amorphous material which separates epithelial cells from their environment, and serves an unknown function. Its chemical composition was largely unknown, its turnover mere speculation, and it was involved in an unknown way in common killing diseases.

It is the purpose of this paper to present data which establishes the idea that epithelial cells synthesize basement membranes, which are composed of tropocollagen and a carbohydrate rich mucoprotein; that injury to the epithelial cells results in synthesis of excessive amounts of basement membrane; and that basement membrane is neither primarily a filter nor an important contributor to the pathological physiology of nephrosis.

I EPITHELIAL BASEMENT MEMBRANE

A. ORIGIN

The basement membrane studied in these experiments was Reichert's membrane, an exceedingly thick basement membrane of the mouse embryo which lies between parietal yolk sac and trophoblastic giant cells of the yolk sac placenta (Snell and Stevens, 1966). Reichert's membrane appears between the 5th and 6th day of fetal life, and attains a thickness of 7 μ or more by the 10th to 12th day (Fig. 3). In the first 10 days of fetal life in rodents, all nutritional elements and wastes are exchanges across the yolk sac placenta, and Reichert's membrane has been the object of extensive study. Histochemically, it was PAS positive, but it stained poorly or not at all with silver stains for reticulin and trichrome stains for collagen (Everett, 1935), and thus it was considered atypical. With the electron microscope, it appeared to be an exceedingly thick, laminated basement membrane, bordered on one side by the plasma membranes of cells of parietal yolk sac and on the other by trophoblast (Schiebler and Knoop, 1959; Wislocki and Dempsey, 1955). Because the partial yolk sac cells were exposed and unable to withstand the vicissitudes of embedding in methacrylate, their ultrastructure was not described in early studies. Even so, the majority of investigators believed Reichert's membrane to be synthesized by trophoblast.

The controversy concerning the origin of Reichert's membrane was settled with the discovery of a parietal yolk sac carcinoma of the mouse (Pierce and Dixon, 1959; Pierce, Midgley, Sri Ram and Feldman, 1962). This highly malignant tumor originated from a testicular teratocarcinoma of strain 129 mice and was characterized by bands of eosinophilic material, not unlike Reichert's membrane, which lay between clumps of tumor cells (Fig. 4). Embedded in this neoplastic basement membrane were the stromal elements of the tumor, blood vessels and fibroblasts, which were inseparable from it.

The role of the tumor cells in the production of the

neoplastic basement membrane was examined first. They could either synthesize the material or induce the stromal elements to do so. Advantage was taken of the ease of growing tumors in vitro to solve this question. When the parietal yolk sac carcinoma was established as a cell line in vitro, it synthesized the material in the absence of connective tissue or its products (Pierce et al., 1962) (Fig. 5). Thus it was established that malignant epithelial cells could synthesize basement membrane, and it was presumed that this was a function of the normal parietal yolk sac which had been carried over in the malignant change.

B. IMMUNOLOGIC RELATIONSHIPS

In an effort to obtain the neoplastic basement membrane free from stroma for immunologic and chemical characterization, the tumor was grown in the ascites, a situation in which tumor cells grow singly or in small clumps in the effusion caused by the presence of tumor cells in the peritoneal cavity. When the parietal yolk sac carcinoma was converted to the ascites, the cells grew in rosettes and synthesized a ball of basement membrane in the center of the rosette (Fig. 6). Although it could not be guaranteed that some connective tissue contamination could not have occurred in this situation, it was minimal and collagen was seldom found when sections of the rosettes were stained with fluorescein-labeled anti-collagen.

The neoplastic basement membrane material (NBM) was prepared as antigen and for chemical analysis by the method of Krakower and Greenspon (1964). The rosettes were separated from erythrocytes and leucocytes by centrifugation, and repeatedly washed in physiologic saline to remove serum proteins. Then the carcinoma cells were destroyed with ultrasound, and the basement membrane, which was resistant to this treatment, was repeatedly washed in 8% sodium chloride, phosphate-buffered saline, distilled water and finally lyophilized after ultrastructural examination failed to reveal evidence of cellular contamination (Pierce, Midgley and Ram, 1963).

Fig. 6. The ascites form of the parietal yolk sac carcinoma. The small cellular aggregates are composed of a central nidus of NBM surrounded by parietal yolk sac carcinoma cells. (X300). (Pierce et al., 1964).

Fig. 7a. Parietal yolk sac carcinoma, frozen section 2 μ in thickness, and stained with fluorescein-labeled anti-NBM. There is a specific fluorescence in NBM and a fine focal intracytoplasmic fluorescence. The nudlei did not fluoresce and appear black. (X500). (Pierce et al., 1964).

Fig. 7b. Mouse placenta stained with fluroescein-labeled anti-NBM. Reichert's membrane is stained brilliantly; the cytoplasm of parietal yolk sac cells focally. (X500). (Pierce et al., 1964).

Fig. 8, Adjacent serial sections of testis of the mouse stained respectively with (a) crude antibody, (b) anti-EBM, and (c) antibody abosrbed with its antigen. In (a), note the staining of testicular tubular basement membranes, the basement membranes of the arteriole and the reaction with collagen of the tunica albuginia. In (b), stained with anti-EBM, note the reaction in testicular tubular membrane only. In (c), the control, there is no reaction. (X300). (Pierce et al., 1964).

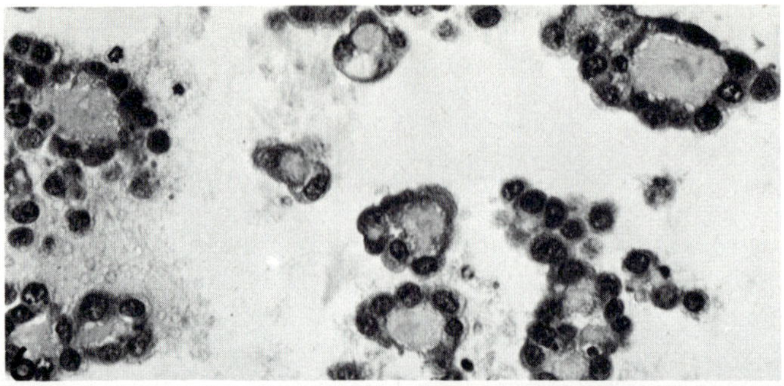
6

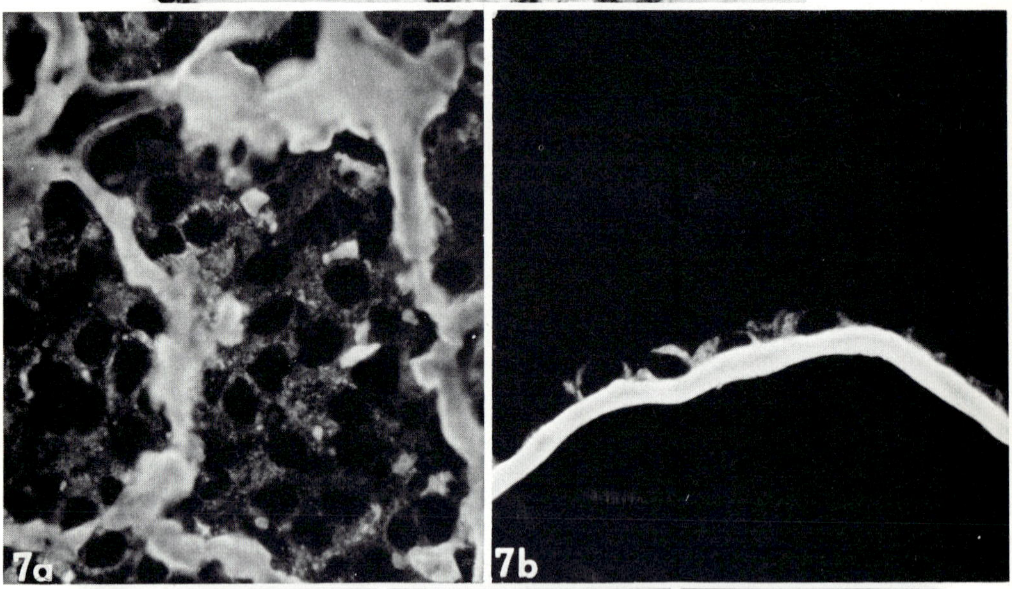
7a
7b

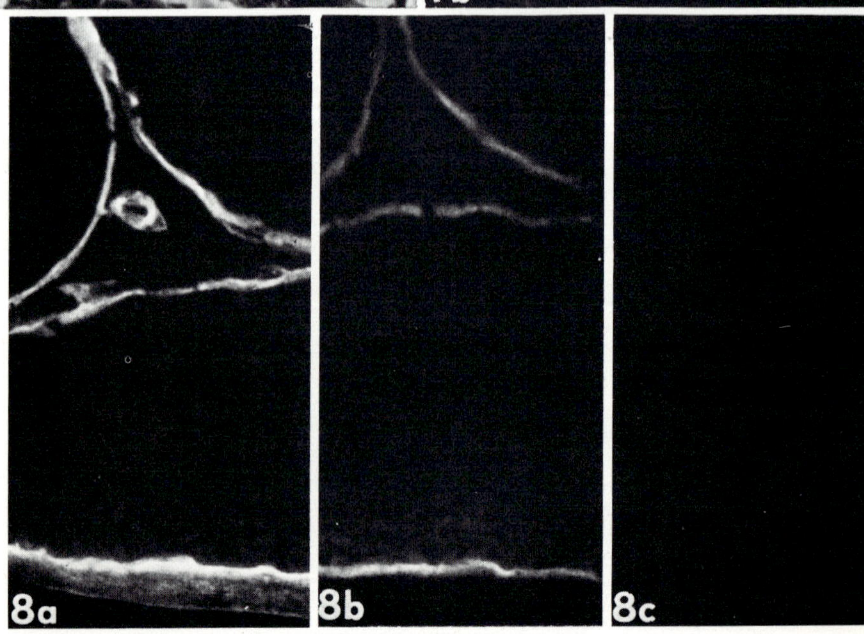
8a
8b
8c

Rabbits were repeatedly immunized with antigen in complete Freund's adjuvant, and the resulting antisera (anti-NBM) were reacted with serum proteins and red blood cells of the host to remove antibodies to these antigens contaminating the preparation. Because of the insolubility of the antigen, it was impossible to prove that the antiserum contained only a single antibody against epithelial basement membrane. Since the antigen was morphologically recognizable in the tissues, we relied upon an extensive series of cross absorptions to establish the specificity of the immunohistochemical reactions as will be detailed below (Pierce et.al.,1963; Pierce, Beals, Ram and Midgley, 1964; Pierce and Nakane, 1967).

The crude anti-NBM was used in the indirect immunohistochemical technique of Coons, in a study to determine whether or not basement membranes produced by the parietal yolk sac carcinoma had antigens similar to those of Reichert's membrane. Anti-NBM localized in the NBM of the tumor and focally in fine droplets in the cytoplasm of the tumor cells (Pierce et al., 1963) (Fig 7a). Since the tissue culture studies had established that these cells synthesized NBM, this intracytoplasmic antigen was considered to be the site of synthesis of the basement membrane. When applied to the placenta, anti-NBM reacted focally in the cytoplasm of the parietal yolk sac cells and with Reichert's membrane, in exactly the same manner as in the tumor.

Since it had never been established that the antiserum contained only antibodies to NBM, it was necessary to prove that the reactions observed represented the localization of similar basement membrane antigens. Thus it was necessary to isolate Reichert's membrane from placentas of the mouse, immunize rabbits with this antigen, and perform cross absorptions between normal and neoplastic systems (Pierce et al. 1964). The results of the experiments are listed in Table I. Briefly, when anti-NBM was absorbed with Reichert's membrane until Reichert's membrane failed to react, the ability of the anti-serum to react with NBM was abolished. This indicated that Reichert's membrane contained antigens capable of neutralizing all of the antibodies produced against NBM. Conversely, absorption of anti-Reichert's membrane with NBM until NBM failed to react, abolished the ability of the antiserum to react with Reichert's membrane. This indicated that NBM contained all of the antigens necessary to neutralize any antibodies that Reichert's membrane could evoke. Thus is was concluded that neoplastic basement membrane and Reichert's membrane contained similar antigens (Pierce et al., 1964).

A study was made to determine whether or not basement membrane synthesized by epithelial cells had specific antigenic markers that could be used for the localization of epithelial basement membrane antigen. To this end, a survey was made of the various tissues of the mouse to determine which structures would react with anti-NBM (Midgley and Pierce, 1963). In addition to reacting with basement membranes of epithelial organs, anti-NBM reacted with vascular basement membranes, the basement membranes of fat and muscle cells, and collagen. Since the spleen was a good source of collagen and endothelial basement membrane uncontaminated with epithelial basement membrane, the anti-NBM was absorbed with splenic pulp until its ability to react with the spleen was exhausted. This absorbed antibody was incapable of reacting with endothelial basement membrane, collagen, or the basement membranes of fat or muscle cells, irrespective of their locations in the body, but it still reacted with neoplastic basement membrane and Reichert's membrane. These observations indicated that this epithelial basement membrane contained an antigen distinct from those of the connective tissues. This antigen was named epithelial specific basement membrane (EBM) (Pierce et. al., 1963; Midgley and Pierce, 1963). Anti-EBM localized specifically in the basement membranes of all epithelia that had basement membrane (Fig. 8a,b,c). When anti-EBM was labeled with peroxidase and used with the electron microscope, the reaction product, denoting epithelial basement membrane, lay in a fine lamella immediately adjacent to the bases of epithelial cells in what the electron microscopist calls the basement membrane

TABLE I

Cross Absorption Study Between anti-NBM and Anti-Reichert's Membrane and Their Respective Antigens

	Tumor		Placenta	
	NBM	Cells	Reichert's membrane	PYS cells
Anti-NBM	++++	+++	++++	+++
Absorbed with NBM	-	-	-	-
Absorbed with Reichert's membrane	-	-	-	-
Anti-Reichert's membrane	++++	+++	++++	+++
Absorbed with NBM	-	-	-	-
Absorbed with Reichert's membrane	-	-	-	-

(Figs. 9 and 10). In these experiments, anti-collagen was used as a control, and it localized on collagenous fibrils but spared the epithelial basement membrane (Fig. 11) (Nakane and Pierce, unpublished data).

The EBM thus localized was species specific in that it did not react with epithelial basement membranes of man or rat. In addition, epithelial basement membrane contained a component that cross reacted with collagen that was species cross reacting (Pierce and Nakane, 1967). To date, this particular antigen has been the only one localized in endothelial basement membrane, and since this is the only antigen present in the glomerulus of the rat (Fig. 12), one can assume with confidence that this is the nephrotoxic antigen described so well by Steblay (1963).

Epithelial basement membrane antigen did not cross react with red blood cells, and it was distinct from the β globulins found in the glomerular basement membrane by Tan and Kaplan (1963). We confirmed the presence of the β globulins in glomerular basement membrane of adult mice, but failed to find them in the glomerular basement membranes of fetal mice before renal filtration had occured (Pierce, 1966). Thus it was concluded that the β globulins were probably not a structural component of basement membrane, but were

Fig. 9. Base of a proximal convoluted tubule of the kidney reacted with peroxidase labeled anti-NBM which reacts with epithelial and endothelial basement membrane. No stains for electronmicroscopy were employed, accounting for the lack of contrast in the cytoplasm. The basement membrane is marked by the dense black amorphous reaction product of the immunohistochemical reaction. (X15,000). (Nakane and Pierce, 1969).

Fig. 10. The base of this proximal convoluted tubule of the kidney was reacted with peroxidase-labeled anti-EBM. Epithelial basement membrane lies in juxtaposition to the epithelial cell, as evidenced by the electron-dense reaction products of peroxidase. The endothelial basement membrane and collagen lying between endothelium (arrow) and EBM, is not stained. No stains for electronmicroscopy were employed. (X22,000). (Nakane and Pierce, 1969).

Fig. 11. The base of this proximal convoluted tubule was reacted with anti-collagen. Note the dense reaction products on the collagen fibers (some of which are artifactually separated from epithelial basement membrane), sparing the epithelial and endothelial basement membrane. No stains for electronmicroscopy were used. (X12,500). (Nakane and Pierce, 1969).

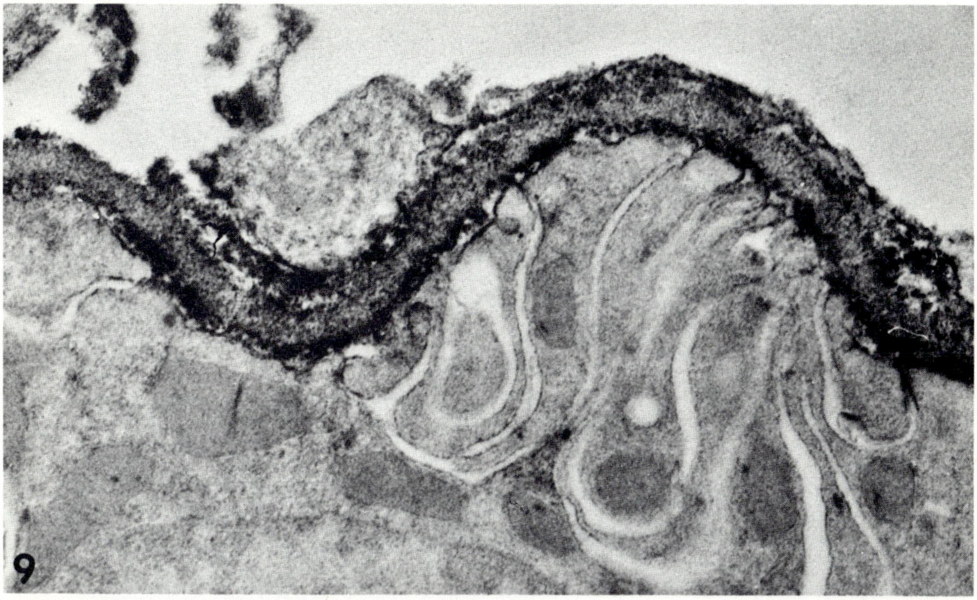

9

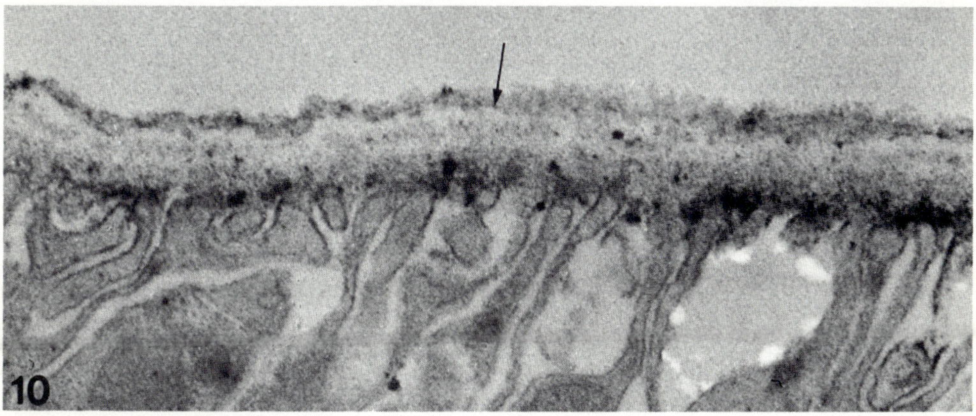

10

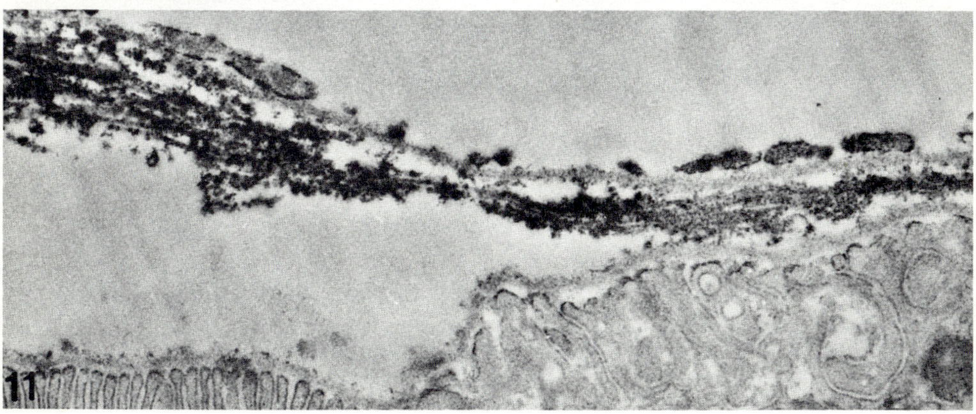

11

Fig. 12a, b. Adjacent serial sections of rat kidney stained respectively with anti-rat collagen and epithelial-specific anti-rat lens capsule. Note that whereas anti-collagen localizes in the glomerular basement membrane (b), anti-rat lens capsule does not localize in the glomerulus (a). Note the epithelial basement membrane antigen around the renal tubules. (a). (X245). (Pierce and Nakane, 1967).

Fig. 13. Electronmicrograph from the margin of a parietal yolk sac cell, illustrating a portion of Reichert's membrane. Note the ribosome encrusted profiles of endoplasmic reticulum distended with EBM. What may be a communication between endoplasmic reticulum and plasma membrane is illustrated at the arrow. (X31.000).

Fig. 14. Electronmicrograph illustrating a portion of Reichert's membrane and a parietal yolk sac cell. Reichert's membrane has a laminar appearance, as though it were laid down in successive layers. The rough surfaced endoplasmic reticulum is well developed as are the Golgi complexes. Only the former contain EBM. There are numerous microtubules. The plasma membrane has many microbilli and the cell has numerous processes adjacent to Reichert's membrane. (X15,000).

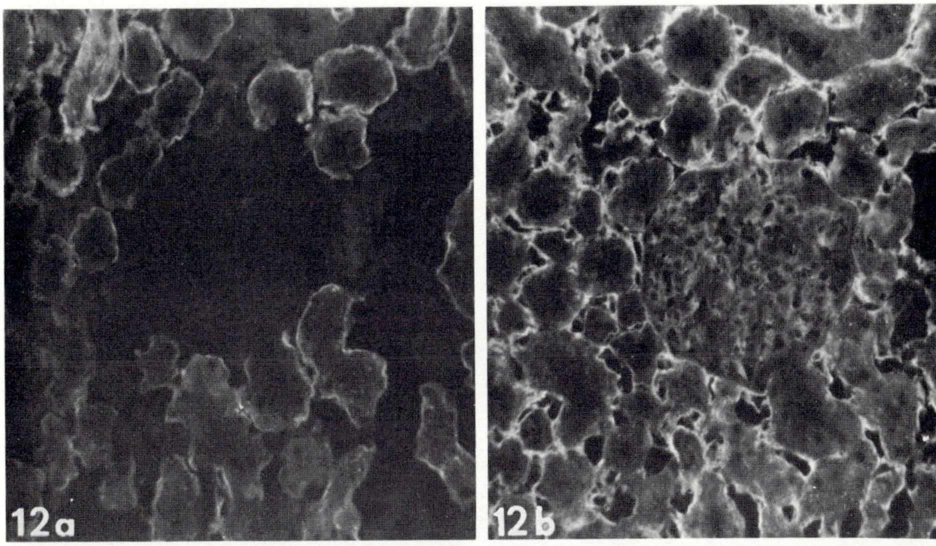
12a
12b

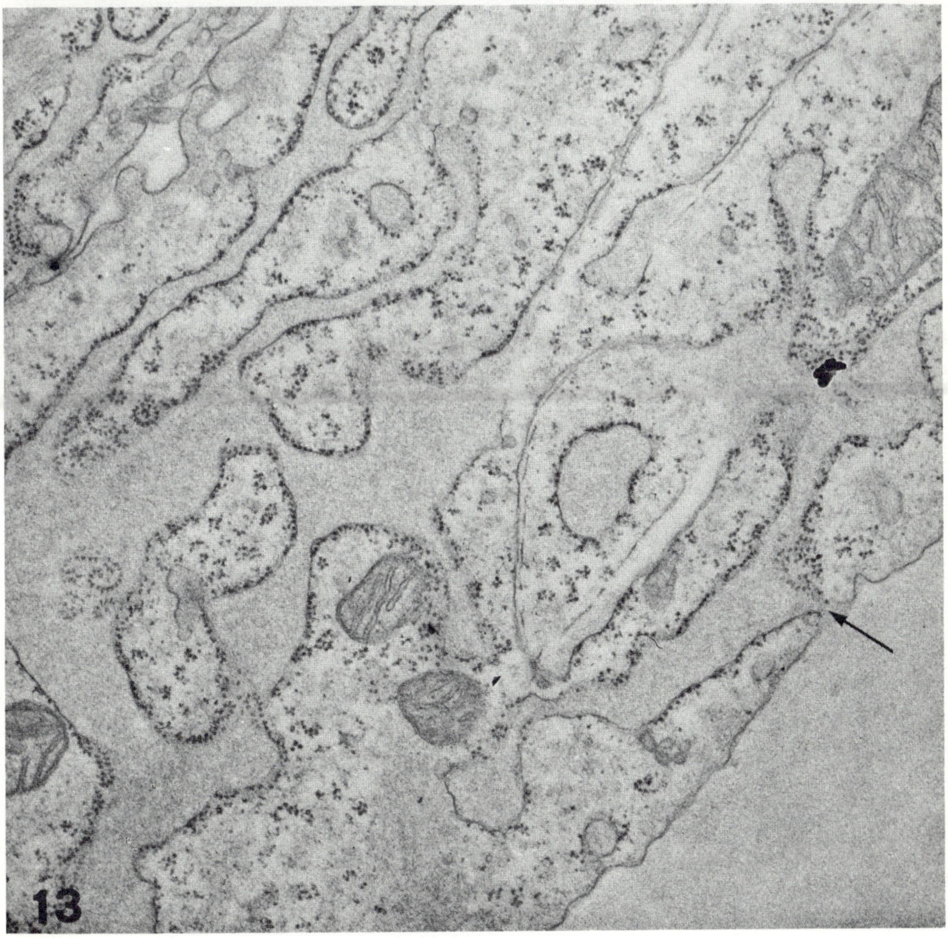
13

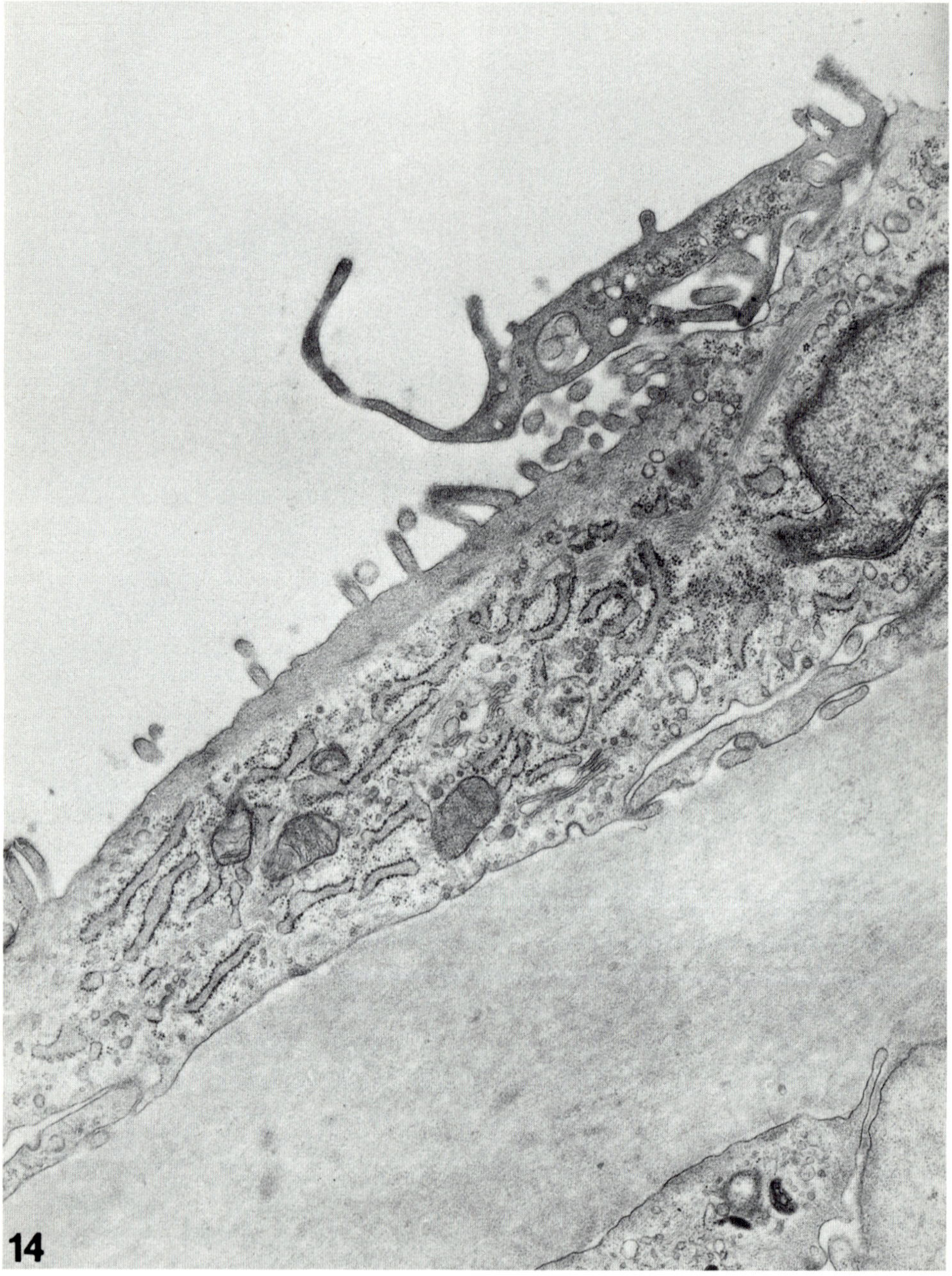

14

adsorbed to it through filtration.

C. LENS CAPSULE AND GLOMERULUS

With the exception of Reichert's membrane, the greatest concentration of epithelial basement membrane antigen was found in the lens capsule (Pierce and Nakane, 1967). This uniquely thick basement membrane was relatively uncontaminated by collagen and was the purest source of epithelial basement membrane antigen in mammals for chemical and immunochemical analyses. The glomerular basement membrane has long been the object of study by chemists. It is clear from our previous studies that glomerular basement membrane of man and mouse contains at least two antigens, one synthesized by epithelium and the other synthesized by endothelium (Pierce and Nakane, 1967). Whether or not this antigenic heterogenity is significant in terms of the biochemical composition of these membranes remains to be seen. Suffice it to say that in the glomerulus of the rat, only endothelial basement membrane antigen can be demonstrated (Fig. 12).

This does not imply that glomerular epithelium of the rat does not synthesize a portion of the glomerular basement membrane, merely that it fails to synthesize the epithelial specific basement membrane antigen found in lens capsule and in Reichert's membrane. In this sense, the glomerulus of the rat is unusual (Pierce and Nakane, 1967).

II SYNTHESIS OF BASEMENT MEMBRANE BY EPITHELIAL CELLS

Although it had been demonstrated that one type of epithelium synthesized a basement membrane antigen distinct from those of the connective tissues, yet present in basement membranes of all epithelia, establishment of the concept that epithelial cells synthesize their basement membranes would require further demonstrations of the phenomenon with additional epithelia. To this end a survey was made of a series of tumors of the mouse to determine which were associated with EBM (Pierce, 1965). With the exception of one tumor that was so anaplastic that its origin was unclear, tumors of epithelial origin all had EBM, but none of the tumors of mesenchymal origin had it. Tumors of the breast and granulosa cell tumors of the ovary contained the most EBM, and were explanted in vitro to determine whether or not they could synthesize this antigen in the absence of connective tissue elements. After repeated subcultures from small numbers of cells, monolayers of these tumor cells were stained with either anti-EBM or anti-collagen. The latter were always negative, but EBM was invariably found on and around the cells stained with anti-EBM (Pierce, 1965).

The demonstration that three types of epithelium synthesize epithelial basement membrane in vitro in the absence of connective tissues, established the concept that epithelial cells in general synthesize at least a portion of their basement membrane. It would also seem logical to suppose that other cells with basement membranes would synthesize their basement membranes.

III EMBRYOLOGIC DEVELOPMENT OF BASEMENT MEMBRANE

Although the concept of synthesis of basement membrane by cells was established, a study employing fluorescein-labeled anti-EBM was performed in the mouse embryo to gain insight into the mode of development of basement membrane and its relationship to collagen in vivo.

The first epithelial basement membrane antigen was observed in the extra embryonic fetal membranes 5 & 1/2 days after fertilization. This was Reichert's membrane. The embryo proper which contained no EBM was composed of an inner mass of embryonic epithelium overlain by a single cuboidal layer of endodermal cells. Since endoderm differentiated from embryonic epithelium in the absence of basement membrane, it can be assumed that EBM probably plays no direct role in differentiation (Pierce, 1966)

The first intra-embryonic epithelial basement membrane antigen was observed between the embryonic epithelium and the endoderm 6 & 1/2 days after fertilization. This occurred at least one day before mesoderm differentiated in the embryo, and suggested that epithelial basement membrane could be formed in vivo in the absence of collagen.

When mesoderm appeared in these embryos, it lay between endoderm, with a newly formed basement membrane, and embryonic epithelium with its original epithelial basement membrane. This newly formed mesoderm lacked collagen. The first collagen, discernible with fluorescein labeled anti-collagen, appeared in the vascular primordia.

With the possible exception of the kidney, epithelial basement membranes were at one time all interconnected, suggesting that basement membranes probably subserve the same function, and have similar chemical compositions irrespective of their locations. For example, the skin differentiates from embryonic epithelium and its basement membrane is a direct continuation of that of embryonic epithelium. In a similar manner, the optic vesicle buds from the brain primordium and carries the epithelial basement membrane from that organ with it (Cohen, 1965; Pierce, 1966). When the optic cup lies beneath the embryonic skin, it induces the latter to form the lens. First the cells of the skin polarize and form a localized, thick patch of cells covered by the basement membrane of the skin. When this lens primordium detaches, it carries the basement membrane with it and retains the ability to synthesize this antigen throughout the life of the animal. One can infer from these studies that environmental signals responsible for initiating differentiation can pass across basement membranes. In addition, it would appear that epithelial basement membrane plays a part in tissue stability, lending strength and support to cells (Pierce, 1966).

IV ULTRASTRUCTURE OF CELLS SYNTHESIZING BASEMENT MEMBRANE

Of the three lines of tumor available for study, parietal yolk sac epithelium was chosen because in approximately 5 days, these cells synthesize Reichert's membrane, a major feat requiring maximal intracellular machinary. Parietal yolk sac epithelial cells were few in number early in the development of the embryo and did not form a complete covering for Reichert's membrane, leaving expanses of the membrane exposed to the yolk cavity. The parietal yolk sac cells lacked hemidesmosomes or other types of membrane specialization, and the impression was gained that they were migratory and moved about synthesizing and depositing basement membrane during their travels.

The cytoplasm was particularly well differentiated (Fig. 13). Profiles of rough-surfaced endoplasmic reticulum were numerous and were distended with material of electron density comparable to that of Reichert's membrane. This rough endoplasmic reticulum budded from the outer membranes of the nuclear envelope, and basement membrane was often observed in the space between the nuclear membranes. Golgi complexes were also highly developed, and one could suppose that they synthesized the carbohydrate-rich moiety of basement membrane, in a manner similar to that described for cartilagenous matrix (Campo and Dziewiatkowski, 1962). Since EBM was not found in the Golgi complexes with labeled antibody, it would appear that the Golgi apparatus does not play a part in secretion of basement membrane. In similar fashion, EBM was never observed in the ground substance of parietal yolk sac carcinoma cells; consequently, it must be secreted directly from the rough endoplasmic reticulum to the exterior via communications with the plasma membrane. Observations compatible with this idea have been made but the point has not been established with high resolution electron microscopy. Figure 14 is a case in point. The plasma membrane appears to reflect back and become continuous with the ribosome-encrusted membranes of the endoplasmic reticulum. Since few such observations have been made, these connections must be exceedingly short-lived or they are broken by methods of fixation. We have incorporated cyanide and phenol in the fixatives in an attempt to obtain exceedingly rapid paralysis, but the incidence of these connections has not been increased. Finally the possibility must be kept in mind, that this observation is nothing more than an artifact of electron-microscopy.

V CHEMICAL COMPOSITION

It will serve no useful purpose to detail the biochemical studies (Mukerjee, Ram and Pierce, 1965; Lee, Blasey, Goldstein and Pierce, 1969) made upon neoplastic basement membrane, because Kefalides (1969) and Spiro (1969) will describe very sophisticated analyses. Suffice it to say, that the material proved to be 75-80% protein, with 12% neutral sugars, 2.5% glucosoamine and 1% lipid. The sugars were glucose, galactose, mannose and fucose-- very little sialic acid was present. With the exception of sialic acid, the molar ratios of carbohydrate components fell within the range of analyses reported by Kefalides and Winzler (1966), Misra and Kaland (1966) and Spiro (1967). Galactosamine and sialic acid, reported in glomerular basement membrane (Spiro, 1967; Lange and Markowitz, 1965), have not been found in NBM, and their presence in glomerular basement membrane is in all probability a reflection of the presence of cell membrane (Mohos and Skoza, 1969) or endothelial basement antigen.

The amino acid composition of NBM is similar to that of glomerular basement membrane. Particularly important, in the amino acid analyses, was the observation that epithelial basement membrane, formed in the absence of connective tissue elements, contained hydroxyproline and hydroxylysine. 7.1% of the amino acid residues were hydroxyproline, 0.1% hydroxylysine, 16.8% lysine, 5.9% proline and 16.8% glycine. X-ray diffraction studies were performed on NBM, lens capsule and tail collagen prepared in similar fashion. The patterns obtained with NBM and lens capsule were identical. In addition to a powder pattern typical of tropocollagen, each had two additional reflections between the 2.9 Å and 4.5 Å reflections (Lee et. al., 1969), in confirmation of Kefalides and Winzler (1966). Thus it was concluded that epithelial basement membrane had a tropocollagen core bonded to an antigenic mucoprotein.

VI TURNOVER OF EPITHELIAL BASEMENT MEMBRANE

Almost nothing is known about the turnover of basement membrane, although most investigators subscribe to the idea that it has a long half-life. The alveoli of the lactating breast are invested by an epithelial basement membrane, and develop and involute with each pregnancy. We examined the resting mammary glands of old female mice that had been used as breeders to see whether or not epithelial basement membrane had been resorbed during involution. None was found in the fat pads which led to the conclusion that the mammal has a mechanism for turning over epithelial basement membrane. The fate of basement membrane during involution was studied using fluorescein-labeled anti-EBM. The process was started by weaning mice 7 days after delivery of a litter. An immediate inflammatory response developed and lasted for about 3 days. During this interval, no changes were noted in the epithelial basement membrane of the alveoli. Subsequently, the alveolar epithelium degenerated and the basement membrane at the bases of the degenerating cells disappeared. This process was complete by the 10th to the 12th day post-involution. It was concluded from these studies that the rapid turnover of epithelial basement membrane is not mediated by inflammatory cells.

Subsequently, ultrastructural studies of the mode of turnover of basement membrane during involution of the breast were made using peroxidase-labeled antibody. As alveolar epithelium underwent degeneration, from the 4th to the 10th day, the basement membrane at the base of the degenerating cells seemed to diffuse toward the adjacent blood vessels. The solubilized antigen was presumably excreted via the blood stream and urine, although we were never able to detect its presence in the glomerular basement membrane of the rat. Epithelial basement membrane is probably removed by enzymatic hydrolysis (Nakane and Pierce, unpublished data), in much the same way that collagenase hydrolyzes collagen (Gross and Lapiere, 1962).

VII BASEMENT MEMBRANE AND INJURY

Since epithelial cells synthesize basement membrane, it was possible to determine some of the factors affecting synthesis of the material. A wide variety of physical, chemical and microbial agents cause fibroblasts to synthesize collagen, and since the epithelial basement membrane molecule contains a collagenous component, the effect of these agents upon the synthesis of epithelial basement membrane was determined (Pierce and Nakane, 1968). The parietal yolk sac carcinoma was injured by the administration of a sublethal dose of x-rays. Large increments in EBM were observed 7 days after exposing the tumor to 5,000 rads. Breast carcinomas of the mouse treated with 5,500 rads also had large increments in epithelial basement membrane about 1 month after treatment.

Two possible mechanisms could explain this observation: either there is an increased synthesis of epithelial basement membrane, or there is decreased removal of the material. We favor the former explanation because x-ray given at the appropriate time is known to increase synthesis of immunoglobulins (Dixon and McConahey, 1963).

It was important to determine whether or not injury might cause increased synthesis of epithelial basement membrane by normal cells. To this end, testes of mice were irradiated, or injected with a crystal of potassium permangenate or with a drop of oily suspension of heat-killed mycobacteria. The radiation produced a generalized atrophy of the testis, the other agents only a local tubular atrophy in the region of the injury. Although it is well known that tubular atrophy in the testis results in a marked infolding of basement membrane (Idänpään-Heikkilä, 1966, Ross and Grant, 1968), the folded basement membranes always remain discreet and never mat to form an apparently thick basement membrane. When treated testes were stained with anti-EBM, marked increments in epithelial basement membrane were noted, and under the electron microscope, multiple lamallae of basement membrane were observed lying parallel to each other

Fig. 15a. Electronmicrograph illustrating the margin of a normal testicular tubule. Tubular epithelium is below and separated by basement membrane (arrow) and fine filaments of collagen from the peritubular cell above. Note the width of the space separating tubular and peritubular cells. (X20,400).

Fig. 15b. The anatomical relationships at the base of a testicular tubule that received 5,000 r 1 month previously. Tubular epithelium is below and has a markedly irregular plasma membrane. The basement membrane is duplicated (arrow) and the twin layers have a tendency to follow the contours of the plasm membrane. Notice the bundles of collagen fibrils separating the basement membrane from the peritubular cell. The space between the tubular epithelium and peritubular cell is at least three times wider than in the control. (X20,400).

Fig. 15c. Multiple lamellae of epithelial basement membrane (arrow) investing atrophic tubules near the site of injection of potassium permanganate crystals in the testis. The space between the base of the testicular tubular epithelium and the peritubular cells is much wider than the control. (X17,300). (Pierce and Nakane, 1969).

Fig. 16a. Section of normal kidney stained with fluorescein-labeled anti-epithelial basement membrane to illustrate the mesangial pattern of epithelial basement membrane in the glomerulus. Note the basement membrane around the bases of renal tubules. (X225).

Fig. 16b. Kidney section from animal which had been x-irradiated at birth, stained with fluorescein-labeled anti-epithelial basement membrane. The glomerulus is larger than the control and contains increased amounts of epithelial basement membrane antigen, particularly in the mesangial regions of the glomerulus. (X225). (Pierce and Nakane, 1969).

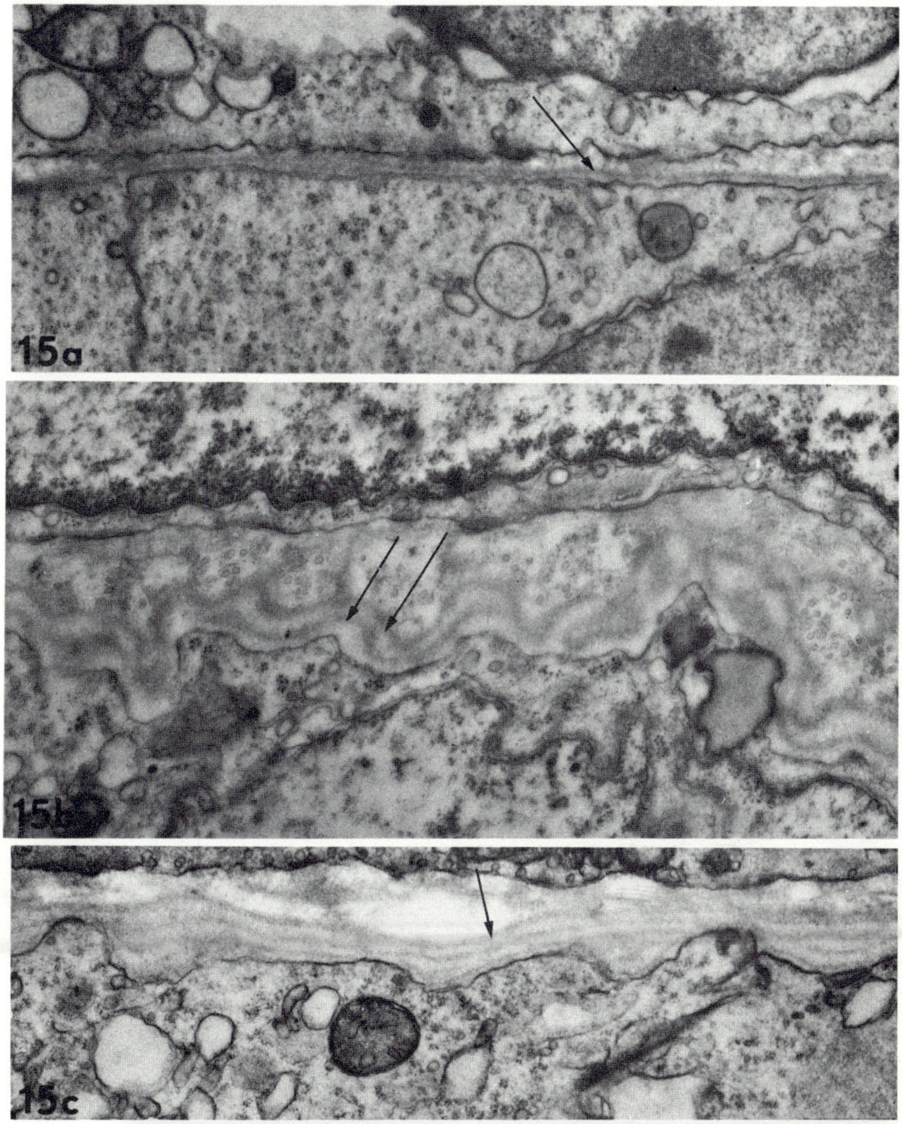
15a
15b
15c

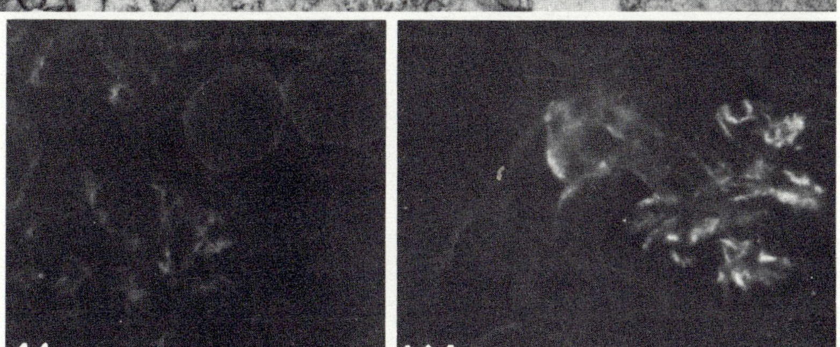
16a
16b

Fig. 17. Part of the mesangial region of a glomerulus from a 4-month-old mouse that received 375 r x-irradiation at birth. Notice the deposits of epithelial basement membrane (EBM) which are continuous with the lamina densa and which project into the mesangium and separate the mesangial cells (M). The texture of the basement membrane varies and in places appears fibrillar or laminated. There is fusion of epithelial cell foot processes. Aside from being widely separated by basement membrane, the mesangial cells are unremarkable. (X12,600). (Pierce and Nakane, 1969).

Fig. 18. Glomerulus of a mouse with an advanced stage of aminonucleoside nephrosis. Notice the thickened capillary basement membrane and the large amounts of epithelial basement membrane (EBM) in the mesangium. The endothelial cytoplasm is thick with many tortuous channels (C) traversing the cytoplasm and apparently connecting capillary lumen with basement membrane. Foot processes of glomerular epithelium have been obliterated and the epithelial cells have microvilli. (X16,800). (Pierce and Nakane, 1969).

Fig. 19. Part of a glomerulus of a nephrotic rat injected intravenously with horse radish peroxidase 2 min prior to death. A histochemical reaction for the enzyme was done and reaction product was found in glomerular basement membrane, the filtration slits (arrow) and adsorbed to the plasma membranes of the foot processes. (X66,000). (Lustig et al., 1969).

Fig. 20. Part of a glomerulus of a nephrotic rat injected intravenously with horse radish peroxidase 2 min prior to death. Foot processes are fused as a result of chemical damage to glomerular epithelial cells and the alternate route of excretion of fluid is between the injured cells and through damaged filtration slits (arrow). Some transport may take place through pinocytotic vesicles. (X44,000). (Lustig et al., 1969).

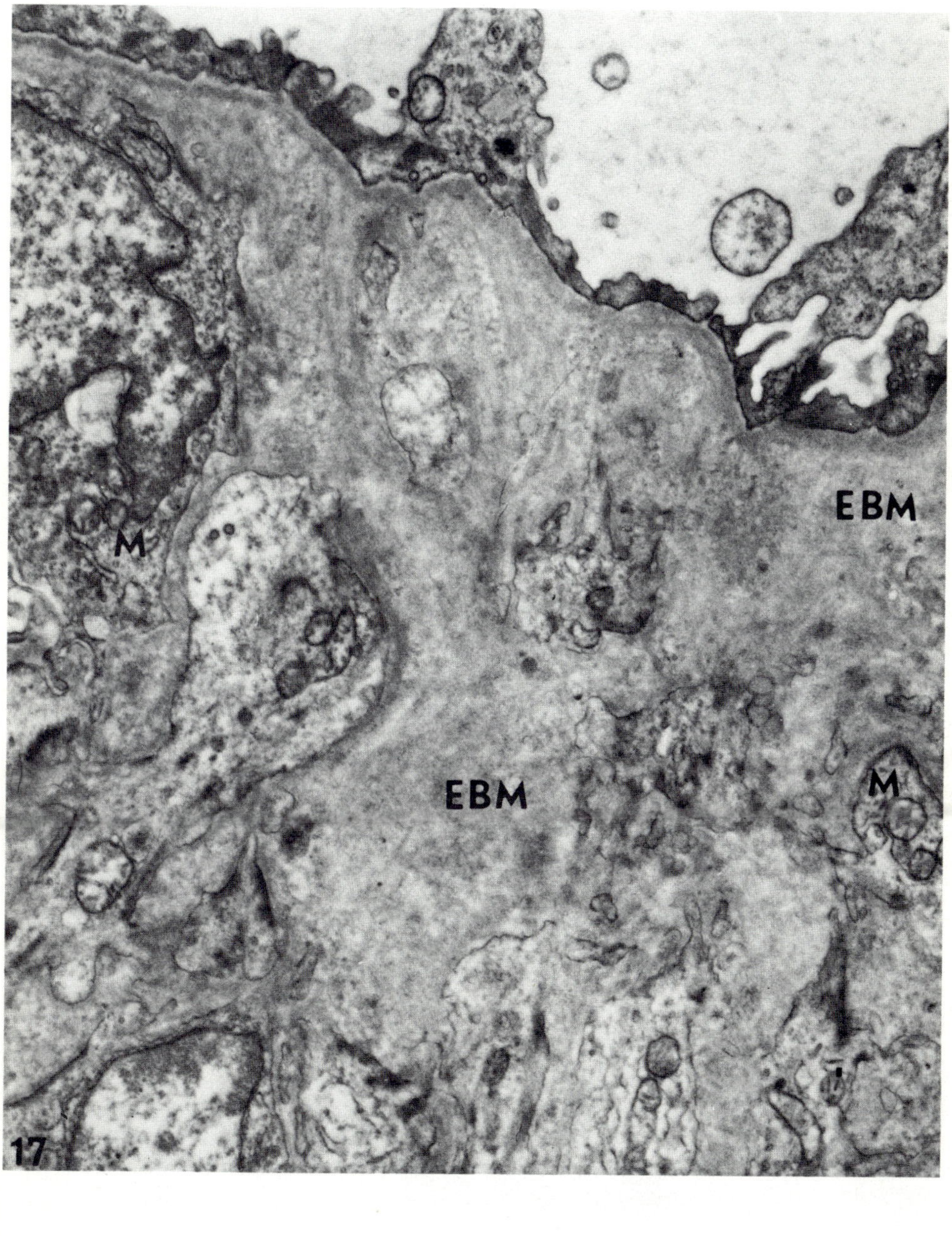
EBM
M
EBM
M
17

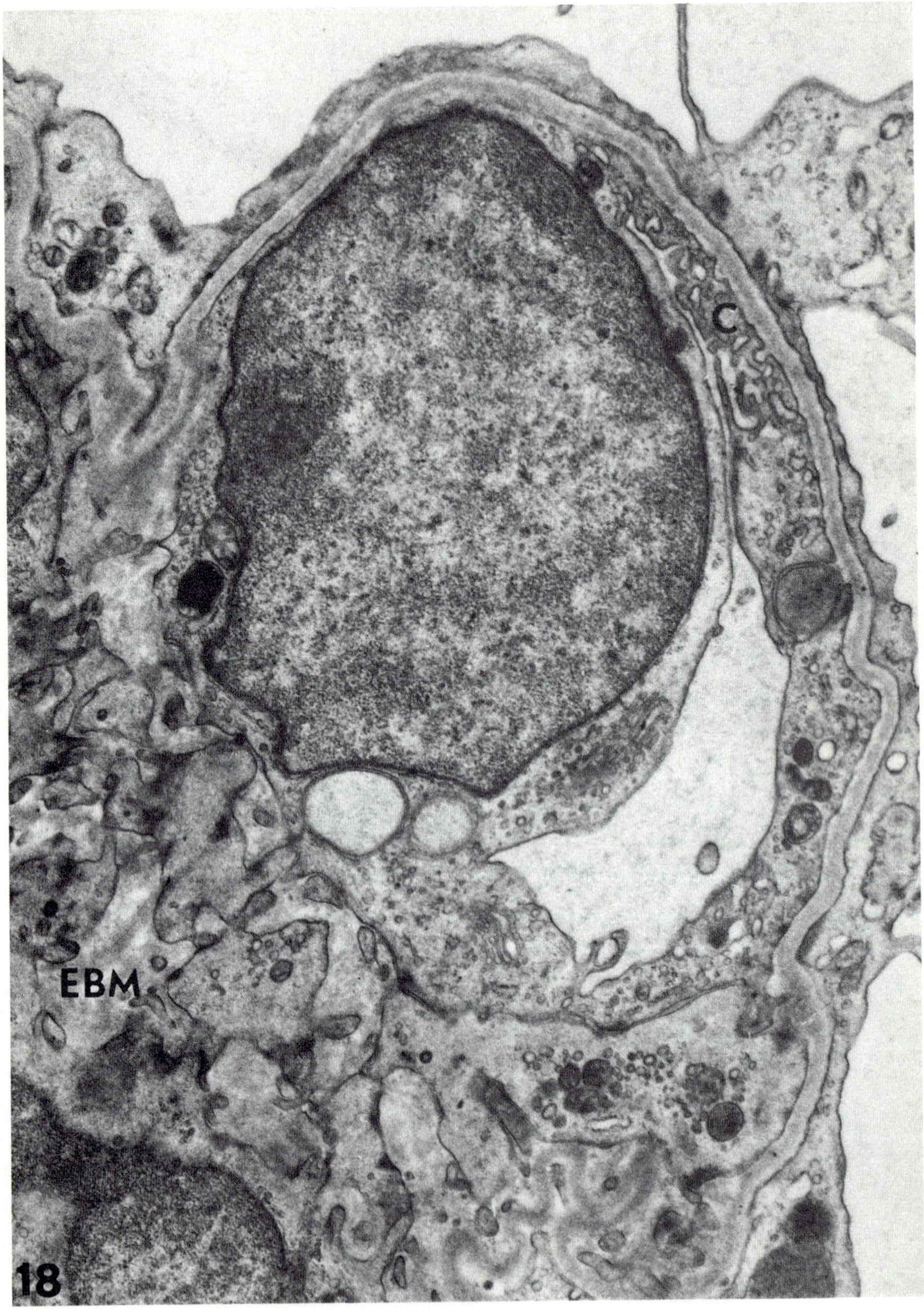
C
EBM
18

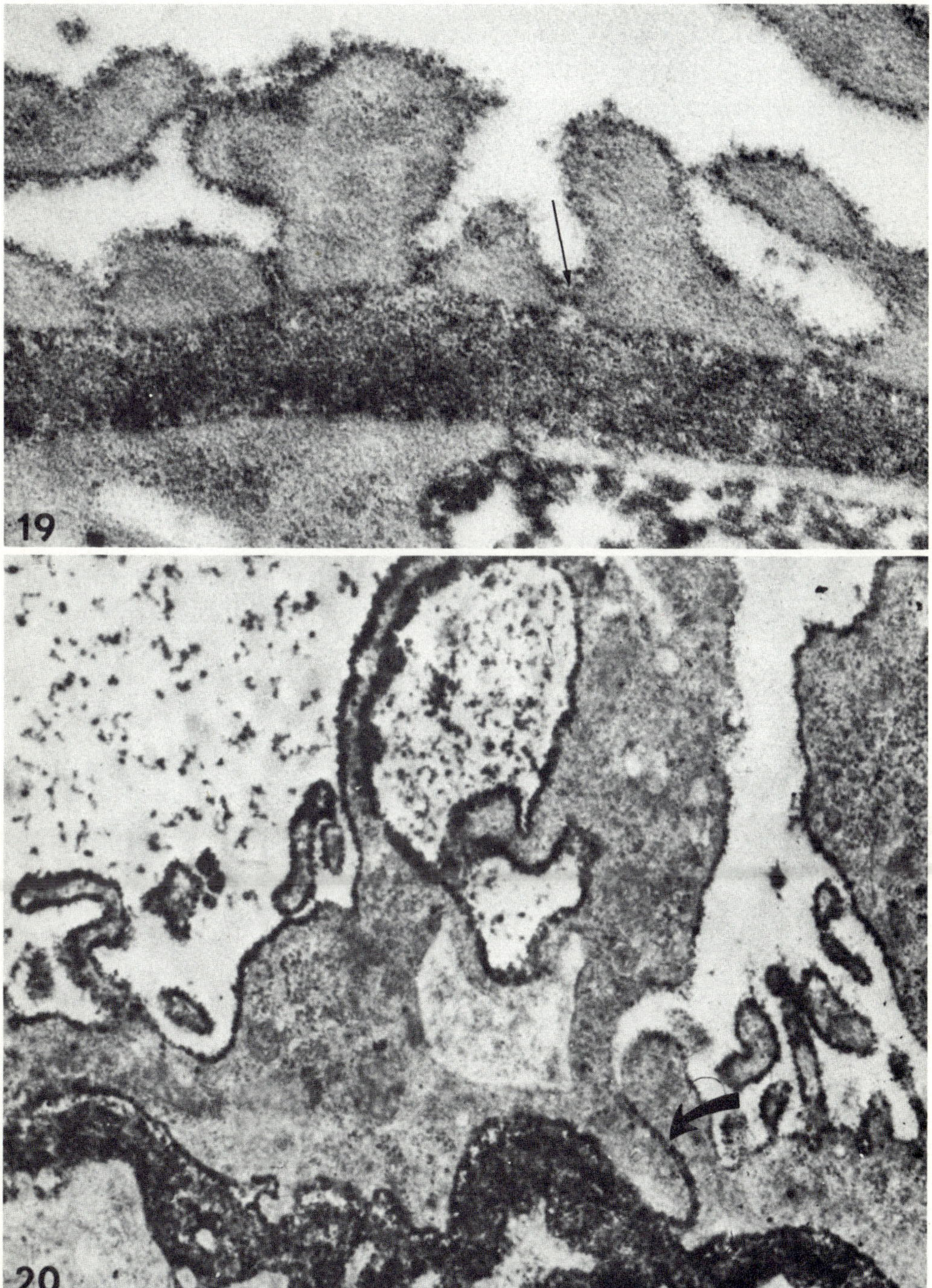

(Fig. 15a,b,c). The conclusion was reached that the injury caused epithelial cells to synthesize additional lamellae of basement membrane (Pierce and Nakane, 1969).

The observation that large amounts of EBM are synthesized in response to injury to epithelium, suggests that cellular injury may be the mechanism for those pathological conditions characterized by the presence of large amounts of hyalin.

There are many diseases characterized by hyalinization of glomeruli. The model of glomerular hyalinization studied by Guttman and Kohn (1960, 1963) was employed in experiments to determine whether or not the hyaline material was epithelial basement membrane. Guttman and Kohn discovered that 375 rads total body irradiation to newborn mice resulted in a severe glomerulosclerotic process of advanced nature 4 months after birth. We analyzed mice so treated by the fluorescein-labeled antibody method and electronmicroscopy, and found that much of the hyaline material was EBM (Fig. 16a,b). The antigen had a mesangial distribution, an observation confirmed by electronmicroscopy (Fig. 17). In the electronmicrographs, some fusion of foot processes was observed over exceedingly thick deposits of basement membrane, but the endoplasmic reticulum and Golgi complexes of the epithelial cells appeared unremarkable. The most notable change was in the basement membranes, all of which were thickened, but those of the mesangium more than the rest. The mesangial cells, which were otherwise unremarkable, were widely separated by masses of epithelial basement membrane (Fig. 17) (Pierce and Nakane, 1969). Some of the basement membrane was in lamellar form and folded on itself. In other areas it had a diffuse light texture. This suggested the possibility that basement membrane produced in response to injury may be physically and chemically different from the normal.

Because we have not as yet identified a specific antigenic marker for endothelial basement membrane, we cannot determine the degree of involvement of endothelium in the production of thickened glomular basement membrane. It must play a part. The experiments demonstrated, however, that physical injury to glomerular epithelium and mesangium resulted in increased deposition of epithelial basement membrane and that one type of glomerular hyalinization was due at least in part to glomerular epithelial injury.

If thickened glomerular basement membrane is the result of injury to glomerular cells, what are the relative roles of the thickened basement membrane, and the glomerular injury on the pathological physiology of the particular disease? For example, are the signs and symptoms of nephrosis due to the changes in the basement membrane or to changes in glomerular cells?

A study of the mechanism of nephrosis was attempted using aminonucleoside nephrosis as the model. A dose of 1.5 mg of the aminonucleosides of puromycin per 100 g of body weight, daily, for 1 week induces nephrosis in 100% of rats (Frenk, Antonowicz, Craig and Metcoff, 1955; Feldman and Fisher, 1959; Vernier, Papermaster and Good, 1959). These animals are characterized by anasarca, extreme proteinuria, hypoproteinemia, hypercholesterolemia, and electronmicroscopically by thickened glomerular basement membranes and fusion of foot processes of glomerular epithelial cells.

Mice proved refractory to the renal effects of aminonucleoside of puromycin (Pierce and Nakane, 1969). Massive doses, 25 mg per 100 g of body weight daily killed all mice by day 12, but none of these animals had either clinical or morphologic evidence of nephrosis. Apparently the animals died of systemic poisoning before they developed nephrosis. It was reasoned that since mice produce little urine, possibly insufficient drug was excreted via the urine to injure the glomerular cells and cause the disease.

In subsequent experiments, animals were given 9 mg of aminonucleosides per 100 g of body weight daily, followed 2 hr later by 2 ml distilled water to promote renal filtration. None of these animals died, and all developed clinical and morphological nephrosis by the 3rd week of the experiment. As in the case of x-ray induced glomerular sclerosis, glomeruli of nephrotic mice contained marked increments in epithelial basement membrane antigen (Fig. 18) (Pierce and

Nakane, 1969). It was concluded from this experiment that development of nephrosis depended upon adequate exposure of glomerular epithelial cells to the injurious agent, after which the cells synthesized additional basement membrane.

Injury also resulted in fusion of foot processes with obliteration of the normal filtration slits. This alters the normal route of passage of fluid through the glomerulus as described by Graham and Karnovsky (1966). Graham and Karnovsky injected horse radish peroxidase intravenously and followed its clearance through the glomerulus. It crossed the basement membrane and entered the urinary space via the filtration slits. Myoperoxidase, with a molecular weight approximately twice that of horse radish peroxidase, was held up temporarily at the filtration slits. Thus it could be deduced that the glomerular epithelial cells were capable of monitoring passage of molecules in excess of a certain size.

To determine the alternate route of flow of fluid in nephrotic animals with obliterated filtration slits, horse radish peroxidase was injected intravenously in nephrotic rats (Figs. 19 and 20) (Lustig, Nakane and Pierce unpublished data). The marker crossed the basement membrane and entered the urinary space between glomerular epithelial cells. Some peroxidase was observed in pinocytotic vesicles. Thus it would seem that macromolecules appear in the urine because the alternate route of flow, between cells, lacks the ability to monitor the molecular size of the constituents of the filtrate as normally occurs in the filtration slits.

ACKNOWLEDGEMENTS

The excellent technical assistance of Mr. Alan Jones is gratefully acknowledged. I wish to thank Drs. Rolla B. Hill and P.K. Nakane for critically reviewing the manuscript.

This work was supported in part by grant E105J from the American Cancer Society and grant AM 13112 from the National Institutes of Health.

REFERENCES

Andres, G.A., Morgan, D., Hsu, K.C., Rifkind, R.A. and Seegal, B.C. (1962). J. Exp. Med. 115, 929.

Campo, R.D. and Dziewiatkowski, D.D. (1962). J. Biol. Chem. 237, 2729.

Cohen, A.I. (1965). Invest. Ophthal. 4, 433.

Everett, J.W. (1935). J. Exp. Zool. 70, 243.

Dixon, F.J. and McConahey, P.J. (1963). J. Exp. Med. 117, 833.

Farquhar, M.G., Wissig, S.L. and Palade, G.E. (1961). J. Exp. Med. 113, 47.

Feldman, J.D. and Fisher, E.R. (1959). Lab. Invest. 8, 371.

Frenk, S., Antonowicz, I., Craig, J.M.and Metcoff, J. (1955). Proc. Soc. Exp. Biol. Med. 89, 424.

Gersch, I. and Catchpole, H.R. (1960). Perspect. Biol. Med. 3, 282.

Graham, R.C. and Karnovsky, M.J. (1966). J. Ext. Med. 124, 1123.

Gross, J. and Lapiere, C.M. (1962). Proc. Nat. Acad. Sci., U.S. 48, 1014.

Guttman, P.H. and Kohn, H.I. (1960). Am J. Pathol. 37, 293.

Guttman, P.H. and Kohn, H.I. (1963). Am J. Pathol. 43, 809.

Idänpään-Heikkilä, P. (1966). Fertil. Steril. 17, 689.

Kefalides, N.A. (1969). This book, p.535.

Kefalides, N.A. and Winzler, R.J. (1966). Biochemistry 5, 702.

Krakower, C.A. and Greenspon, S.A. (1964). In Small Blood Vessel Involvement in Diabetes Mellitus, p. 161. Ed. by Siperstein, M.D., Colwell, A.R., Sr. and Meyer, K. American Institute of Biological Science, Wash. D.C.

Kurtz, S.M. (1958). Exp. Cell Res. 14, 355.

Lange, C.F., Jr. and Markowitz, A.S. (1965). Biochim.Biopys. Acta 101. 217.

Lee, P., Blasey, K., Goldstein, I.J. and Pierce, G.B. (1969). J. Mol. Exp. Pathol. 10, 323.

Midgley, A.R. and Pierce, G.B. (1963). Am. J. Pathol. 43, 929.

Misra, R.P. and Kalant, N. (1966). Nephron 3, 84.

Mohos, S.C. and Skoza, L. (1969). Science 164, 1519.

Mukerjee, H., Sri Ram, J. and Pierce, G.B. (1965). Am J. Pathol. 46, 49.

Pierce, G.B. (1965). Cancer Res. 25, 656.

Pierce, G.B. (1966). Develop. Biol. 13, 231.

Pierce, G.B., Beals, T.F., Sri Ram, J. and Midgley, A.R. (1964). Am. J. Pathol. 45, 929.

Pierce, G.B. and Dixon, F.J. (1959). Cancer 122, 584.

Pierce, G.B., Jr.Midgley, A.R., Jr., Sri Ram, J. and Feldman, J.D. (1962). Am. J. Pathol. 41, 549.

Pierce, G.B., Midgley, A.R. and Sri Ram, J. (1963). J. Exp. Med. 117, 339.

Pierce, G.B. and Nakane, P.K. (1967). Lab. Invest. 17, 499.

Pierce, G.B. and Nakane, P.K. (L968). Fed. Proc. 27, 411.

Pierce, G.B. and Nakane, P.K. (1969). Lab. Invest. 21, 27

Robbins, S.L. (1968). Pathology, 3rd ed., p. 986. W.B. Saunders & Co.

Ross, M.H. and Grant, L. (1968). Exp. Cell. Res. 50, 277.

Schiebler, T.H. and Knoop. A. (1959). Ztschr. Zellforsch. 50, 494.

Snell, G.D. and Stevens, L.C. (1966). In Biology of the Laboratory Mouse, p. 205. Ed. by Green, E.L. McGraw Hill Inc., New York.

Spiro,R.G. (1969). This book, p. 511.

Spiro, R.G. (1967). J. Biol Chem. 242, 1915.

Steblay, R.W. (1963). Lab. Invest. 12, 432.

Tan, E.M. and Kaplan, M.H. (1963). Immunology 6, 331.

Vernier, R.L., Papermaster, B.W. and Good, R.A. (1959). J. Exp. Med. 109, 115.

Wislocki, G.B. and Dempsey, E.W. (1955). Anat. Rec. 123, 33.

SYMMETRICAL FIBRILS ASSOCIATED WITH BASEMENT MEMBRANES

Romaine R. Bruns

Since 1960 unusual banded fibrils have been observed near basement membranes in a variety of tissues, notably in the skin of the toad (Brody, 1960; Palade and Farquhar, 1965; Younes, Steele, Robertson and Bencosme, 1965; Susi, Belt and Kelly, 1967; Carroll and Kuwabara, 1968; Swanson and Helwig, 1968; Bruns, 1969; Rowlatt, 1969). The detailed structure of these fibrils and their relation to the basement membrane have been difficult to establish because the fibrils are usually curved and occur along folded basement membranes. Recently, however, well-oriented fibrils were found in the tail of the bullfrog tadpole along the outer surface of the smooth basement membrane covering the notochord. In this favorable location, it was established that: 1) the notochord fibrils have a symmetrical banded structure (Fig. 1); 2) they are attached at both ends to the basement membrane; and 3) they appear occasionally between the basement membrane and the notochord cells, and within the notochord sheath among the collagen fibrils (Bruns, 1969). On the basis of these observations and on the finding of symmetrical fibrils in other locations (uterus (Rowlatt, 1969); skin of tadpole and toad (Bruns, 1969)) it was proposed that the banded fibrils associated with basement membranes consitute a single new class of extracellular fibrils and that the symmetrical type of fibril is the fundamental fibril of this class.

Other than these morphological characteristics, little is known about the fibrils. Their transverse band pattern bears no obvious similarity to the transverse bands on nearby collagen fibrils or to other banded objects reported

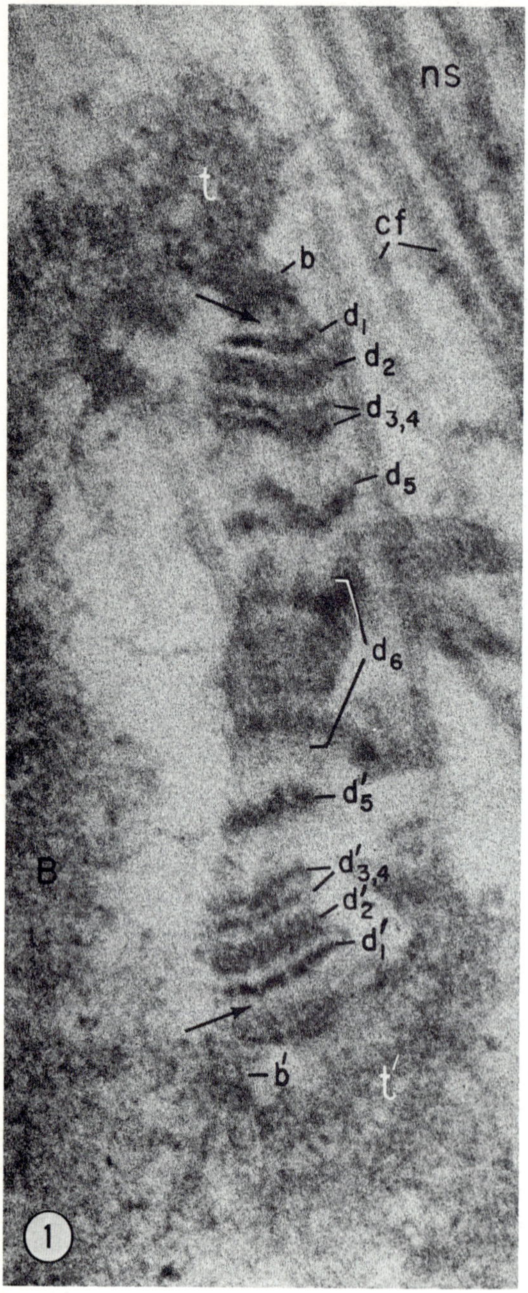

Fig. 1. A symmetrical banded fibril found at the periphery of the notochord in the tail of a Rana catesbeiana tadpole. The fibril consists of a banded stem (between arrows) having short branches (b, b′) and basement membrane-like material (t, t′) at both ends. Note that the stem (~ 4, 500 Å long) shows a long symmetrical central band, d_6 (~ 1,000 Å long) and that the transverse bands d_1-d_5 are mirror images of bands $d'_5$5-d'_1. The plane of this section grazes the junction of the notochord basement membrane, B, and the overlying collagenous notochord sheath, ns (collagen fibrils are marked cf). (X200,000).

in the literature. But it should be mentioned that in overall length and in the presence of a long central band, the stems of the symmetrical fibrils resemble certain tropocollagen aggregates found among vitrosin fibrils (Olsen, 1965). With regard to function, it has been proposed that the fibrils in skin secure the folds of basement membrane in micropapillae and assist in anchoring the basement membrane to the underlying tissue (Palade and Farquhar, 1965). In other sites, however, where the fibrils attach at both ends to a smooth basement membrane (e.g. at the notochord basement membrane (Bruns, 1969) and in the uterus (Rowlatt, 1969)), anchoring may not be an important function. The origin of the fibrils is unknown, but their presence between the notochord cells and the overlying basement membrane suggests that here they are products of the notochord cells. Finally, it is interesting to note that the fibrils have not been found on basement membranes in glomeruli or blood vessels.

ACKNOWLEDGMENTS

This is publication No. 490 from the Robert W. Lovett Memorial Group for Diseases Causing Deformities, Department of Medicine, Harvard Medical School at the Massachusetts General Hospital, Boston, Mass. This investigation was supported by Public Health Service Grants AM12785 and AM 3564 from the National Institute of Arthritis and Metabolic Diseases awarded to Professor J. Gross.

REFERENCES

Brody, I. (1960). J. Ultrastruct. Res. 4, 264.

Bruns, R. R. (1969). J. Cell Biol. 42, 418.

Carroll, J. M. and Kuwabara, T. (1968). Arch. Ophthal.,80, 683.

Olsen, B. R. (1965). J. Ultrastruct. Res. 13, 172.

Palade, G. E. and Farquhar, M. G. (1965). J. Cell Biol. 27, 215.

Rowlatt, C. (1969). J. Ultrastruct. Res. 26, 44.

Susi, F. R., Belt, W. D. and Kelly, J. W. (1967). J. Cell Biol. 34, 686.

Swanson, J. L. and Helwig, E. B. (1968). J. Invest. Derm. 50, 195.

Younes, M. S., Steele, H. D., Robertson, E. M. and Bencosme, S. A. (1965). Am. J. Obstet. Gynec. 92, 163.

BIOCHEMISTRY OF BASEMENT MEMBRANES

Robert G. Spiro

Basement membranes are extracellular membranes which are widely distributed in animal tissues. Their intense reaction with the periodic acid-Schiff stain makes them readily discernible in tissue sections and indicates their glycoprotein nature (McManus, 1948; Lillie, 1952; Leblond, Glegg and Eidinger, 1957). Basement membranes are found in the glomeruli and tubules of the kidney, the lining of the capillaries of the vascular tree, the alveoli of the lungs, and the follicles of the thyroid. They are moreover important structural components of the eye in the form of the lens capsule, Descemet's and Bowman's membranes of the cornea, and Bruch's membrane of the retina.

Studies using immunofluorescent antibodies have indicated that basement membranes have common antigenic determinants and that tagged antibodies against the renal glomerular basement membrane will deposit on the basement membrane of other tissues (Cruickshank and Hill, 1953; Roberts, 1957). Chemical studies performed on a number of basement membranes have shown that they belong to the collagen family of proteins. However, when viewed under the electronmicroscope, they are amorphous and do not show the fibrillar structure nor the axial banding of the classical collagens from tissues such as tendon and skin.

An important biological function performed by basement membranes is that of a selective filter. They also act as a supportive structure upon which cells can rest, forming thereby a microskeleton. The renal glomerular basement membrane best exemplifies the function of basement membranes as a physiological filter, as it constitutes the only complete barrier between the plasma and its filtrate. The other two components of the glomerular capillary wall, the endothelial and epithelial cells are discontinuous, being interrupted by either filtration pores or slits (Farquhar, 1964; Vernier, 1961). It is likely that the glomerular basement membrane serves as a passive filter and that its porosity is determined by the organization of the peptide chains. This concept makes a study of the chemistry of this membrane challenging, since a key to its function would reside in an understanding of its structure. The glomerular basement membrane is believed to undergo alteration in a variety of disease states, including diabetic microangiopathy, leading to a resultant loss of its selective filtration function.

Despite their wide distribution, the isolation of basement membranes in pure form poses great technical problems because of the presence in most tissues of other insoluble proteins, such as collagen and elastin. This is evident, for example, with such an important basement membrane as found in the alveoli of the lung, which is found surrounded by collagen and elastic tissue. A few membranes, however, are located in anatomically advantageous situations and can be obtained in pure form for chemical study. These include the renal glomerular basement membrane (Krakower and Greenspon, 1951; Spiro, 1967a), the lens capsule of the eye (Fukushi and Spiro, 1969), Descemet's membrane of the cornea (Dohlman and Balazs, 1955), and Reichert's membrane from neoplastic yolk sac cells (Pierce, Beals, Sri Ram and Midgley, 1964).

Our investigations of basement membranes have been carried out on glomerular basement membranes from bovine and human kidneys and lens capsules from calf and cow eyes. For the isolation of glomeruli, sieves of varying mesh were employed for the disruption of the tissue and also for the separation of the glomeruli from the other components (Spiro, 1967a). From the isolated glomeruli, highly purified basement membranes could be obtained after ultrasonic disruption, and th membranes could be shown to be free of cellular contaminants by chemical analysis.

Approximately 10% of the weight of the membrane is made up of carbohydrate in the form of glucose, galactose, mannose, fucose, hexosamines and sialic acids (Table I).

TABLE I

Amino Acid composition of the Bovine Glomerular Basement Membrane and Anterior Lens Capsule

Component	Glomerular basement membrane *	Anterior lens capsule+
	Residues per 1000 total amino acid residues	
Glycine	208	267
Alanine	61	40
Valine	38	30
Isoleucine	29	31
Leucine	59	57
Proline	69	71
Phenylalanine	28	31
Tyrosine	18	11
Tryptophan	6.0	3.6
Serine	55	45
Threonine	37	28
Half-cystine	31	17
Methionine	14	12
Lysine	27	12
Histidine	16	12
Arginine	49	36
Aspartic acid	68	54
Glutamic acid	96	88
Amide	68	68
Hydroxyproline	68	111
Hydroxylysine	22	45

* Data taken from Spiro (1967a).

\+ Data taken from Fukushi and Spiro (1969).

The remainder of the membrane consists of peptide, and its amino acid composition is shown in Table II. Noteworthy is the occurrence of substantial amounts of hydroxyproline and hydroxylysine, as well as the presence of approximately one-fifth of the total amino acid residues as glycine. This composition indicates that the glomular basement

TABLE II

Carbohydrate Composition of the Bovine Glomerular Basement Membrane*

Monosaccharide	Percentage of dry weight of membrane	Residues per 1000 total amino acid residues
Glucose	2.47	16.4
Galactose	3.05	20.2
Mannose	0.77	5.1
Fucose	0.22	1.6
N-acetylglucosamine	1.86	10.0
N-acetylgalactosamine	0.27	1.4
N-glycolylneuraaminic acid	0.72	2.6
N-acetylneuraminic acid	0.47	1.8

* Data taken from Spiro (1967a).

membrane is a member of the collagen family, albeit a very specialized and carbohydrate-rich member distinct from the classical fibrillar collagens.

The glomerular basement membrane is insoluble under physiological conditions and cannot be solubilized by techniques which extract fibrillar collagen, such as treatment with neutral salt or with citrate buffer at pH 3.7. However, treatment with mild alkali causes complete solubilization (Table III). While buffered urea itself has no solubilizing effect, complete solubilization can be achieved by thiols in the presence of urea. Substantial digestion and solubilization occured with various proteolytic enzymes (Table III), and over 90% of the carbohydrate and peptide portions could be solubilized with either collagenase or Pronase.

In studying the structure of this membrane, we first undertook to characterize the carbohydrate portion in regard to the size, number and structure of its units, as well as the linkages which attach these to the peptide portion.

TABLE III

Effect of Various Treatments on the Solubility of the Bovine Glomerular Basement Membrane

Agent	Length of treatment (hr)	Temperature (°C)	Percent solubilized	
			Carbohydrate	Peptide
Pepsin	51	37	59	76
Trypsin	42	37	64	68
Collagenase	48	37	93	89
Pronase	93	37	100	98
0.1 N NaOH	8	37	97	95
8 *M* urea (*p*H 8.0)	48	37	<10	<10
Thiols + 8 *M* urea (*p*H 8.0)	24	22	100	100

We were also interested in attempting to determine the relationship of the carbohydrate units to each other in terms of their distribution on the peptide chains.

In order to obtain the carbohydrate units with a minimum number of amino acids attached, the membrane was digested with collagenase and the material solubilized by this treatment was further treated with Pronase. This digest was then submitted to gel filtration on Sephadex G-25 and further fractionated on Sephadex G-50 (Spiro, 1967b). In this manner, three distinct glycopeptide fractions could be obtained which differed markedly in composition (Table IV). One group of glycopeptides penetrated Sephadex G-25, (Sephadex G-25, peak 2) and contained as their monosaccharides only glucose and galactose, which were present along with hydroxylysine in equimolar amounts. These glycopeptides were further chromatographed on Dowex-50 X 2 and were shown to contain a 2-*O*-α-*D*-glucosylgalactose disaccharide linked by a β-glycosidic bond to the hydroxyl group of hydroxylysine (Spiro, 1967b,c). The studies

TABLE IV

Composition of the Glycopeptide Fractions Obtained by Gel Filtration of the Collagenase-Pronase Digest of the Bovine Glomerular Basement Membrane

Component	Sephadex G-50 Peak 1	Sephadex G-50 Peak 2	Sephadex G-25 Peak 2
	(Residues per 100 amino acid residues)		
Hydroyx-proline	12.2	0	4.65
Aspartic acid	5.52	16.8	9.31
Theronine	2.63	9.06	2.80
Serine	3.30	9.40	4.65
Glutamic acid	8.45	7.56	14.6
Proline	6.05	10.25	6.52
Glycine	30.7	10.25	26.9
Alanine	2.35	7.56	3.33
Valine	2.21	4.02	1.73
Methionine	0.37	1.01	0.26
Isoleucine	3.36	2.33	1.73
Leucine	4.40	2.53	2.13
Tryosine	1.23	1.34	0
Phenylalanine	2.46	1.51	0.53
Hydroxylysine	5.21	0	13.3
Lysine	0.67	2.69	1.60
Histidine	1.17	2.85	1.20
Arginine	4.23	3.35	2.66
Half-cystine	3.20	7.20	2.26
Galactose	6.60	38.4	13.1
Glucose	4.65	0	13.1
Mannose	2.35	31.6	0
Fucose	0.84	7.21	0
Sialic acids	0.59	21.7	0
Hexosamines	4.77	43.5	0

which were used to establish to establish this structure are reviewed in another section of this book (Spiro, 1969b).

Another group of glycopeptides which were excluded from Sephadex G-25 but penetrated Sephadex G-50 (Sephadex G-50, peak 2) contained sialic acid, fucose, galactose, mannose, hexosamines, but no glucose (Table IV). They were rich in aspartic acid and other polar amino acids and contained no hydroxyproline or hydroxylysine. The third group of glycopeptides was excluded from both gels (Sephadex G-50, peak 1) and had a very unusual composition, containing all of the sugars present in the original basement membrane, but at a concentration about three and a half times that of the native membrane. In addition, it contained almost one-third of its residues as glycine and very high amounts of hydroxylysine and hydroxyproline. The hydroxylysine to lysine ration was 7.8 compared to 0.83 in the native membrane, while the hydroxyproline to proline ration was 2.0 instead of 0.99 as in the native basement membrane. In addition, these glycopeptides contained a large number of half-cystine residues.

The glycopeptides which were excluded from Sephadex G-25 but entered Sephadex G-50 (Sephasex G-50, peak 2)

TABLE V

Carbohydrate Composition of Glomerular Basement Membrane Glycopeptides Obtained by DEAE-Cellulose Chromatography of Material in Sephadex-50, peak 2 *

Glycopeptide	Molar Ratio to Fucose			
	Galactose	Mannose	Hexosamines	Sialic acid
1	3.6	2.8	4.4	0.3
2	3.0	2.9	4.1	1.4
3	4.2	3.2	4.5	2.1
4	4.2	3.5	5.6	2.8
5	3.8	3.8	5.5	3.0
6	4.4	3.2	4.9	2.9
7	4.3	3.8	4.5	3.0
8	4.3	3.9	5.3	3.6
9	3.5	3.6	5.0	3.6
10	4.3	3.4	5.3	4.3

* Data taken from Spiro (1967b).

could be further fractionated by chromatography on DEAE-cellulose into peaks for which analyses are shown in Table V. These glycopeptides all contained sialic acid, galactose, mannose, fucose, and hexosamines, and manifested the microheterogeneity which is characteristic of complex carbohydrate units of this type. The average molecular weight of the carbohydrate portion of these glycopeptides, determined by sedimentation equilibrium, was 3500 (Spiro, 1967b). Further studies have shown that these glycopeptides contain branched heteropolysaccharide units similar to those previously described for fetuin (Spiro, 1962 a,b; 1964), thyroglobulin (Spiro, 1965), and the α_2-macroglobulin (Dunn and Spiro, 1967), in which oligosaccharide chains consisting of the sequence sialic acid (or fucose) →galactose → N-acetylglucosamine are linked to an internal portion of mannose and N-acetylglucosamine (Fig. 1). The heterogeneity of this type of carbohydrate unit arises from the existence of variable numbers of chains in different stages of completion. C-1 of the most internal sugar of these basement membrane glycopeptides is linked to the peptide chain by what appears to be a glycosylamine type of linkage to an asparagine residue.

Table VI summarizes the information about the two types of carbohydrate units present in the basement membrane. One type is the glucosylgalactose disaccharide, while the other is a branched heteropolysaccharide consisting on an average of 4 residues of galactose, 3 of mannose, 5 of hexosamines, 3 of sialic acid, and 1 of fucose, but containing no glucose. The molecular weight of the disaccharide is 324, while the average molecular weight of the heteropolysaccharide calculated from the sum of the sugar residues is 3170. The heteropolysaccharide shows marked microheterogeneity, while the disaccharide unit appears to be of only

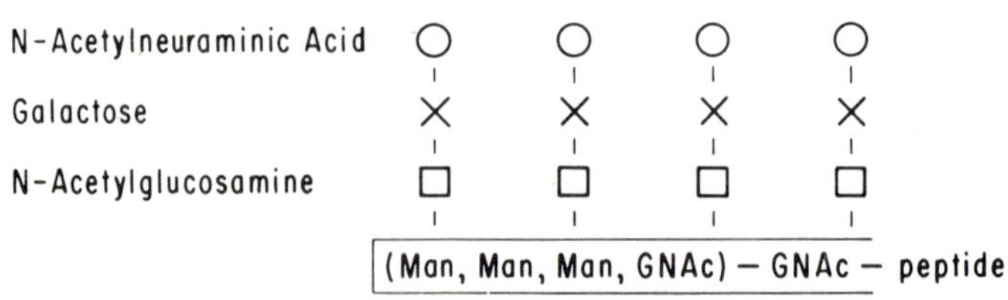

Fig. 1. Schematic representation of heteropolysaccharide unit. From studies on fetuin. (Spiro, 1962a,b,; 1964).

TABLE VI

Carbohydrate Units of the Bovine Glomerular Basement Membrane *

Carbohydrate unit	Residues per unit							
	Glucose	Galactose	Mannose	Hexosamines	Sialic acids	Fucose	Molecular weight	Amino Acid of glycopeptide bond
Disaccharide	1	1	---	---	---	---	324	Hydroxylysine
Heteropolysaccharide +	--	4	3	5	3	1	3170	Asparagine

* Data taken from Spiro (1967b).

\+ Average composition of glycopeptides containing this carbohydrate unit.

one type. The carbohydrate of the membrane is about evenly divided by weight between these two types of units, and there are approximately 10 of the disaccharide units for every heteropolysaccharide present. The disaccharide is linked glycosidically to hydroxylysine, while the heteropolysaccharide is believed to be attached to asparagine residues in the peptide chain.

In order to determine if there are common structural features among basement membranes, a study of the lens capsule of the eye of the calf and cow was undertaken (Fukushi and Spiro, 1969; Spiro and Fukushi, 1969). The lens capsule is a representative basement membrane and is present as an amorphous structure which encloses the lens. It can be readily obtained in pure form by mechanical means. Its carbohydrate portion had been previously studied by Pirie (1951) and also by Dische and his collaborators (Dische and Borenfreund, 1954; Dische, Zelmenis and Rothschild, 1967).

We found that approximately 11% of the weight of the lens capsule consists of carbohydrate, and Table VII shows the monosaccharide analyses of the anterior and posterior portions of the calf and cow lens capsules. In many respects, these sugar analyses are similar to those of the glomerular basement membrane, with a predominance of glucose and galactose. The lens capsules, however, contain small amounts of hexuronic acids, which are completely absent in the glomerular basement membrane. From these analyses, distinct topographical and age differences in the sugar compositions can be noted.

The amino acid composition of the cow anterior lens capsule is shown in Table I where it is compared to that of the glomerular basement membrane. After collagenase-Pronase digestion of the calf and cow lens capsules, similar groups of glycopeptides as described for the glomerular basement membrane could be obtained by gel filtration, indicating the presence of hydrosxlysine-linked disaccharide units, heteropolysacchride units consisting of sialic acid, fucose, mannose, hexosamines, and galactose, and high

TABLE VII

Carbohydrate Composition of Anterior and Posterior Parts of Calf and Cow Lens Capsule*

Monosaccharide	Residues per 1000 total amino acid residues+			
	Calf		Cow	
	Anterior	Posterior	Anterior	Posterior
Glucose	28.5	23.8	38.8	31.7
Galactose	33.0	27.5	40.0	36.2
Mannose	5.1	5.2	3.7	4.0
Fucose	1.9	2.0	2.0	2.2
Hexosamines	11.2	16.9	5.3	7.0
Sialic acids	1.3	2.7	0.4	0.9
Hexuronic acids	2.1	8.9	0.4	1.4

* Data taken from Fukushi and Spiro (1969).

\+ The total residue weights of carbohydrate in g per 100g of dry capsule were as follows: calf anterior capsule 11.2; calf posterior capsule 11.5; cow anterior capsule 11.3; cow posterior capsule 10.9.

molecular weight crosslinked fragments (Spiro and Fukushi, 1969).

When the alkaline hydrolysate of the lens capsule was placed on the amino acid analyzer, a very large new component appeared which could be identidied as glucosylgalactosylhydroxylysine (Fig. 2). This was present in even greater amounts than in the glomerular basement membrane. Paper chromatography of the alkaline hydrolysate of the lens capsule glycopeptides indicated the presence of a large component which migrated to the same position as the glucosylgalactosylhydroxylysine from the glomerular basement membrane (Fig. 3). Only very small amounts of galactosylhydroxylysine were evident in the lens capsule, just as in the glomerular basement membrane.

Structural studies of the disaccharide units from the lens capsule employing periodate oxidation, methylation,

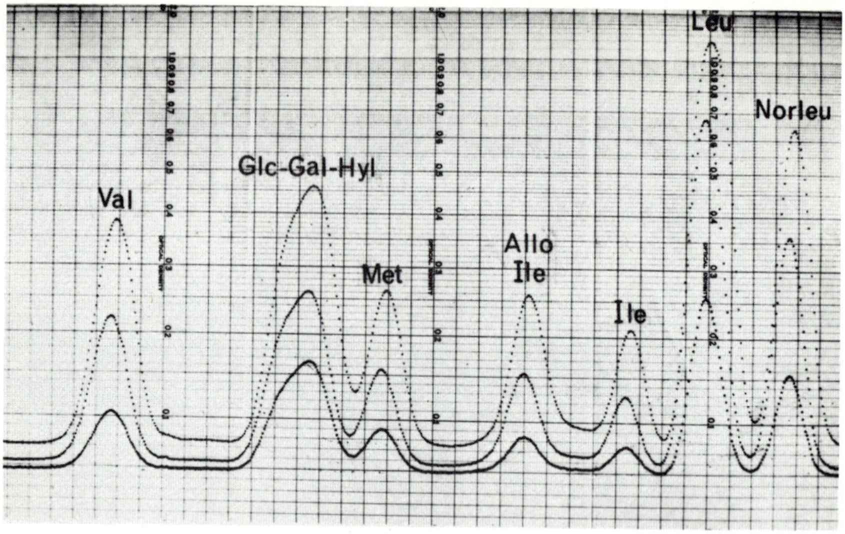

Fig. 2. Segment of an elution diagram from an alkaline hydrolyzate of cow anterior lens capsule on the amino acid analyzer (Technicon). The glucosylgalactosylhydroxylysine (Glc-Gal-Hyl) is seen ahead of the methionine. Taken from Spiro and Fukushi (1969).

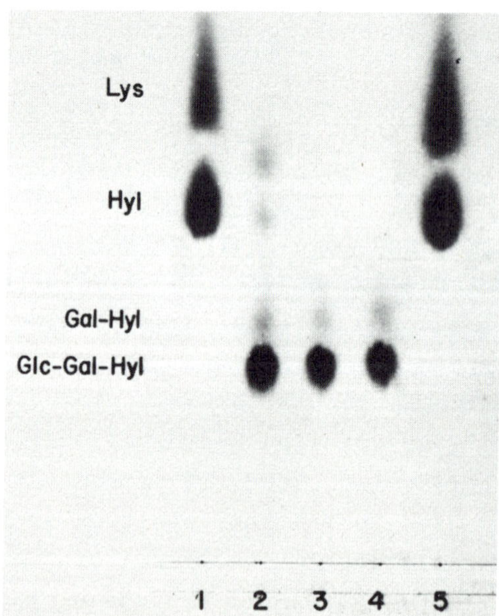

Fig. 3. Comparison of paper chromatographic migration of hydroxylysine-linked carbohydrate of lens capsules and glomerular basement membrane. The chromatogram shows the alkaline hydrolysate of glycopeptides containing glucose and galactose from bovine glomerular basement membrane (2), anterior calf lens capsule (3), and posterior calf lens capsule (4). 1 and 5 are amino acid standards. The solvent system was n-butanol-acetic acid-water (4:1:5) run for 110 hr. Taken from Spiro and Fukushi (1969).

graded acid hydrolysis, and enzymatic treatment, revealed the structure of this unit to be identical with that present in the glomerular basement membrane and fibrillar collagens, that is, 2-O-α-D-glucosylgalactose linked by a β-glycosidic bond to the hydroxyl group of hydroxylysine (Spiro and Fukushi, 1969). As in the glomerular basement membrane, approximately 80% of the hydroxylysine residues are glycosidically substituted. However, there are about twice as many disaccharide units in the cow lens capsule as in the glomerular basement membrane from this species (Table VIII) because of the large amount of hydroxylysine in the capsule (Table I). The lens capsule has a greater percent of its carbohydrate weight in the form of disaccharide than the glomerular basement membrane (Table VIII), and a higher content of the disaccharide unit with increasing age.

An important consideration in regard to the carbohydrate of the basement membrane is the positions on the peptide chains to which the two different carbohydrate units are attached and the relationship of these two units to each other in the intact membrane. From the analyses of the glycopeptide fractions obtained after collagenase-Pronase digestion (Table IV), it is obvious that the amino acid composition in the immediate vicinity of the attachment of the carbohydrate units is quite different for the disaccharide and heteropolysaccharide units. However, since these glycopeptides have been obtained after very extensive proteolytic digestion and have only a small segment of the peptide chain attached, their composition gives little information in regard to their position in the overall structure of the basement membrane.

It is of value to make a comparison of the compositions of the two basement membrane which we have studied, the glomerular basement membrane, and the lens capsule, with that of a soluble fibrillar collagen (skin collagen), whose structure is understood somewhat better. From Table IX it may be noted that in addition to the much greater amount

TABLE VIII

Distribution of Carbohydrate of Glomerular Basement Membrane and Lens Capsule between Disaccharide and Heteropolysaccharide Units

Membrane	Residue weight		Carbohydrate distribution by weight	
	Disaccharide	Heteropolysaccharide	Disaccharide	Heteropolysaccharide
	(g/100 g dry membrane)		(%)	
Cow glomerular basement membrane*	4.44	4.49	50	50
Lens capsules+				
Calf anterior	7.34	3.23	69	31
Calf posterior	5.80	3.14	65	35
Cow anterior	9.54	1.68	85	15
Cow posterior	7.94	2.41	77	23

*Data taken from Spiro (1967b).

+Data taken from Spiro and Fukushi (1969).

TABLE IX

Comparison of the Amino Acid Patterns and Hydroxylysine-linked Carbohydrate of the Glomerular Basement Membrane, Lens Capsule and Skin Collagen

Component	Glomerular basement membrane (bovine)*	Anterior lens[+] capsule (bovine)	Skin collagen[°] (calf)
	(Residues/1000 total amino acid residues)		
Glycine	208	267	320
Imino acids	137	182	232
Hydroxyamino acids	210	240	158
Acidic amino acids	164	142	117
Amide groups	68	68	46
Basic amino acids	115	104	89
Aromatic amino acids	52	46	16
Sulfur-containing amino acids	45	30	4.3
Hydroxylysine	22	45	7.4
Glucoslygalactosylhydroxylysine#	17	35	1.2
Galactosylhydroxylysine#	0.5	2.3	1.1

* Data taken from Spiro (1967a).
+ Data taken from Fukushi and Spiro (1969).
° Data taken from Piez and Gross (1960).
Data taken from Spiro (1969).

of carbohydrate which the basement membranes contain, they also consist of a greater number of polar amino acids than the collagen. Moreover, they are richer in hydroxylysine, and contain significant amounts of sulfur amino acids, particularly cystine, an amino acid which is not found in fibrillar collagens. On the other hand, the basement membranes contain substantially less glycine than the collagen, with one-fifth to one-fourth rather than one-third of their total amino acids being made up of this component.

The difference between the composition of these membranes and fibrillar collagen could be the result of the membranes having two types of chains, one "collagen-like" and the other rich in polar amino acids, or their containing on the same chain extensive peptide regions which are rich in polar amino acids and different from the helical portions. Small segments of such polar regions have been shown to occur in fibrillar tropocollagen (Kang, Bornstein, and Piez, 1967).

Several schemes can be proposed to explain the relationship of the two types of carbohydrate units to each other, presuming that the hydroxylysine-linked disaccharide unit is in a more "collagen-like" portion of the membrane and the heteropolysaccharide unit is in a more polar region (Fig. 4). In model 1, two different proteins, a collagen and another glycoprotein are held together by noncovalent bonds. Although this scheme has been hypothesized (Kefalides, 1966), no separation of the units can be achieved without extensive degradation of the peptide portion and breakage of covalent bonds by either chemical or proteoly-

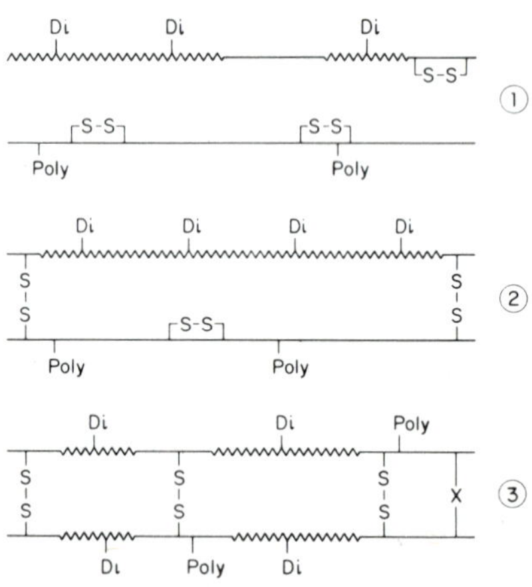

Fig. 4. Representation of three hypothetical models of the glomerular basement membrane showing the possible relationship of the disaccharide (Di) and heteropolysaccharide (Poly) units to each other and the peptide chains. The jagged line represents "collagen-like" portions of the peptide chains while the straight line indicates polar regions. Disulfide bonds are shown and (X) represent possible other crosslinks between the peptide chains.

tic treatment. Moreover, such agents as urea, which might be presumed to breakup a noncovalent union, cause no solubilization of the membranes (Table III). In fact we have found that no separation of two such hypothetical proteins can even be achieved after solubilization of the basement membrane by reduction and alkylation of the disulfide bonds. Model 2 shows two different types of peptide chains, one containing the disaccharide and the other containing the heteropolysaccharide, which are held together by disulfide and possibly other covalent bonds, while model 3 shows the units on the same chains, with alternating regions of collagen-like and polar characteristics. Possibilities 2 and 3 are difficult to distinguish and require the isolation of pure peptide fragments containing both types of units.

Some information about the relationship of the two types of units was obtained by further studying the high molecular weight glycopeptide fraction (Sephadex G-50, peak 1) (Table IV) obtained after collagenase-Pronase digestion of the glomerular basement membrane. This high moleuclar weight material could be further fractionated on agarose gels and shown to consist of three major fractions ranging in moleuclar weight from 1 to 5 million. No separation of the two types of units could be obtained. Both the sugar and amino acid composition of these fractions were similar and they continued to show the presence of both the disaccharide and heteropolysaccharide units. Amino-terminal analyses indicated that these high molecular fragments consist of numerous small peptides which are cross-linked by covalent bonds. When performic acid oxidation of this high molecular weight material (Sephadex G-50, peak 1) was performed in order to split its disulfide bonds, gel filtration of the oxidized material indicated that most of it had been broken into several small molecular weight components which now entered the Sephadex G·50 gel (Fig. 5). The peak which penetrated the gel most deeply (fractions 3 and 4) had as its monosaccharide components only glucose

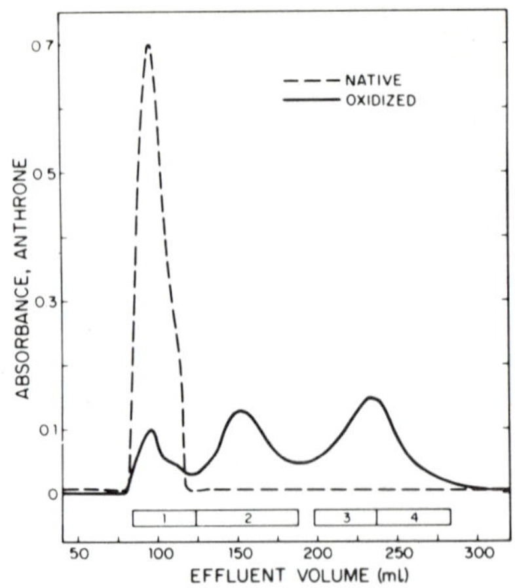

Fig. 5. Gel filtration of Sephadex G-50 of performic acid oxidized (——) high molecular weight glycopeptide fraction (Sephadex G-50, peak 1) from collagenase-Pronase digest of bovine glomerular basement membrane. Position of elution of glycopeptides prior to performic acid treatment is shown (--). Column size was 2.1 x 86 cm. Elution was performed with 0.1 M pyridine acetate buffer, pH 5.0.

and galactose, while the peak which penetrated the gel to a smaller extent (fraction 2) contained primarily the heteropolysaccharide unit. Reduction and alkylation of the high molecular weight fraction (Sephadex G-50, peak 1) followed by gel filtration similarly resulted in a marked decrease in its size. These experiments clearly indicated that disulfide bonds represent important crosslinks in the glomerular basement membrane and that the high molecular weight material obtained after collagenase-Pronase digestion represents a highly crosslinked core which is resistant to complete digestion by the proteolytic enzymes used.

The problem of the relationship of the two carbohydrate units of the basement membrane was also approached in a different manner by digesting the basement membrane with highly purified collagenase alone. When this type of digest was separated by gel filtration on agarose columns, all the fractions contained the sugars of both types of carbohydrate units. Substantial amounts of the disaccharide were found again in the high molecular weight fraction, but of greater interest was the fact that sialic acid-containing glycopeptides (Fig. 6), penetrated deeply into the gel, being

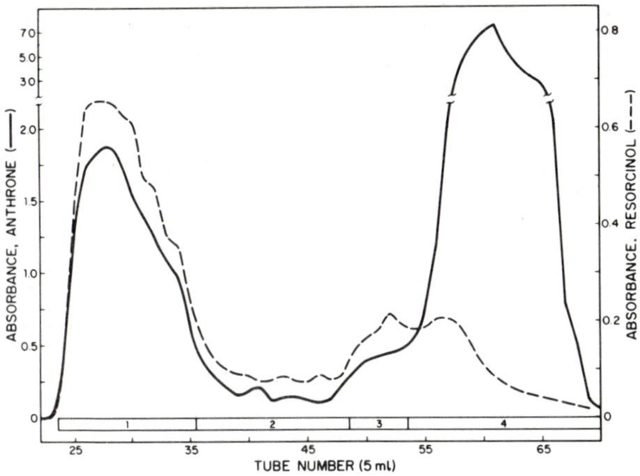

Fig. 6. Gel filtration on Bio-Gel A-0.5 m of collagenase digest of bovine glomerular basement membrane. Elution diagram shows sialic acid by resorcinol method and hexose by anthrone method. Column size was 2.1 x 85 cm. Elution was performed with 0.10 N sodium phosphate buffer at pH 8.0.

found in fractions 3 and 4, and indicating that the heteropolysaccharide unit is present at least to a certain extent in regions which could be extensively split by the very specific enzyme collagenase.

A portrayal of a section of the basement membrane is depicted in Fig. 7. The disaccharide and heteropolysaccharide units have been placed on different regions of the same chains, although they could also occur on separate but covalently linked chains. Disulfide bonds predominate as crosslinks, but other crosslinking agents may also occur. The carbohydrate units constitute bulky hydrophilic substituents on the peptide chains and may affect the spacing of the chains in their vicinity. In a section of the basement membrane containing about 600 amino acids, one would find one heteropolysaccharide, 10 disaccharide units, and approximately 10 disulfide bonds. Upon collagenase and Pronase digestion of this membrane, one obtains small glycopeptides containing either the disaccharide or heteropolysaccharide unit and large molecular weight glycopeptides that contain both units, which consist of many peptide chains crosslinked primarily by disulfide bonds. Those peptides which are crosslinked

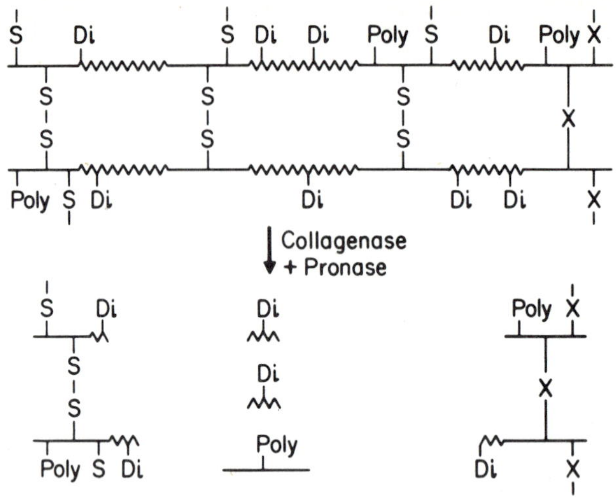

Fig. 7. Schematic representation of the effect of collagenase and Pronase digestion on glomerular basement membrane. A hypothetical segment of the basement membrane is shown with disaccharide (Di) and heteropolysaccharide (Poly) units attached to peptide chains which are crosslinked by disulfide bonds and possible other (X) crosslinking compounds. The jagged lines represent "collagen-like" regions of the peptide chains while the straight lines indicate the more polar regions.

by disulfide bonds can be significantly reduced in size by performic acid oxidation or reduction and alkylation.

It is apparent that the biosynthesis of this membrane is a very complicated process involving beyond the synthesis of the peptide chains, several other steps, including the hydroxylation of lysine and proline, the assembly of both types of carbohydrate units, and the formation of crosslinks.

We have recently studied the enzymes which are responsible for the assembly of the hydroxylysine-linked carbohydrate unit (Spiro and Spiro, 1968c), and found them to consist of a glucosyl- and galactosyltransferase with high degrees of specificity. These enzymes have been isolated from rat kidney cortex, but are also present in other tissues which synthesize basement membranes or collagens containing this hydroxylysine-linked carbohydrate unit.

The glucosyltransferase serves to transfer glucose from UDP-glucose to hydroxylysine-linked galactose, either in high or low molecular weight substrates. Galactose itself, or galactose linked to other sugars or amino acids, will not serve as an acceptor. Collagens, with their large number of galactosylhydroxylysine units are good acceptors for this enzyme. Basement membrane, which has no galactosylhydroxylysine, serves as an acceptor only after selective removal of the glucose. For this enzyme to be active the ε-amino group of the hydroxylysine of the acceptor must be unsubsituted.

The second enzyme is a galactosyltransferase, which functions to transfer galactose from UPD-galactose to hydroxylysine in high molecular weight substrates. It will not transfer galactose to free hydroxylysine or to hydroxylysine in small peptides. Collagens with their large percentage of unsubstituted hydroxylysine residues are good acceptors for this enzyme, while basement membranes, where few hydroxylysine residues remain unsubstitutted, are acceptors only after the disaccharide unit is removed by Smith degradation. This enzyme, like the glucosyltransferase, requires a positive charge on the ε-amino group of the hydroxylysine of the acceptor in order to function.

The various steps involved in the biosynthesis of basement membranes (or collagens) are schematically depicted in Fig. 8. First the peptide is synthesized on the ribosomes presumably by the usual machinery for protein synthesis. Next the hydroxylation of lysine (and proline) residues takes place. In this step 45% of the lysines of the glomerular basement membrane, 79% in the lens capsule, and 21% in skin collagen, are hydroxylated. Subsequently, hydroxylysine becomes the site of attachment of the galactose residues. Approximately 80% of the hydroxylysine residues in basement membranes become glycosylated, while a much smaller percentage become substituted with galactose in fibrillar collagens. The glucosyltransferase then attaches glucose to all of the hydroxylysine-linked galactose residues in the basement membranes to form the α-(1→2)-linked disaccharide. However, 15 to 45% of the galactose residues do not become substituted by glucose in the fibrillar collagens. At the

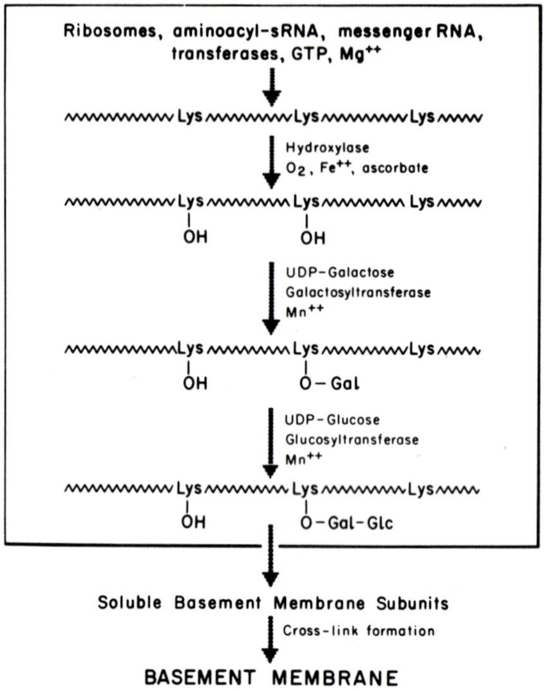

Fig. 8. Schematic representation of steps involved in the synthesis of basement membrane (or collagen). All of the events in the assembly of the membrane are presumed to take place intracellularly except for the establishment of crosslinks to form the insoluble membrane.

same time that the disaccharide unit is being put together, the heteropolysaccharide linked to asparagine is being assembled on another part of the peptide chains through the stepwise action of a series of glycosyltransferases, presumably similar to those which have been described in the thyroid for the synthesis of thyroglobulin (Spiro and Spiro, 1968a,b). The chains with the carbohydrate attached are then presumed to pass to the outside of the cell where crosslinks forming the insoluble membrane or collagen are established.

It is of interest that several steps in the synthesis of these complex moleucles are not directly coded and can therefore be controlled by such forces as enzyme specificity, substrate availability, cofactors, and other environmental variables. These steps could therefore serve as points at which physiological regulation can be imposed, or at which pathological factors may influence the synthesis of these molecules.

ACKNOWLEDGEMENTS

This work was supported by grants AM 05363, AM 10428 and HE 11306 from the National Institutes of Health, Public Health Service.

REFERENCES

Cruickshank, B. and Hill, A.G.S. (1953). J. Pathol. Bacteriol. 66, 283.

Dische, Z. and Borenfreund, E. (1954). Am. J. Ophthalmol. 38, 165.

Dische, A., Zelmenis, G. and Rothschild, C. (1967). Arch. Biochem. Biophys. 121, 685.

Dohlman, C.H. and Balazs, E.A. (1955). Arch. Biochem. Biophys. 45, 445.

Dunn, J.T. and Spiro, R.G. (1967). J. Biol. Chem. 242, 5556.

Farquhar, M.G. (1964). In Small blood involvement in diabetes mellitus. p. 31. Ed. by Siperstein, M.D., Colwell, A.R. Sr., and Meyer, K. American Institute of Biological Sciences,Washington,D.C.

Fukushi, S. and Spiro, R.G. (1969). J. Biol. Chem. 244, 2041.

Kang, A.H., Bornstein, P. and Piez, K.A. (1967). Biochemistry 6, 788.

Kefalides, N.A. (1966). Biochem. Biophys. Res. Commun. 22, 26.

Krakower, C.A. adn Greenspon, S.A. (1951). A.M.A. Arch. Pathol. 51, 629.

Leblond, C.P., Glegg, R.E. and Eidinger, D. (1957). J. Histochem. Cytochem. 5, 455.

Lillie, R.D. (1952). Lab. Investigations 1, 30.

McManus, J.F.A. (1948). Am. J. Pathol. 24, 643.

Pierce, G.B., Jr., Beals, T.F., Sri Ram, J. and Midgley,

A.R., Jr. (1964). Am. J. Pathol. 45, 929.

Piez, K.A. and Gross, J. (1960). J. Biol. Chem. 235, 995.

Pirie, A. (1951). Biochem. J. 48, 368.

Roberts, D. St. C. (1957). Brit. J. Ophthalmol. 41, 338.

Spiro, M.J. and Spiro, R.G. (1968a). J. Biol. Chem. 243, 6520.

Spiro, M.J. and Spiro, R.G. (1968b). J. Biol. Chem. 243, 6529.

Spiro, R.G. (1962a). J. Biol. Chem. 237, 382.

Spiro, R.G. (1962b). J. Biol. Chem. 237, 646.

Spiro, R.G. (1964). J. Biol. Chem. 239, 567.

Spiro, R.G. (1965). J. Biol. Chem. 240, 1603.

Spiro, R.G. (1967a). J. Biol. Chem. 242, 1915.

Spiro, R.G. (1967b). J. Biol. Chem. 242, 1923.

Spiro, R.G. (1967c). J. Biol. Chem. 242, 4813.

Spiro, R.G. (1969a). J. Biol. Chem. 244, 602.

Spiro, R.G. (1969b). This book, p. 195.

Spiro, R.G. and Fukushi, S. (1969). J. Biol. Chem. 244, 2049.

Spiro, R.G. and Spiro, M.J. (1968c). Fed. Proc. 27, 345.

Vernier, R.L. (1961). In Ciba Foundation Symposium on Renal Biopsy. p. 4. Ed. Wolstenholme, G.E.W. and Cameron, M.P., Little Brown and Co., Boston.

COMPARATIVE BIOCHEMISTRY OF MAMMALIAN BASEMENT MEMBRANES

Nicholas A. Kefalides

Basement membranes are extracellular matrices found in numerous tissues of the body. Histologically they appear to be homogeneous, amorphous structures. Morphologic alterations in basement membranes have been observed in a number of diseases, including post-streptococcal glomerulonephritis, nephrotic syndrome, diabetes mellitus, lupus erythematosus and others. It is because of this relationship in disease that a number of investigators began to study the nature of basement membranes.

Basement membranes have been examined from various points of view: a) morphologic, b) compositional, c) structural, d) immunologic and e) functional.

Among the various types of basement membranes, the one isolated from the glomerulus has been studied most extensively, and from chemical studies it appears that it is composed of at least three carbohydrate-rich protein moieties, one a collagen and the others a small molecular weight and a large molecular weight non-collagen glycoproteins. The chemical nature of these components, their structural characteristics and their mode of interaction are aspects which need further study, especially when one considers the existence of basement membranes of different cellular origin and function.

The purpose of this article is to review the available information from our laboratory and others on the chemical composition and structure of isolated basement membranes from representative tissues, to discuss the nature of the collagen component and to present data on the chemistry of the antigenic components of basement membranes. References will also be made to some of their morphologic aspects.

I MORPHOLOGIC ASPECTS

The presence of basement membranes in tissues was recognized as early as 1848, when Todd and Bowman (1857), in a discussion of the histologic appearance of synovial and serous membranes, stated that their epithelium rests "immediately on a continuous basement membrane of excessive tenuity, apparently identical with that which supports the epithelium of mucous membranes." In a description of capillaries, they reported that "in most mucous membranes, the basement membrane is placed between them (the capillaries) and the epithelium."

The electronmicroscope made it possible to study the ultrastructure of basement membranes. I shall refer to only a few of the many excellent studies that have been reported.

Kurtz and McManus (1959), Vernier (1964) and Farquar (1964) studied the ultrastructure of the glomerular basement membrane. These authors support the view that the glomerular basement membrane contains a fine, partially oriented feltwork of fibrils 30-40 Å in diameter associated with an amorphous matrix. The ultrastructure of muscle capillaries has been investigated by Palade and Bruns (1964) and that of skin capillaries by Fawcett (1963), and Friederici, Tucker and Schwartz (1966). The basement membrane of muscle capillaries appears to contain a feltwork of fibrils, about 30-40 Å in diameter, which cross each other at random and are embedded in a matrix of moderate density. The basement membranes of skin capillaries also contain fine filaments embedded in an amorphous matrix but at times they exhibit an additional feature; they may be lamellated or stratified. Karrer (1956) and Weibel (1963) examined the basement membrane of alveolar capillaries. Here, again, similar ultrastructural features are noted.

The ultrastructure of Descemet's membrane and of the anterior lens capsule was studied by Jakus (1964). Unlike other epithelial or endothelial (capillary) basement membranes, Descemet's membrane and the lens capsule exhibit a more fibrillar structure with high degree of orientation. In sections of human, bovine and owl monkey corneas, portions of Descemet's membrane show a regular banding measuring about 1100 Å. It should be pointed out here that, in all normal specimens examined so far, collagen fibrils with their typical 600-700 Å periodic structure have not been demonstrated within the basement membrane proper. Collagen-like fibrils have been observed, however, in the mesangial matrix between the intercapillary cells and the basement membrane of normal rat glomeruli (Latta, 1961), and in a pathological specimen of human anterior lens capsule (Jakus, 1964).

If we examine basement membranes in terms of the type of cell with which they are associated, we could divide them into three categories, as shown in Table I.

TABLE I

Classification of Basement Membranes by Cell-Type Association

Cell type	Examples of tissue
Epithelial	Anterior lens capsule; (Posterior lens capsule has no cellular attachment in the mature animal); Bowman's Capsule; respiratory, intestinal and glandular epithelium. Kidney tubules.
Endothelial	Capillaries of skin, muscle and choroid plexus*. Descemet's membrane of cornea.
Epithelial and Endothelial	Capillaries of glomerulus and alveolar septum.

*Adjacent to the capillary network of the choroid plexus there is an ependymal layer of epithelial cells but its basement membrane is separate and distinct from that of the capillaries.

In the first category are included the basement membranes of the respiratory, intestinal, kidney tubular, and glandular epithelium, the lens capsule and Bowman's capsule. The anterior and posterior lens capsules derive embryologically from ectoderm (McKeehan, 1951), but only the anterior retains its single epithelial cell layer in the mature animal. Bowman's capsule, composed of a layer of epithelial cells and a basement membrane, is separated from the glomerular capillary tuft by the Bowman's space.

The basement membrane of the glomerular capillary tuft is associated with two types of cells, epithelial cells with their foot processes and endothelial cells of the capillary wall. The glomerulus is thought to derive from differentiated mesenchymal tissue (Davies, 1950). A third cell, the mesangial cell, located in the axial region of glomerulus, is in contact with basement membrane material. The mesangial cell is also thought to be of mesenchymal origin (Suzuki, 1959). In the alveolar septa, the basement membrane forms, for the most part, a continuous layer. It is in contact with the epithelial cells at its outer surface and with the capillary endothelial cells at its inner surface. At intervals, an intermembranous space is formed, resulting in the separation of the basement membrane into an epithelial and an endothelial component.

The basement membranes of capillaries of skin, muscle and choroid plexus are associated with cells of mesenchymal origin--the endothelial cell and the pericapillary cell or pericyte. Adjacent to the capillaries of the choroid plexus there is an ependymal layer of epithelial cells with their own basement membrane which is separated from that of the capillaries by loose connective tissue. Descemet's membrane overlies a single layer of endothelial cells at the inner surface of the cornea (Jakus, 1964).

II THE CHEMISTRY OF BASEMENT MEMBRANES

A. SOLUBILITY PROPERTIES

Isolated basement membranes are insoluble in water.

Basement membranes associated with capillaries are relatively insoluble in weak acids and alkalis at 4°C (Kefalides and Winzler, 1966). Descemet's membrane is likewise insoluble in weak solutions of HCl or Na OH (Dohlman and Balazs, 1955). Glomerular basement membrane can be solubilized with 60% trichloroacetic acid at 25°C for 6 hr (Krakower, Greenspon and Warren, 1957). Extraction with 5% trichloroacetic acid at 90°C for 45 min results in the separation of the collagenous component of basement membranes. This procedure leads to denaturation of the collagen (Kefalides, 1966). Five per cent trichloroacetic acid at 90°C will dissolve Descemet's membrane in a few hours (Dohlman and Balazs, 1955). The solubility of certain basement membranes in a number of solvents appears in Table II. Solubilization of over 60% of glomerular basement membrane and anterior lens capsule, and 22% of Descemet's membrane has been accomplished in our laboratory by reduction and alkylation of disulfide bonds in 8 M urea (Kefalides and Winzler, 1966, and unpublished data). This procedure does not alter the antigenicity of the basement membranes. About 30-35% of bovine or dog anterior lens capsules can be solubilized by extracting with 0.3 M acetic acid to 4°C for 72 hr. Similarly, 8 M urea in 1 M Tris-HCl buffer, pH 8.4, at 40°C will solubilize 30% of anterior lens capsule.

TABLE II

Solubility Properties of Basement Membranes

(Per cent dry weight)

Solvent	GM	ALC	DM
0.3 M Acetic acid (4°C, 48 hr)	1	32	1.4
8 M Urea, pH 7.2 (40°C, 48 hr)	35	33	15%
ME*, IAA+, pH 8.4 (40°C, 24 hr)‡	60	60	22
0.1 M CaAcetate, pH 7.2 (20°C, 24 hr)	0.5	0.5	0.5
0.5 M NaCl, 0.05 $PO_4^{=}$, pH 7 (4°C, 48 hr)	<0.5	<0.5	<0.5

*ME=mercaptoethanol; +IAA=iodoacetamide, ‡in 8 M urea.

It appears, therefore, that glomerular basement membrane and Descemet's membrane differ structurally from the basement membrane of lens capsule since about one-third of the latter is soluble in 0.3 m acetic acid, whereas practically none of the former are soluble in the same solvent.

Variable amounts of basement membrane can be solubilized by proteolytic enzymes, including collagenase, depending on temperature and length of incubation (Kefalides, 1968a, 1969b; Spiro, 1967b). When we treated glomerular basement membrane with collagenase for 48 hr at 37°C, 90% of the hydroxyproline, 87% of the hexose and 90% of the hexosamine were found in the soluble fraction. When anterior lens capsule was treated similarly, 97% of the hydroxyproline, 88% of the hexose and 88% of the hexosamine were found in the soluble fraction (unpublished data).

B. COMPOSITIONAL STUDIES

1. Amino Acid Composition

Early studies by Goodman, Greenspon and Krakower (1955) demonstrated the presence of significant amounts of hydroxyproline and carbohydrate in canine glomerular basement membrane. The authors concluded that collagen must be one of the components in this substance. Pirie (1951) analyzed bovine lens capsule and found 10% hexose, 1% hexosamine and significant amounts of hydroxyproline, proline and glycine. Later, Dische and Borenfreund (1954) reported that glucose and galactose were the main carbohydrate components of anterior and posterior lens capsule with a ratio of 3:4. Hexosamine was found in trace amounts and there was no hexuronic acid or fucose. However, upon reexamination of bovine lens capsule by Dische, Zelenis and Rothschild (1967) and of rabbit lens capsule by Dische (1964) the presence of hexuronic acid, hexosamine, mannose, fucose and sialic acid was demonstrated. Quantitative determinations of the amino acid and carbohydrate content of bovine lens capsule were reported by Kefalides (1969a). These studies show that glycine makes up 27.5%, hydroxyproline 7.5%, proline 6.8% and hydroxylysine 3.5% of all the amino acid residues. Half-cystine accounts for 2.8% of the amino acid residues. There is 5.1% glucose, 5.4% galactose, trace of mannose, 1.0% hexosamine, 0.62% fucose and 0.5% sialic acid by weight. The composition of calf and cow anterior and posterior lens capsule was reported recently by Spiro (1969).

The amino acid and carbohydrate composition of glomerular basement membrane has been established by a number of investigators in various species. Markowitz and Lange (1964) and Lazarow and Speidel (1964) studied human, Kefalides and Winzler (1966) canine, and Spiro (1967a) bovine glomerular basement membranes.

Descemet's membrane was examined by Dohlman and Balazs (1955). They reported the presence of 9.8% hydroxyproline, 11-13% reducing sugar and 2% hexosamine. Glucose, galactose, mannose and fucose were identified by paper chromatography.

In all these studies it appears that there is considerable similarity in terms of amino acid and carbohydrate composition among basement membranes from various tissues and species.

Since the presence of collagen in basement membrane has been suggested by the presence of significant amounts of hydroxyproline, it will be necessary to mention the physicochemical criteria which define collagen. According to Ramachandran, Sasisekharan and Thathachari (1962), a protein is defined as collagen when glycine accounts for about 33% of the amino acid residues and the sum of proline and hydroxyproline for about 22%. Furthermore, the protein must exhibit a triple helical structure in which three polypeptide chains are aggregated to form a molecule.

The various studies on glomerular basement membrane showed that the content of glycine and the sum of hydroxyproline plus proline are much lower than that found in connective tissue collagen. This led to the assumption (Kefalides and Winzler, 1966) that in addition to collagen, other protein components, non-collagen in nature, must be present. This assumption is further supported by the presence of significant amounts of mannose, hexosamine, sialic acid and fucose, carbohydrates which are not present in soluble collagens.

Since basement membranes are secreted by cells differing in their embryologic origin and are found in tissues which perform different functions, we felt it sould be of interest to compare their chemical and immunologic properties.

Lens capsule offered an excellent example of epithelial basement membrane, while Descemet's membrane represented a membrane derived from mesenchymal cells--both found in non-vascular tissue. Alveolar basement membrane, choroid plexus and glomerular basement membrane represented membranes of mesenchymal cell origin--all associated with capillaries. Soluble collagen was prepared from canine tendon and analyzed for comparison. With these preparations, we set out to answer a number of questions regarding the nature of basement membranes: a) are they all alike in terms of amino acid and carbohydrate compositions? b) what is the nature of their macromolecular components and how are they related to connective tissue collagen? c) what are some of their structural characteristics? d) are they related immunologically? e) can we correlate the available chemical and structural data with their possible function?

Table III summarizes the amino acid composition of glomerular basement membranes from human, canine, bovine and rat kidneys. It can be seen that there are many similarities and few differences among the glomerular basement membranes from various species. They are characterized by a high content of hydroxylysine which accounts for 2.5% of all the amino acid residues. The hydroxylysine content of glomerular basement membrane is four times higher than that of tendon collagen (Kefalides, 1968a). Glycine accounts for about 23% of the amino acid residues compared with 33% in tendon collagen. The sum of hydroxyproline plus proline is lower than that of tendon collagen, 12.9% and 13.4% respectively, for the human and canine basement membranes compared with 22.6% for tendon collagen. Basic amino acids account for about 9.1%, while acidic amino acids account for 17% of all amino acid residues. The alanine content is about 50% lower than that in skin or tendon collagen. Phenylalanine on the other hand accounts for almost 2.9% of the amino acid residues which is twice the amount found in tendon collagen.

TABLE III

Amino Acid Composition of Glomerular Basement Membranes*
(Residues/1000 residues)

Amino Acid	Human	Canine+	Ovine	Rat
Hydroxylysine	24.5	25.0	22.5	21.8
Lysine	26.4	26.0	27.0	40.0
Histidine	18.7	14.4	18.5	21.0
Arginine	48.3	48.2	50.5	52.6
3-Hydroxyproline	12.0	8.5	7.0	7.0
4-Hydroxyproline	53.0	56.5	56.0	50.0
Aspartic	70.0	70.0	72.0	70.0
Threonine	40.3	40.5	41.5	45.5
Serine	54.2	49.0	54.5	62.8
Glutamic	101.3	97.0	98.0	100.0
Proline	64.1	69.8	66.0	62.0
Glycine	225.2	229.0	220.0	200.0
Alanine	58.6	65.0	60.0	67.0
Half-Cystine	22.0	22.7	20.0	20.4
Valine	36.0	36.0	38.0	43.0
Methionine	7.0	5.0	7.5	11.0
Isoleucine	28.6	28.1	29.5	30.0
Leucine	60.3	60.2	59.0	60.0
Tyrosine	20.5	22.0	23.0	17.0
Phenylaline	28.3	26.8	28.0	19.0

*Kefalides, unpublished data

+Kefalides, 1968a

Table IV shows the amino acid composition of the anterior lens capsule from various species. Embryologically, lens capsule derives from ectodermal tissue and in the adult animals, the anterior portion is associated with only one layer of epithelial cells, while no cells are attached to the posterior capsule.

The characteristic feature of the various anterior lens capsules is the presence of large amounts of hydroxylysine. The hydroxylysine content varies from 32 residues per 1000 residues in the dog to 39 residues in the sheep. The hydroxyproline content is also high and ranges between 99.5 in canine and 123 in ovine lens capsule.

Since the hydroxylysine and hydroxyproline content

TABLE IV

Amino Acid Composition of Anterior Lens Capsule

(Residues/1000 residues)

Amino Acid	Human*	Canine[+]	Bovine[+]	Ovine[‡]
Hydroxylysine	34.5	32.0	35.0	39.0
Lysine	19.4	11.0	13.2	12.3
Histidine	15.2	12.0	10.2	11.6
Arginine	39.5	38.3	43.0	37.0
3-Hydroxyproline	21.3	19.5	15.0	19.0
4-Hydroxyproline	85.0	80.0	85.0	104.0
Aspartic	57.0	57.8	55.0	55.0
Threonine	31.0	31.0	29.0	29.0
Serine	43.4	48.0	42.0	44.0
Glutamic	94.4	95.0	92.5	92.0
Proline	67.3	66.0	68.0	68.8
Glycine	260.0	288.0	275.0	266.0
Alanine	40.6	46.0	42.8	44.7
Half-Cystine	21.0	18.0	28.0	12.0
Valine	33.2	35.0	30.0	30.0
Methionine	5.0	6.2	8.0	5.0
Isoleucine	32.0	30.0	28.8	26.0
Leucine	57.7	56.5	58.0	62.0
Tyrosine	13.0	11.0	10.0	11.0
Phenylalanine	29.8	29.0	32.0	28.0

*Kefalides, unpublished data

[+]Kefalides, 1969a

[‡]Kefalides and Denduchis, 1969

reflect the amount of collagen present in a tissue component, then we must conclude that the proportion of collagen in lens capsule is higher than that in glomerular basement membrane; the remainder of the protein content must be contributed by non-collagen polypeptides.

The amino acid composition of canine and ovine Descemet's membrane are shown in Table V. Descemet's membrane derives embryologically from mesenchymal tissue and represents an avascular basement membrane. The amino acid composition of canine and ovine Descemet's membranes is very similar. It is interesting to note that in terms of the amino acid composition Descemet's membrane resembles more glomerular basement membrane than lens capsule.

TABLE V

Amino Acid Composition of Descemet's Membrane

(Residues/1000 residues)

Amino Acid	Canine*	Ovine+
Hydroxylysine	20.0	19.0
Lysine	24.0	24.8
Histidine	11.6	12.0
Arginine	39.5	40.0
3-Hydroxyproline	6.8	7.0
4-Hydroxyproline	77.0	78.0
Aspartic	58.0	60.0
Threonine	36.4	35.0
Serine	42.0	41.0
Glutamic	94.0	95.0
Proline	95.0	90.0
Glycine	230.0	224.0
Alanine	53.0	53.5
Half-Cystine	11.0	10.0
Valine	45.0	50.0
Methionine	8.2	8.0
Isoleucine	28.5	30.0
Leucine	75.2	77.0
Tyrosine	21.0	20.0
Phenylalanine	25.0	26.0

*Kefalides, unpublished data

+Kefalides and Denduchis, 1969

What is surprising, however, is the high proline content. There is 50% more proline in Descemet's membrane than in either lens capsule or glomerular basement membrane. This high value is maintained even in the isolated collagen component.

These data imply that lens capsule and Descemet's membrane which embryologically derive from different cell lines are also distinct biochemically.

The amino acid composition of choroid plexus and alveolar basement membranes appears in Table VI.

It will be seen that both choroid plexus and alveolar basement membrane contain amounts of hydroxylysine and hydroxyproline which are lower while the content of proline and glycine is very

TABLE VI

Amino Acid Composition Choroid Plexus and Alveolar Basement Membrane

(Residues/1000 residues)

Amino Acid	Canine*		Ovine+
	ABM[a]	CP[b]	CP
Hydroxylysine	6.8	9.0	8.0
Lysine	41.5	41.0	49.3
Histidine	12.6	16.0	15.4
Arginine	50.0	61.0	58.4
3-Hydroxyproline	Trace	Trace	Trace
4-Hydroxyproline	35.0	48.3	54.0
Aspartic	68.6	68.0	73.0
Threonine	38.8	39.0	38.0
Serine	57.7	52.0	53.0
Glutamic	78.0	94.0	100.0
Proline	77.0	69.0	69.0
Glycine	222.6	235.6	236.0
Alanine	97.8	104.5	100.0
Half-Cystine	12.0	10.0	9.0
Valine	57.7	37.0	45.5
Methionine	4.6	9.4	5.0
Isoleucine	32.4	22.5	28.0
Leucine	67.0	50.0	60.0
Tyrosine	10.4	12.0	13.7
Phenylalanine	29.3	21.5	22.8

[a]Alveolar basement Membrane

[b]Choroid plexus

*Kefalides and Denduchis, 1969

+Kefalides, unpublished data

similar to that found in other membranes. On the basis of amino acid composition, therefore, vascular basement membranes differ among themselves and from avascular basement membranes whether of epithelial or mesenchymal origin.

2. Carbohydrate Composition

The carbohydrate composition of the various basement membranes appears in Table VII. The same sugars are present in all basement membranes. However, significant differences are noted among them not only in terms of

TABLE VII

Carbohydrate Composition of Basement Membranes

(g/100g)

Carbohydrate	Human* GM[a]	Human* ALC[b]	Canine[+] GM[‡]	Canine[+] ALC	Canine[+] DM[c]	Canine[+] AL[d]	Canine[+] CP[e]
Hexose	6.8	11.8	7.0	10.5	8.2	4.8	4.0
Glucose	2.5	5.5	2.4	5.0	3.5	1.8	1.4
Galactose	2.6	5.6	2.5	5.1	3.7	2.0	1.85
Mannose	1.7	0.7	2.1	0.4	2.0	1.0	0.75
Glucosamine	1.7	0.8	1.2	0.85	1.2	0.7	1.1
Galactosamine	0.3	0.2	0.3	0.15	0.3	0.2	0.5
Fucose	0.7	0.6	0.75	0.6	0.6	0.2	0.2
Sialic acid	1.5	0.5	2.0	0.4	0.7	0.8	1.5
Uronic acid	-	-	-	0.4	0.5	-	-

[a]Glomerular, [b]Anterior lens capsule, [c]Descemet's membrane
[d]Alveolar, [e]Choroid Plexus
*Kefalides, unpublished data
+Kefalides and Denduchis, 1969
‡Kefalides, 1968a

total carbohydrate but also in the relative amounts of the individual sugars. Neutral hexose is higher in anterior lens capsule compared to Descemet's membrane (10.5% compared with 8.2%). Descemet's membrane contains twice as much hexose as does choroid plexus basement membrane. Glomerular basement membrane contains one third more hexose than does alveolar basement membrane. The ratio of glucose to galactose varies slightly from 1 in all basement membranes. Both glucosamine and galactosamine are present. Glucosamine accounts for about 80% of the total hexosamine content. Fucose does not vary significantly among basement membranes from lens capsule, Descemet's membrane and glomerulus; however, the choroid plexus contains about one third the amount found in the above basement membranes. Significant variability was noted in the sialic acid content of the various basement membranes. Uronic acid was determined in both anterior lens capsule and Descemet's membrane and was found to be 0.4% and 0.5% respectively.

C. CHARACTERIZATION OF BASEMENT MEMBRANE COLLAGEN

One of our major tasks in the study of basement membranes was to isolate and characterize the collagen component. It was not only enough to know its composition but we had to learn certain of its physical properties. Since extraction with hot 5% trichloroacetic acid produced a collagen material which was unsuitable for physical characterization (Kefalides, 1966), we resorted to the use of proteolytic digestion at very low temperatures. Davison, Bumps and Schmitt (1966), had demonstrated that pronase at 20°C for 12 hr acted upon soluble skin tropocollagen by cleaving peptide appendages with an amino acid composition unlike that of collagen. Furthermore, under the same conditions, pronase solubilized insoluble skin collagen. An important observation in this study was that treatment with Pronase did not alter the physical properties of the collagen. We modified this method and adapted it for the solubilization of basement membrane collagen (Kefalides, 1968a).

Glomerular basement membrane, Descemet's membrane, anterior lens capsule and basement membrane from the alveolus and choroid plexus were treated in a similar manner.

Limited digestion with pronase at 4°C and at pH 7.2 results in the solubilization of variable amounts of basement membrane depending upon its source (Kefalides and Denduchis, 1969). Dialysis of the solubilized portion against 0.05% acetic acid at pH 3.7 results either in a precipitate and a soluble fraction, only a soluble fraction, or only a precipitate in the dialysis bag. From the fraction which remains soluble at pH 3.7 a collagen can be precipitated with 15% KCl. The fraction which is soluble at pH 7.2 but precipitates at pH 3.7 is designated Precipitate-A in Table VIII. Precipitate-B is obtained upon addition of 15% KCl to the fraction which remains soluble at both pHs. Glomerular basement membrane and Descemet's membrane yield both Precipitate-A and -B, anterior lens capsule only Precipitate-B and alveolar and choroid plexus

TABLE VIII

Amino Acid Composition of Fractions Obtained from Basement Membranes after Treatment with Pronase at 4°C for 24 hr*

Amino Acid	ALC[c]	DM[c]		GM[c+]		AL[c]
	Ppt. B[a]	Ppt. A[b]	Ppt. B[a]	Ppt. A[b]	Ppt. B[a]	Ppt. A[b]
HO-Lysine	41.0	37.6	40.0	36.6	42.0	18.0
Lysine	11.0	28.0	15.0	25.0	7.0	25.3
Histidine	9.0	16.5	7.0	16.0	9.2	12.1
Arginine	33.8	34.0	29.8	47.0	27.0	44.3
3-HO-Prol.	23.0	8.0	6.0	16.7	18.0	Trace
4-HO-Prol.	118.7	81.0	135.7	83.1	134.0	77.0
Aspartic	51.6	61.0	41.1	65.8	52.0	69.0
Threonine	23.0	43.0	21.3	37.2	23.1	35.3
Serine	38.0	47.0	31.4	50.0	42.8	49.6
Glutamic	80.0	86.0	83.5	86.3	79.0	86.5
Proline	65.5	85.0	88.0	65.6	62.0	80.0
Glycine	313.0	220.0	310.0	236.0	322.4	284.0
Alanine	32.0	50.0	36.0	50.4	33.4	80.0
Half-Cystine	9.3	18.0	4.3	31.3	6.0	28.5
Valine	24.0	45.0	31.0	38.4	27.0	21.1
Methionine	9.4	7.0	7.1	7.0	7.6	5.0
Isoleucine	26.1	31.0	27.9	28.0	27.3	18.5
Leucine	58.0	65.0	57.9	54.2	51.0	39.0
Tyrosine	6.3	12.0	5.5	13.9	4.0	9.0
Phenylal.	27.7	25.0	22.3	27.9	25.2	16.3

[a]Fraction which is soluble at pH 3.7 and 7.2 and precipitates with 15% KCl. [b]Fraction which remains insoluble at pH 3.7, but soluble at pH 7.2. [c]For explanation see Table VII.

*Kefalides and Denduchis, 1969 +Kefalides, 1968a

basement membranes only Precipitate-A. Both Precipitate-A and -B contain significant amounts of hydroxylysine, hydroxyproline and glycine but only Precipitate-B meets the chemical and physical criteria for collagen (Kefalides, 1968a).

1. Amino Acid Composition

When we examine the fraction designated Precipitate-B which is the basement membrane collagen, we note that glycine makes up about one-third of the amino acid residues, while the sum of proline plus hydroxyproline accounts for about 20% of the amino acids. The hydroxylysine content is high and makes up about 4% of the amino acid residues. The high content of hydroxylysine is a unique characteristic of the collagens from basement membranes regardless of the source. The large amount of hydroxylysine is also reflected in the high amounts of glucose and galactose which are linked to hydroxylysine as a disaccharide, glucosyl-galactose and a monosaccharide, galactose (Spiro, 1967b, Kefalides, 1969a). The lysine content is proportionately low and the sum of lysine plus hydroxylysine accounts for 5% of the total amino acid content. The proline content is similar in the collagen from the glomerular basement membrane and lens capsule but is higher in the collagen from Descemet's membrane and reflects the high amount found in the intact membrane (Table V). Half-cystine is present in all and varies from 4.3 residues per 1000 residues in the collagen from Descemet's membrane to 9.3 residues in the collagen from anterior lens capsule. Another feature which distinguishes basement membrane collagen from tendon collagen is the low alanine content (33 residues per 1000 vs. 112). The phenylaline content is twice that found in tendon collagen while the tyrosine content does not differ significantly.

The fraction which precipitates in 0.05% acetic acid (Precipitate-A, Table VIII) appears to be a mixture of at least two protein moieties. Although it contains significant amounts of hydroxylysine, hydroxyproline and glycine, their content is much lower than that in Precipitate-B.

There are greater similarities in the amino acid composition between Precipitate-A from Descemet's membrane and glomerulus than between these two tissues and alveolus.

2. Carbohydrate Composition

The carbohydrate composition of the collagen (Precipitate-B) from three basement membranes appears in Table IX. Striking similarities are present in the hexose content which accounts for about 10% of dry weight. Glucose and galactose exist in almost equimolar amounts and account for all the hexose. No other sugars are present. Precipitate-B from lens capsule contains about 0.2% hexosamine. Except for vitreous, the collagen isolated from the citreous humor of the eye (Gross, Maltoltsy and Cohen, 1955), no other mammalian collagen has such high hexose content.

TABLE IX

Carbohydrate Composition of Fractions Obtained from Basement Membranes after Treatment with Pronase at 4°C for 24 hr*

(g/100 g)

Carbohydrate	ALC[c]	DM[c]		GM[c+]		AL[c]
	Ppt. B	Ppt. A	Ppt. B	Ppt. A	Ppt. B	Ppt. A
Hexose[a]	10.4	11.5	10.0	9.4	10.4	9.3
Glucose	5.0	3.5	5.0	3.2	5.1	2.2
Galactose	5.2	6.0	5.2	3.4	5.25	2.2
Mannose[b]	Trace	2.0	0.0	2.8	0.00	1.6
Glucosamine	0.2	6.4	Trace	2.2	Trace	1.0
Galactosamine	0.0	1.6	0.0	0.4	0.0	0.4
Fucose	0.0	0.2	0.0	0.1	0.0	0.2
Sialic Acid	0.0	1.5	0.0	3.0	0.0	2.3

[a]Corrected for contribution of fucose

[b]Value obtained by difference between total hexose and the sum of glucose and galactose

[c]For explanation see Table VII

*Kefalides and Denduchis, 1969

+Kefalides, 1968a

The carbohydrate composition of Precipitate-A (Table IX) from three basement membranes differs qualitatively and quantitatively from Precipitate-B. In addition to glucose and galactose, mannose hexosamine, fucose and sialic acid are present. Furthermore, differences are noted in the total hexose content and the relative amounts of the various sugars of Precipitate-A among the three types of basement membranes. The hexosamine content of this fraction from Decemet's membrane is three to five times higher than that from the other two sources. The sialic acid content varies from 1.5% to 3%.

It would appear from these data that in basement membranes in addition to collagen there are polypeptides with an amino acid and carbohydrate composition unlike that of the collagen. Furthermore, a portion of the collagen is linked to these polypeptides in such a manner that it is not rendered soluble in acetic acid after limited digestion with pronase, while a portion becomes soluble. It is also apparent that the proportion of the acid soluble collagen varies from one basement membrane to another; for example, all the collagen in anterior lens capsule is rendered acid soluble after limited digestion with pronase or pepsin, while only about 16% becomes soluble in glomerular basement membrane and Descemet's membrane and none appears to become soluble in basement membranes from alveolus or choroid plexus.

3. Physical Characteristics

The physical characteristics of the collagen (Precipitate-B) isolated from various basement membranes are given in Table X. The specific optical rotation $[\alpha]_D^{24}$ of the collagen from three types of basement membranes is -360°. The intrinsic viscosity of these collagens is lower than that observed with pronase-treated calfskin tropocollagen (Davison and Drake, 1966). The collagen from glomerular basement membrane has an intrinsic viscosity of 5.2 dl/g; the value for Descemet's membrane collagen is 5.4 dl/g, and the value for anterior lens capsule collagen 5.4 dl/g. However, digestion with pronase for only 10 hr at 4°C or with pepsin for 16 hr at 4°C yields collagens with intrinsic viscosities of 10 and 13 dl/g respectively. These data indicate that digestion with pronase for 24 hr results in

TABLE X

Physical Properties of Basement Membrane Collagens*

	GM[+]	ALC	DM
Specific optical rotation (deg) $[\alpha]_D^{24}$	-360	-360	-360
Intrinsic viscosity, $[\eta]$ (dl/g)	5.2	5.4(10)[a] (13.2)[b]	5.4
Sedimentation coefficient, $S^{\circ}_{20,w}$	4.0	4.2	4.1
Diffusion coefficient, $D_{20,w}$	1.35	1.28	-----
Molecular weight S-V	268,000	279,000	279,000
S-D	250,000	274,000	-----
Molar ellipticity, $[\theta](10^{-4}$ (deg cm^2)/dmole)	+0.46(+0.475)[c] -3.4(-3.7)[c]	-----	-----

[a]Intrinsic viscosity after digestion with pronase for 10 hr

[b]Digestion with pepsin in 0.01 N HCl, pH 2, for 16 hr yields a fraction with an intrinsic viscosity of 13.2.

[c]Values in parentheses are for native calfskin tropocollagen

*Kefalides and Denduchis, 1969

[+]Kefalides, 1968a

cleavage of the molecular proper.

The sedimentation coefficient, $S_{20,w}$, determined at 4°C is 4.0 S for glomerular basement membrane collagen. The value obtained for anterior lens capsule collagen is 4.2 S, and the value for Descemet's membrane collagen is 4.1 S. These are values for the collagens obtained after 24 hr digestion.

Circular dichroism studies of basement membrane collagen gave molar ellipticity values similar to those obtained with native calfskin tropocollagen (Table X). The spectra for the two collagens appear in Fig. 1. There is a positive band at 223 mμ with an amplitude of 0.46 x 10^{-4} (deg cm^2)/dmole for basement membrane collagen and 0.475 x 10^{-4} (deg cm^2)/dmole for calfskin tropocollagen. A negative band forms at 198 mμ with an ellipticity value of 3.4 x 10^{-4} (deg cm^2)/dmole for basement membrane col-

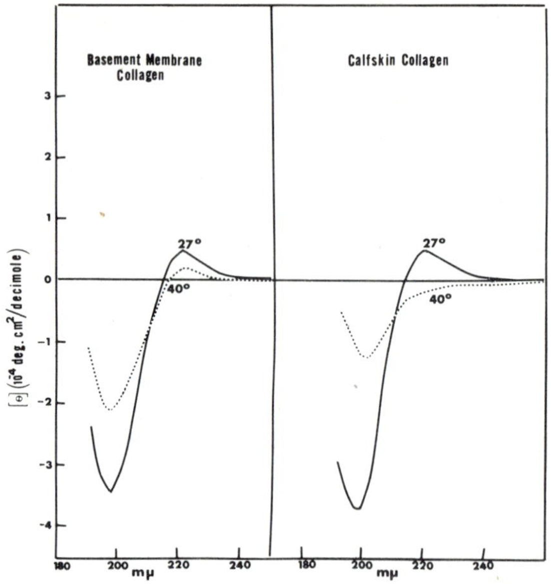

Fig. 1. Circular dichroism of basement membrane collagen and calfskin tropocollagen. Basement membrane collagen: 0.00133 g/ml of 0.05% acetic acid. Calfskin tropocollagen: 0.002 g/ml of 0.05% acetic acid. Temperature 27°C. Continuous line before heat denaturation; broken line after heat denaturation at 40°C for 10 min.

lagen and 3.7 x 10^{-4} (deg cm^2)/dmole for calfskin tropocollagen. The circular dichroism spectra of the two collagens reported here are almost identical with that for calfskin collagen reported by Timasheff, Susi, Townsend, Stevens, Gorbunoff and Kumosinski (1967). On conversion of the native collagen structure to random coil by heating at 40°C for 10 min (Fig. 1) the positive Cotton effect disappears in the case of the calfskin tropocollagen but it is reduced only by 50% in the case of the basement membrane collagen. Similarly, the negative Cotton effect is reduced by 70% in the case of calf skin tropocollagen and only by 20% in the case of the basement membrane collagen. These data indicated that the origin of the positive and negative Cotton effects is largely conformation-dependent and that the collagen from basement membrane exhibits a higher degree of conformational stability under the experimental conditions.

The molecular weight determinations for the collagens from various basement membranes are based on material with low intrinsic viscosity. From the values for molecular weight the contribution of hexose (10-12% by weight) must be subtracted if comparison with skin tropocollagen is to be made. When this is done, the molecular weight approaches 240,000 and corresponds roughly to 80% of the weight of skin tropocollagen.

4. Acrylamide Electrophoresis

The electrophoretic pattern of basement membrane collagen from the glomerulus, lens capsule and Descemet's membrane appears in Fig. 2. It separates into three fast components, two components with intermediate mobility and one with the least mobility. All bands stain for protein and carbohydrate. The similarities among the collagens from three different sources is evident.

5. Reconstitution of Collagen

The collagen from glomerular basement membrane was dissolved in 0.05% acetic acid and examined in the electronmicroscope after negative staining with phosphotungstic acid. Only a filamentous structure could be observed. Addition of ATP to basement membrane collagen resulted in the formation of SLS-type aggregates with periodic structure (Fig. 3). Certain fibers measure about 1660 Å while most measure 3250 Å. The latter appear to be aggregates of the 1660 Å fibers (Kefalides, 1968a).

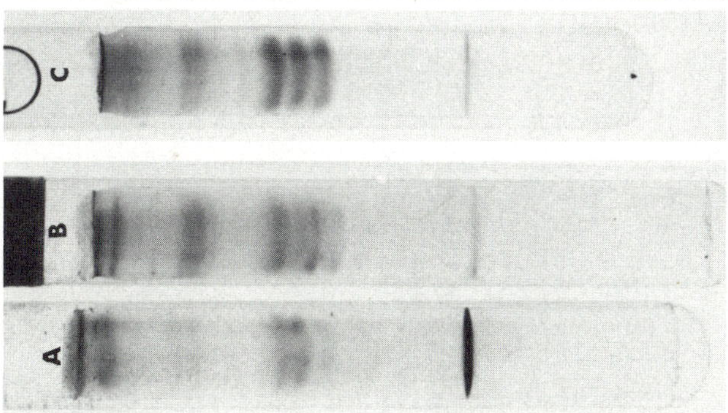

Fig. 2. Disc electrophoresis of basement membrane collagen, 0.04m acetic acid - 0.23 m glycine buffer (pH 4.0). A from Descemet's membrane; B from lens capsule; C from glomerulus (from Kefalides and Denduchis, 1969).

D. NATURE OF THE CARBOHYDRATE UNITS

The structure and linkage of the carbohydrate units of skin collagen and basement membranes have been investigated in several laboratories. Butler and Cunningham (1966) and later Cunningham and Ford (1968) showed that in guinea pig skin collagen the neutral hexose units are composed of the disaccharide, glucosyl-galactose and the monosaccharide, galactose, linked by an o-glycosidic bond to hydroxylysine. Spiro (1967c) isolated the disaccharide from bovine glomerular basement membrane and determined its sequence and linkage. The disaccharide unit has the following structure: 2-o-α-D-glucopyranosyl-o-β-D-galactopyranosyl-hydroxylysine. In our laboratory we have isolated both the disaccharide and monosaccharide units from canine, rat and human glomerular basement membrane, from bovine and canine anterior lens capsule and sheep choroid plexus (Kefalides, 1967, 1968b, 1969). Both neutral hexose units are linked to hydroxylysine of the collagen component of basement membrane. The predominant moiety is the disaccharide and accounts for about 95% of all the hexose (Table XI). Recently we characterized the carbohydrate units in Descemet's membrane. The glycopeptides were prepared by a modification of the alkaline hydrolysis method of Butler and Cunningham (1966). After hydrolysis of the Descemet's membrane, the hydrolysate was neutralized with hydrochloric acid and passed through Dowex-50 H^+. Elution was accomplished with NH_4OH. The eluate was passed through a column of Sephadex G-10 and the hexose was measured in all fractions. The glycopeptides emerged in a symmetrical hexose-containing peak (Fig. 4). Aliquots from the fractions con-

Fig. 3. SLS-type aggregates of glomerular basement membrane collagen precipitated with 1% ATP. Negative staining with phosphotungstic acid. (Electronmicrograph, X45,000) (From Kefalides, 1968a).

Fig. 5. High voltage electrophoresis of fractions from hexose-containing peak following Sephadex G-10 filtration (See Fig. 4). Aliquot from tube 51 was hydrolyzed with 2 N HCl, at 100°C for 2 hr. Solvent, pyridine:acetic acid: water (1:10:289, v/v), pH 3.7. Ly = Lysine; HOLy = Hydrolysine.

3

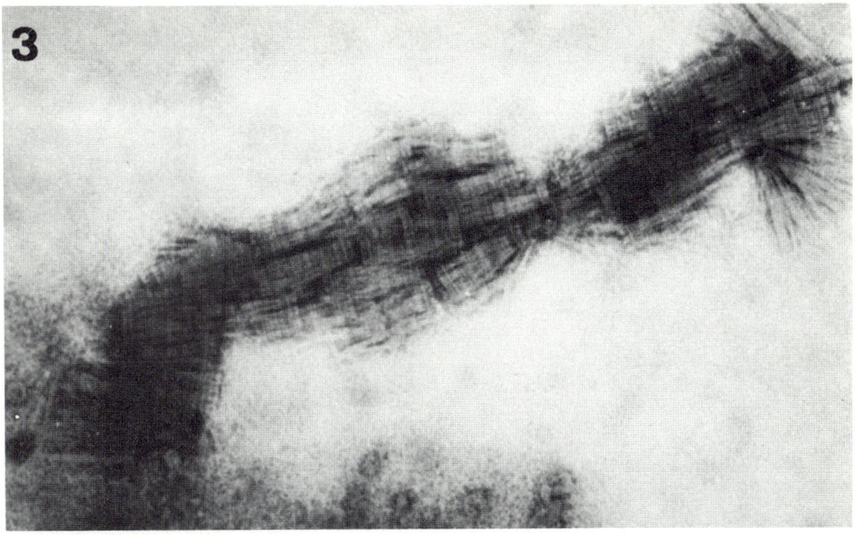

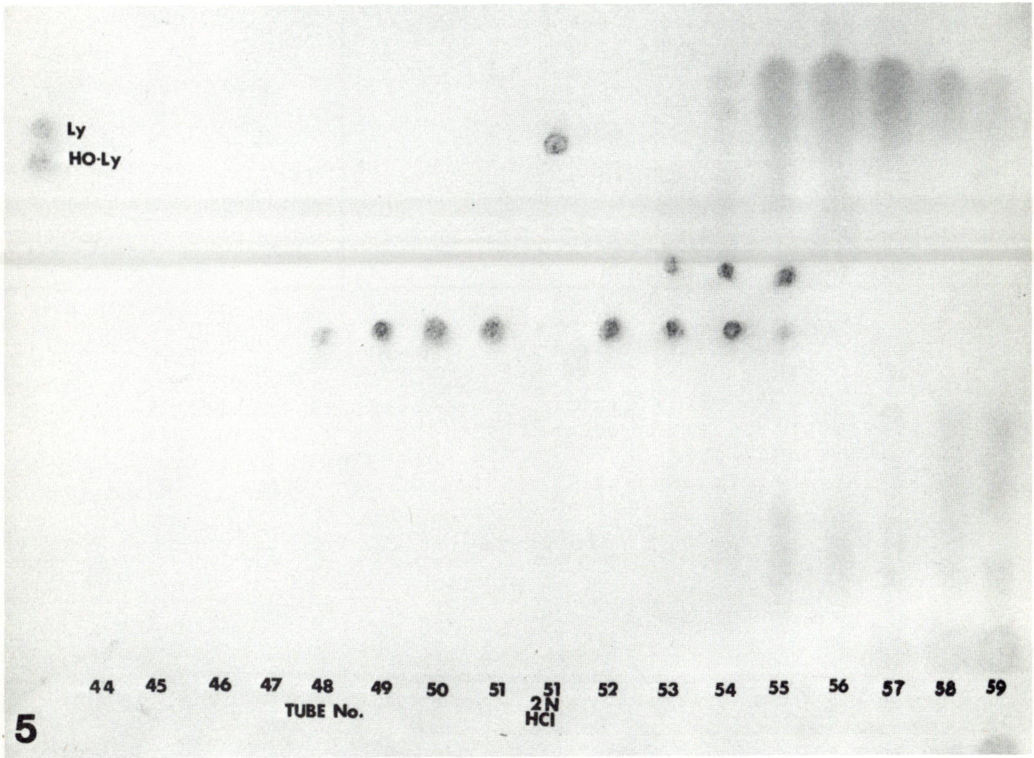
Ly
HO·Ly
44 45 46 47 48 49 50 51 51 52 53 54 55 56 57 58 59
TUBE No.
2N
HCl

5

TABLE XI

Hydroxylysine-bound Carbohydrate Units of Canine Basement Membranes*

Basement membrane	No. of units per 1000 a.a. residues	Substituted hydroxylysine (% of total)	Glu-Gal-HOLys.	Gal-HOLys.
			(% of total units)	
Glomerular	18.7	75	95	5
Ant. lens capsule	33.0	80	95	5
Descemet's membrane	16.0	80	94	6

*Kefalides, unpublished data

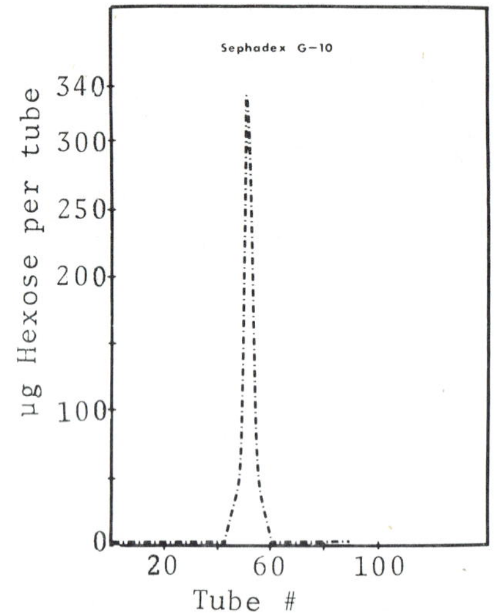

Fig. 4. Gel filtration on a column of Sephadex G-10 of glycopeptides from Descemet's membrane following alkaline hydrolysis and Dowex-50, 8 x (H^+) chromatography. Elution buffer, 0.1 m pyridine-acetic acid, pH 5.

tained within the peak were characterized by high-voltage electrophoresis. The results are shown in Fig. 5. Fractions from the ascending portion of the peak contained only the glucosyl-galactosyl-hydroxylysine unit, while the descending portion contain the galactosyl-hydroxylysine unit as well as the disaccharide unit

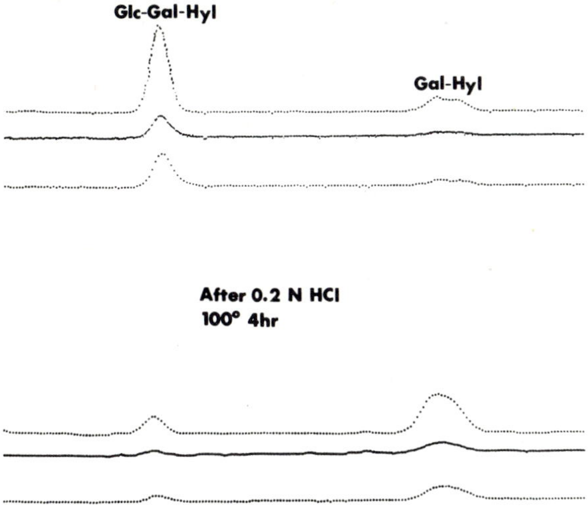

Fig. 6. Elution diagram from amino acid analyzer of aliquots from hexose-containing peak (tube 54) from Sephadex G-10 column. Upper, before hydrolysis; Lower, after hydrolysis with 0.2 N HCl, at 100°C for 4 hr. The Glc-Gal-Hyl unit has been converted to Gal-Hyl.

(fractions 53-55, Fig. 5). Mild acid hydrolysis of the disaccharide unit with 0.2 N HCl for 4 hr at 100°C splits off the terminal glucose and yields the monosaccharide unit (Fig. 6), while hydrolysis with 2 N HCl for 2 hr at 100°C splits off both sugars and releases hydroxylysine (tube 51, Fig. 5). Fig. 7 is a paper chromatogram for sugars showing the release of only glucose under mild acid hydrolysis, while both glucose and galactose are released when the disaccharide unit is hydrolysed with 2 N HCl for 2 hr at 100°C. Since the galactosyl-hydroxylysine linkage is not labile to mild acid hydrolysis, we resorted to oxidative deamination of the hydroxylysine by the use of HNO_2, on Dr. J. A. Cifonelli's suggestion. This procedure destabilizes the bond and the disaccharide, glucosyl-galactose can be split off by hydrolysing with 0.1 N HCl for 4 hr at 90°C (Fig. 8). The linkage and sequence of the disaccharide unit in Descemet's membrane has been shown to be the same as in other basement membranes (Kefalides, unpublished data).

If we accept the molecular weight of acetic acid soluble collagen from basement membrane as 275,000, and its hexose content as 11%, then the number of disaccharide units would equal 79 and the monosaccharide units 8. Assuming

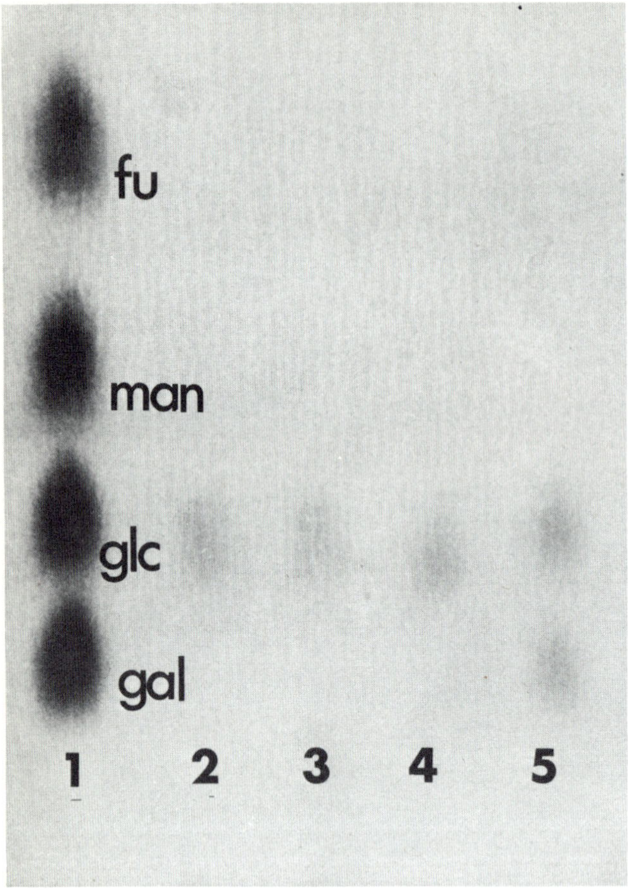

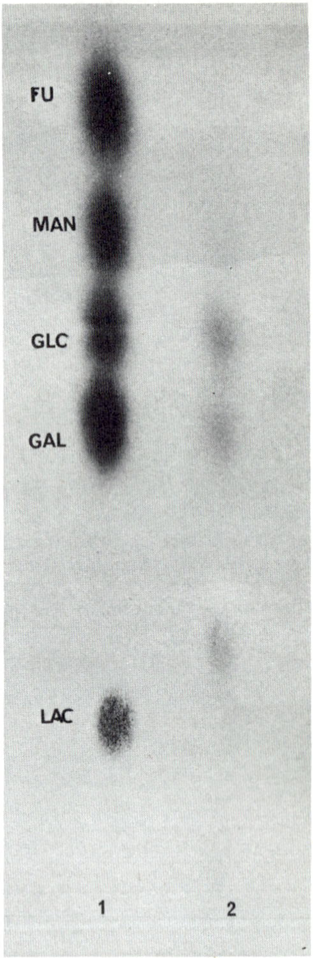

Fig. 7. Paper chromatogram of glycopeptide Glc-Gal-Hyl. Solvent, ethylacetate:pyridine:water (10:4:3, v/v). 1. Standards: galactose, glucose, mannose, fucose. 2,3, and 4 after hydrolysis of Glc-Gal-Hyl with 0.2 N HCl, 100°C for 30, 60 and 120 min. respectively. 5. After hydrolysis with 2 N HCl at 100° for 2 hrs.

Fig. 8. Paper chromatogram of glycopeptide Glc-Gal-Hyl after treatment with HNO_2 and hydrolysis with 0.1 N HCl at 90° for 4 hrs to release the disaccharide glucosyl-galactose. The disaccharide migrates just ahead of lactose. 1. Standards. 2. Glycopeptide. Ethyl acetate:pyridine:water (10:4:3, v/v).

that hydroxylysine accounts for 6.4% by weight of the protein, then there should be 108 residues of hydroxylysine per molecule of basement membrane collagen. Since about 80% of the hydroxylysine is resistant to periodate oxidation, then about 86.5 residues of hydroxylysine must be involved in glycosidic linkage. This value approaches that of the sum of 79 disaccharide and 8 monosaccharide units.

The carbohydrate unit of glomerular basement membrane which contains hexosamine, galactose, mannose, fucose and sialic acid has only partially been characterized. Spiro (1967b) isolated glycopeptides from collagenase and pronase digests of bovine glomerular basement membrane containing these sugars with the following ratios: glucosamine 5; galactose 4; mannose 3; fucose 1; sialic acid 3. It is suggested that this polysaccharide is linked to asparagine (Spiro, 1967b). The presence of a similar polysaccharide has been reported to occur in human glomerular basement membrane by Dische, Pappas and Dische (1965). In our laboratory we have isolated similar polysaccharides from canine glomerular basement membrane and anterior lens capsule. At present, it is not quite clear how the protein moiety to which the polysaccharide is attached interacts with the collagen molecule in basement membrane.

III IMMUNOCHEMICAL CHARACTERISTICS

The immunologic reactivity of basement membranes has been studied by several investigators (Cruickshank and Hill, 1953; Goodman, et. al., 1955; Krakower and Greenspon, 1964; Loewi, 1967; Pierce, Beals, Sri Ram and Midgley, 1964; Roberts, 1957; Rothbard and Watson, 1961, 1967; Steblay and Rudofsky, 1968; Yagi, Korngold and Pressman, 1956). A number of these studies have demonstrated immunologic cross-reaction among homologous basement membranes derived from different tissues and between heterologous glomerular basement membranes. Recent studies by Krakower and Greenspon (1964) show that epithelial and mesenchymal basement membranes possess at least two types of antigens. One is related to collagen. The second antigenic component is shared by all these basement membranes. Basement membranes from capillaries and venules appear to possess a third antigenic component, the so-called "nephrotoxic" one, which according to Krakower and Greenspon, is not identical with the second antigen but would seem to be related to it. Rothbard and Watson (1961, 1967) demonstrated that antibodies to rat and human collagen became fixed in glomerular basement membrane of the rat and human kidney, respectively.

Recently, data became available on the isolation and chemical characterization of the antigenic components from isolated basement membranes. Shibata et. al. (1967) have isolated a glycoprotein from rat kidney cortex. Antiserum to this protein localizes in the region of glomerular basement membrane, as demonstrated by immunofluorescence, and gives rise to experimental glomerulonephritis. The amino acid composition of this protein is puzzling. In terms of mole per cent, it contains, among other amino acids, glycine 37.76, cysteic acid 4.5, alanine 3.99, and proline 8.59. It contains only a trace of hydroxyproline and no hydroxylysine. We know of no proteins which contain one-third glycine outside the collagen group and we know of no collagen with only a trace of hydroxyproline. Total hexose accounts for 12.45% of their protein, half of which is glucose. Since, from our studies (Kefalides, 1967, 1969) and those of others (Spiro, 1967c), all the glucose in glomerular basement membrane is part of a disaccharide, glucosyl-galactose, linked to hydroxylysine of the collagen component, it is difficult to understand the amino acid analysis of the protein isolated by Shibata, Naruse, Nagasawa, Takuma and Miyakawa (1967). I can only offer one explanation. At times, if buffer and pH conditions are not exact, the hydroxyproline peak may be partly or completely masked by that of the aspartic acid in the chromatogram.

Huang and Kalant (1968) identified antigenic components in rat glomerular basement membrane. One of these is a

FIGURE 9

FRACTIONATION OF GLOMERULAR BASEMENT MEMBRANE

Basement Membrane

Tris HCl 0.05 M pH 7.4
0.01 M $CaCl_2$
Collagenase, 37°, 120 hrs.
Centrifuge 34,800 g, 30'

Residue

tion & Alkylation
Sephadex G-200
Single Peak (Vo)

Supernatant

Dialyze vs. H_2O

Retentate
Sephadex G-200

Dialysate

Peak A (Vo) Peak B ≃(Vo) Peak C Retarded Peak D Peak E Peak F

Fig. 9. Fractionation of glomerular basement membrane.

TABLE XII

Partial List of the Amino Acid Composition of Glomerular Basement Membrane Fractions after Digestion with Collagenase*

(Residues/1000 residues)

Sephadex G-200

		Peaks			
	Residue	A	B	C	D
HO-Lysine	Trace	8	20.	Trace	Trace
Lysine	53.6	38.7	43.2	50.0	58.5
HO-Proline	Trace	23.7	52.5	0	0
Proline	55.3	56.8	56.2	61.7	67.3
Glycine	93.0	124.0	195.0	99.3	110.3
Aspartic Acid	91.0	88.7	66.2	85.5	100.0
Glutamic Acid	112.0	130.3	100.5	110.4	108.7
Arginine	66.4	73.2	71.0	68.3	51.0
Half-Cystine	22.0	35.0	32.0	35.5	36.2
Hexose (%)	6.0	8.45	8.2	5.0	4.5
Hexosamine	0.8	3.9	2.1	1.35	2.0

*Kefalides, unpublished data

glycoprotein which lacks hydroxyproline and hydroxylysine, contains 10.6% carbohydrate and gives rise to nephrotoxic antibodies.

In our laboratory, we have solubilized dog basement membranes from the glomerulus, alveolus and anterior lens capsule by reduction and alkylation of disulfide bonds in 8 M urea (Kefalides, 1969). Antisera were prepared in rabbits to the glomerular and anterior lens capsule material. Using the immunodiffusion technique, two precipitin lines of identity were demonstrated when material from lens capsule and glomerular basement membrane was allowed to react with antiserum to the former and vice versa. Similarly, two lines of identity were obtained when antiserum to glomerular basement membrane was allowed to react with solubilized glomerular and alveolar basement membrane (Fig. 11, I). Solubilized glomerular basement membrane completely absorbed out antibodies directed against anterior lens capsule.

Digestion of glomerular basement membrane with collagenase for 120 hrs results in two main fractions (Fig. 9). One is an insoluble undigestible residue which can be solubilized by reduction and alkylation in 8 M urea. Upon gel filtration with Sephadex G-200 it emerges as a single peak with the void volume. Amino acid analysis reveals the absence of hydroxylysine and hydroxyproline (Table XII). It contains 6% hexose, composed of glucose, galactose, mannose and fucose, 0.8% hexosamine and 1.5% sialic acid. The second fraction is the soluble undialyzable portion of the collagenase digest which after gel filtration of Sephadex G-200 separates into six peaks (Fig. 10). Of these, only peaks A, B, C and D give precipitin lines with the antiserum to reduced and alkylated basement membrane (Fig. 11, II), and only peaks A and B contain hydroxyproline and hydroxylysine (Table XII). Peaks A, B, C and D give lines of identity among themselves and with the fast diffusing component of the reduced and alkylated basement membrane, while the undigested residue gives a line of identity with the fast diffusing component (Fig. 11, III). More recently we have demonstrated a cross-

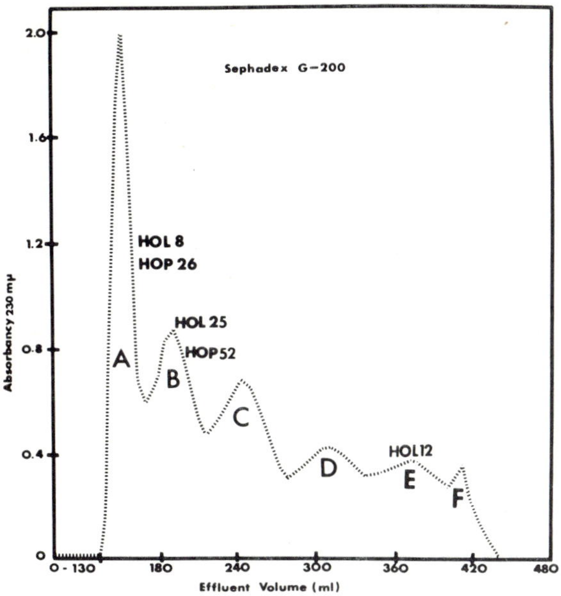

Fig. 10. Gel filtration on Sephadex G-200 of the soluble, undialysable fraction of glomerular basement membrane after digestion with collagenase. HOL = hydroxylysine; HOP = hydroxyproline. Numbers refer to residues per 1000 residues.

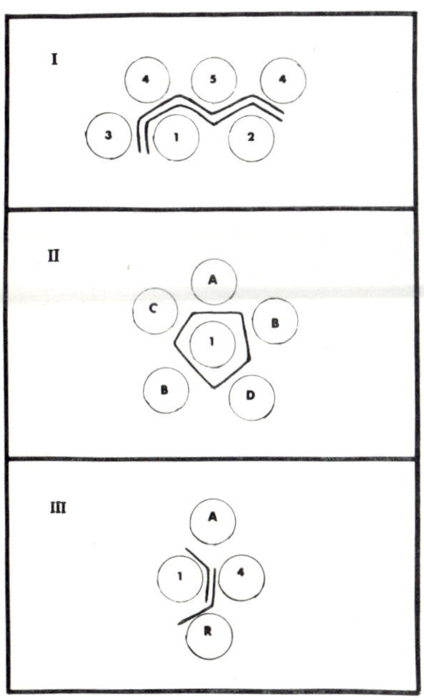

Fig. 11. Immunodiffusion pattern of antisera against dog reduced and alkylated glomerular basement membrane and reduced and alkylated anterior lens capsule. I. Well 1 contains antiserum to reduced and alkylated glomerular basement membrane. Well 2 contains antiserum to reduced and alkylated anterior lens capsule. Well 3 contains reduced and alkylated alveolar basement membrane, Well 4 reduced and alkylated glomerular basement membrane, Well 5 reduced and alkylated lens capsule. II. Well 1, same as I. Wells A,B,C and D contain material from fractions A,B,C and D of Sephadex G-200 (Fig. 10). III. Wells 1 and 4, same as I. Well A contains material from fraction A of Sephadex G-200. Well R contains material from the undigested residue after collagenase digestion of glomerular basement membrane (Fig. 9).

reaction between solubilized Descemet's membrane and antiserum to reduced and alkylated glomerular basement membrane and lens capsule. The isolated collagen from basement membranes also gives rise to precipitating antibodies when injected into rabbits (unpublished data).

It can be concluded that in the basement membranes examined so far at least three chemically distinct antigenic components are present. One of these is represented by polypeptides with an amino acid composition unlike that of the collagen molecule proper, which, however, appear to be linked to the collagen molecule (telopeptides, Fig. 12). The other is a large molecular weight glycoprotein, unlike collagen and is represented by the undigested residue (Fig. 12). The third antigenic component is represented by the collagen molecule proper. These antigenic components are shared by both the epithelial and mesenchymal basement membranes.

IV STRUCTURAL CHARACTERISTICS

There is little doubt that the intact basement membrane possesses a complex chemical structure. Our present knowledge of its structural organization is scanty. Some

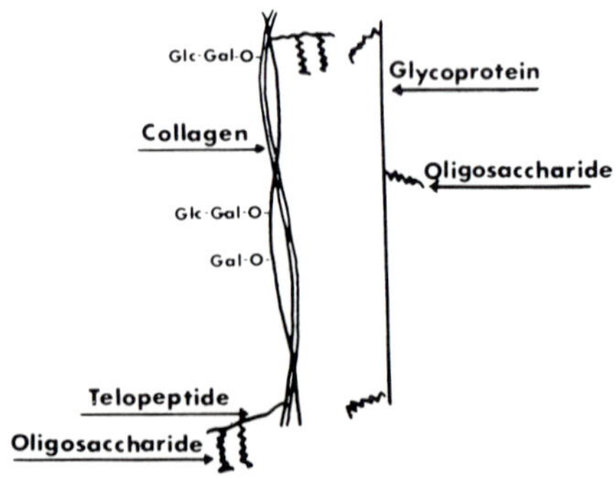

Fig. 12. A schematic representation of the relationship of the antigenic components of glomerular basement membrane. The undigested residue is represented by the large molecular weight glycoprotein. The telopeptides correspond to peaks C and D and the telopeptides with portions of the collagen molecule proper still attached correspond to peaks A and B (Fig. 10).

insight into the structural characteristics of basement membranes has been obtained from studies of these substances from a number of approaches: 1) use of solubilizing agents which are known to break specific chemical bonds, 2) isolation of macromolecules and characterization of their structure by physical means, and 3) enzymatic degradation of whole basement membrane and of its collagen component followed by structural analysis of peptides.

Isolated glomerular basement membrane is practically insoluble in 0.3 M acetic acid at 4°C (about 1% by weight becomes soluble), while about one-third of lens capsule is soluble (Table II). The amino acid and carbohydrate composition of the acetic acid soluble fraction from lens capsule is very similar to that of the intact capsule (Kefalides, unpublished data). The intrinsic viscosity of this material is about 10 dl/g and on acrylamide gel electrophoresis it separates into γ, β and α components, characteristic of mammalian collagens. The residue which remains insoluble in acetic acid becomes swollen to an almost gel-like state in both the case of glomerular basement membrane and lens capsule. These observations suggest that the organization of macromolecules differs in the two types of basement membrane. Furthermore, the swelling of glomerular basement membrane in dilute acid without concomitant solubilization suggests the presence of a continuously crosslinked network of protein molecules which could interact either by covalent or hydrogen bonds. The partial solubilization of lens capsule in weak acetic acid with swelling of the insoluble residue suggests that a portion of the macromolecules must interact with each other by weak forces which do not involve covalent or hydrogen bonds.

Solubilization of about one-third of either glomerular basement membrane or lens capsule with 8 M urea at pH8, at 40°C (Table II) suggests that hydrophobic type bonds must be involved in the interaction of macromolecules. The urea extractable fraction lacks hydroxyproline and hydroxylysine and contains hexosamine, galactose, mannose, fucose and sialic acid.

The solubilization of glomerular basement membrane and lens capsule by reduction with mercaptoethanol followed by alkylation with sodium iodoacetate suggests that disulfide bonds are involved in the interaction of macromolecular components. The presence of disulfide bonds in glomerular basement membrane has already been reported (Kefalides and Winzler, 1966).

Some insight into the structural features of the individual macromolecules has been gained from the characterization of the collagenous component from glomerular basement membrane, anterior lens capsule and Descemet's membrane. The collagen which is rendered soluble in weak acetic acid after limited treatment with pronase at 4°C (Table VIII has a triple helical configuration characteristic of other mammalian collagens (Fig. 1).

It can be stated, however, with some certainty that basement membranes are polymers of two dissimilar subunits. Preliminary studies suggest that a collagen molecule containing approximately 79 glucosyl-galactose and 8 galactose units is associated with one or more non-collagen polypeptides which contain a polysaccharide composed of hexosamine, galactose, mannose, fucose and sialic acid. In addition, there is large molecular weight glycoprotein associated with the collagen molecules. This protein can be extracted with 8 M urea and corresponds to the undigestible residue after treatment of basement membrane with collagenase (Fig. 12). Basement membranes of different structural organization have emerged from the association of different proportions of these subunits. The differences in structural organization are probably related to the functional properties of the particular basement membrane.

V CONCLUSIONS

Basement membranes appear to be a specialized form of connective tissue. Embryologically they derive from ectodermal and mesenchymal tissue and in the adult they are associated with epithelial cells, endothelial cells or both.

Basement membranes appear to have two main functions: they offer support and participate in the differential permeability to molecules across capillary walls and epithelial surfaces.

On the basis of their amino acid and carbohydrate composition, basement membranes show qualitative similarities but differ quantitatively from one another. Vascular basement membranes show a wide variation in their amino acid and carbohydrate composition as do nonvascular basement membranes. However, the amino acid and carbohydrate composition of Descemet's membrane resembles more that of the glomerulus than of the anterior lens capsule.

Structurally, basement membranes appear to be composed of dissimilar protein subunits rich in carbohydrate. These subunits appear to interact by covalent and hydrogen bonds and by weak forces which involve neither of the above types of bonds. One of these is a collagen characterized by high amounts of hydroxylysine and hydroxyproline. Unlike other mammalian collagens it contains half-cystine. It contains from 10-12% carbohydrate which exists mainly as a disaccharide, glucosyl-galactose and to a small extent as a monosaccharide, galactose, linked glycosidically to hydroxylysine. The same type of carbohydrate units have been identified in other mammalian collagens but the total amount of hexose is about 20 times less. Depending on the embryologic origin and tissue localization of the basement membrane variable amounts of this collagen can be removed by limited proteolytic digestion of the basement membrane. In lens capsule all the collagen isolated is soluble in weak acetic acid while only 16% of it is acid soluble in glomerular basement membrane and Descemet's membrane; the remainder is insoluble in acid pH and appears to be associated still with non-collagen polypeptides rich in hexosamine, galactose, mannose, fucose and sialic acid. One of the non-collagen polypeptides has a molecular weight of about 55,000 and is linked to the collagen by disulfide bonds. The second non-collagen polypeptide has a molecular weight of over 200,000. The latter interact with each other by hydrogen bonds and with the collagen by disulfide bonds.

On the basis of immunochemical studies, basement membranes possess three antigenic components. One is represented by the collagen, another by the small molecular weight glycoprotein and a third by the large molecular weight glycoprotein.

ACKNOWLEDGEMENTS

This investigation was supported by U. S. Public Health Grant AM-11634.

REFERENCES

Butler, W.T. and Cunningham, L.W. (1966). J. Biol. Chem. 241, 3882.

Cruickshank, B. and Hill, A.G.S. (1953). J. Pathol. Bacteriol. 66, 283.

Cunningham, L.W. and Ford, J.D. (1968). J. Biol. Chem. 243, 2390.

Davies, J. (1950). J. Anat. 84, 95.

Davison, P.F. and Drake, M.P. (1966). Biochemistry 5, 313.

Dische, Z. (1964). In Small Blood Vessel Involvement in Diabetes Mellitus, p. 201. Ed. by Siperstein, M.D., Colwell, A.R. and Meyer, K. American Institute of Biological Sciences, Washington, D.C.

Dische, Z. and Borenfreund, E. (1954). Am. J. Ophthalmol. 38, 165.

Dische, R.M., Pappas, G.D. and Dische, Z. (1965). Biochem. Biophys. Res. Commun. 20, 63.

Dische, Z., Zelmenis, G. and Rothschild, C. (1967). Arch. Biochem. Biophys. 121, 685.

Dohlman, C.H. and Balazs, E.A. (1955). Arch. Biochem. 57, 445.

Drake, M.P., Davison, P.F., Bumps, S. and Schmitt, F.O. (1966). Biochemistry 5, 301.

Farquar, H.G. (1964). In Small Blood Vessel Involvement in Diabetes Mellitus, p. 31. Ed. by Siperstein, M.D., Colwell, A.R. and Meyer, K. American Institute of Biological Sciences, Washington, D.C.

Fawcett, D.W. (1963), In The Peripheral Blood Vessels, p. 17. Ed. by Orbison, J.L. and Smith, D.E. Williams and Wilkins, Baltimore.

Friederici, H.H.R., Tucker, W.R. and Schwartz, T.B. (1966). Diabetes 15, 233.

Goodman, M., Greenspon, S.A. and Krakower, C.A. (1955). J. Immunol. 75, 96.

Gross, J., Matoltsy, A.G. and Cohen, C. (1955). J. Biophys. Biochem. Cytol. 1, 215.

Huang, F., and Kalant, N. (1968). Can. J. Biochem. 46, 1523.

Jakus, M.A. (1964). Ocular Fine Structure. Little, Brown, Boston.

Karrer, H.E. (1956). J. Biophys. Biochem. Cytol. 2, 241.

Kefalides, N.A. (1966). Biochem. Biophys. Res. Commun. 22, 26.

Kefalides, N.A. (1967). 154th National Meeting of the American Chemical Society (Chicago, Ill. Sept.).

Kefalides, N.A. (1968a). Biochemistry 7, 3103.

Kefalides, N.A. (1968b). 156th National Meeting of the American Chemical Society. (Atlantic City, N.J., Sept.).

Kefalides, N.A. (1969a). In Proceedings, Sixth Congress of the International Diabetes Federation (Stockholm, 1967), p. 307. Excerpta Medica Foundation, Amsterdam.

Kefalides, N.A. (1969b). Fed. Proc. 28, 699.

Kefalides, N.A. and Winzler, R.J. (1966). Biochemistry 5, 702.

Kefalides, N.A. and Denduchis, B. (1969). Biochemistry, 8, 4613.

Krakower, C.A., Greenspon, S.A. and Warren, H.M. (1957). Exptl. Cell Res. 13, 230.

Krakower, C.A. and Greenspon, S.A. (1964). In Small Blood Vessel Involvement in Diabetes Mellitus, p. 161. Ed. by Siperstein, M.D., Colwell, A.R. and Meyer, K. American Institute of Biological Sciences, Washington, D.C.

Kurtz, S.M. and McManus, J.F.A. (1959). Am. Heart J. 58, 357.

Latta, H. (1961). J. Ultrastruct. Res. 5, 364.

Lazarow, A. and Speidel, E. (1964). In Small Blood Vessel Involvement in Diabetes Mellitus, p. 127. Ed. by Siperstein, M.D., Colwell, A.R. and Meyer, K. American Institute of Biological Sciences, Washington, D.C.

Loewi, G. (1967). Ann. Rheum. Dis. 26, 544.

Markowitz, A.S. and Lange, C.F., Jr. (1964). J. Immunol. 92, 565.

McKeehan, M.S. (1951). J. Exptl. Zool. 117, 31.

Palade, G.E. and Bruns, R.R. (1964). In Small Blood Vessel Involvement in Diabetes Mellitus, p. 39. Ed. by Siperstein, M.D., Colwell, A.R. and Meyer, K. American Institute of Biological Sciences, Washington, D.C.

Pierce, G.B. Jr., Beals, T.F., Sri Ram, J. and Midgley, A.R. (1964). Am. J. Path. 45, 929.

Pirie, A. (1951). Biochem. J. 48, 368.

Ramachandran, G.N., Sasisekharan, V. and Thathachari, Y.T. (1962). In Collagen, p. 81. Ed. by Ramanathan, N. Interscience Publishers, New York.

Roberts, D. St. C. (1957). Brit. J. Ophthalmol. 41, 338.

Rothbard, S. and Watson, R.F. (1961). J. Exptl. Med. 113, 1041.

Rothbard, S. and Watson, R.F. (1967). J. Exptl. Med. 125, 595.

Shibata, S., Naruse, T., Nagasawa, T., Takuma, T. and Miyakawa, Y. (1967). J. Immunol. 99, 454.

Spiro, R.G. (1967a). J. Biol. Chem. 242, 1915.

Spiro, R.G. (1967b). J. Biol. Chem. 242, 1923.

Spiro, R.G. (1967c). J. Biol. Chem. 242, 4813.

Spiro, R.G. (1969). J. Biol. Chem. 244, 2041.

Steblay, R.W. and Rudofsky, U. (1968). Science 160, 204.

Suzuki, Y. (1959). Keio J. Med. 8, 129.

Timasheff, S.N., Susi, H., Townsend, R., Stevens, L., Gorbunoff, M.J. and Kumosinski, T.F. (1967). In Conformation of Biopolymers, p. 173. Academic Press, New York.

Todd, R.B. and Bowman, W. (1857). The Physiological Anatomy and Physiology of Man, pp. 129, 523 and 660. Blanchard and Lea, Philadelphia.

Vernier, R.L. (1964). In Small Blood Vessel Involvement in Diabetes Mellitus, p. 57. Ed. by Siperstein, M.D., Colwell, A.R. and Meyer, K. American Institute of Biological Sciences, Washington, D.C.

Weibel, E.R. (1963). Morphometry of the Human Lung, Academic Press, New York.

Yagi, Y., Korngold, L. and Pressman, D. (1956). J. Immunol. 77, 287.

THE ROLE OF GLOMERULAR BASAL LAMINA IN RENAL DISEASE

Giuseppe A. Andres, Lidia Accinni, Konrad C. Hsu
and Beatrice C. Seegal

The concept that antibodies to renal tissue may provoke glomerulonephritis was first proposed at the beginning of this century, when Lindemann (1900) demonstrated the nephritogenic properties of heterologous anti-kidney antibodies. Subsequent work on nephrotoxic nephritis (also called Masugi nephritis) has provided precise information concerning the nature and potency of these heterologous nephritogenic antibodies. Additional information has been accumulated on the localization and immunochemical characteristics of the glomerular antigen (s)--mainly of the antigens of the basal lamina (BL)--and some of the mediators of the inflammation activated by antigen-antibody reactions.

A further step in the study of the immunologic mechanisms involved in nephritis was achieved by Steblay (1962) who showed that sheep immunized with homologous or heterologous glomerular basal laminae (GBL) could develop glomerulonephritis. The demonstration of antibody to GBL in the serum and kidneys of such animals and the passive transfer of this form of nephritis to normal homologous recipients, provided definitive evidence that an animal could, upon appropriate immunization, form nephritogenic anti-GBL antibodies capable of producing an "autoimmune" glomerulonephritis.

More recently Lerner, Glassok and Dixon (1967) have shown that anti-GBL antibodies may be formed spontaneously in man, in Goodpasture's disease and in certain forms of progressive glomerulonephritis, and that these antibodies are responsible for the nephritis. The antibodies react with GBL antigens in vitro and in vivo. On passive transfer they induce immediate glomerulonephritis in recipient monkeys.

The role of anti-GBL antibodies in the pathogenesis of some instances of both human and experimental glomerulonephritis is well established. It has been shown, however, that there are at least two quite distinct and independent mechanisms which may operate in the genesis of the disease. First--as we have already mentioned--antibodies against antigens fixed to, or part of, the GBL are pathogenic. Second, circulating soluble antigen-antibody (Ag-Ab) complexes, immunologically unrelated to the glomeruli, may produce tissue lesions. The antigens of such complexes may be exogenous, as for example, LCM virus in mice or endogenous, as DNA in lupus glomerulonephritis, which are unrelated to the filtering structures of the body, mainly GBL (Dixon, 1968).

The morphologic, immunofluorescent and immunoelectronmicroscopic patterns of the glomerulonephritis produced by circulating Ag-Ab complexes are different from those produced by antibodies attached to, or part of, the GBL. In the immune complexes glomerulonephritis the antigens, their specific antibodies and complement are usually localized, in scattered and granular fashion, on both sides of the GBL which obviously is not the protagonist, but a passive target (Fig. 1).

I NEPHROTOXIC GLOMERULONEPHRITIS (MASUGI)

Let us examine now the immunopathology of the glomerular injury produced by antibodies directed against antigens fixed in the GBL: the so-called nephrotoxic nephritis or Masugi nephritis.

In this model the GBL from animal of species A is injected into an animal of species B. Then the serum of the immunized animal of species B is injected back into a normal animal of species A. Almost immediately the antibody is removed from the circulation and fixed in the GBL and, to a slight degree, in non-glomerular BL. Within the first 2 hr after fixation of antibodies in the GBL, polymorphonuclear leukocytes collect in the glomeruli apparently attracted by the antigen-antibody-complement reaction. The nephrotoxic antibody can be seen in immunofluorescence to be evenly distributed in a ribbon-like pattern along the GBL (Fig. 2, inset), in contrast to the irregular, granular distribution of complexes immunologically unrelated to glomeruli. The nephrotoxic antibody localizes also in the basal lamina-like material collected in the cisternae of the epithelial endoplasmic reticulum (Figs. 2 and 3). This observation indicates the presence of similar antigens in the cisternae of the epithelial endoplasmic reticulum and in GBL thus lending support to the hypothesis that the epithelial endoplasmic reticulum contains components of the BL and may be concerned with synthesis, intracellular transport and storage of these components (Andres, Morgan, Hsu, Rifkind and Seegal, 1962).

The recipient of injected nephrotoxic globulin elaborates antibody to the heterologous globulin and this host antibody reacts with nephrotoxic globulin fixed in the glomeruli, thus increasing the glomerular damage. By immunofluorescence the host γ globulins can be seen distributed in the GBL in the same manner as the heterologous nephrotoxic globulin. During the time that this secondary host antibody response continues the immunologic inflammatory reaction in the glomeruli progresses. The polymorphonuclear leukocytes play an important role producing endothelial changes and coming in direct contact with the BL itself (Fig. 4). The polymorphonuclear leukocytes are probably directly responsible for damage to the BL by activation of lysosomes and liberation of their cathepsin, or by some proteolytic process (Hawkins and Cochrane, 1968). Morphologic damage of the GBL has not yet been demonstrated, despite high resolution electron microscopy, but it can be clearly conceived from the immunologically recognizable pieces of GBL that appear in the urine.

Fig. 1. The picture illustrates glomerular capillaries from a patient with lupus glomerulonephritis. Thickening of glomerular capillary walls and electron opaque subepithelial deposits (arrows) are visible. CL indicates the capillary lumens and EP the epithelium. (x5,000). The inset shows a glomerulus from the kidney of a rabbit with chronic serum sickness glomerulonephritis produced by circulating BSA-antiBSA immune complexes. The section was stained with anti-BSA serum labeled with fluorescein. Irregular, granular fluorescence, corresponding to the foreign deposits of immune complexes in the glomerular capillary walls, is observed. (x250)

Fig. 2. Electronmicrograph which shows a small portion of a glomerular basal lamina (BL) in a rat, and part of a podocyte (EP). In the epithelial cytoplasm a large "cisterna" of the rough endoplasmic reticulum (C) contains material morphologically similar to the basal lamina. In the peripheral part of the cisterna the material is more electron dense. (x13,000). The inset illustrates the localization of a rabbit anti-rat-GBL serum in the glomerulus of a rat. The nephrotoxic antibody is bound, in a linear manner, in the GBL and in the epithelial cisternae of the endoplasmic reticulum (arrows). (x550)

Fig. 3. A micrograph illustrating a kidney from a rat made nephritic with rabbit anti-rat-GBL serum and then treated with ferritin-conjugated antibody to rabbit globulin. In the cytoplasm of this epithelial cell (EP) a distended cisterna contains basal-lamina-like material which is concentrated in a peripheral zone. Numerous ferritin granules are present in this area.

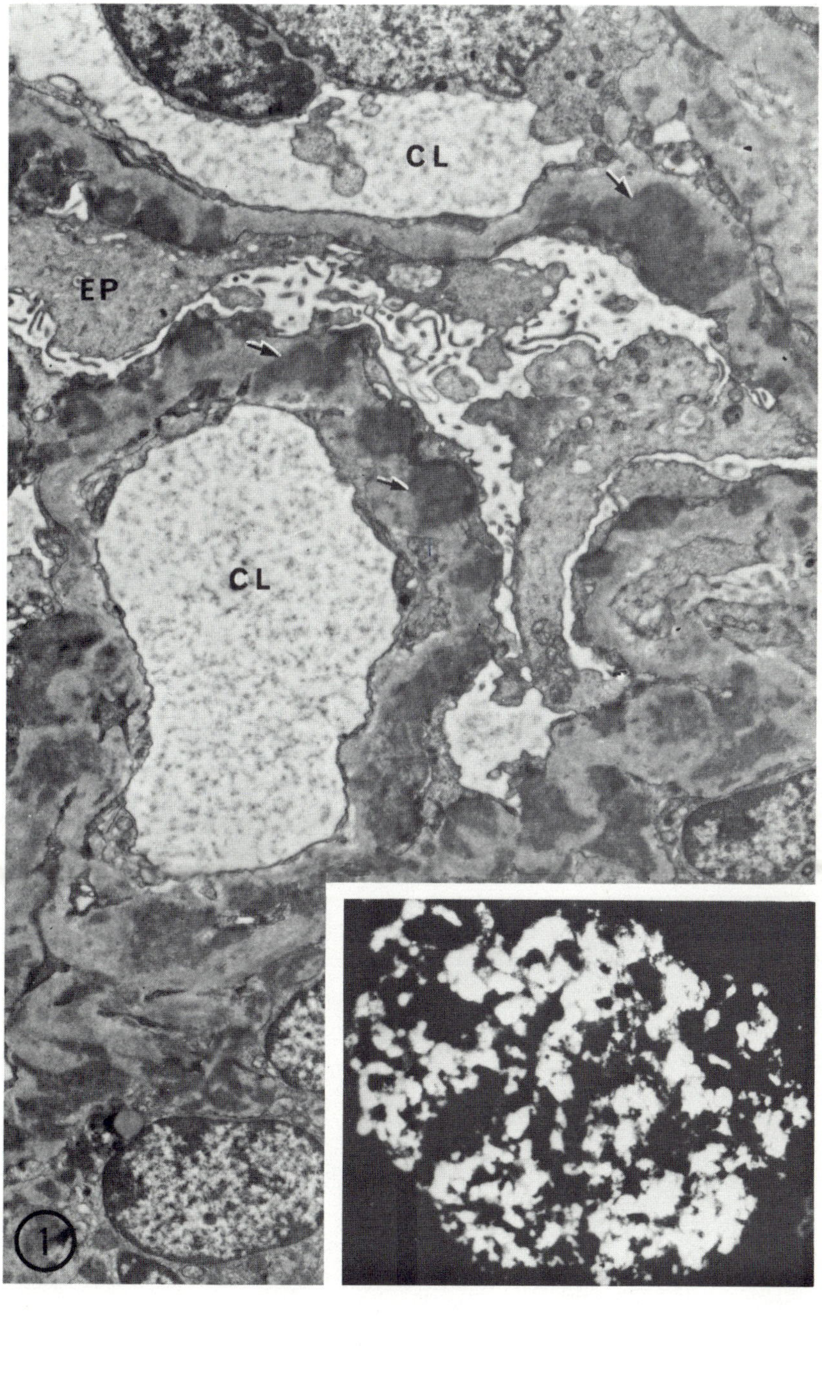
CL
EP
CL
1

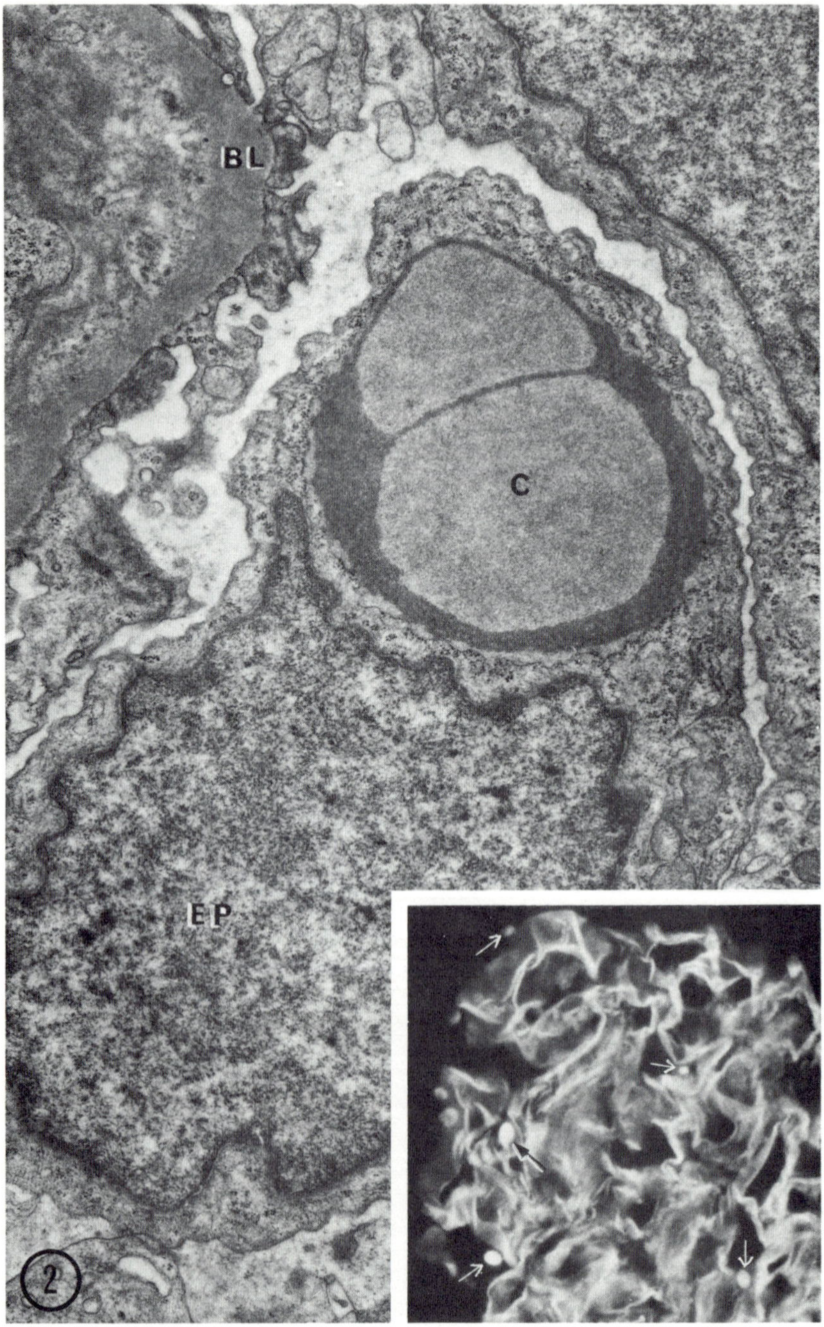
BL
C
EP
2

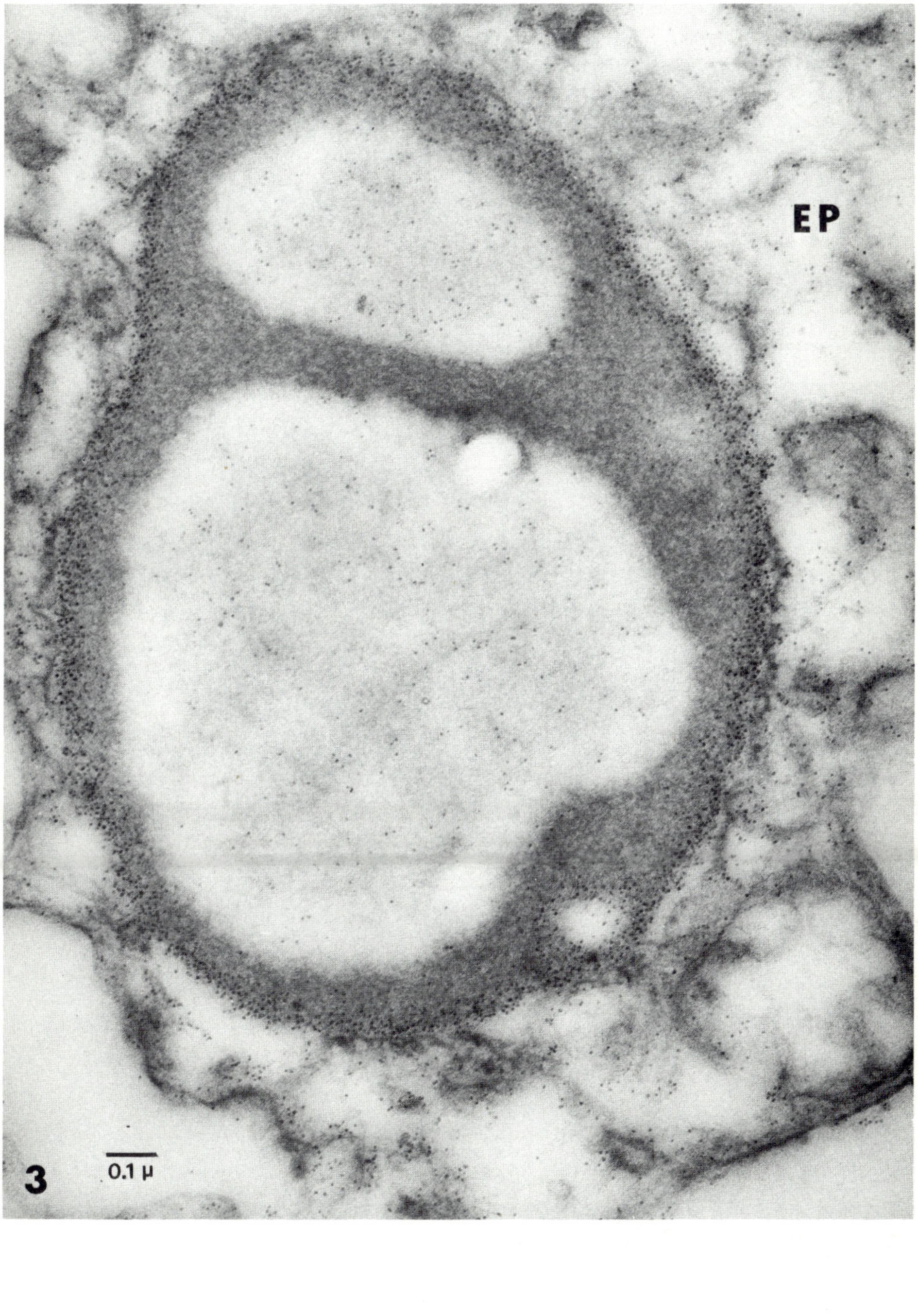
EP
3
0.1 μ

II "AUTOIMMUNE" GLOMERULONEPHRITIS (STEBLAY, 1962)

A second experimental model in which GBL antigens play a fundamental role is the "autoimmune" nephritis induced in sheep by injection of heterologous (usually human) GBL in Freund's adjuvant (Steblay, 1962). The sheep form antibodies against the GBL which cross-react with their own GBL, causing progressive, severe glomerulonephritis. These antibodies localize in a linear fashion in the GBL together with complement and polymorphonuclear leukocytes and thus an inflammatory reaction is produced. Circulating anti-GBL antibodies can be found in bilaterally nephrectomized sheep and may produce nephritis when injected into normal animals. Bilateral nephrectomy is necessary because the kidneys, with their GBL exposed to the circulation via endothelial pores, are extremely efficient in removing antibodies from the blood. The lack of strict species-specificity of these antibodies indicates that there is considerable antigenic cross-reactivity among mammalian GBL.

III GOODPASTURE'S DISEASE

Injection of sheep with human lung basal laminae in Freund's adjuvant induces progressive glomerulonephritis indicating common antigens in the BL of lung and kidney. This finding is useful in explaining the pathogenesis of Goodpasture's disease, which is the most characteristic example of human glomerulonephritis produced by anti-BL antibodies. This rare disease usually has a clinical history of initial lung hemorrages, followed by a rapidly progressive proliferative glomerulonephritis (Benoit, Rulon, Theil, Doolan and Watten, 1964). Linear deposition of gamma-globulin and complement is found in the GBL (Fig. 5) and in the BL of the lung alveoli (Fig. 6) which show ultrastructural lesions similar to those observed in the GBL (Fig. 7). Acid buffer elution of both lung and kidney reacted with BL of either organs but fail to react with BL of organs other than kidney or lung (Koffler, Sandson, Carr and Kunkel, 1969). Similar anti-GBL antibodies have been eluted from the kidney of patients with progressive--non-Goodpasture's--glomerulonephritis.

It has been established that the primary cause of this tissue-specific type of glomerulonephritides is due to the deposition of antibodies against some component(s) of GBL. The mechanism stimulating the production of these antibodies is unknown. How does the patient become immunized against his own GBL? It may be that 1) the GBL proteins have been altered in some way so that the lymphocytes react to them as foreign proteins. This is known to happen with erythrocytes in some viral infections with development of autoimmune hemolytic anemia; 2) another possibility is the anatomic displacement of GBL antigens. This might occur if the GBL components, (present in the urine both in normal and pathologic conditions) were somehow brought into contact with lymphoid cells; 3) the lymphocytes may have undergone some mutational changes of their own; and 4) it is also possible that the initiating antigen may come from outside, a foreign protein which happens to resemble the GBL sufficiently to make such immunologic cross-reaction possible. This has been suggested by Kaplan (1963) in rheumatic heart disease.

The identification of types of glomerulonephritis with reference to antibody to GBL is most important. While the pathogenetic role of anti-GBL antibodies in Goodpasture's disease seems established, it is difficult to ascertain the incidence of this mechanism in adult human glomerulonephritis. The present method of testing sera for anti-GBL antibody may underestimate the presence of this antibody in nephritis for several reasons. First, the anti-GBL antibody seems to be detectable in the sera only after bilateral nephrectomy as observed in sheep with autoimmune experimental nephritis. Second, the sera from nephrectomized chronic glomerulonephritics may well have a much lower level of antibody because of loss of glomerular antigenic stimulation and the immunosuppressive effect due to uremia. Moreover, chronic sclerotic glomeruli are scarcely useful for elution

Fig. 4. The electronmicrograph shows a section of a glomerular capillary from a patient with acute glomerulonephritis. Two polymorphonuclear leukocytes (PMN) are present within the lumen (CL). One of the polys is in close contact with the GBL and seems to discharge the content of its lysosomal granules (1) into the basal lamina (arrow). EP indicates the epithelium, EN the endothelium and BS the Bowman's space. (x12,000)

Fig. 5. Micrograph illustrating the linear localization of an anti-human IgG globulin fluorescein-conjugated in the GBL of a patient with Goodpasture's disease. (x350)

Fig. 6. Lung of the same patient illustrated in Fig. 5. The fluorescent antibody to human IgG binds in the alveolar septal basal laminae. (x130)

Fig. 7. The picture shows parts of two lung capillaries (CL) in a patient with Goodpasture's disease. The basal lamina (BL) is thickened and contains collagen fibrils (arrows). RBC indicates part of a red blood cell, EP the epithelium and AL the alveolar lumen. (x9,000)

Fig. 8. Localization of ferritin-conjugated antibody to human IgG in the glomerular basal lamina (BL) of an human renal allograft. CL indicates the capillary lumen and EP the epithelial foot processes. (x40,000). In the inset linear staining of the glomerular basal lamina in renal tissue obtained from a human allograft and treated with fluorescein-conjugated antibody to human IgG. (x350)

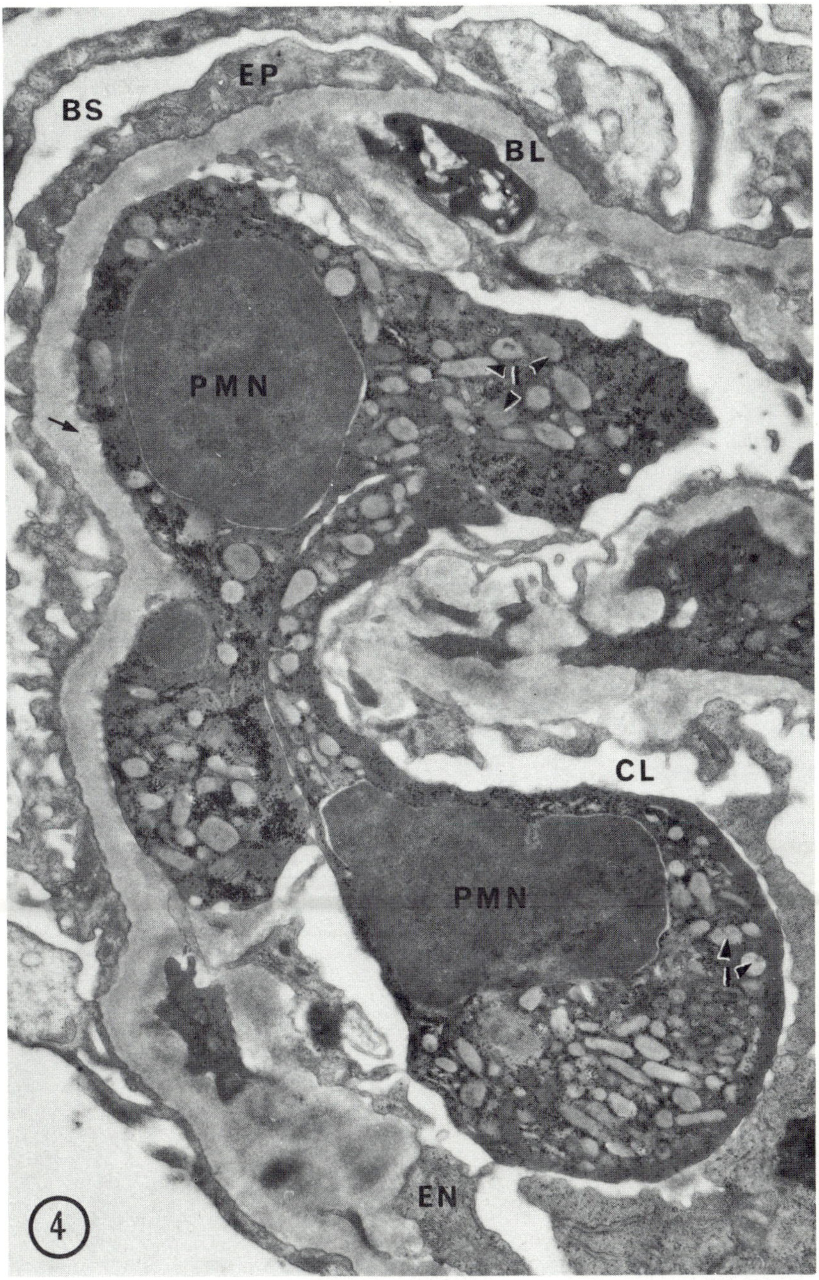
EP
BS
BL
PMN
CL
PMN
EN
4

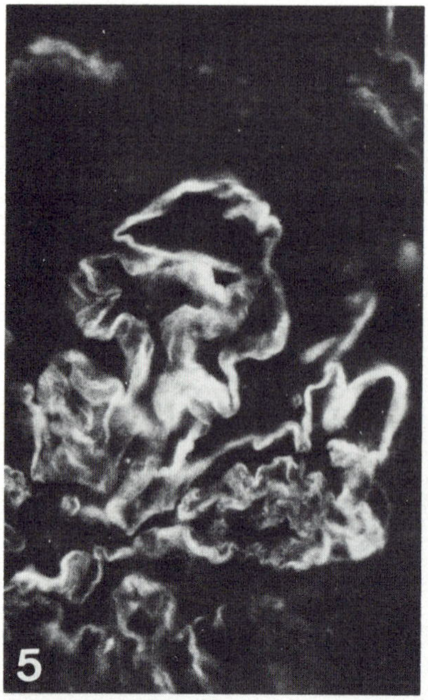
5

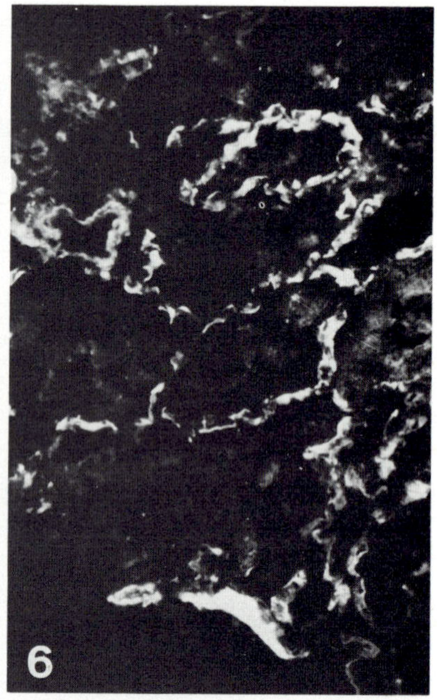
6

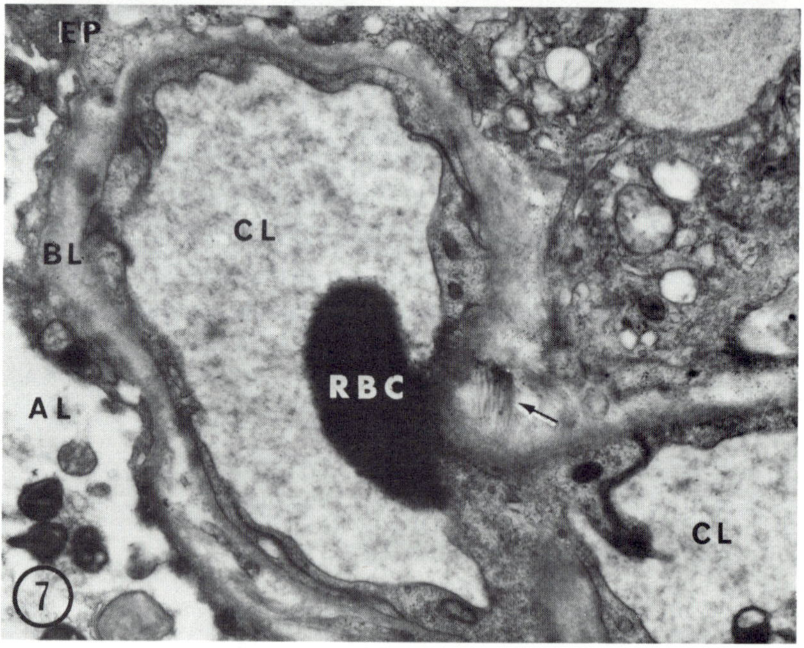
EP
CL
BL
RBC
AL
CL
7

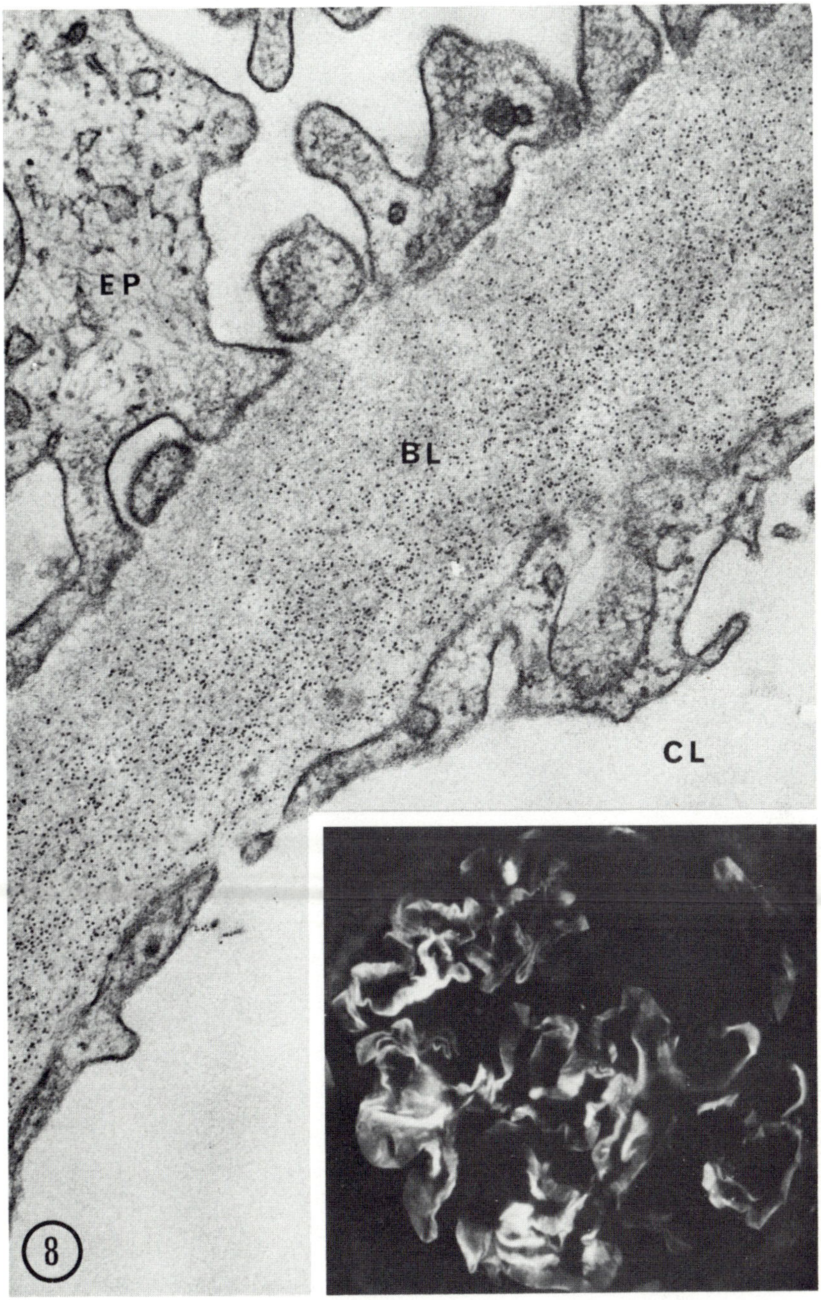
EP
BL
CL
8

procedures. Third, the test for anti-GBL antibodies is not the most sensitive nor is it certain that the antigen employed contains all the GBL determinants.

Perhaps the better method of detecting anti-GBL antibody is by the use of immunofluorescence and immunoelectronmicroscopic staining for host IgG and β1C in renal biopsies taken during early or active glomerulonephritis.

IV ANTIBODY TO GLOMERULAR BASAL LAMINA AND KIDNEY TRANSPLANTATION

The interest in the anti-GBL antibody in human pathology has been greatly increased by the study of the immunologic mechanisms affecting kidney transplants. Detectable circulating anti-GBL antibodies appear in the sera of some patients after bilateral nephrectomy prior to transplantation during the anephric period of chronic dialysis. With the implantation of a renal allograft in such a patient the antibody promptly disappears from the circulation, and host IgG (presumably antibody) and β1C accumulate in a linear pattern along the GBL of the graft (Fig. 8). Concurrently the kidney develops proliferative glomerulonephritis (Dixon, 1968).

It is obvious that there is much more to be learned about the pathogenesis of anti-GBL glomerulonephritis. These investigations have been greatly facilitated by materials made available in transplantation units. In the near future serologic, electronmicroscopic, immunofluorescence, and immuneolectronmicroscopic studies may give us the data necessary to more efficiently manage patients with this type of glomerular disease.

ACKNOWLEDGEMENTS

These studies were supported by Grants 115/0815/1365 and 115/0815/4677 from the Consiglio Nazionale delle Ricerche (C.N.R.) Italy and by United States Public Health Service Grants AI-04527, HE-03929, and AM-13200.

REFERENCES

Andres, G.A., Morgan, C., Hsu, K.C., Rifkind, R.A. and Seegal, B.C. (1962). J. Exp. Med. 115, 929.

Benoit, F.L., Rulon, D.B., Theil, G.B., Doolan, P.D. and Watten, R.H. (1964). Am. J. Med. 37, 424.

Dixon, F.J. (1968). Am. J. Med. 44, 493.

Hawkins, D. and Cochrane, C.G. (1968). J. Immunol. 14, 665.

Kaplan, M.H. (1963). J. Immunol. 90, 595.

Koffler, D., Sandson, J., Carr, R. and Kunkel, H.G. (1969). Am. J. Pathol. 54, 293.

Lerner, R.A., Glassock, R.J., and Dixon, F.J. (1967). J. Exp. Med. 126, 989.

Lindemann, W. (1900). Ann. Inst. Pasteur 14, 49.

Steblay, R.W. (1962). J. Exp. Med. 116, 253.

Chapter IV

Chemistry and Properties of Elastin

ISOLATION AND CHARACTERIZATION OF ELASTIN

S.M. Partridge

First we should try to define, in general terms, what we mean by elastin. Elastic fibres have long been recognised histochemically, by their specific staining properties and general morphology. They are known to play a functional role in connective tissues which relates to their mechanical properties; in particular to the endowment of a collagenous network with the capacity for rubber-like recoil and a complete recovery after extension.

It has long been known that the yellow fibres of elastic tissue are rarely homogeneous. It is easy to demonstrate that they contain occluded collagen and that they are contaminated to some extent or other with all the usual components of the ground-substance together with lipids and lipo-proteins. In all discussions of elastic tissues we must therefore be careful to distinguish between "elastic fibres" on the one hand and the protein "elastin" on the other. By elastin we mean the component of elastic fibres which appears amorphous in the light microscope and the electron microscope at low powers: which takes up specifically "elastin stains" as defined by the early microscopists; and finally which endows the fibre with the characteristic property of rubber-like extension and elastic snap on recoil.

All synthetic elastomers appear to be built in the same way. Long polymer chains, which must have little kinetic restriction to rotational or translational movement, are crosslinked together by firm chemical bonds to form a 3-dimensional network. If the elastomer is a protein the structure so formed is a gel which swells in water to an extent depending, among other things, on the degree of crosslinking.

I METHODOLOGY AND CRITERIA OF PURITY

For the chemical study of a protein, purity is essential. This is particularly valid for an insoluble fibrous protein like elastin, since we are interested, among other things, in the nature of the crosslinkages which probably represent at the most some 2% of the dry weight of the protein. How then can we be sure that, in our isolation procedures, we can separate all of the crosslinked elastin network from other contaminating peptide structures which may be very intimately associated and probably occluded within the elastin gel? If we use vigorous reagents, such as hot dilute alkali, we may be able to remove all material which is not firmly bound to the gel by stable covalent crosslinkages: but in doing so there is the danger that severe extraction procedures will themselves result in changes in composition and properties (Gotte, Stern, Elsden and Partridge, 1963). The answer is that there is no general method for the isolation of a homogeneous protein elastomer called elastin, and we have to choose our isolation procedure in relation to the kind of experiment we wish to perform and the kind of information we require.

The problem can be illustrated by some very recent work by Dr. Russell Ross and his colleagues about which we shall hear more later in this session. Dr. Ross, I think, started from electron microscope investigations, and observed that around young and growing elastic structures there is always a fringe of microfibrils which stain well with heavy metals. These microfibrils are very intimately associated with the amorphous, relatively nonstaining elastin, and are often occluded in structures of true elastin. The microfibrils present a quite different appearance from the proteoglycans (PG) of the ground-substance and they also make their appearance in all sorts of connective tissue structures, particularly in very young or foetal material. Quite vigorous chemical procedures have to be used to separate the microfibrils from the amorphous component of the fibre which is true elastin. Ross and Bornstein

(1969) have shown that dilute sodium hydroxide will effect this separation, but a more effective method is to solubilize the microfibrils with reducing thiols in 5 M guanidine solution.

The behaviour of the microfibrils is very similar to that of the glycoproteins which have been separated from human thoracic aorta, (Barnes and Partridge, 1968). Part of the glycoproteins can be separated from the elastic structures of the aorta with cold dilute sodium hydroxide but to remove all the glycoprotein fraction requires hot alkali. The amino acid composition of the glycoprotein fraction and the microfibrils is quite similar, and I understand from Dr. Ross that his microfibrilllar protein also contains neutral sugars. However, what is important to our present argument is that the observation of the microfibrils (and the glycoproteins) explains why it has always been so difficult to isolate chemically homogeneous elastin from the foetus or the embryo. In foetal tissue the insoluble and chemically resistant microfibrillar or glycoprotein fraction represents a considerable part of the newly formed elastic structures and is correspondingly difficult to remove. It was probably for this reason then that the early chemists, searching for elastin of authentic purity, tended to avoid foetal tissue and to concentrate exclusively on elastin from the ligamentum nuchae or the aorta of postnatal young animals.

Again the chemist meets difficulties when he attempts to isolate elastin from old or senile animals. The parts of the aorta near the atheromatous plaques in elderly humans is nearly always found to contain an elastin of slightly changed composition, and the same is true of human skin which has been exposed for years to ultraviolet light. Both these materials frequently contain an excess of polar amino acids which cannot be removed except by procedures so vigorous as to risk degradation of the elastin network itself. We know almost nothing about the origin of this extra peptide material which seems to become attached to the elastin network over a long period of time; however, we know that elastin is biologically very inert and after cessation of growth its turnover rate is vanishingly small (Walford, Carter and Schneider, 1964). It may be that it is for this reason that chemical changes can be observed in senile elastin that are not apparent in cellular proteins which are replaced and renewed throughout the lifetime of the animal.

In spite of our uncertainties about the chemical composition of developing elastic fibres and elastic structures in the senile animal I think it is true to say that we still have some assurance that, by utilising a variety of extraction methods, it is possible to separate a chemically defined elastin from collagen and other closely associated components of the fibre. I do not propose to attempt a detailed comparison of all the various extraction procedures for elastin that have been devised. Nevertheless, it is the concern of all of us to know if any part of the now accepted amino acid analysis of elastin isolated by the classical methods really belongs to some other component which cannot be regarded as part of the amorphous elastomer we know as "elastin". I think this kind of information will eventually come from researches such as those by Carnes and his colleagues at Salt Lake City. This group has isolated what appears to be a soluble protein precursor of elastin, now called "tropoelastin", from the aortas of copper deficient pigs. The soluble elastin precursor has a composition in general very similar to "standard pig elastin" but contains, as would be expected, a large excess of lysine (Smith, Weissman and Carnes, 1968; Sandberg, Hackett and Carnes, 1969). I am sure that Dr. Franzblau will discuss the formation of elastin crosslinkages from the side chains of lysine in his paper which is to follow.

Apart from the utilization of lysine during the formation of elastin crosslinks the question has remained as to whether elastin contains or does not contain hydroxyproline. We already know with certainty that the composition of elastin is unusual in that it contains very large amounts of glycine, proline and alanine. It also contains more valine than any other known protein. Large sections of the peptide chains of elastin must therefore be composed almost entirely of nonpolar amino acids.

In a recent paper Petruska and Sandberg (1968) compared a whole range of amino acid analyses carried out on elastin preparations of varying purity. The measurements were then extrapolated using increasing glycine content as a parameter of increasing purity. If the rather drastic assumption was made that elastin contains no hydroxyproline, then the result of the mathematical analysis was that bovine elastin could be comprised of a very simple polypeptide framework containing no methionine, cystine, serine, tryptophan, histidine, arginine or aspartic acid. Presumably we would have to assume that the demands of a protein elastomer are so specific that selection pressure has eliminated all mutations tending to introduce any of these seven amino acids into the structure of the elastin gel. However, the assuption that proline is not hydroxylated in elastin, as it is in collagen, appears to have no particular biological virtue. We ourselves have purified ligament elastin with hot sodium hydroxide to the point when hydrolysis rendered the material soluble. We then continued to fractionate the soluble product. On comparing the amino acid analyses of all the fractions, the results were extrapolated, <u>not</u> to hydroxyproline equals zero, but to a value for hydroxyproline of about 1.6%. Bentley and Hanson (1969) also came to the same conclusion after treating α-elastin with collagenase. There was no loss of hydroxyproline and it was concluded that this amino acid is indeed a constituent of elastin in which it occurs as a collagenase-resistant polypeptide sequence. A careful study by Steven and Jackson (1968), in which a combination of enzyme digestions were used to avoid the use of hot alkali, showed that the resulting elastins had much the same composition as standard alkali-treated elastin and contained about the same amount of hydroxyproline.

Finally, the soluble protein precursor of elastin, "tropoelastin", is reaching a state of high purity (Sandberg et al., 1969); however, the most recent analysis I have so far seen still shows an amino acid composition similar to that of standard insoluble pig elastin, except for the absence of the small amounts of methionine and histidine usually quoted. The molecular weight is given as 67,000 and the hydroxyproline content is 11.2 residues per thousand residues, which is about the same as for insoluble pig elastin. Desmosine, isodesmosine and lysinonorleucine are, of course, absent and the lysine content is 48 residues per thousand instead of about 8 residues per thousand in insoluble elastin.

The uncertainty of an amino acid analysis of an extracellular protein such as elastin arises because not all the amino acids are coded directly by DNA. Thus we must not expect each peptide unit to be an exact replica of a standard model. Proline hydroxylation within the confines of the cell may proceed to a variable extent and the extracellular oxidation of lysine to aldehyde, which is specific for some only of the lysine residues, may proceed to a variable extent in the formation of crosslinks. In addition, we know that other reactions such as glutamyl transaminations may occur in the connective tissue space and also that in older animals free radical scissions and additions may proceed irregularly as aspect of advancing age.

II AMINO ACID CROSSLINKS UNIQUE TO ELASTIN

It is scarcely possible to talk about the characterization of elastin without some mention of the crosslinking system and the biosynthetic process by which it arises. If elastin is hydrolysed with a series of proteolytic enzymes, in order to reduce it to small peptides, it is found that some of the peptides contain amino acids which are unique to this protein and which absorb strongly in ultraviolet light. Two amino acid isomers, desmosine and isodesmosine, have been isolated (Partridge, Elsden and Thomas, 1963; Thomas, Elsden and Partridge, 1963) and were found to contain a pyridinium ring which in both cases united four aliphatic side chains bearing α-amino acid terminals. The steric formulae of the desmosines are given in Fig. 1. It is evident that these amino acids are capable of cross-bridging up to four separate peptide-chains in the intact protein, and since they occur in peptide combination they were regarded as forming part of the crosslinking system of the protein elastomer.

The empirical formula of the desmosine isomers is $C_{24}H_{40}N_5O_8$ and this suggested that they could have arisen from four molecules of lysine with elimination of three ammonia residues. In the years 1961-64 several groups of workers in the United States reported that copper deficiency in chicken, turkeys and pigs results in aortic ruptures and physical and chemical changes in elastin. Copper deficient elastin swells more readily and is more easily soluble during partial hydrolysis with dilute sodium hydroxide, but the amino acid composition is similar except that it contains about three times the normal amount of lysine. These results suggest that, during fibrogenesis, some lysine side chains on a soluble proelastin are oxidised under the influence of a copper enzyme.

The information from the nutritional studies led us to begin collaboration with Dr. Albert Dorfman and his colleagues at Chicago in an attempt to study the biosynthesis by use of labelled amino acids. The results (Partridge et al., 1964, 1966) made it clear that four molecules of lysine are incorporated into the desmosine crosslink. The biosynthetic

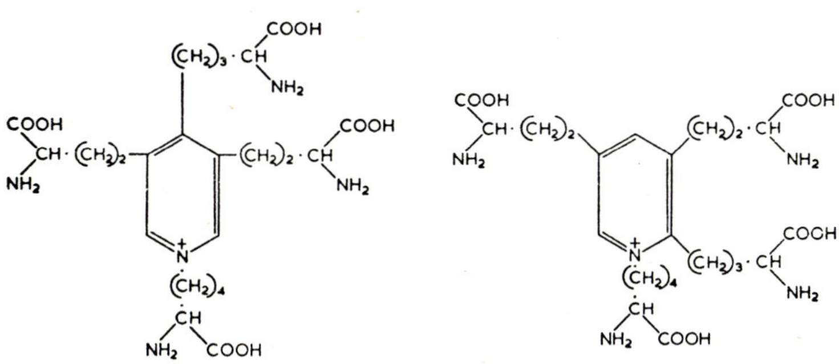

I - DESMOSINE

II - ISODESMOSINE

Fig. 1.

process is an uncommonly slow one and in the growing rat requires up to 17 days for completion. While this work was in progress a similar approach was made by Miller, Martin and Piez (1965) and their work gave similar results to our own.

We have already seen that copper is involved in some way in the process of crosslink formation and this suggests that the enzyme concerned in the preliminary oxidation of the ε-amino side chains of lysine may be similar to the amine oxidases that have been isolated from many animal tissues and are known to contain copper. It has also long been known that if lathyrogenic compounds are fed to young animals, there follows a marked reduction in the strength of collagenous tissues throughout the body. Reports by a number of workers have now shown that there are degenerative changes in the elastin of the aorta and a reduction in the amount of elastin in the blood vessels as a result of feeding β-aminopropionitrite (BAPN) (Dasler and Milliser, 1957; Savage, Bird, Reynolds and O'Dell, 1966). This might suggest that the lathyrogenic compounds act as metabolic inhibitors in the process of desmosine biosynthesis. Accordingly, the action of BAPN on the incorporation of lysine into desmosine was studied using aortas from ducklings grown in organ culture. The results (O'Dell et al., 1966) showed that the lathyrogen had no effect on the specific activity of lysine but the incorporation of lysine into the desmosines was markedly inhibited. Closely similar results have been obtained independently by Dr. Karl Piez and his colleagues at Bethesda (Miller et al., 1965).

In elastin from the aortas of copper deficient and lathyritic chicks the lysine content of the protein is much higher than normal, while the desmosine is the same or slightly reduced. The sum of lysine + quarter desmosine is not constant and in both lathyrism and copper deficiency is greatly in excess of the normal value. This suggests that in normal growing elastin there are present intermediates of desmosine synthesis, derived from lysine, which do not normally appear in the amino acid analysis of the hydrolysate. One of these intermediates is undoubtedly α-aminoadipic semialdehyde since we were able to isolate 6-hydroxynorleucine from elastin which had been reduced with borohydride. However, the amount of hydroxynorleucine isolated accounted for only about 1/20 of the discrepancy and there must be other intermediates, derived from lysine, which have not yet been identified.

In an attempt to trace some of the intermediate steps in desmosine biosynthesis the aortas of day old ducklings were labelled with [^{14}C]lysinein tissue culture. Figure 2 (a) shows the pattern obtained from normal growing aorta tissue. The position of the lysine-labelled peaks due to the unknown intermediates of desmosine biosynthesis can be exactly logged by reference to the position of the normal amino acids found in the same fractions. Some of the labelled peaks formed arise by degradation reactions occurring during the hydrolysis of the elastin with 6 N hydrochloric acid. It was thought however that degradation reactions of this sort could be avoided by reducing the elastin with sodium borohydride before acid hydrolysis in order to convert aldols, aldehydes and Schiff bases to more stable compounds. The hydrolysis products of reduced elastin are shown in Fig. 2b. During the reduction with borohydride desmosine and isodesmosine form reduced products which migrate with a rather higher elution volume in the buffers used. The most striking effect however is a reduction in the counts associated with free lysine and unidentified intermediates and replacement by a new peak which occupied a position somewhat overlapping lysinonorleucine.

In view of the possible importance of this new amino acid as a derivative of lysine, its isolation was attempted from a large quantity (1 kg) of elastin purified by alkali extraction from the <u>ligamentum nuchae</u> of young heifers and steers (Starcher, Partridge and Elsden, 1967). I will not attempt to detail the isolation procedure, but we obtained just over 80 mg of material which we thought was pure. This quantity was very small, but a few chemical procedures were possible. The best empirical formula we could obtain

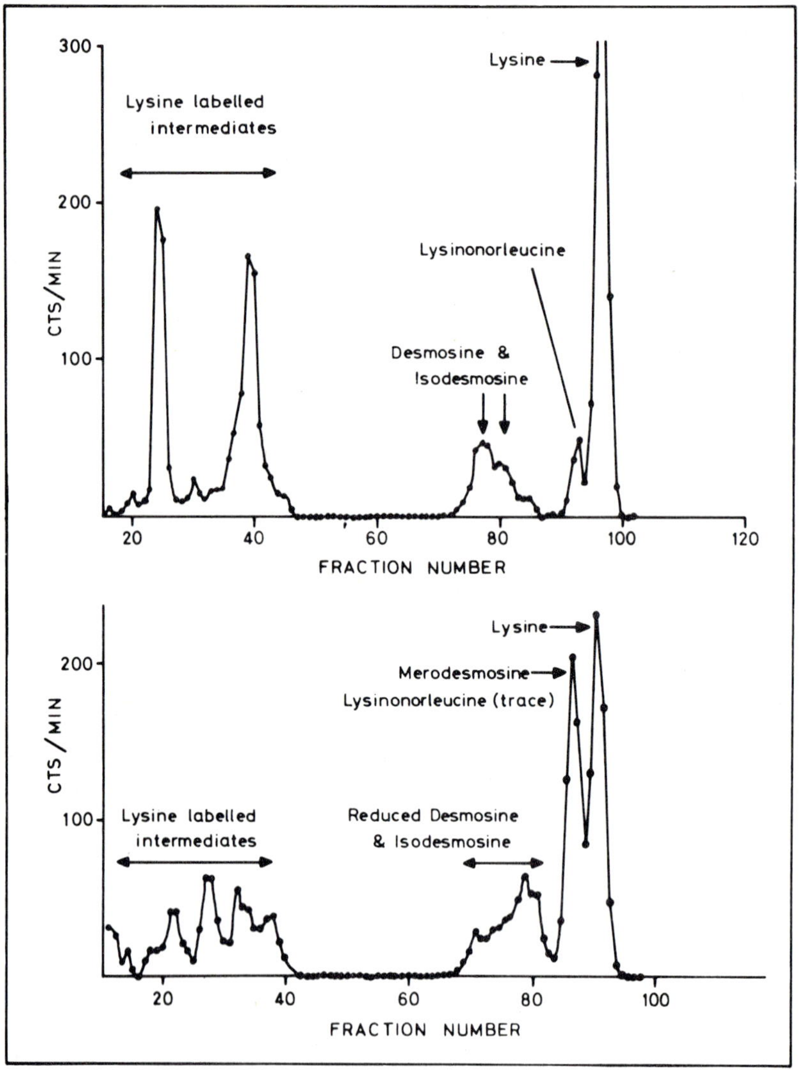

Fig. 2. (a) Chromatographic separation of the hydrolysis products of elastin labelled with [^{14}C]lysine in tissue culture. Fractions 20-50 contain compounds arising from lysine, which are believed to be derived from intermediates in desmosine biosynthesis. (b) Chromatogram of the hydrolysis products of elastin after reduction with unlabelled borohydride. The appearance of the new lysine-labelled amino acid "merodesmosine" is dependent upon prior treatment of the elastin with alkali, and is accompanied by a reduction in the amount of labelled lysine and lysine-derived intermediates.

by combustion was $C_{18}H_{34}O_6N_4H_2O$ from which molecular weight (calc.) was 420. The molecular weight found by use of a vapor pressure osmometer was 436.

Since the new compound (now called "merodesmosine") incorporated the lysine label and had 18 carbon atoms it seemed possible that it could be derived from three molecules of lysine. No evidence of a heterocyclic ring could be found from ultraviolet, infrared or NMR spectra, and it was concluded that the compound was aliphatic. Comparison of its electrophoretic mobility with lysine, lysinonorleucine and desmosine suggested that the compound contained three potential negative charges and four potential positive charges.

There was some difficulty in finding a derivative which was volatile enough and stable enough to give a good mass spectrum but eventually we found that the derivative produced by N-acylation with trifluoracetic anhydride and esterification with butanol was suitable. In the mass spectrum the highest recorded ion occurred at m/e 954, which corresponds to the molecular ion expected for the tetra-N-acyl tributyl ester.

An exact mass measurement was made of this molecular ion and gave a value 954.3628±.009 for which the only reasonable result is $C_{38}H_{54}N_4F_{12}O_{10}$. This confirms that the derivative is indeed the expected tetra-N-trifluoroacetyl tri-N-butyl ester and the formation of this derivative locates the four nitrogen atoms in merodesmosine as primary or secondary amino residues, and the six oxygen atoms as three carboxyl residues. The results as a whole allow a partial characterization of mesodesmosine as follows:

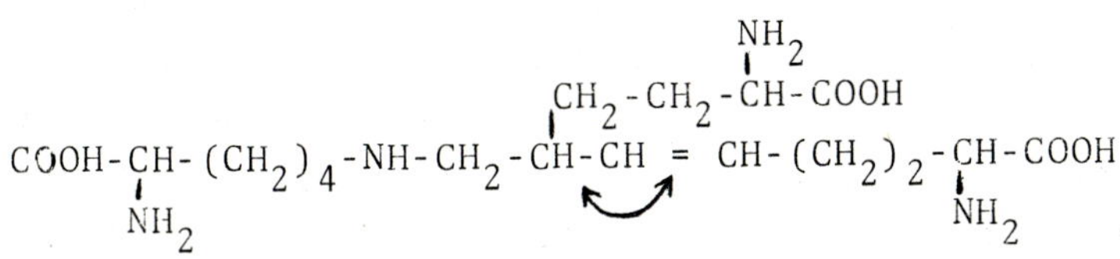

Merodesmosine

We do not know the exact position of the double bond but the two most probable positions are shown.

Figure 3 shows a possible interpretation of the biosynthetic reactions leading to the desmosines. Although many details of the biosynthetic pathway still require elicidation it seems clear that the process is a slow one, requiring many steps, and that during a period of time before the formation of a permanent chemical link, by cyclization to the desmosine ring, the situation can best be described as a dynamic equilibrium of reversible aldols and Schiff bases.

We believe that the importance of this result lies in the demonstration that the first products in the process of desmosine formation are labile Schiff bases and aldols some of which can easily be reversed by variations in pH or by the presence of aldehyde reagents or lathyrogens such as penicillamine. There now seems no doubt that aldols and Schiff bases from lysine and hydroxylysine are also the first steps in collagen crosslinkage formation, and it is easier to understand the reversal of early crosslinkage by lathyrogens and indeed the remodelling which occurs during the growth of collagenous and elastic tissues. The basic principle which appears to be emerging is that both with collagen and elastin the first corsslinkages to be formed are labile and reversible, and as the tissue matures these temporary links are afterwards consolidated by a further chemical change.

When either BAPN or low concentrations of semicarbazide are added to aorta tissue cultures given a pulse dose of [^{14}C]lysine as in the experiments of Fig. 2, the label appears in the chromatogram of the elastin hydrolysate only as free lysine. Thus both types of reagent completely inhibit the formation of desmosine intermediates, without significantly reducing the incorporation of lysine into the growing elastin. Since no other radioactive amino acids were found, the effect must be due to the inhibition of the first step in the train of desmosine intermediates; the initial oxidation of lysine to α-aminoadipic semialdehyde.

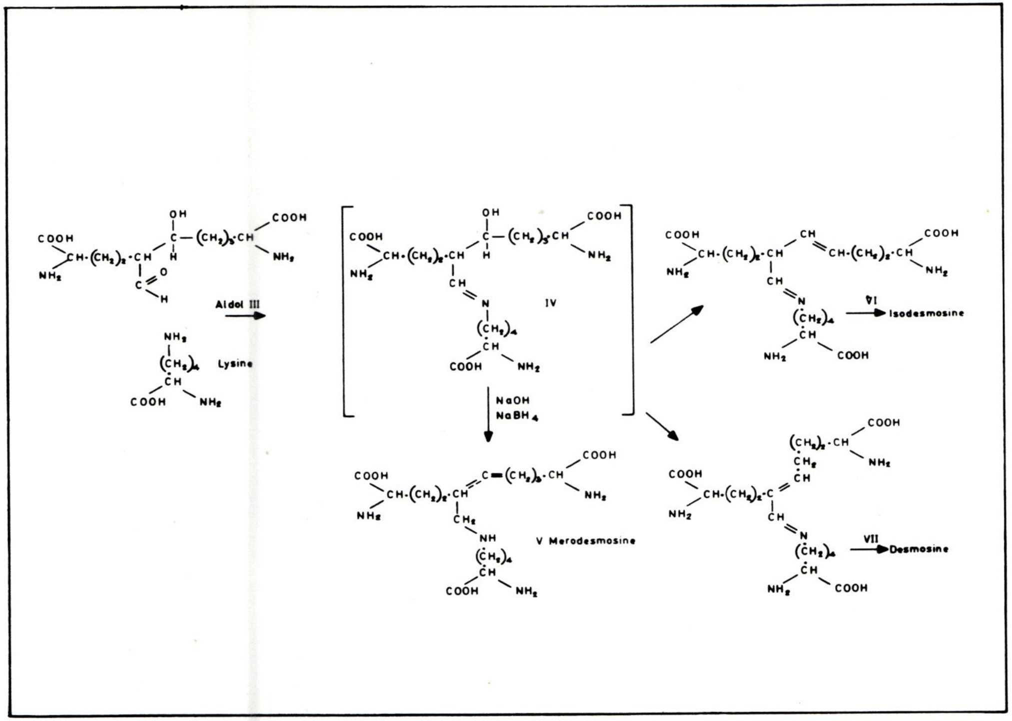

Fig. 3. Scheme proposed for part of the biosynthetic route to the desmosine isomers. The formation of the stable reduced compound merodesmosine V from the system of labile intermediates is favoured by alkaline conditions. The structure of the unstable compound IV is deduced from the isolation of merodesmosine. Dehydration of IV on either side of the carbinol hydroxyl yields a pair of isomers which form desmosine or isodesmosine when cyclized with a third oxidized lysine side-chain.

III CHARACTERISATION OF ELASTIN

Turning now more specifically to the question of the characterisation of elastin of course any property, chemical or physical, can be used to characterise a protein. In general, methods for the characterization of elastin by the description of its physical properties have not received much attention. This may be due largely to the difficulties of making measurements with a protein which is quite insoluble in any solvent. However, various ways of circumventing this are now beginning to appear and our first crude models of elastin, based almost entirely on rubber theory, are being replaced by rather more sophisticated models to accommodate an increasing amount of reliable data.

An approach of this sort was made by ourselves two or three years ago, when we attempted to estimate "an equivalent diameter" for the size of the pores in the water-swollen elastin gel. This was done by packing a filtration tube with elastin fibres and using it as a gel filtration column. The elastin column was used for the chromatography of sugars, glycols and alcohols of different molecular weight (Partridge, 1967a). This is not the place to go into details of this technique, but the results of the work indicated that water-swollen elastin could be regarded as a gel containing pore spaces equivalent to cylinders of 32 Å in diameter: or alternatively, within the accuracy of the measurements, it may be regarded as a structure with about 55% free water and composed of randomly disposed hydrated rods about 16 Å in diameter. The water between the hydrated rods behaved as "free-water" and was available for the solution of solutes up to a molecular weight of about 1,000 (Partridge, 1967b).

It seems to me that the importance of this information lies in the fact that it tells us what the structure of elastin <u>is not</u>. The structure is not that of a network of substantially independent hydrated peptide chains such as might be expected, for instance, in a gelatin gel crosslinked with a bi-functional aldehyde; and it is not a structure of formed anisometric units of fibrillar dimensions. In fact the structural elements found are of intermediate size and are small enough to account for the amorphous appearance of elastin under the light microscope and at low magnifications in the electron microscope. Actually electron microscope pictures of negatively stained elastin particles by Cox and O'Dell (1966) and other later workers have agreed rather well with this concept of structure, though it should be borne in mind that with the staining techniques adopted we are looking at the dried, collapsed gel. Figure 7a and b shows recent electronmicrographs, prepared by C.A. Voyle in my laboratory, which compare the elastin fibre and the coacervate precipitated from soluble α-elastin. Half of the figure is a particle of elastin, negatively stained and dried, and the other half is a droplet of soluble α-elastin, precipitated at 37°C, and negatively stained and dried as before. It will be seen that the two structures have a basic similarity: both appear to be composed of a basketwork of short bent rods. In the dried elastin fibre these rods are about 12-15 Å in diameter. The coacervate of soluble elastin appears to have a looser structure, and this may be because it is a very thin film precipitated on to the surface of the grid from dilute solution at 37°C. It is impossible to say at the present time if this difference in appearance is related to differences in film thickness or if it represents a difference in conformational form.

Although the material of the elastin fibre always presents the same uniform, fine-grained structure when examined at magnifications of the order 1,000,000 details of the structure (in so far as they are resolved), appear to be sharply dependent upon the procedure used for staining and preparation. The electron microscope pattern is particularly sensitive to the degree to which the structure has collapsed on drying out. In collaboration with Dr. Sylvia Fitton Jackson and Miss Judy Goldstein we attempted to avoid collapse of the structure by filling the water spaces with a polyglycol (Fitton Jackson, Goldstein and Partridge, 1967). It was found that the structure then presents a different appearance and takes the form of a rather disordered array of spheroidal particles about 40-50 Å in diameter. This is illustrated in Fig. 7c in which lightly stained elastin fibres were equilibrated with a series of polyglycols prior to fine-grinding and application to the grid.

It should perhaps be mentioned at this point that when elastic fibres are reduced to very fine particles by ultrasonic irradiation, electronmicroscopic observation of the smaller particles reveals the presence of fibrillar structures of varying diameter and appearance (Gotte and Serafini-Fracassini, 1963; Serafini-Fracassini and Tristram, 1966). It is thought that these structures may arise from local configurational changes brought about by superstretching under the influence of an intense force-field. If this is so, the fibrilllar conformation of elastin should be regarded as a manifestation of a form of denaturation brought about by mechanical stress, and its existence may have important biological implications.

Considerations deriving from the biogenesis of fibrous elastin from a soluble globular precursor; from the dimensions of the water spaces as revealed by the molecular exclusion studies; and finally from the structure as revealed by the electron microscope have together led us to suggest a model for the structure of elastin based on the presence of regions of hydrophobic interaction relatively free from water. These regions were assumed to derive directly from the corpuscular molecules of the soluble tropoelastin synthesized by the cell.

Figure 4 is the model drawn in two-dimensions. It is assumed that when elastin is swollen in water, the centre part of the spheres is largely hydrophobic with a hydrated interface between the rather globular particles and the water spaces surrounding them. The concept is similar in principle to that of Richards and Knowles (1968) who studied the reactions of glutaraldehyde with protein crystals. It

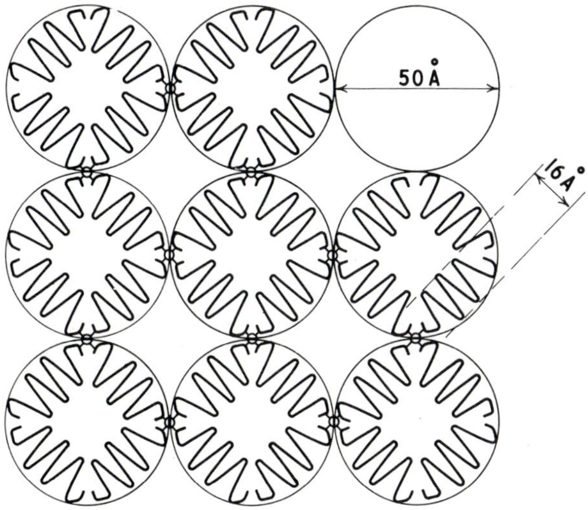

Fig. 4. Two-dimensional representation of a model for the structure of elastin incorporating measurements from the electronmicrographs and gel filtration experiments. Reproduced from page 245 of Fibrous Proteins (Butterworth, Australia, 1968) by permission of the editors.

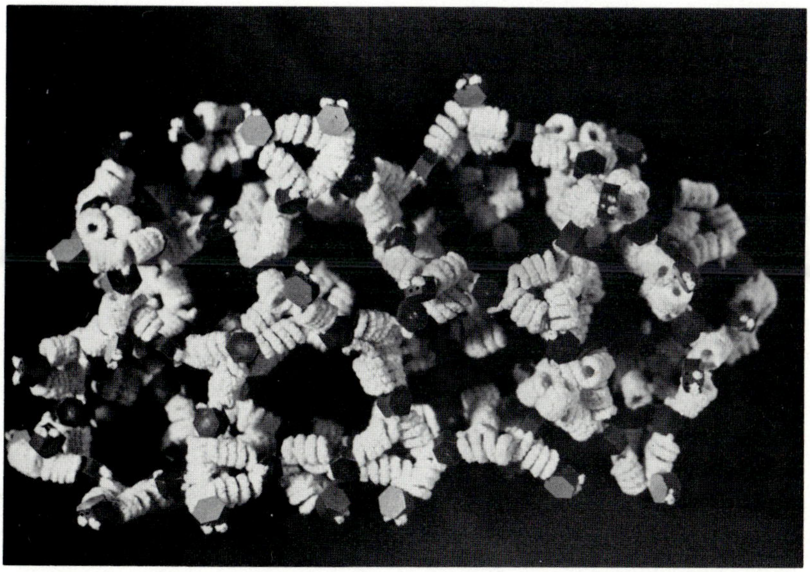

Fig. 5. Photograph of a three-dimensional model constructed on the basis of Fig. 4.

was observed that glutaraldehyde crosslinks occurred at the interface of the globular protein molecules in such a way as to render the whole material of the crystal insoluble. For several proteins the reaction did not disorder the crystal structure and very similar single-crystal X-ray defraction patterns resulted from treated and untreated protein. In other cases some disordering did occur, presumably because the crosslinks themselves resulted in the enforcement of new conformations. It is evident that, if such a crosslinked structure is dried out, the water interface disappears and the globular shape of the particle is lost, although it may be recovered again on rehydration. Figure 5 shows a three-dimensional model representing, in a tentative way, the kind of structure proposed. Of course these models are intended at the present time solely as a summary of the rather sparce information at present available and as a means of formulating further research ideas.

It will be observed that models of the kind indicated above contain the possibility of almost unlimited continuous conformational change and are also capable of a sharply discontinuous change involving penetration of the hydrophobic centres by water. In envisaging such a model we make the assumption that the entropy change due to elastic stretching and recoil may be accounted for in part by a change in conformational entropy and in part by the change in the area of the internal water interfaces. However, the problem of elasticity and structure will be treated in some detail later both by Professor Weis-Fogh and by Professor Volpin.

IV CONFORMATIONAL CHANGES IN THE STRUCTURE OF ELASTIN

A structure consisting of free water spaces and hydrophobic centres also offers an explanation for the phenomenon of coacervation observed with α-elastin. The coacervate phase has a water content a little less than elastin fibres swollen in the same buffer. Phase separation of the coacervate occurs on raising the temperature to about 37°C, and may be due to a conformational change involving hydration of the hydrophobic centres and a reduction in the water of swelling. It was thought possible that such a conformational change would result in a corresponding change in the circular dichroism pattern during the act of coacervation. Professor Gotte and his colleagues at Padua had already reported a change in the circular dichroism pattern of α-elastin brought about by the addition of ethanol (Mammi, Gotte and Pezzin, 1968) and postulated a continuous increase in helix content as the alcohol content of the solvent is increased.

In collaboration with Drs. Urry and Starcher in Chicago, (Urry, Starcher and Partridge, 1969) the circular dichroism of the solution phase and the coacervate phase of soluble α-elastin was compared. Figure 6 shows the results. The spectrum of the solution phase resembles that of disordered proteins and peptides, whereas the spectrum of the coacervate phase is characteristic of those obtained for highly helical proteins and polypeptides. The dotted curve in Figure 6 is the curve for the coacervate corrected for absorption flattening due to particulate systems, using the method of Urry and Ji (1968). This curve is typical of a protein with about 50% α-helix content. Unfortunately at present we have no means of knowing if the elastin in the elastic fibre resembles α-elastin in solution at 10°C or α-elastin as a coacervate at 40°C.

In the last two or three years there have been numerous observations of the physical properties of elastin which confirm the presence in this protein of substantial centres of hydrophobic interaction. Thus Robert and Poullain (1963) and Kornfeld-Poullain and Robert (1968) have observed a marked increase in the rate of alkaline hydrolysis of elastin in the presence of the lower alcohols. From analysis of the data they conclude that the effect is due to penetration of the hydrophobic centres by the water-alcohol mixture. I understand that Dr. Robert will be telling us about this work in more detail later.

A similar conclusion was reached in some very recent

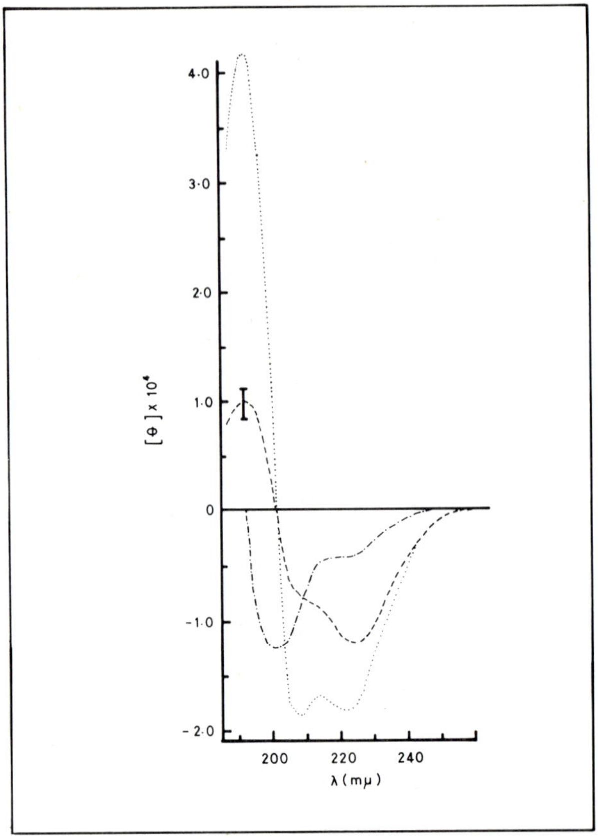

Fig. 6. Circular dichroism curves for elastin preparations. The mean residue ellipticity [θ] was calculated using a mean residue molecular weight of 80.7 — — —, solution spectrum; - - - coacervate film spectrum; . . . coacervate film spectrum after making corrections for absorption flattening and dispersion distortions.

Fig. 7.a)Elastin fibres were stained with phosphotungstic acid (PTA) at pH 6.75, washed thoroughly with water and ground wet in an agate mortar. The electron micrograph shows the edge of a thin particle. Instrument magnification 100,000. Magnification as at (c)

b)α-Elastin was allowed to coacervate at 37°C and a thin film of the coacervate collected on a grid. Film stained at 37°C with PTA (pH 6.9) magnification as (c).

c)Stained and washed elastin fibres were equilibrated with glycerol followed by a range of polyethyleneglycols up to MW 1000. The fibres were then ground in glycol suspension in an agate mortar and a droplet of the slurry applied to the grid. Excess glycol was removed by standing over night on blotting paper. Bar = 300 Å.

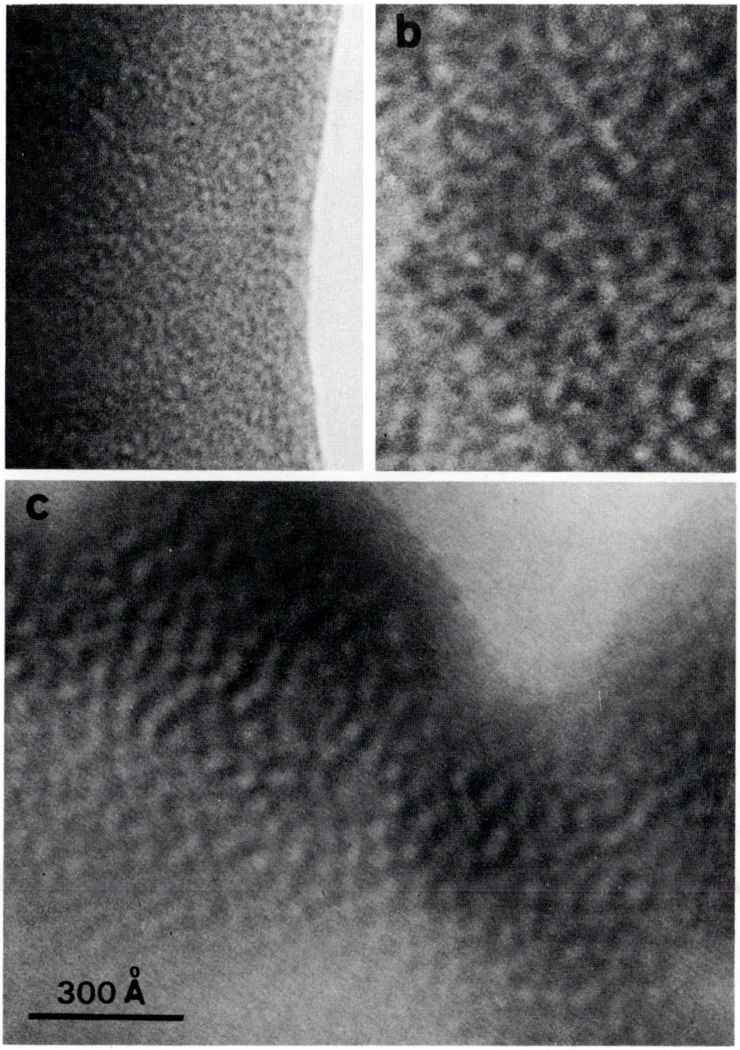
b
c
300 Å

work by Hoffman and Mukherjee (1969) in which a fresh attempt was made to estimate the molecular weight of the kinetically free portion of the chains between crosslinks. In the older work (cf. Hoeve and Flory, 1958) the stress/strain curves were measured either in water or glycol-water mixtures, and under these conditions the between-crosslink molecular weight was estimated at about 3,400. This chain weight would indicate the presence of considerably more crosslinks in elastin than are found chemically on the basis of desmosine, isodesmosine and lysinonorleucine content. However, Hoffman and Mukherjee (1969) found that if they swelled the elastin in formamide or formamide-water mixtures then the between-crosslink molecular weight rose to about 8,000. The effect of formamide increased to a maximum at a formamide-water ratio of about 40% and then flattened off.

The value for the between-crosslink molecular weight found in formamide solution correlates very well with the known content of the desmosines and lysinonorleucine assuming a model of the kind indicated in Figs. 4 and 5. The explanation of the effect of formamide-water given by Hoffman and Mukherjee (1969) was that the solution parameters of the 40% mixture were closely similar to the solubility parameters of the more hydrophobic peptide sequences. This would be expected to result in the abolition of hydrophobic interactions which enforce additional constraints on the peptide chains in elastin samples swollen in pure water. The gradual conformational change brought about by increasing concentrations of formamide was not quite reversed when the elastin was attacked by pancreatic elastases at a much faster rate than elastin which had never been exposed to formamide.

REFERENCES

Barnes, M.J. and Partridge, S.M. (1968). Biochem. J. 109, 883.

Bentley, J.P. and Hanson, A.N. (1969). Biochim. Biophys. Acta 175, 339.

Cox, R.W. and O'Dell, B.L. (1966). J.Roy. Microsc. Soc. 85, 401.

Dasler, W. and Milliser, R.V. (1957). Proc. Exptl. Biol. Med. 96, 171.

Fitton Jackson, S., Goldstein, J. and Partridge, S.M. (1967). Reported by Partridge, S.M. In Symposium on Fibrous Proteins, P. 245. Butterworths, Australia (1968).

Gotte, L., Stern, P., Elsden, D.F. and Partridge, S.M. (1963). Biochem. J. 87, 344.

Gotte, L. and Serafini-Fracassini, A. (1963). J. Atheroscher. Res. 3, 247.

Hoeve, S.A.J. and Flory, P.J. (1958). J. Am. Chem. Soc. 80, 6523.

Hoffman, A.S. and Mukherjee, D.P. (1969). In Mukherjee, D.P., Thesis submitted for the degree of D.Sci. Massachusetts Institute of Technology, Boston, January 1969.

Kornfeld-Poullain, N. and Robert, L. (1968). Bull. Soc. Chim. Biol. 50, 759.

Mammi, M., Gotte, L. and Pezzin, G. (1968). Nature 220, 371.

Miller, E.J., Martin, G.R., Mecca, C.E. and Piez, K.A. (1965). Nature 209, 401 (1966).

Miller, E.J., Martin, G.R., and Piez, K.A. (1965). Fed. Proc. 24 (Pt. 1) 359 (Abstr. No. 1271).

O'Dell, B.L., Elsden, D.F., Thomas, J., Partridge, S.M., Smith, R.H. and Palmer, R. (1966). Nature 209, 401.

Partridge, S.M. (1967a). Nature (Lond.) 213, 1123.

Partridge, S.M. (1967b). Biochim. Biophys. Acta 140, 132.

Partridge, S.M., Elsden, D.F. and Thomas, J. (1963). Nature 197, 1279.

Partridge, S.M., Elsden, D.F., Thomas, J., Dorfman, A., Telser, S. and Pei-Lee Ho (1964). Biochem. J. 93, 30c.

Partridge, S.M., Elsden, D.F., Thomas, J., Dorfman, A., Telser, A. and Pei-Lee Ho (1966). Nature 209, 399.

Petruska, J.A. and Sandberg, L.B. (1968). Biochem. Biophys. Res. Comm. 33, 222.

Richards, F.M. and Knowles, J.R. (1968). J. Mol. Biol. 37, 231.

Robert, L. and Poullain, N. (1963). Bull. Soc. Chim. Biol. 45, 1317.

Ross, R. and Bornstein, P. (1969). J. Cell Biol. 40, 366.

Sandberg, L.B., Hackett, T.N. and Carnes, W.H. (1969). Biochim. Biophys. Acta 181, 201.

Savage, J.E., Bird, D.W., Reynolds, G. and O'Dell, B.L. (1966). J. Nutr. 88, 15.

Serafini-Fracassini, A. and Tristram, G.R. (1966). Proc. Roy. Soc. Edinburgh. Section B. 69, 334.

Smith, D.W., Weissman, N. and Carnes, W.H. (1968). Biochem. Biophys. Res. Comm. 31, 309.

Starcher, B.C., Partridge, S.M. and Elsden, D.F. (1967). Biochemistry 6, 2425.

Steven, F.S. and Jackson, D.S. (1968). Biochim. Biophys. Acta 168, 333.

Thomas, J., Elsden, D.F. and Partridge, S.M. (1963). Nature 222, 795.

Urry, D.W. and Ji, T.H. (1968). Arch. Biochim. Biophys. 128, 802.

Urry, D.W., Starcher, B. and Partridge, S.M. (1969). Nature 222, 795.

Walford,R.L., Carter, P.K. and Schneider, R.B. (1964). Arch. Pathol. 78, 43.

CHEMISTRY AND BIOSYNTHESIS OF CROSSLINKS IN ELASTIN

C. Franzblau, B. Faris, R. W. Lent, L. L. Salcedo, B. Smith,
R. Jaffe and G. Crombie

I DESMOSINES

Little is known of the amino acid sequence and three-dimensional structure of elastin but a great deal has been learned about the chemistry and biosynthesis of the cross-links. We owe much of the pioneering work on these cross-links to Partridge and his collaborators. As reported at the NATO conference five years ago (Partridge, Thomas and Elsden, 1965) these workers were able to isolate from an acid hydrolysate of elastin two new polyfunctional amino acids which they designated as desmosine and isodesmosine. Each of these amino acids were shown to contain a pyridine nucleus alkylated in four positions including the ring nitrogen. They differed only in the position of ring substitution. The structure of these amino acids are shown in Fig. 1.

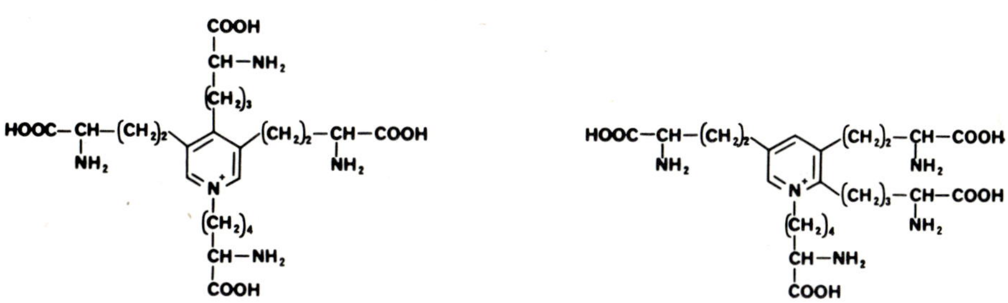

Fig. 1. Structure of desmosine (left) and isodesmosine (right).

On the basis of their structures and the nature of the peptides in which they were contained, it was proposed by the group in Cambridge (Thomas, Elsden and Partridge, 1963) that desmosine and isodesmosine are involved in the cross-linking of elastin. The number of peptide chains cross-linked by these unusual amino acids is still unknown. As illustrated in Fig. 2, it is possible for two, three or four peptide chains to be crosslinked by one desmosine or isodesmosine molecule.

To gain more insight into the nature of the crosslinking in elastin we attempted to isolate, from various proteolytic digests of elastin, peptides enriched in desmosine and isodesmosine. In the course of this study, we observed that such peptides could be obtained but that they contained yet another undescribed amino acid, which we originally designated as X_4 (Franzblau, Sinex and Faris, 1965a).

II LYSINONORLEUCINE

This amino acid was isolated from a total acid hydrolysate of elastin by the usual chromatographic techniques.

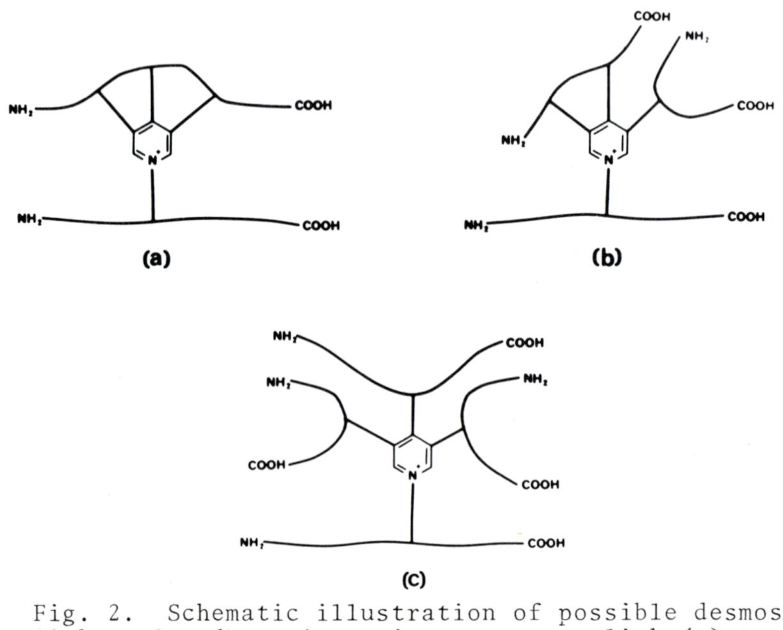

Fig. 2. Schematic illustration of possible desmosine crosslinks. One desmosine moiety may crosslink (a) two peptide chains, (b) three peptide chains, or (c) four peptide chains.

In contrast to the desmosines, the purified material did not absorb ultraviolet light over the range 220 to 340 mμ. The infrared spectrum was typical of an amino acid and additional studies which included potentiometric titrations, NMR spectra among others suggested the presence of two primary and one secondary group. These data, together with determination of α-amino groups by a manometric ninhydrin method, total amino groups by a nitrous acid method, total nitrogen, and total carbon, led to formulation of the structure shown in Fig. 3. Proof of structrue of this compound was confirmed by synthesis and we suggested the trivial name, lysinonorleucine (Franzblau, Sinex, Faris and Lampidis, 1965b). A more efficient method for the synthesis of lysinonorleucine has recently been employed (Franzblau, Faris and Papaioannou, 1969). This procedure is a modification of that used by Speck, Rowley and Horecker (1963) for the synthesis of N-ε-glyceryllysine. Briefly, 5-δ-bromobutylhydantoin is refluxed with N-α-benzoyllysine ethyl ester in tetrahydrofuran. The reaction mixture is concentrated and then treated with alkali to form lysinonorleucine. The polyfunctional structure of lysinonorleucine suggests that it, like the desmosines, also serves a crosslinking function in elastin. As illustrated in Fig.4, a lysinonorleucine residue is capable of crosslinking two peptide chains.

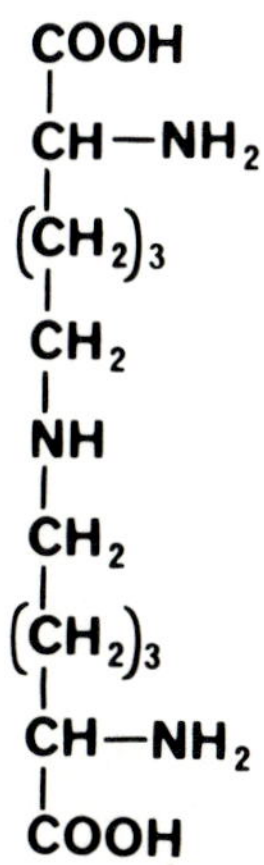

Fig. 3. Structure of lysinonorleucine.

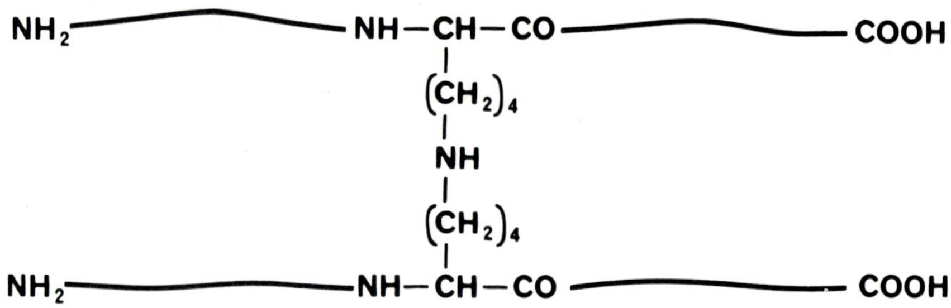

Fig. 4. Schematic illustration of lysinonorleucine crosslink.

III ALDOL CONDENSATION PRODUCT OF α-AMINOADIPIC-δ-SEMIALDEHYDE

Most recently our studies on the reduction of elastin with sodium borohydride have led to the isolation of what we believe to be still another crosslinking amino acid in elastin (Lent, Smith, Salcedo, Faris and Franzblau, 1969). To obtain this compound, reduced bovine elastin was hydrolyzed in 2 N NaOH and the resulting hydrolysate placed on an amino acid analyzer. The compound which eluted in the region between leucine and tyrosine on the analyzer was collected in fractions, desalted, and its ethyl ester prepared. The mass spectrum of the derivative was consistent with the structure of the reduced aldol condensation product of two molecules of α-aminoadipic acid-δ-semialdehyde (Fig. 5). However, the value obtained for the molecular ion needs further explanation.

A. STRUCTURE

If one examines the structure of the compound shown in Fig. 5, one would have expected a molecular ion of 330 for the diethyl ester derivative. However, a molecular ion of 358 was obtained. It appears, therefore, that under the conditions of esterification employed not only were the carboxyl groups esterified but additionally the α,β unsaturated

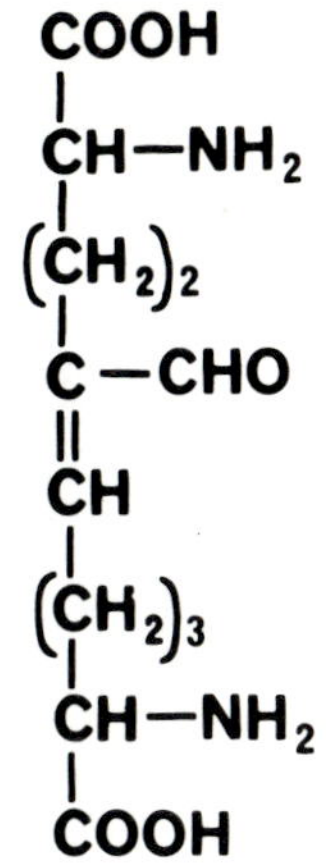

Fig. 5. Aldol condensation product of two molecules of α-aminoadipic-δ-semialdehyde.

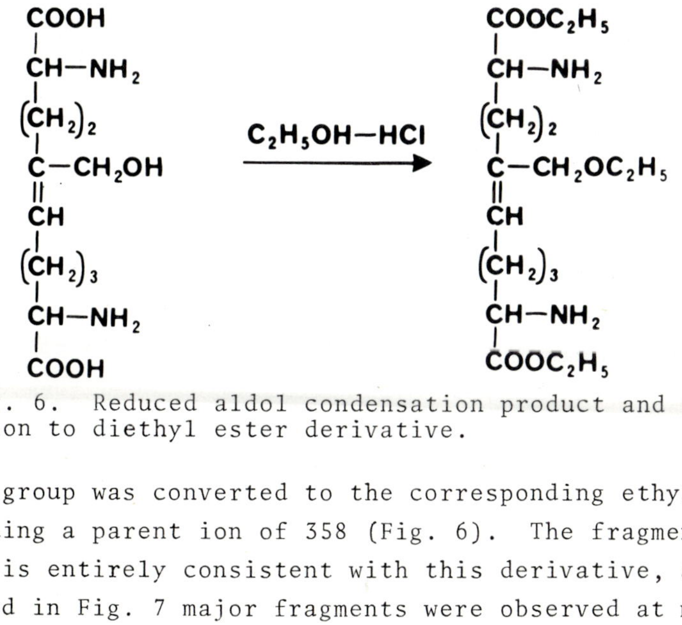

Fig. 6. Reduced aldol condensation product and its conversion to diethyl ester derivative.

alcohol group was converted to the corresponding ethyl ether yielding a parent ion of 358 (Fig. 6). The fragmentation pattern is entirely consistent with this derivative, and as indicated in Fig. 7 major fragments were observed at m/e of 313, 312, 299, 285, 239 and 83. The most plausible structures for this fragmentation pattern are also illustrated in Fig. 7, along with the parent ion itself. As can be seen, the fragment of m/e 313 results from the loss of O C_2H_5; that of 312 results from the loss of C_2H_5OH; that of 299 results from the loss of $CH_2OC_2H_5$ and that of 239 results from the loss of C_2H_5OH + $COOC_2H_5$. The fragment of 83

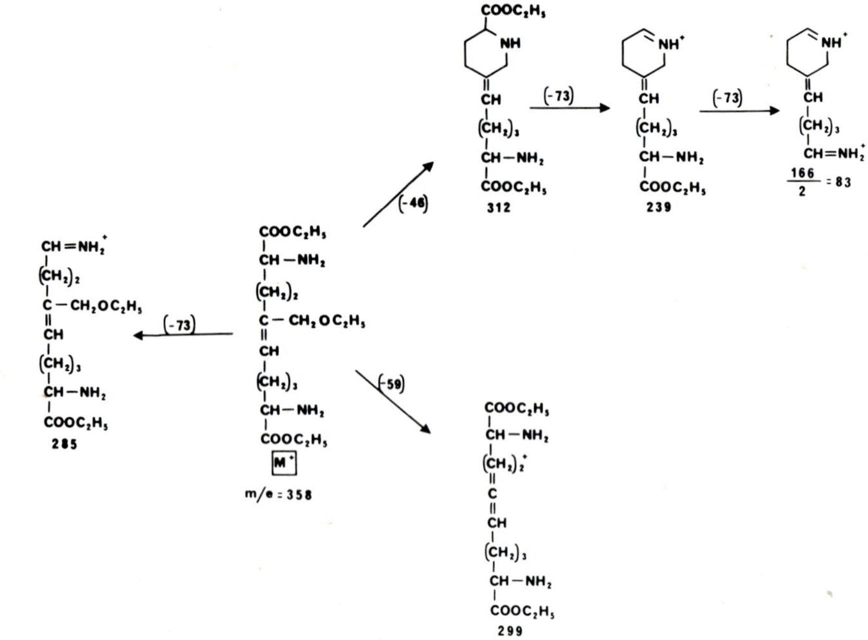

Fig. 7. Schematic illustration of major fragments obtained in the mass spectrometer from reduced derivatized aldol condensation product.

most likely arises from the formation of a diamine fragment which is also illustrated in the figure.

Further proof of the structure given in Fig. 5 comes from data obtained from periodate-permanganate oxidation studies. According to the procedure followed (Lemieux and von Rudloff, 1955) oxidation of 1 mole of an allylic alcohol should result in the appearance of 1 mole of formaldehyde and 2 moles of carboxylic acid. This is schematically illustrated in Fig. 8. If the two R groups in the allylic alcohol are different then oxidation will result in formation of two different carboxylic acids. If oxidation is not complete, as we found to be true, one will obtain instead of carboxylic acids, the corresponding aldehydes. Examine the possible products of a periodate-permanganate oxidation of the reduced aldol condensation product mentioned above. As seen in Fig. 9, depending upon where one places the double bond, oxidation would yield the following results. If

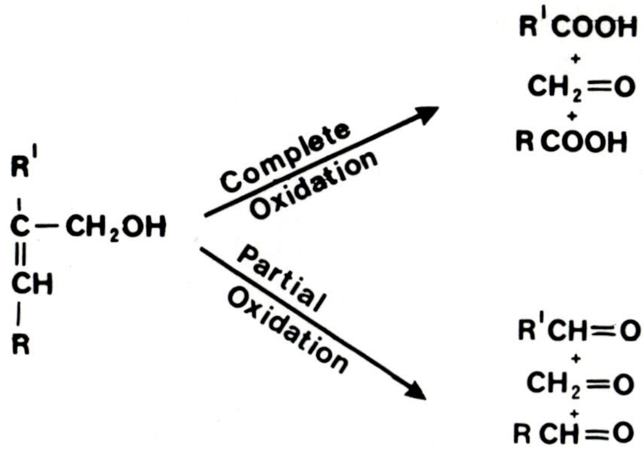

Fig. 8. Periodate-permanganate oxidation of an allylic alcohol.

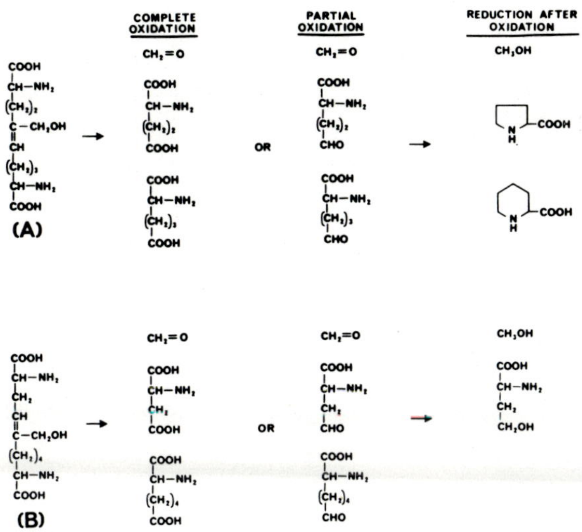

Fig. 9. Periodate-permanganate oxidation of the reduced aldol condensation product of two molecules of α-aminoadipic-δ-semialdehyde. See text for details.

the double bond is located as illustrated in structure (A) of Fig. 9, complete oxidation would yield 1 mole formaldehyde, 1 mole of α-aminoadipic acid and 1 mole of glutamic acid. If oxidation is not complete then one mole of the compound would yield 1 mole of formaldehyde, 1 mole of glutamic γ-semialdehyde, and 1 mole of adipic acid-δ-semialdehyde. These resulting semialdehydes are then capable of cyclizing to their corresponding Schiff bases and subsequent reduction should result in the formation of proline and pipecolic acid respectively. If these compounds are reduced with $NaBT_4$ then one should obtain radioactive proline and radioactive pipecolic acid. If the double bond is located as illustrated in Structure (B) of Fig. 9, complete oxidation of the aldol condensation product should result in the formation of 1 mole of formaldehyde, 1 mole of aspartic acid and 1 mole of α-aminopimelic acid. If oxidation is not complete, then one would obtain in addition to 1 mole of formaledhyde, 1 mole each of aspartic acid β-semialdehyde and the ε-semialdehyde of α-aminopimelic acid. Reduction of these latter compounds would yield homoserine and most likely the corresponding 7-carbon hydroxyamino acid. The results of our oxidation studies are summarized in Fig. 10. For every mole of amino acid oxidized we obtained 0.92 moles of formaldehyde. Amino acid analyses of the oxidation reaction mixture indicated the presence of aspartic acid, glutamic acid and α-aminoadipic acid. Reduction of the oxidation reaction mixture with $NaBT_4$ resulted in the formation of radioactive proline and radioactive pipecolic acid. From these data it is not certain where the double bond actually exists. The data suggests a possibility that the compound may exist in both forms. It is noted that the location of the double bond in merodesmosine (Starcher,

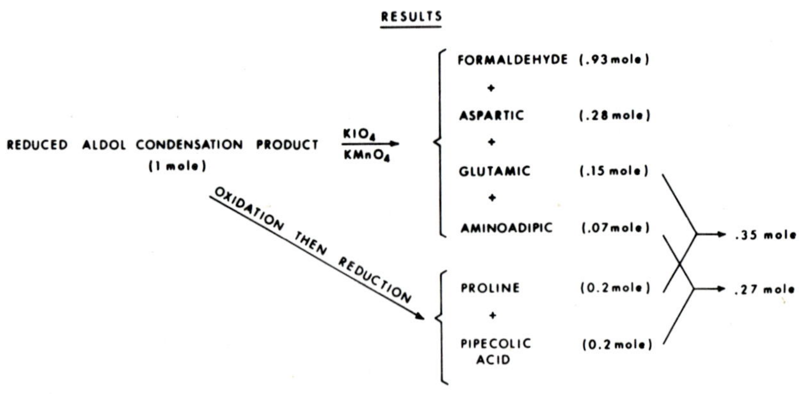

Fig. 10. Results of periodate-permanganate oxidation of reduced aldol condensate.

Partridge and Elsden, 1967), is also not well defined. However, we have not been able to obtain any evidence for the formation of α-aminopimelic acid and therefore favor Structure (A) in Fig. 9. The appearance of aspartic acid in our reaction mixtures might well have occurred from a possible enolization of an intermediate which arises during the oxidation procedure resulting in the cleavage of that carbon-carbon bond which would result in the formation of aspartic acid.

Because we employed tritiated sodium borohydride to reduce the protein the reduced aldol condensation product isolated after hydrolysis and chromatography was radioactive. Calculating the specific activity of the isolated amino acid we concluded that one tritium atom per molecule of aldol was present. This result is entirely consistent with the structure proposed in Fig. 5.

B. AMOUNT

The most remarkable finding was the fact that in mature bovine elastin there exists 4-5 residues of the aldol condensation product per 1,000 amino acid residues. This is equal to or greater than the number of residues of desmosine, isodesmosine and lysinonorleucine combined. Since the concentration of the reduced aldol condensation product is of such magnitude in a mature animal ligament, we suggest that this compound in its non-reduced form also serves as a crosslinking compound in elastin. In addition to this function it does, in all probability, function as a precursor for the crosslinking amino acids, desmosine and isodesmosine. This point will be discussed below. One should note that employing these same procedures to collagen, namely reduction with $NaBT_4$ and hydrolysis in 2 N NaOH resulted in the presence of the reduced aldol condensation product in hydrolysates of collagen (Paz et al., 1969). Most recently, in collaboration with Dr. A. H. Kang (Kang, Faris and Franzblau, 1969) we have shown that the intramolecular crosslink in a β_{12} chain from chick skin collagen is the aldol condensation product. This result serves to strengthen the hypothesis that such a compound can serve as a crosslinking amino acid. A schematic illustration of the crosslink is shown in Fig. 11. It is still not certain whether the aldol condensation product, in vivo, is in the hydrated or dehydrated form.

IV LYSINE AS PRECURSOR OF CROSSLINKS

Treatment of desmosine or isodesmosine with a mild oxidizing agent such as alkaline ferricyanide results in formation of a significant amount of lysine, which suggested to Partridge, Elsden and Thomas (1963) that the biosynthesis of the desmosines could be from lysine. Independent studies by Miller, Martin and Piez (1964) on chick embryo aorta and by Partridge, Elsden, Thomas, Dorfman, Telser, and Ho (1966) on rat aorta indeed have confirmed that lysine is the precursor of both desmosine and isodesmosine. Uniformly labeled [^{14}C]lysine was supplied to chick aortas in tissue culture, and the specific activity of the desmosine in the elastin isolated subsequently was found to be four times that of lysine. This would suggest that four lysine residues are incorporated into one desmosine or isodesmosine molecule.

That lysine is also the precursor of lysinonorleucine was proposed by Franzblau et al.(1965b). In studies ex-

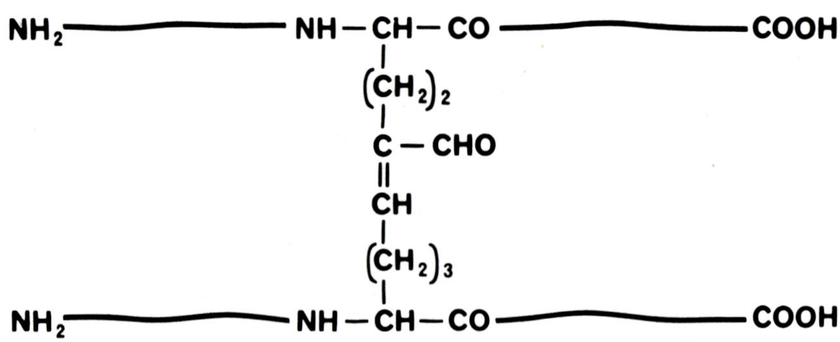

Fig. 11. Schematic illustration of crosslink involving the aldol condensation product of two residues of α-aminoadipic acid-δ-semialdehyde.

tending those of Miller et al. (1964) on developing chick embryos, the concentration of lysinonorleucine in aortic elastin was found to increase at the same rate as that of the desmosines. Results obtained by using 12-day-old chick embryo aortas in tissue culture substantiated the hypothesis that two lysine residues are incorporated into one lysinonorleucine molecule. Briefly, [^{14}C]lysine was added to the tissue culture medium for 1 day and chased with non-radioactive medium for an additional 8 days. Elastin was isolated from the organ culture and hydrolyzed, and the hydrolyzate was placed on an amino acid analyzer equipped with a stream-splitting device. The portion of the eluant not analyzed with ninhydrin reagent was counted in a liquid scintillation device. The specific activities obtained for lysine, the desmosines, and lysinonorleucine are given in Table I. The data confirm the results of other laboratories that four lysine molecules are incorporated into the desmosines. It is also evident from these data that two lysine molecules are condensed to form one lysinonorleucine. Sandberg and Cleary (1968) obtained similar results by feeding [^{14}C]lysine to growing chicks.

TABLE I

Specific Activities of Several Amino Acids Obtained from [^{14}C]Lysine Labeled Elastin

Amino acid	Not reduced (cpm/μM*)	Reduced (cpm/μM*)
Lysine	34,000	31,000
Desmosine	27,000	44,000
Isodesmosine	31,000	
Lysinonorleucine	33,000	37,000
Merodesmosine	---	31,000

*Based on lysine equivalents: (a) assuming desmosine and isodesmosine equal to four lysine equivalents, (b) merodesmosine equal to three lysine equivalents, and (c) lysinonorleucine equal to two lysine equivalents.

V BIOSYNTHESIS OF CROSSLINKS

A. PROPOSED REACTIONS

Knowing that lysine is the precursor of these special amino acids, one may then ask how they are synthesized. The cell or cell type responsible for the biosynthesis of elastin has never been well defined. At present there appears to be two schools of thought--one implicates the muscle cells and the other fibroblasts. However, Dr. R. Ross at this conference has displayed convincing electron-microscopic evidence of a smooth muscle cell line in tissue culture that is apparently synthesizing elastic fibers. In either case the first step in the biosynthesis of elastin would require formation of a soluble "pro-elastin", which should be recognizable by its amino acid composition. Compared with mature elastin, a "pro-elastin" should contain less desmosine, isodesmosine, and lysinonorleucine, but relatively more lysine. A recent article by Sandberg, Weissman and Smith (1969) has reported the isolation and characterization of such a soluble elastin, designated tropoelastin, which contains relatively high concentrations of lysine with little or no desmosine or isodesmosine. The tropoelastin was isolated from the aortic tissue of copper-deficient pigs, a condition which inhibits the biosynthesis of the crosslinkages of elastin.

The tropoelastin could be incorporated into an insoluble elastic fiber through the following series of events: (1) an enzymatic deamination of the ε-amino groups of specific lysine residues along the polypeptide chain leading to formation of residues of α-aminoadipic acid-δ-semialdehyde. (2) Three of the aldehyde residues, arising either on different chains or on the same chain, brought into juxtaposition with a fourth intact lysine residue, condense to form the carbon and nitrogen skeleton of the demosines. The condensation may occur stepwise or in a concerted fashion. That is to say that two of these aldehydes may combine to form a stable intermediate and then combine in turn with either another semialdehyde residue or a lysine residue or it may in fact combine with the Schiff base which arises from the joining of a lysine residue to an adipic acid-δ-semialdehyde residue. All of these pathways are possible. (3) If any of the three aldehyde residues implicated or the intact lysine residue is present in the insoluble fiber initially, the soluble tropoelastin would then by this process be incorporated into the insoluble elastic network. The possibility is not precluded that additional desmosine crosslinks can be formed in the insoluble elastin fiber by the same mechanism.

The synthesis of lysinonorleucine could occur with certain similarties. The proposed biosynthetic scheme would include: (1) enzymatic deamination of the ε-amino group of <u>one</u> residue of lysine to yield a residue of α-amino adipic acid-δ-semialdehyde; (2) condensation of the aldehyde residue with the ε-amino group of a second residue of lysine to form a Schiff base (i.e., a residue of $\Delta^{6,7}$-dehydrolysinonorleucine) resulting in crosslinking of two elastin chains or two segments of a single chain, thus being the same Schiff base proposed as a possible intermediate in the desmosine synthesis; and (3) reduction of the aldimine function of the Schiff base to produce the final crosslinking residue of lysinonorleucine.

The synthesis of the aldol condensation product would occur in a similar fashion. <u>Two</u> lysine residues either on the same chain or different chains would be deaminated and condensed to form the aldol. This compound also is implicated above as an intermediate in the biosynthetic pathway of desmosine or isodesmosine.

B. CHEMICAL EVIDENCE

In support of the above scheme for the biosynthesis of lysinonorleucine, we have obtained evidence that the proposed Schiff base intermediate is present in elastin and can be reduced chemically to lysinonorleucine according to the reactions shown in Fig. 12 (Lent and Franzblau, 1967). Since sodium borohydride can reduce carbonyl compounds to alcohols, Schiff bases to secondary amines, and

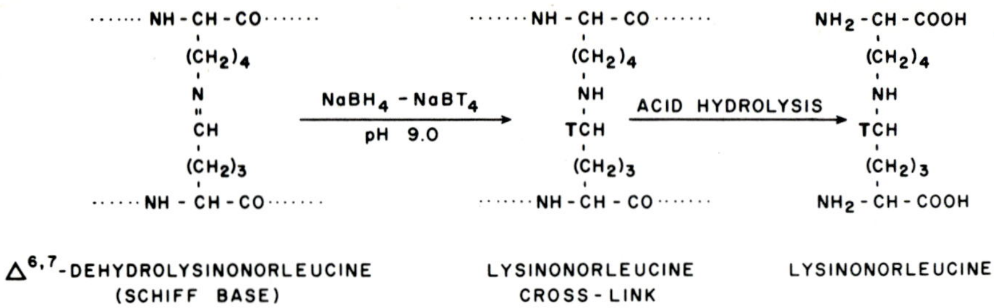

Fig. 12. Reduction of $\Delta^{6,7}$ dehydrolysinonorleucine to lysinonorleucine.

pyridinium compounds to dihydropyridine compounds, the use of this reagent would lead to formation of derivatives more stable than the parent intermediates. The use of tritiated sodium borohydride ($NaBT_4$), as described by Blumenfeld and Gallop (1966), has the additional advantages of providing a means of quantitating the extent of reduction and of adding a radioactive marker to the components in question. Thus, treatment of elastin with $NaBT_4$ followed by hydrolysis resulted in the introduction of tritium into fractions, separable on the column of our amino acid analyzer, containing lysinonorleucine. Indeed an increase of total content of lysinonorleucine was observed as compared with the amount in a control (non-reduced) elastin, which specifically demonstrated the initial presence of the Schiff base precursor.

In the same manner, as mentioned above, we were also able to isolate the reduced derivative of the aldol condensation product. In this latter case, however, we found that it was necessary to hydrolyze the reduced elastin in 2 N NaOH rather than the more generally used acid treatment, because the reduced aldol condensation product is degraded or converted to another compound in 6 N HCl at 105°C. It is of interest to note that the desmosines also were reduced by the borohydride treatment and when $NaBT_4$ was used the desmosines were converted to reduced derivatives which were radioactive.

If bovine elastin was treated first with 2,4-dinitrophenylhydrazine (2,4-DNPH), subsequent treatment with $NaBT_4$ did not cause incorporation of tritium into lysinonorleucine; in fact only the desmosines were reduced and labeled. Conversely, if reduced elastin was subequently treated with 2,4-DNPH, little or no hydrazone formation occurred. Reduction caused about 25% increase in the content of lysinonorleucine determined chromatographically. The magnitude of this increase is highly significant because the extent of radioactivity incorporated into the lysinonorleucine also indicated a 25% increase in lysinonorleucine content.

Reaction of 2,4-DNPH with elastin before reduction should produce DNP-hydrazones of carbonyl and Schiff base components present in the protein if these are accessible to the reagent. Treatment of the DNP-hydrazone derivative of elastin with sodium borohydride, in contrast to elastin per se, would not result in reductive formation of alcohols and secondary amines since the precursor aldehydes and Schiff bases, respectively, would be present as DNP-hydrazone derivatives.

These results support the conclusion that carbonyl and Schiff base components are present in the bovine elastin preparation utilized. Reduction of desmosine or isodesmosine must occur in the pyridinium portion of the molecule, since treatment of elastin with 2,4-DNPH had no apparent effect on the extent of this reduction. Incorporation of tritium in the desmosine fractions is accompanied by a skewing of chromatographic peaks obtained subsequently, so that discrete desmosine and isodesmosine peaks are no longer observed. Also absorption of light at 275 mμ decreases significantly compared with that shown by the desmosines before borohydride treatment.

It should be apparent that the first step in the synthesis of all the crosslinks in elastin results in the conversion of certain specific lysine residues to α-aminoadipic acid-δ-semialdehyde residues. Indeed, the work of Martin, Pinnell and their collaborators has led to the isolation and partial characterization of an enzyme system which is capable of catalyzing this reaction. Their results are reported elsewhere in this symposium. That residues of α-aminoadipic acid-δ-semialdehyde do exist in elastin preparations has been shown by several laboratories including ours. Miller, Pinnell, Martin and Schiffman (1967) have reported that performic acid oxidation of elastin labeled with [^{14}C]lysine by tissue culture procedures resulted in formation of [^{14}C]α-aminoadipic acid. We have found that by reducing elastin with $NaBT_4$ we could obtain radioactive ε-hydroxynorleucine. Unexpectedly, however, we found that under the conditions of 6 N HCl normally employed for protein hydrolysis approximately 70% of the ε-hydroxynorleucine residues are converted to ε-chloronorleucine residues (Lent et al., 1969). These, in turn may be converted to pipecolic acid on treatment with mild alkali. We found that hydrolysis of reduced elastin in 2 N NaOH yields only radioactive ε-hydroxynorleucine. Therefore, by hydrolyzing reduced elastin in 2 N NaOH we could obtain not only the concentration of ε-hydroxynorleucine but also the concentration of the aldol condensation product of two residues of α-aminoadipic acid-δ-semialdehyde. We estimate from these results that there exists in mature bovine elastin approximately 2-3 residues of α-aminoadipic acid-δ-semialdehyde per 1000 amino acid residues. It should be noted that Tanzer and Mechanic have reported at this meeting that hydrolysis of ε-hydroxynorleucine in 3 N HCl minimizes the amount of ε-chloronorleucine found.

C. INCORPORATION OF LYSINE IN TISSUE CULTURE

In an attempt to learn more about the relative rates of formation of the various intermediates in the desmosine synthesis, we followed the fate of [^{14}C]lysine in cultures of chick embryo aorta and measured its incorporation into α-aminoadipic acid-δ-semialdehyde and its aldol condensation product. [^{14}C]lysine was pulsed for 2 days and then chased for an additional 10 days. Figs. 13, 14 and 15 describe the percentage of total counts present as lysine, ε-hydroxynorleucine and the reduced aldol condensation

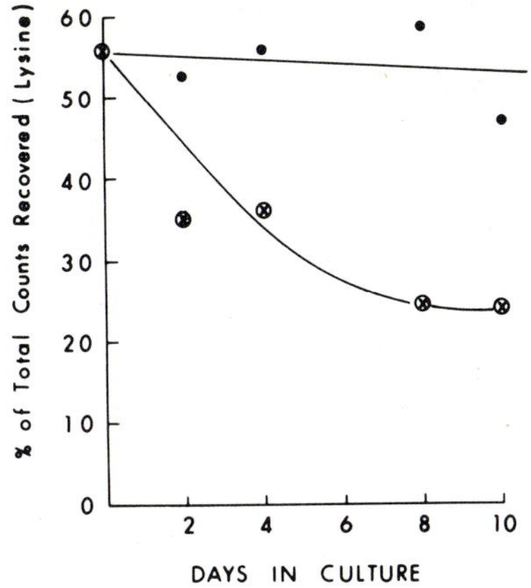

Fig. 13. Percentage of total counts in lysine versus time in tissue culture. No BAPN (crossed circles); BAPN added (open circles).

product after the elastin was isolated, reduced and hydrolyzed in alkali. Zero day in these figures actually represents the time after the 2-day pulse. One notes immediately the striking amount of total radioactivity that is found in the aldol at the zero day. This amount continues to increase steadily through the entire experiment. If one adds β-aminopropionitrile (BAPN) after the two day pulse (in zero day), no further incorporation into the aldol occurs. The specific activities of lysine and the reduced aldol condensation products are given in Table II. The percentage of total counts in ε-hydroxynorleucine does not vary much throughout the experimental period. It almost appears to be at a steady state concentration. That is to say, when a residue of α-aminoadipic acid-δ-semialdehyde is formed from a residue of lysine, it rapidly participates, either spontaneously or enzymatically, in an aldol condensation with another semialdehyde residue. If BAPN is added no α-aminoadipic acid-δ-semialdehyde is formed, but little or no α-aminoadipic acid-δ-semialdehyde is depleted either. Lysine as expected does increase both in total counts and specific activity.

Since the overall concentration (not radioactivity)

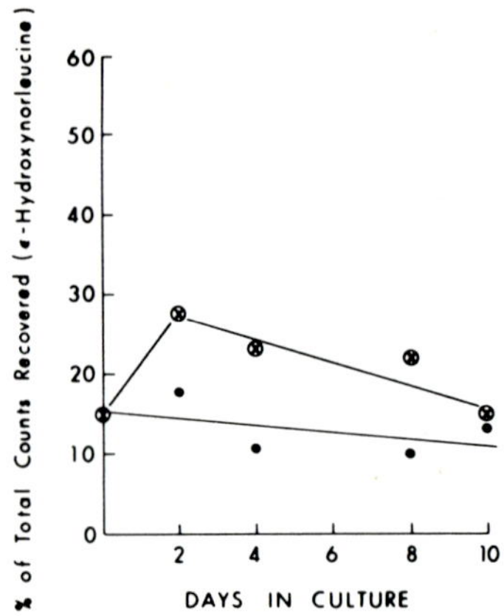

Fig. 14. Percentage of total counts in ε-hydroxy-norleucine versus time in tissue culture. No BAPN (crossed circles); BAPN added (open circles).

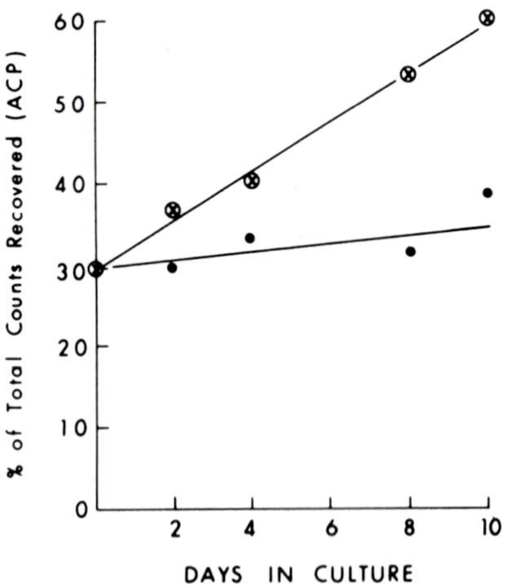

Fig. 15. Percentage of total counts in reduced aldol condensation product versus time in tissue culture No BAPN (crossed circles); BAPN added (open circles).

of the aldol condensation product does not change significantly throughout the tissue culture experiment it suggests that a portion is probably being utilized for the formation of the desmosines. The amount of radioactive desmosines obtained in these experiments is small because both reduction and alkaline hydrolysis tend to destroy the integrity of these amino acids. It is possible that not only is the α-aminoadipic acid-δ-semialdehyde at

TABLE II

Specific Activities of Reduced ACP and Lysine After Isolation from Tissue Culture

Days in culture following pulse	Lysine		Reduced ACP	
	[cpm/μMole(10^{-3})]			
	No BAPN	BAPN	No BAPN	BAPN
0	46.0	46.0	21.8	21.8
2	39.7	38.0	26.5	24.0
4	29.2	43.5	25.8	24.8
8	26.6	37.0	30.7	22.5
10	22.5	26.0	43.1	23.1

a steady state level, but also the aldol condensation product may be in a steady-state condition. Of course, further work remains to be done to clarify this point.

If we examine the aortas during the pulse period and calculate the ratio of counts in ε-hydroxynorleucine to counts in the reduced aldol condensation product, then one clearly sees a change in the ratio which ranges from 1.5 after 2 hr to 0.5 after 48 hr (Table III).

Knowing the concentration of all the lysine derived amino acids in mature bovine elastin, it is of interest to estimate the lysine equivalents that can be accounted for by these unusual components. The results are given in Table IV. Sandberg et al. (1969) have found that the tropoelastin isolated from copper deficient pigs contains

TABLE III

Ratio of Counts in ε-Hydroxynorleucine to Counts in Reduced Aldol Versus Time in Tissue Culture

Time	Ratio
6	1.71
12	1.11
24	0.78
48	0.52

TABLE IV

Summary of Lysine Derived Amino Acids in Bovine Elastin

Amino Acid	Res/1000 res	Lys equiv/1000 res
Lysine	4	4
Aminoadipic semialdehyde	2-3	2-3
Aldol condensate	4-5	8-10
Desmosines	3	12
Lysinonorleucine	1	2
Merodesmosine	--	--
TOTAL	14-16	28-31

47 lysine residues per 1000 amino acids. We can now account for 28-31 lysine equivalents in bovine elastin. It is tempting to suggest the possibility that one other lysine-derived compound may be present (possibly a double aldol condensation or a merodesmosine). On the other hand, this variation may simply be explained by species and tissue differences. We are not able to detect merodesmosine in mature bovine elastin unless, as stated by Starcher et al. (1967) we treat the protein first with alkali and then reduce with $NaBH_4$. However, small amounts of merodesmosine are detectable in chick embryo elastin, which had been reduced but not pretreated with alkali.

D. EFFECT OF PENICILLAMINE

Finally, I would like to mention some observations we have made concerning the reaction of elastin with penicillamine (Jaffe and Franzblau, unpublished data). It had been shown previously by Pinnell, Martin and Miller (1968) that penicillamine injected into chick embryos inhibits the formation of the desmosines. Similar inhibition of crosslinkages in collagen (not desmosines) had been noted earlier by Nimni and Bavetta (1965). From their data, the group at the NIH proposed that penicillamine in some manner, blocks the conversion of α-aminoadipic

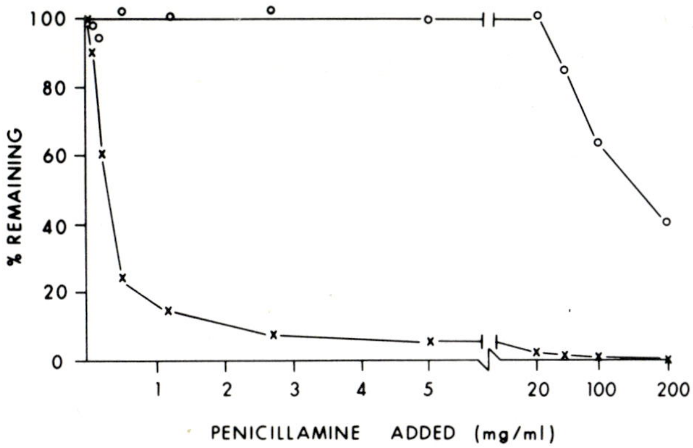

Fig. 16. Interaction of penicillamine with elastin in vitro. See text for details. Reduced aldol condensation product (o——o); ε-hydroxynorleucine (x——x).

acid-δ-semialdehyde residues to the crosslinks of elastin, most probably by the formation of a thiazolidine ring. We examined the interaction of bovine elastin with penicillamine, in vitro, in the following manner. We reasoned that since we had two types of aldehyde residues in elastin, namely α-aminoadipic acid-δ-semialdehyde and its aldol condensation product, we could examine the integrity of each of these after incubating elastin with varying concentrations of penicillamine. This could be achieved by reducing the treated elastin with $NaBT_4$ and examining the radioactivity in the two fractions, the ε-hydroxynorleucine and the reduced aldol condensation product. We found that at relatively low concentrations, penicillamine reacts specifically with α-aminoadipic acid-δ-semialdehyde residues in elastin. This is shown in Fig. 16. At extremely high concentrations of penicillamine some interaction with the aldol condensation product is apparent. As pointed out by Deshmukh and Nimni (1969) in their studies on collagen, the penicillamine effect is reversible. We have shown similar results by simply washing the penicillamine-elastin complex and recovering the theoretical quantity of ε-hydroxynorleucine. If, however, reduction of the elastin-penicillamine complex preceeds washing, the ε-hydroxynorleucine is not recoverable. This indicates to us that reduction has caused the formation of a stable covalent bond between the penicillamine and elastin, most likely derived from a Schiff base. We are at present pursuing the nature of this product.

VI CONCLUSIONS

In summary, we believe that there exists in elastin at least three different types of crosslinks all derived from lysine residues originally incorporated in the backbone of a tropoelastin. The most abundant of these, the aldol condensation product of two residues of α-amino-adipic acid-δ-semialdehyde, which has been isolated and characterized as the reduced derivative, probably plays a dual role. In addition to serving as a crosslink, it probably acts as a precursor to the desmosines as well.

ACKNOWLEDGEMENTS

This investigation was supported by grants from the U.S. Public Health Service (AM-07697) and from the American Heart Association (68-777).

REFERENCES

Blumenfeld, O.O. and Gallop, P.M. (1966). Proc. Natl. Acad. Sci. U.S. 56, 1260.

Deshmukh, K. and Nimni, M.E. (1969). J. Biol. Chem. 244, 1787.

Franzblau, C., Faris, B. and Papaioannou (1969). Biochemistry **8**, 2833.

Franzblau, C., Sinex, F.M. and Faris, B. (1965a). Nature 204, 802.

Franzblau, C., Sinex, F.M., Faris, B. and Lampidis, R. (1965b). Biochem. Biophys. Res. Commun. 21, 575.

Kang, A.H., Faris, B. and Franzblau, C. (1969). Biochem. Biophys. Res. Commun. 36, 345.

Lemieux, R.U. and van Rudloff, E. (1955). Can. J. Chem. 33, 1710.

Lent, R.W. and Franzblau, C. (1967). Biochem. Biophys. Res. Commun. 26, 43.

Lent, R.W., Smith, B., Salcedo, L.L., Faris, B. and Franzblau, C. (1969). Biochemistry 8, 2837.

Miller, E.J., Martin, G.R. and Piez, K.A. (1964). Biochem. Biophys. Res. Commun. 17, 248.

Miller, E.J., Pinnell, S.R., Martin, G.R. and Schiffman, E. (1967). Biochem. Biophys. Res. Commun. 26, 132.

Nimni, M.E. and Bavetta, L.A. (1965). Science 150, 905.

Partridge, S.M., Elsden, D.F. and Thomas, J. (1963). Nature 197, 1297.

Partridge, S.M., Elsden, D.F., Thomas, J., Dorfman, A., Telser, A. and Ho, P.-L. (1966). Nature 209, 399

Partridge, S.M., Thomas, J. and Elsden, D.F. (1965). In Structure and Function of Connective and Skeletal Tissue, p. 88. Ed. by Fritton Jackson, S. et al. Butterworth and Co., London.

Paz, M.A., Lent, R.W., Faris, B., Franzblau, C., Blumenfeld, O.O. and Gallop, P.M. (1969). Biochem. Biophys. Res. Commun. 34, 222.

Pinnell, S.R., Martin, G.R. and Miller, E.J. (1968). Science 161, 465.

Sandberg, L.B. and Cleary, E.G. (1968). Biochim. Biophys. Acta 154, 411.

Sandberg, L.B., Weissman, N. and Smith, D.W. (1969). Biochemistry 8, 2940.

Speck, J.C., Rowley, P.T. and Horecker, B.L. (1963). J. Am. Chem. Soc. 85, 1012.

Starcher, B.C., Partridge, S.M. and Elsden, D.F. (1967). Biochemistry 6, 2425.

Thomas, J., Elsden, D.F. and Partridge, S.M. (1963). Nature 200, 651.

STUDIES OF THE COMPONENTS OF THE ELASTIC FIBER

Russell Ross and Paul Bornstein

Electronmicroscopic observations of elastic fibers in arteries, tendons, and elastic ligaments of mature animals have demonstrated that these fibers contain two morphologically different components (Greenlee, Ross and Hartman, 1966; Fahrenbach, Sandberg and Cleary, 1966; Greenlee and Ross, 1967; Ross, 1968). One of these components consists of microfibrils (110-120 Å in diameter); the second is amorphous in appearance in the electronmicroscope. The latter component may not truly be amorphous, although it demonstrates little clearly defined structure (Figs. 1 and 2). The microfibrils have an affinity for cationic stains such as lead or uranyl acetate, whereas, the amorphous component has an affinity for anionic stains such as phosphotungstic acid (Greenlee et al., 1966).

Both the microfibrils and the amorphous component are integral constituents of the mature elastic fiber and are usually aggregated so that the amorphous component is surrounded by an envelope of the microfibrils. Many microfibrils are also found to be dispersed within the interstices of the amorphous component (Figs. 1 and 2).

During the embryogenesis of elastic tissues, the first observable structure that can be identified as an elastic fiber consists of only a single component, the microfibrils (Karrer, 1960, 1961; Low, 1962; Greenlee et al., 1966). These nicrofibrils form parallel aggregates or bundles in the first recognizable, or immature, elastic fibers. They are usually found extracellularly in close association with the surface of smooth muscle cells in blood vessels, or near the surface of fibroblasts in tendons and elastic ligaments. With increa-

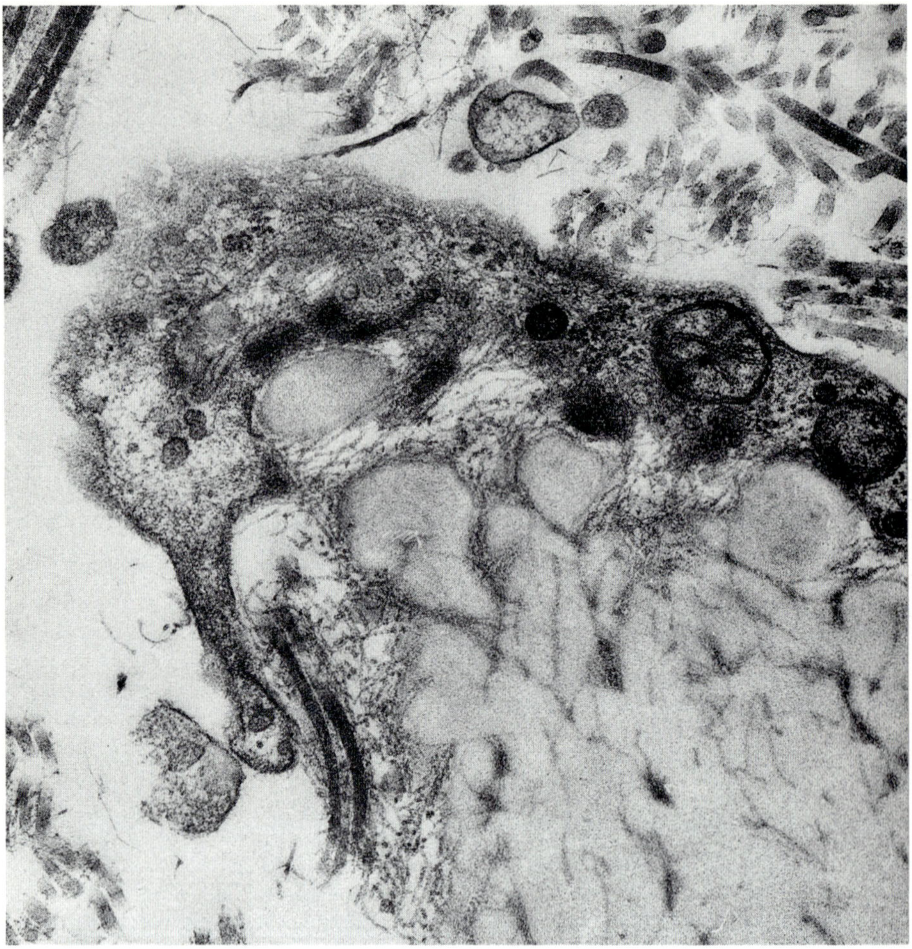

Fig. 1. This electron micrograph demonstrates several elastic fibers in guinea pig aorta. Cell processes can be seen to surround the elastic fibers which are intermixed with collagen fibrils. The microfibrils surround the periphery of the elastic fiber and are also embedded within its interstices. (X34,000).

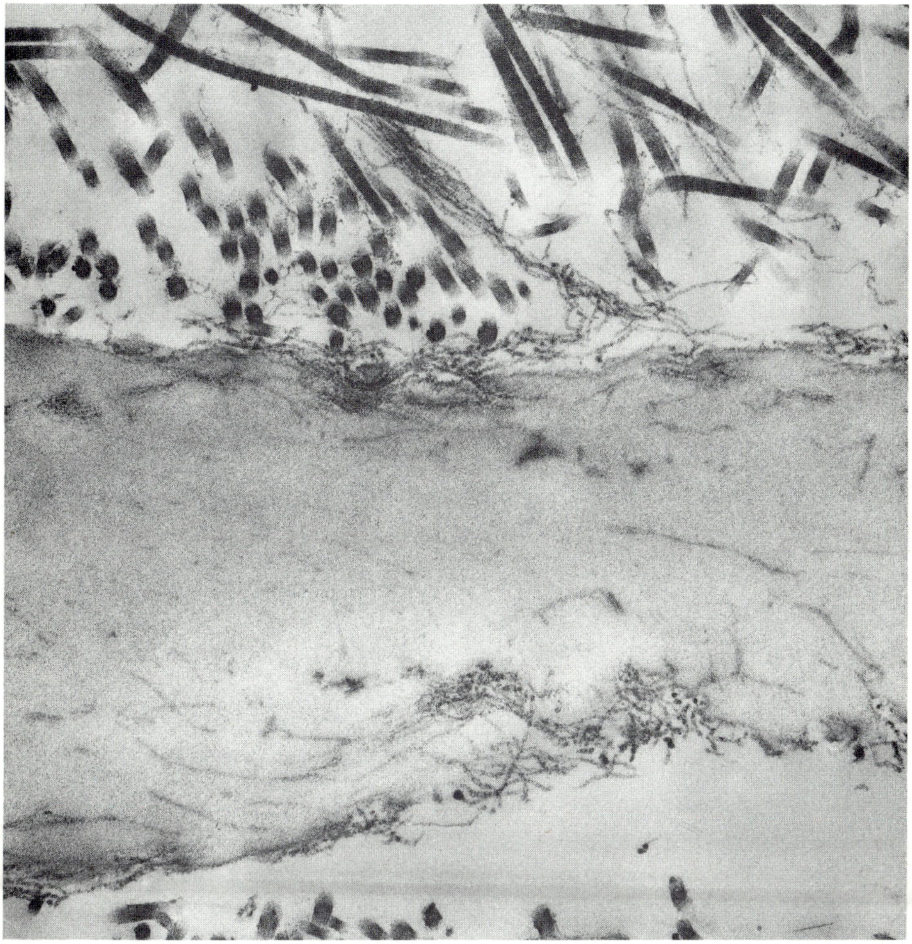

Fig. 2. Another view of a portion of an elastic fiber from a developing guinea pig aorta. The beaded appearance of the microfibrils, which are part of the elastic fiber, can be more readily seen in this electronmicrograph. A few collagen fibrils from this tissue are also visible. (X33,000).

sing age, the amorphous component is secreted by the cells and is deposited between and around the microfibrils. At maturity the elastic fibers are several microns in diameter and consist largely of the amorphous component together with a relatively small volume of microfibrils (Haust, More, Bencosme and Balis, 1965, Greenlee et al.,1966; Ross and Greenlee, 1966).

Because of these differences in morphology and affinity for stains, a series of studies was initiated to isolate and characterize each of the components of the elastic fiber (Ross and Bornstein, 1969).

I MATERIALS, METHODS, AND RESULTS

Ligamentum nuchae from term fetal calves was homogenized in 5 M guanidine and extracted in 5 M guanidine, pH 7, for 72 hr. This procedure yielded a pellet of elastic fibers and collagen fibrils. The pellet was thoroughly washed with both buffer and distilled water and subsequently digested with collagenase for 24 hr. When pellets treated in this manner were examined in the electronmicroscope, they were found to consist of essentially pure preparations of intact elastic fibers in which both components of the fibers were present in the same morphologic relationship seen in vivo (Figs. 3 and 4). These extraction studies substantiated the notion that both the microfibrils and the amorphous component were integral parts of the elastic fiber.

Fig. 3. This electronmicrograph represents part of a pellet obtained from a term fetal calf ligamentum nuchae after homogenization and extraction with 5 M guanidine followed by digestion with collagenase and treatment with sodium dodecyl sulfate. The pellet consists of a relatively pure preparation of elastic fibers in which both the microfibrils and the amorphous component can be seen to have the same morphologic relationship as that demonstrated in vivo in Figs. 1 and 2. (X22,500)

Similar preparations of purified elastic fibers were used for a subsequent series of studies. The first of these tested the susceptibility of each elastic fiber component to enzymes.

Elastic fibers were digested with either trypsin, chrymotrypsin, hyaluronidase, β-glucuronidase, pepsin, or elastase. Treatment with hyaluronidase and β-glucuronidase had no effect upon either component of the elastic fiber. Trypsin, chymotrypsin, and pepsin selectively digested the microfibrillar component leaving the amorphous component devoid of these structures. Electronmicrographs of isolated pellets of elastic fibers treated with chymotrypsin illustrate the selective removal of the microfibrillar component (Figs. 5 and 6).

Treatment with elastase for relatively short periods of time demonstrated that after 15 or 30 min of digestion with this enzyme the amorphous component was more susceptible to elastase than were the microfibrils. Treatment for longer periods of time resulted in digestion of both components.

The greater susceptibility of the amorphous component of the elastic fiber to elastase digestion suggested that it was elastin. However, it is well known that elastase possesses general proteolytic as well as elastolytic activity. Therefore, final identification required amino acid analysis of this component. The marked susceptibility of the microfibrils to the other proteolytic enzymes, together with the opposite staining affinities of these two structures strongly suggested that the microfibrils were a different protein.

The observation that the microfibrils could be cleaved by proteolytic enzymes permitted their separation and solubilization for a preliminary study of their amino acid composition. Analyses were performed on a chymotryptic digest obtained from elastic fibers in which chymotrypsin represented less than 1% of the dry weight of the microfibrillar component of the intact fibers. These analyses demonstrated that the microfibrillar protein contained a markedly different amino acid composition from that of either elastin or collagen. The protein was rich in polar amino acids, relatively poor in neutral and basic amino acids, contained no hydroxyproline, hydroxylysine, desmosine, or isodesmosine, and was rich in cystine. The presence of relatively large amounts of cystine suggested that disulfide bonds might play

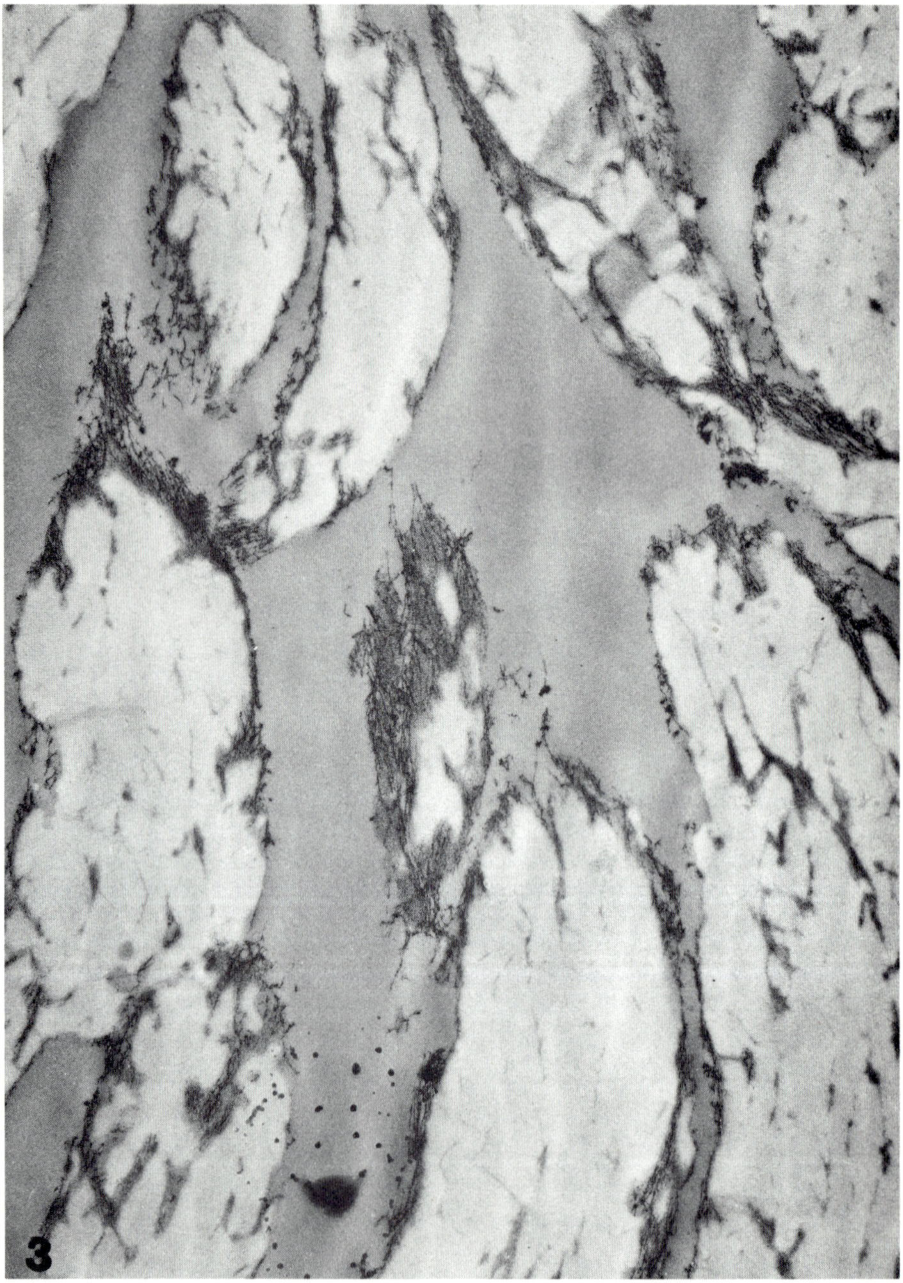
3

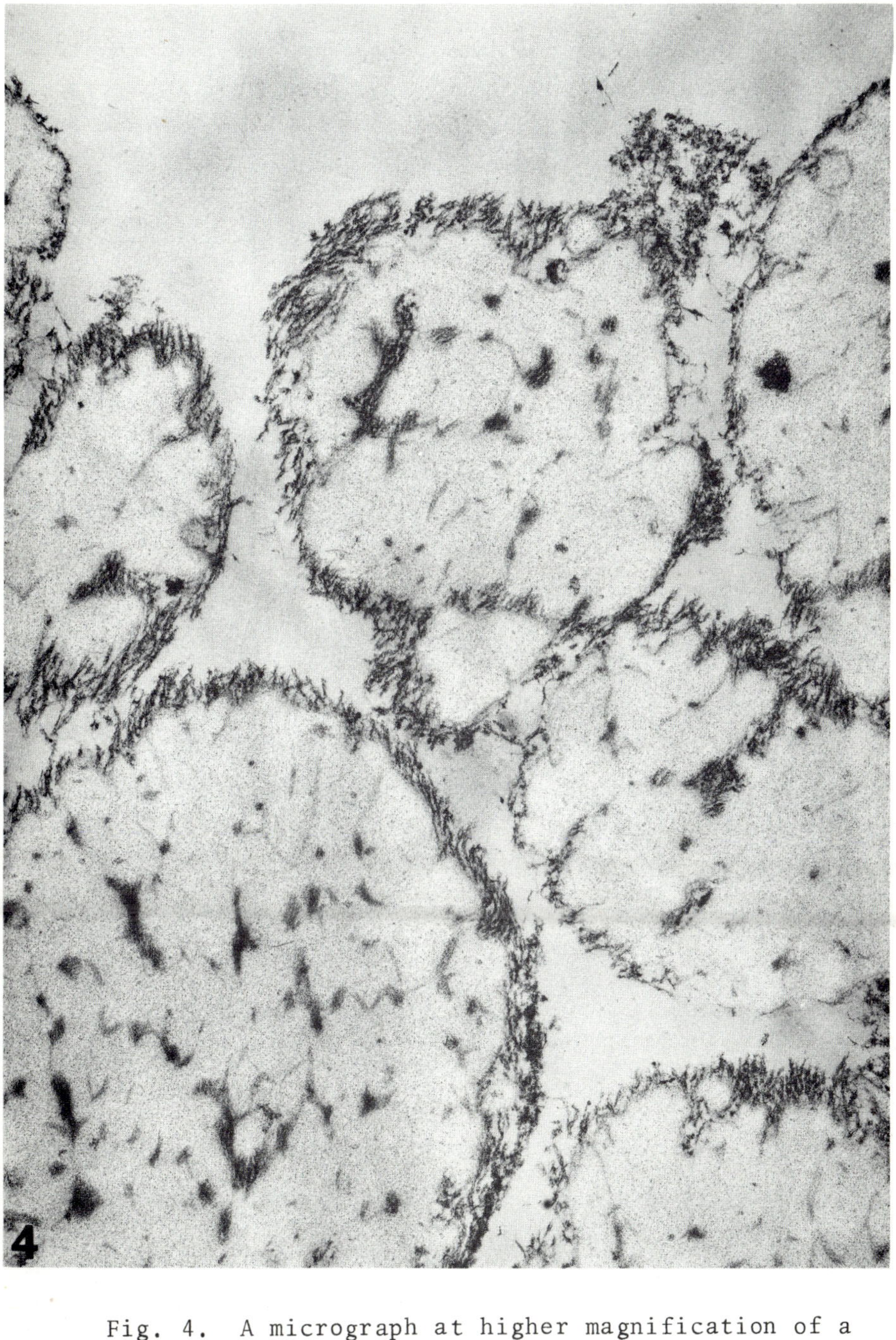

Fig. 4. A micrograph at higher magnification of a portion of an elastic fiber pellet prepared as noted in the legend of Fig. 3. (X34,000)

an important role in the stability of the microfibrillar protein.

These observations led to a subsequent series of studies in which a disulfide bond reducing reagent (dithiothreitol) was used to solubilize the microfibrillar protein so that both it and the amorphous component could be studied individually by amino acid analysis. Fig. 8 summarizes the procedures used in the separation of the components of the elastic fiber.

In later studies, preparations of elastic fibers were further purified by extraction with sodium dodecyl sulfate. The isolated and further purified elastic fibers were suspended in 6 M guanidine containing 0.1% EDTA, and 0.1 M Tris buffer, pH 9.5. Sufficient dithiothreitol was added to prepare a .05 M solution and reduction was performed under nitrogen for 15 hr at 37°C. Following centrifugation, the pH of the supernatant was lowered to 8. A volume of ethylenimine, sufficient to provide a 50-fold molar excess over available sulfhydryl groups was added in aliquots over a 30-minute period. Hydrochloric acid was added simultaneously to maintain the pH at 8. At the completion of the reaction, the pH was lowered to 6 and the solution was dialyzed exhaustively against water. The microfibrillar protein remained in solution and was concentrated by lyophilization. The pellet of reduced elastic fibers lacked the microfibrillar component as seen in the electron micrograph in Fig. 7.

Fig. 5. A portion of a preparation of elastic fibers similar to those demonstrated in Figs. 3 and 4 which has been subsequently treated with chymotrypsin. In this micrograph, it can be seen that the microfibrils have been selectively digested and removed from the elastic fibers. (X13,000)

Fig. 6. X11,000; and Fig. 7. X34,000. These two micrographs represent respectively a low and high-power magnification of a preparation of elastic fibers in which the microfibrils have been selectively solubilized by reduction with dithiothreitol. After centrifugation, the pellet of elastic fibers is identical in appearance with elastic fibers which had been treated with either trypsin or chymotrypsin in which the elastic fiber microfibrils have been selectively solubilized.

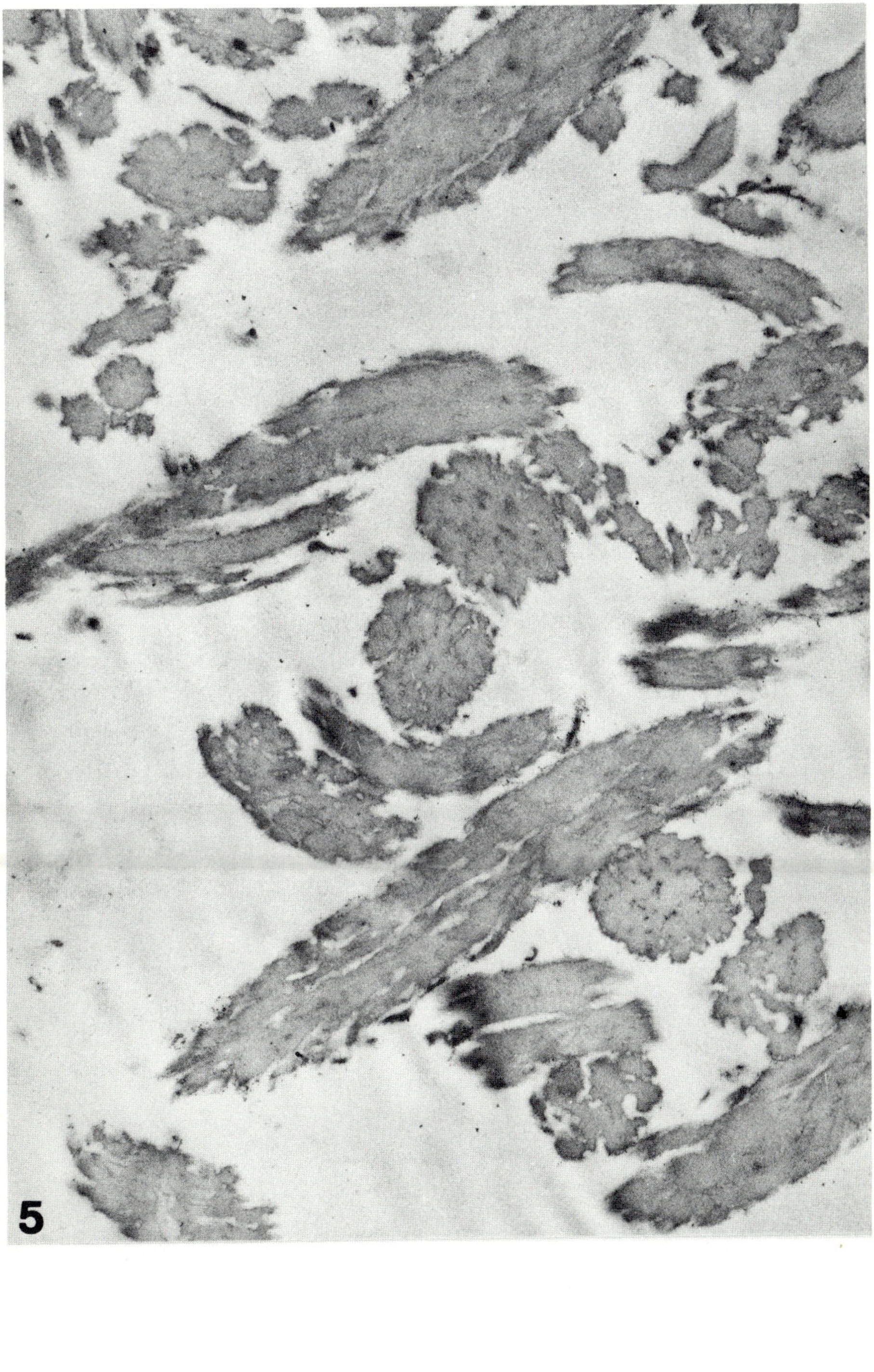

5

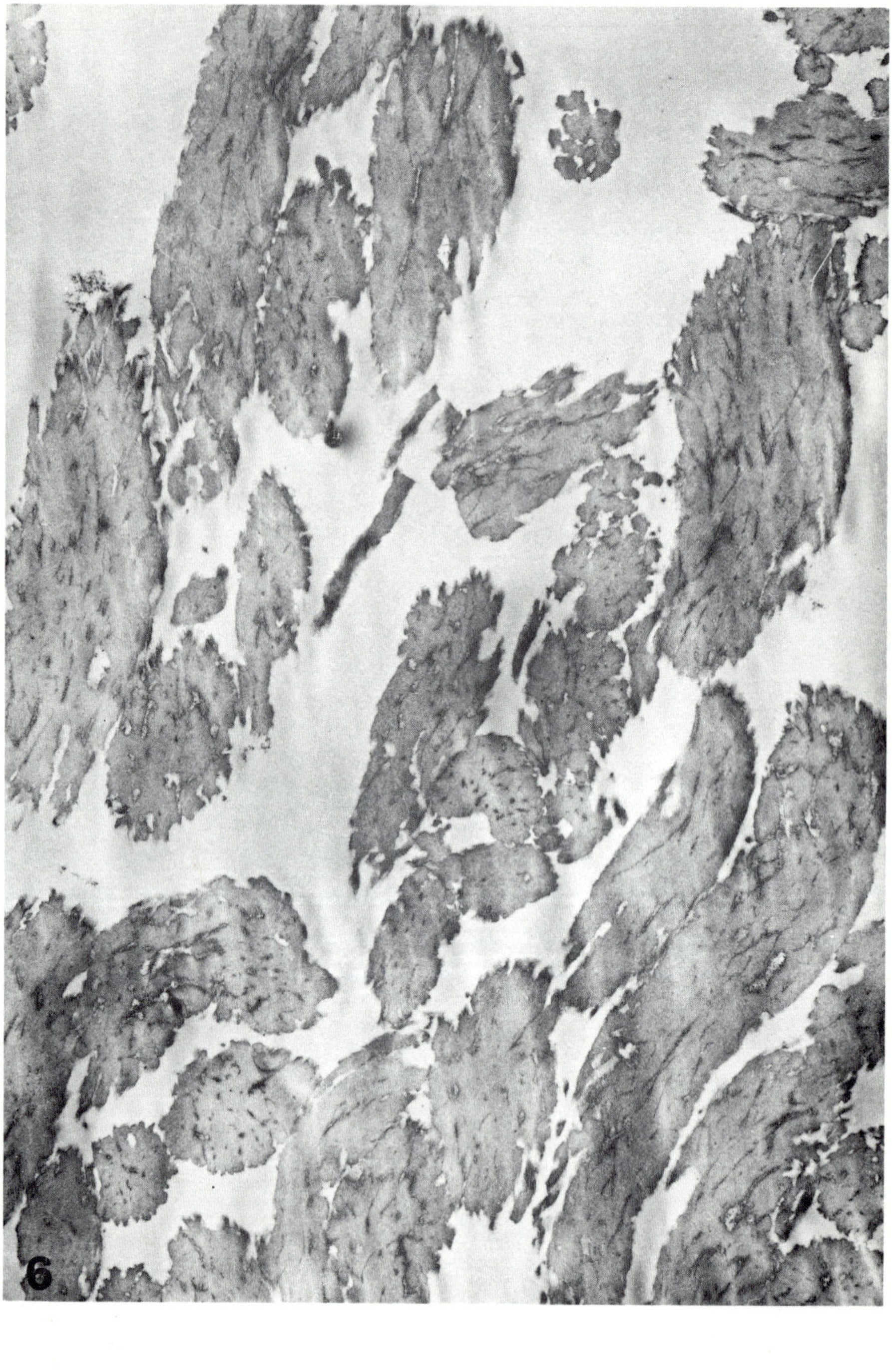
6

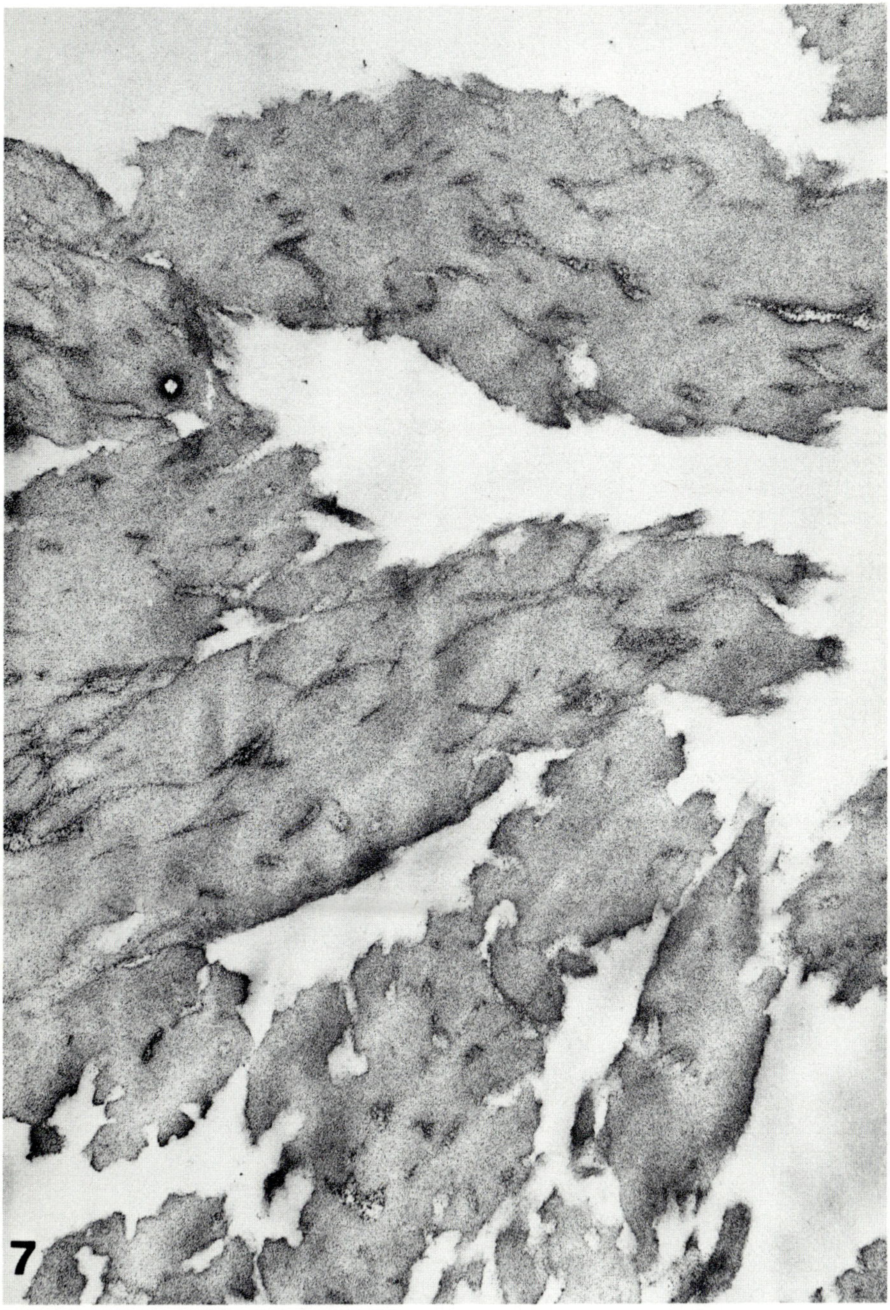
7

TABLE I

Amino Acid Composition of the Elastic Fiber and its Components

Residues/1000

	Elastic fiber	Elastin	Microfibrils	Microfibrils (alkylated)
Hydroxyproline	16.4	10.7	---	---
Aspartic acid	16.1	6.4	114	127
Threonine	13.8	8.9	55.9	65.0
Serine	16.1	9.9	62.2	77.5
Glutamic acid	24.6	15.0	114	136
Proline	90.2	120	63.5	60.5
Glycine	305	324	110	106
Alanine	212	223	65.1	63.0
Cystine/2	10.2	4.1	48.2	---
Valine	130	135	56.3	60.5
Methionine	0.7	---	15.6	13.5
Isoleucine	29.6	25.5	47.7	51.6
Leucine	60.3	61.1	68.6	74.2
Tyrosine	9.4	7.1	36.0	33.7
Phenylalanine	34.4	30.1	37.7	39.3
Desmosine/4	9.4	7.9	---	---
S-aminoethyl cysteine	---	---	---	24.8
Lysine	11.9	7.4	45.0	39.3
Histidine	3.7	0.6	15.4	10.2
Tryptophan	n.c.	n.c.	n.c.	24.8
Arginine	11.1	5.4	45.2	54.0

Fig. 8

Procedure for Separating Components of Elastic Fiber

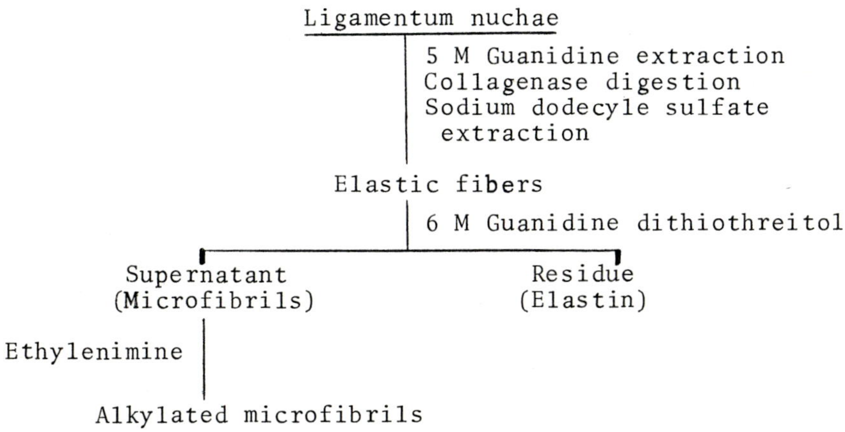

Amino acid analyses of the residual amorphous component following reduction and removal of the microfibrillar protein, and of the microfibrillar protein which was solubilized by reduction and alkylation with ethylenimine, are listed in Table I. S-β-aminoethyl cysteine results from the reaction of cysteine with ethylenimine. These analyses demonstrate that the compositions of microfibrillar protein previously solubilized by enzymatic digestion or by reduction and alkylation with iodoacetamide were very similar to that obtained with the above procedure. The amorphous component was strikingly different in amino acid composition from the microfibrillar protein, but was identical with elastin as previously reported from other laboratories.

Preliminary studies of carbohydrate content of the microfibrillar protein have been made. These indicate that the microfibrils contain 4-7% by weight of hexose, as determined with the anthrone reagent, and approximately 0.7% hexosamine, as determined by ion exchange chromatography. Further studies of the glycoprotein nature of the microfibrillar protein are in progress.

Since the microfibrils appear first during elastic fiber formation, they may be important in the morphogenesis of the elastic fiber and may play a role in determining both the shape and direction of the elastic fiber. This is suggested by the observation that in aggregate the microfibrils assume the shape in ligamentum nuchae and tendon (that of a cylinder) taken by mature elasticfibers containing both components. The same is true for the formation of young aortic elastic fibers which in aggregate form a flat, fenestrated sheet.

II SUMMARY

These studies of isolated elastic fibers from ligamentum nuchae have demonstrated that the mature elastic fiber consists of at least two different proteins. The first of these to form embryologically is the microfibrillar protein. The microfibrils appear to consist of a glycoprotein rich in polar amino acids and cystine, relatively poor in basic and neutral amino acids, and lacking hydroxyproline, hydroxylysine, and the desmosines. The microfibrillar protein must, therefore, be a separate protein of the connective tissue that is neither an elastin nor a collagen precursor.

The amorphous-appearing component appears, on the basis of its amino acid composition, to be identical with what has eventually forms the major proportion of the elastic fiber in the adult animal, although at all times it is seen in association with the microfibrillar protein.

ACKNOWLEDGEMENTS

These studies were supported in part by grants from the U.S. Public Health Service, Nos. DE-01703 and AM-11238. The authors gratefully acknowledge the technical assistance of Marcia Usui and Felicia Arguelles, and the personnel of the electron microscope laboratory of the Department of Pathology.

REFERENCES

Fahrenbach, W.H., Sandberg, L.B. and Cleary, E.G. (1966). Ant. Rec. 155, 563.

Greenlee, T.K., Jr. and Ross, R. (1967). J. Ultrastruct. Res. 18, 354.

Greenlee, T.K., Jr., Ross, R. and Hartman, J.L. (1966). J. Cell Biol. 30, 59.

Haust, M.D., More, R.H., Bencosme, S.A. and Balis, J.V. (1965). Exp. Mol. Pathol. 4, 508.

Karrer, H.E. (1960). J. Ultrastruct. Res. 4, 420.

Karrer, H.E. (1961). J. Ultrastruct. Res. 5, 1.

Low, F.N. (1962). Anat. Rec. 142, 131.

Ross, R. (1968). In Treatise on Collagen, vol. 2, p. 1 Ed. by Gould, B.S. Academic Press, New York

Ross, R. and Bornstein, P. (1969). J. Cell. Biol. 40, 366.

Ross, R. and Greenlee, T.K., Jr. (1966). In Electron Microscopy, vol. 2, p. 561. Proc. 6th Int. Cong. Electron Microscopy. Ed. by Uyeda, R. Maruzen Co., Ltd., Tokyo

RELATIONSHIP BETWEEN THE ANTIGENICITY AND CHEMICAL COMPOSITION OF COMPONENTS OF ELASTIN DIGESTS

Ines Mandl, Stephen Keller and Michael Levi

We previously reported a comparative study of the hydrolysis of bovine ligamentum nuchae elastin by various specific enzymes and by various specific enzymes and by alcoholic KOH (Keller and Mandl, 1965). These methods were found to yield soluble products in all cases, but with important differences in molecular weight distributions and amino acid compositions. In this paper we intend to investigate possible relationships between the composition of isolated fractions of the elastin molecule and some biological properties of elastin such as elasticity, antigenicity and stability. To study this we have fractionated the digests on DEAE-Sephadex columns, and have compared the isolated components as to their chemical and immunological properties.

I MATERIALS AND METHODS

A. PREPARATION AND FRACTIONATION OF THE DIGESTS

Bovine ligamentum nuchae elastin was used in this study. Ligament was freed from fascia, ground into small pieces, refluxed 1 hr with methanol and 1 hr with ether, dried, extracted with 0.1 N NaOH at 93-98°C for 45 min, washed with water, air-dried and ground to 40 mesh. This material was characterized by amino acid analysis (Table I), lipid content (1.4% extractable lipid) and carbohydrate analysis (0.33% as glucose).

The resulting elastin was solubilized either by

pancreatic elastase or by the use of ethanolic KOH (Robert and Poullain, 1963). For the first method, 5 g elastin was digested with 15 mg of crystalline bovine pancreatic elastase (Worthington) at 37°C in a 0.01 M Tris-HCl buffer at pH 8.8. After 3 days the digestion mixture was centrifuged and the supernatant was dialyzed for 5 days against daily changes of distilled water. The second method involved digestion of 5 g elastin with 100 ml of 1 M KOH in 80% v/v ethanol at 37°C for 18 hr. After centrifugation the supernatant was dialyzed and the retentate was lyophilized. Approximately 50% of the original weight of the elastin was recovered in each case after drying.

The non-dialyzable portions of the digests were then fractionated on DEAE-Sephadex A-50. Columns 1.7 x 30 cm in size were filled with a suspension of the exchanger in 0.005 M phosphate buffer, pH 8.0. After equilibration of the packed columns with this buffer for 18 hr, 1.6 g of digest was applied to the column in 10 ml of the starting buffer. The separation proceeded at room temperature with the following buffer sequence:

(a) 0.005 M sodium phosphate, pH 8.0;
(b) 0.005 M sodium phosphate, pH 6.8;
(c) gradient to 0.1 M NaH_2PO_4 in 0.5 M NaCl;
(d) 0.1 M NaH_2PO_4 in 1 M NaCl

Fractions of 10 ml per tube were collected at 15-min intervals and examined for peptide content with a Beckman DU-2 spectrophotometer at 272 mμ. The tubes corresponding to the peaks were pooled, dialyzed and lyophilized.

Fraction I from the chromatography of the elastase digest was fractionated further on a 1.7 x 100-cm column of Sephadex G-200, using a 0.1 M Tris-HCl buffer, pH 8.0 in 1 M NaCl. This was done to remove the small amount of a desmosine and isodesmosine containing peptide which was still present in this fraction as a contaminant, possibly from peak II. The elution profiles obtained after DEAE Sephadex chromatography of the two preparations are shown in Fig. 1A and B.

The similarity between the two curves is striking and

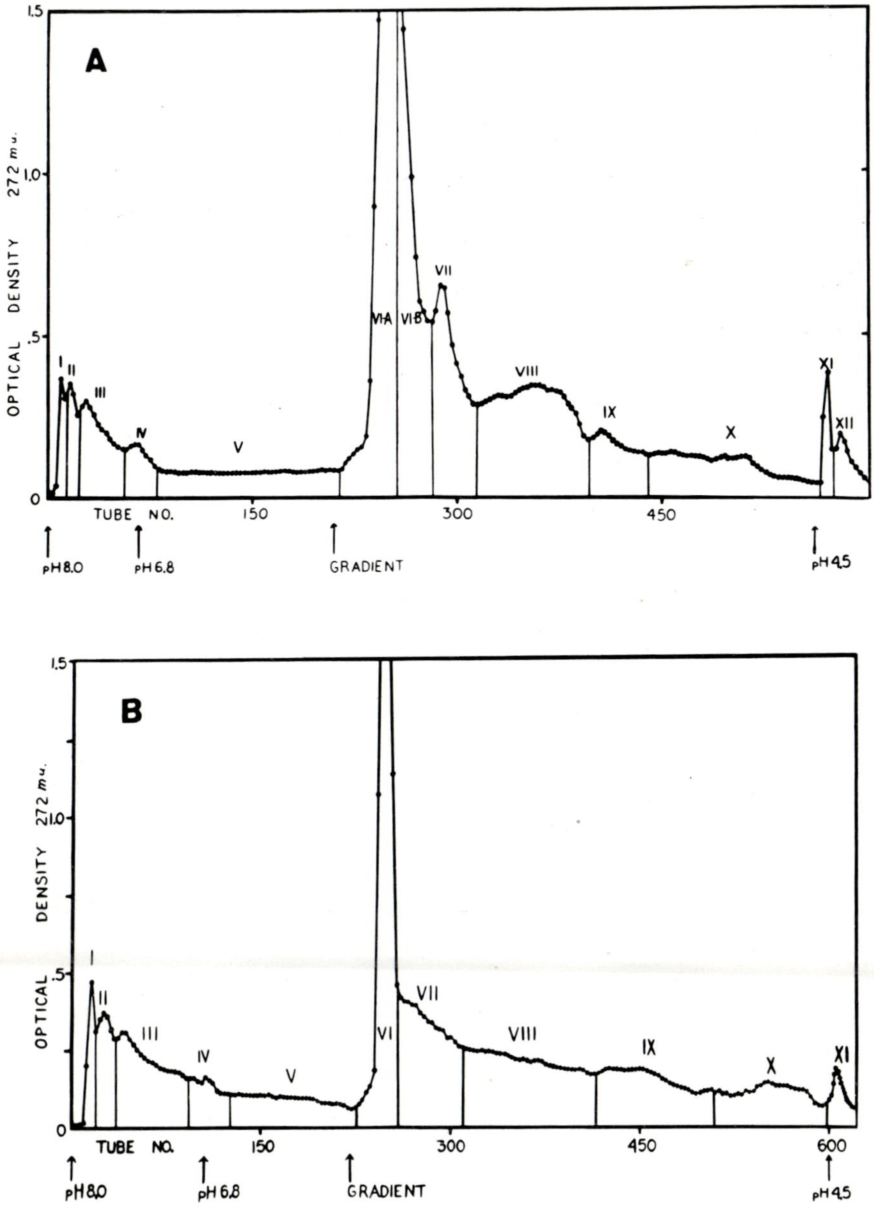

Fig. 1. Elution profiles obtained after DEAE-Sephadex chromatography of the non-dialyzable portions of (A) a pancreatic elastase digest and (B) an ethanolic KOH digest of *ligamentum nuchae* elastin.

is borne out further by comparison of the amino acid composition of the areas under the main peaks.

B. CHEMICAL ANALYSES OF THE FRACTIONS

Fractions I, VIA and X as well as the whole elastin used as starting material were subjected to amino acid analysis on a Technicon Auto-Analyzer with 0.8 mg of 18 hr acid hydrolyzates. Analyses for sugar and lipid were done as reported elsewhere (Keller, Levi and Mandl, 1969). Chain length determinations were performed on the fractions by comparing the ninhydrin test values before and after complete acid hydrolysis in 6 N HCl.

C. IMMUNOLOGICAL INVESTIGATIONS

Rabbits were immunized by three consecutive weekly injections with 100 mg of a dialyzed pancreatic elastase-elastin digest in 1 ml saline plus 1 ml Freund's complete adjuvant as described elsewhere (Keller et al., 1969). Reactivity with the circulating antibodies obtained was determined by Ouchterlony double gel agar diffusion. For this we employed 1% Special Noble Agar in saline-phosphate buffer at pH 7.0. The spacing between the central well and peripheral wells was kept at 1 cm. Both 10 and 50 mg per ml concentrations of the fractions were employed in the peripheral wells. A plate was also set up to test reactivity of the antiserum against the elastase digest at 50 mg/ml in one well, and the elastase itself in concentrations from 10 to 0.8 mg/ml.

II RESULTS

A. COMPOSITION OF THE FRACTIONS

Table I reports the amino acid composition and the average chain lengths of the respective fractions from the two digests.

It can be seen that there are marked differences in composition among the various fractions in a single digest, whereas corresponding fractions of different digests have

TABLE I

Amino Acid Analysis of Elastin Fractions

	I		VI		X		Elastin
	Elastase	KOH	Elastase	KOH	Elastase	KOH	
Mole %							
Hyp	4.10	3.55	1.43	0.79	1.67	0	1.14
Asp	0.15	0.09	0.37	0.63	3.43	3.34	0.52
Thr	0.12	0.07	0.63	0.50	2.45	1.10	0.39
Ser	0.49	0.28	1.06	0.69	2.64	1.17	0.61
Glu	0.31	0.19	1.59	1.86	1.61	4.00	1.38
Pro	15.70	15.30	12.00	11.62	13.50	11.23	12.20
Gly	38.20	39.20	29.40	25.70	27.20	22.70	32.60
Ala	2.87	4.45	30.20	35.20	24.80	31.10	23.20
Val	35.90	32.60	9.97	10.52	4.71	8.80	13.00
Cys	0	0	0	0	TR	0	0.11
Met	0	0	TR	0	0.31	0	TR
Isl	0.41	0.51	1.33	1.42	1.73	1.94	2.33
Leu	0.52	2.28	4.75	4.69	3.80	5.70	6.35
Tyr	TR	0.06	0.80	0.93	2.14	1.55	0.50
Phe	0.97	1.11	3.60	3.06	3.93	3.22	4.41
Isd	0	0	0.29	0.23	0.22	0.19	0.11
Des	0	0	0.45	0.51	0.31	0.69	0.17
Hyl	0	0.14	0.57	0.16	0	0	0.02
Orn	0.15	TR	0.22	0.05	0.21	0.17	0.18
Lnl	0	0	0.19	0.16	0.13	0.10	0.10
Lys	0.10	0.07	0.60	0.57	2.26	1.15	0.27
His	0.06	0	0.05	0.04	0.63	0.33	0.05
Arg	0.08	0.12	0.72	0.72	2.55	1.60	0.39
μM/mg	8.50	8.67	8.14	9.20	3.97	5.23	8.69
Av.No. Res.	32.2	23.2	12.5	12.9	8.8	17.5	

very similar contents of amino acids. The percentage of valine, for example, in both fractions I is even higher than in whole elastin, which in itself has been considered high in this amino acid; on the other hand, fraction X contains less valine than whole elastin. Both fractions I are devoid of the crosslinks desmosine, isodesmosine and lysinonorleucine, while the fractions VI are enriched in those materials. It can be seen from such comparisons that the various fractions investigated, although they have been isolated by only one or two fractionation procedures, do have compositions which appear significantly unique. This is evident in spite of some apparent overlap or mixing to be inferred from Fig. 1. Lipids account for approximately 50% of the weight of the fraction X derived from the elastase digest, and 33% in the alcoholic KOH product. The carbohydrate was found to be 7% of the total weight in the elastase derived fraction X, and 5% in the alcoholic KOH fraction.

B. LOCALIZATION OF ANTIGENICITY IN DIGEST FRACTIONS

When the antiserum against the elastase digest of elastin was reacted by the immunodiffusion technique against the fractions of the same digest, it was observed that X gave the strongest reaction, while fraction VIA gave a line when the antigen concentration was raised to 50 mg/ml. It is of importance that when this same serum was reacted against the fractions of the alcoholic KOH digest, fraction X also gave a precipitin reaction. This is significant since the alcoholic KOH digest contained no enzyme, so that any precipitin lines observed with the KOH fractions against the serum cannot be due to enzyme-antibody interaction but must be due to the reaction with the elastin fractions themselves. Additional proof was adduced by immunoelectrophoresis, which gave no reaction between antiserum and enzyme, and the non-identity of the precipitin lines on Ouchterlony plates between antiserum and elastase and antiserum and fraction X.

III DISCUSSION

A. DISTRIBUTION OF THE AMINO ACIDS AMONG THE VARIOUS FRACTIONS

In the first fraction from both digests (Table I) the three neutral amino acids glycine, valine and proline together comprise 87-90% in a molar ratio of 2:2:1. The valine content is almost three times that of whole elastin, and the hydroxyproline is enriched four-fold. On the other hand, the remaining neutral amino acids are greatly reduced along with the polar amino acids, and the crosslinking agents are completely absent. Fraction I, therefore, appears to be a large fragment of a non-polar region of the elastin molecular complex; Sephadex G-200 fractionation indicated a molecular weight of the order of 20,000.

Fraction VI in comparison with elastin is enriched in the crosslinking agents desmosine, isodesmosine and lysinonorleucine, slightly lower in valine, and 30-50% higher in alanine. This amplifies our previous assumption that alanine predominates in the same regions of elastin as the desmosines, whereas valine may be one of the major constituents of an outer non-polar envelope responsible for both the elasticity and insolubility of the elastin (Keller and Mandl, 1969).

Fraction X, compared with elastin, is enriched in the polar amino acids approximately five times; in addition there is a four-fold increase of tyrosine and slightly increased amounts of the crosslinking agents. The alcoholic KOH fraction X in comparison with its enzymatic homologue has a longer average chain length (17.5 residues vs. 8.8), a greater amount of protein material (5.23 μM amino acids/mg vs. 3.97) and a lesser amount of lipid (33% vs. 50%) and carbohydrate (5% vs. 7%). This we believe reflects a difference in the number of amino acid residues attached to and possibly enveloping the carbohydrate and lipid moieties. Apparently under the conditions of digestion, the enzyme was more thorough in removing the amino acid residues from the lipid and carbohydrate.

B. RELATION BETWEEN ANTIGENICITY AND COMPOSITION

The results of this study indicate that the primary determinant of elastin antigenicity must be a component uniquely present in the polar fractions of both preparations, rather than in the crosslinked or non-polar fractions. It appears likely that the charge and the lipid content play an essential role in determining antigenicity and that the enrichment in polar amino acids, especially aspartic acid, and the relatively high content of serine and threonine parallel concentrations in the antigenic moiety of collagen reported earlier by Seifter (1965) and more recently by Leroy (1969). However, as pointed out by Sela (1969) the spatial configuration and the relative positioning of the amino acid side chains in the backbone of a protein must be considered before the requisites for antigenic sites can be established.

REFERENCES

Grabar, P. and Burtin, P. (1960). Analyse Immunoelectrophoretique.

Keller, S., Levi, M. and Mandl, I. (1969). Arch. Biochem. Biophys. 132, 565.

Keller, S. and Mandl, I. (1965). In Structure and Function of Connective and Skeletal Tissue, p. 119. Ed. by Fitton Jackson, S. et al. Butterworth and Co., London.

Keller, S. and Mandl, I. (1969). Biochem. Biophys. Res. Comm. 35, 687.

LeRoy, E.C. (1969). J. Immunol. 102, 919.

Robert, L. and Poullain, N. (1963). Bull. Soc. Chim. Biol. 45, 1317.

Seifter, S. (1965). In Structure and Function of Connective and Skeletal Tissue, p. 417. Ed. by Fitton Jackson, S. et al. Butterworth and Co., London.

Sela, M. (1969). Naturwiss. 56, 206.

STUDIES ON THE STRUCTURE OF ELASTIN AND THE MECHANISM OF ACTION OF ELASTOLYTIC ENZYMES

B. Robert and L. Robert

The study of the tertiary structure and conformation of elastin is facilitated by the availability of controlled degradation methods giving large peptides. Such methods were proposed (Partridge, Davis, and Adair, 1955) and some interesting information could be obtained already with these peptides (Partridge and Davis, 1955: Mammi, Gotte and Pezzin, 1968; Kornfeld-Poullain and Robert, 1968). We want to report here briefly on some recent studies we have undertaken in order to gain insight into the structure of purified elastin and in the mechanism of its enzymatic degradation. Iodine labelled elastin was prepared and used as a substrate for the study of kinetics and mechanism of action of elastolytic enzymes and for the preparation of kappa-elastin and its fractionation (Robert and Robert, unpublished data).

I. PROPERTIES OF IODINE-LABELLED ELASTIN

Elastin labelled with ^{125}I or ^{131}I having a specific activity of 2 to 10.10^3 C/m/mg was prepared and degraded to kappa-elastin by incubation at 37°C with 1 $\underline{M}$ KOH in 80% aqueous ethanol (Robert and Poullain, 1963). This kappa-elastin was then fractionated on a DEAE-Sephadex column using an ammonium formate buffer for elution (Robert and Robert, unpublished data). Fig. 1 shows the fractionation obtained. The first major peak (comprising fractions I, II, III) has a specific radioactivity of 5100 C/min/mg

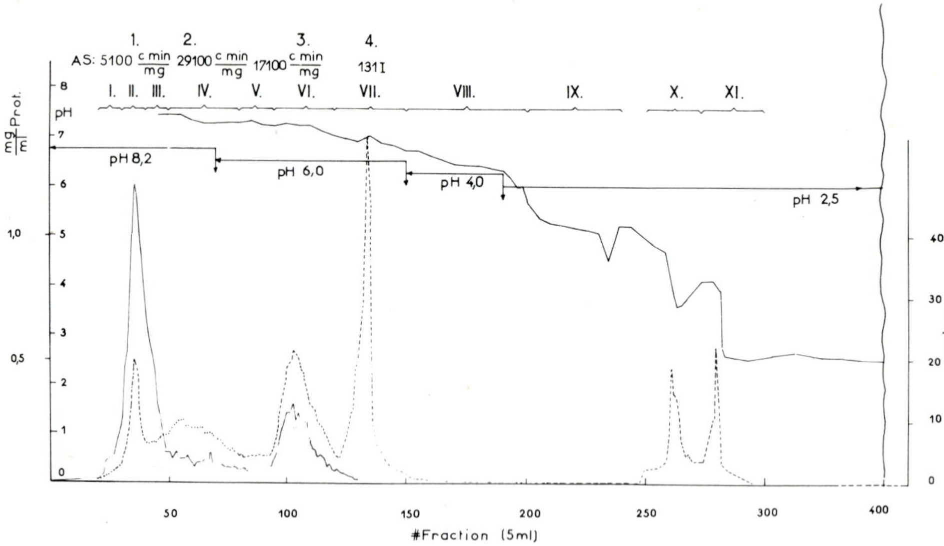

Fig. 1. Elution profile of kappa-elastin prepared from a ^{131}I -labelled elastin (NaOH purified, bovine ligamentum nuchae 12400 C/min/mg) on DEAE-Sephadex-A50 (47x2.5 cm). Stepwise elution with ammonium formate buffer 0.05 M of the pH is indicated. The specific activity of peaks 1, 2 and 3 are indicated at the top. (A.S.). Roman numbers indicate the fractions which were separately analysed. Ordinate on the left indicates the protein concentration of the fractions and on the right the radioactivity. Proteins, ———— ; radioactivity, --------- . The continuous decreasing curve indicates the pH-gradient.

protein and comprises the major portion of elastin peptides. It coacervates at pH 4.5 above 25° C, as does α-elastin (Partridge et al., 1955). It is followed by a second minor (fractions IV-V) and third major peaks (fraction VI) having a much higher specific activity (3 to 6 times higher than for the first peak). After the peak of free iodine, (fraction VII) a yellow band still firmly adheres sticking to the column and can be eluted only with a strongly acid buffer or with HCl at pH 2.5. In this fraction are found two close radioactive peaks that do not react to the Biuret and Folin reagent (fractions X-XI) and a final peak which has no radioactivity and absorbs at 280 mμ (fraction not shown in Fig. 1). These fractions, derived from the yellow pigment, contain lipidic material

(Robert and Robert, unpublished data). The yield of iodination of elastin being quite low ($\lesssim 10^{-3}$ g/atom of ^{125}I/g mole tyrosine), it appears that peptides of fractions IV to VI are preferentially iodinated. Together with the chemical, physical, metabolic and immunological properties of these fractions, these results were interpreted as signifying a heterogenous composition of elastin. It appears quite possible that some of the peptides present in peaks IV to VI are derived from the structural glycoprotein fraction strongly attached to elastin (Robert, Robert, Moczar and Moczar,1968). These glycoproteins are more accessible than the hydrophobic elastin fibers to iodination; they are also richer in tyrosine (Robert and Comte, 1968). This conception could also explain the attack on elastin fibers by enzymes unable to entirely "solubilise" in vitro purified elastin, as the blood platelet enzyme which recently was shown to attack iodine-labelled elastin (Robert, Pignaud, Legrand, Caen and Robert, 1969). Such enzymes may play an important role in the pathological degradation of elastin.

II MECHANISM OF ACTION OF PANCREATIC ELASTASE ON IODINE-LABELLED ELASTIN

A. EXISTENCE OF SPECIFIC FIXATION SITES FOR ELASTASE

Using ^{125}I-labelled elastin as a substrate we could follow the kinetics of its "solubilisation" by crystalline pancreatic elastase parallel to the splitting of peptide bonds as determined from the pH-stat-recording (Robert and Robert, unpublished data). It was shown that there is a rapid and first-order splitting of peptide bonds during the lag phase of the solubilisation curve. This is followed by a rapid "solubilisation" of elastin as shown by the appearance of radioactive peptides in the supernate. During this rapid solubilisation phase the peptide bond splitting slows considerably and follows a zero-order reaction with no apparent plateau. The considerable slowing of the peptide bond splitting is interpreted to be a result of the disappearance of specific fixation sites during the rapid hydrolysis which takes place during the lag period of solubilisation. The disappearance of specific fixation sites for the enzyme on the surface of the fibers could be due to conformational changes of the peptide chains consecutive to the hydrolysis of a limited number of critical peptide bonds. This contention is supported by the absence of the rapid first-order hydrolysis-phase when soluble kappa-elastin is used as a substrate. The hydrolysis of kappa-elastin appears as a slow zero-order process on the pH-stat-recording with a velocity quite close to the one observed with fibrous elastin during the last zero-order phase of the reaction.

B. ADSORPTION OF ELASTASE ON ELASTIN

The existence of such specific fixation sites for elastase on the surface of the elastic fibers is strongly supported by the following experiments: 50-200 hg of crystalline elastase is added to 10 mg of ^{125}I-labelled elastin in 0.005 M, ph 4.5, acetate buffer. After 10 min of incubation the elastin suspension is washed three times on a centrifuge and resuspended in 0.1 M, pH 8.6, Tris-HCl buffer. Figure 2 shows the kinetics of "solubilisation" of this elastin suspension, due to the strongly adsorbed elastase, which could not be removed by washing. The speed of "solubilisation" of elastin by the adsorbed enzyme is quite comparable to that obtained with freshly added enzyme (Fig. 2). The time for 50% "solubilisation" is even shorter with the pre-adsorbed elastin-elastase complex. When ^{131}I-labelled elastin is added to a ^{125}I-elastin-elastase adsorption complex the kinetics of degradation of both elastin can be followed. Figure 3 shows that the ^{125}I-elastin to

Préabsorbtion at pH 4.5 on Elastin – ^{125}I

Enzyme conc.	t 50% min. with	t 50% min. without
50 μg	55	66
100 μg	30	48
200 μg	17	34

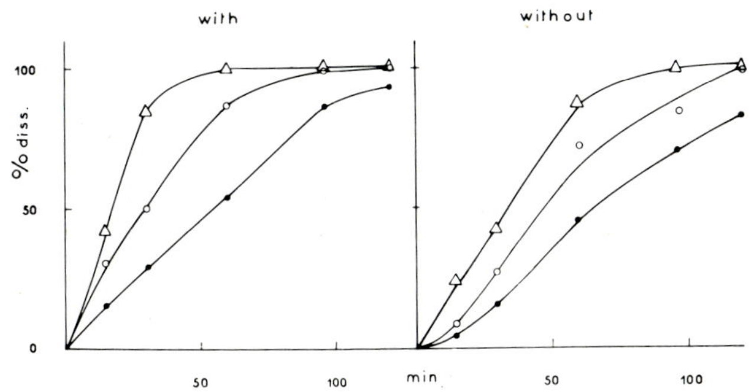

Fig. 2. Kinetics of "solubilisation" of 10 mg of ^{125}I-labelled elastin in the presence of 50, 100 and 200 ug pancreatic elastase. Left: with preabsorption followed by washing as described in the text. Right: without preabsorption, by adding the enzyme directly to elastin. "Solubilisation" was determined on aliquots taken at time intervals and determining radioactivity in the filtrate. The table above the figure indicates the time for 50% "solubilisation" of elastin with and without preabsorption of elastase.

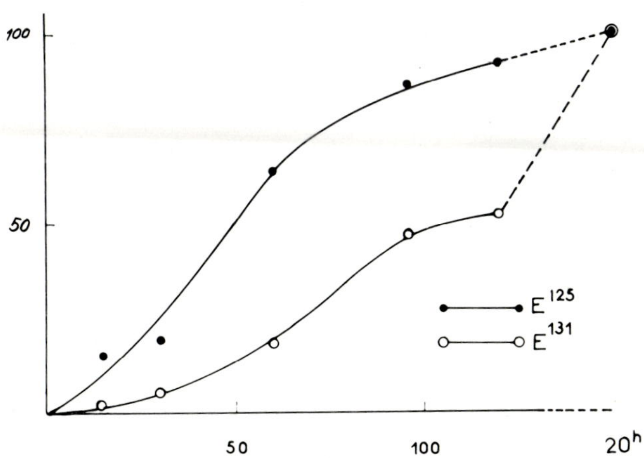

Fig. 3. Kinetics of dissolution of ^{131}I and ^{125}I-labelled elastin. 50 ug elastase was preabsorbed on ^{125}I-elastin, washed and mixed with ^{131}I-elastin. Ordinates: per cent dissolution. Abscissa: time of incubation at 37°C.

which elastase was adsorbed is degraded at a much faster rate. The diffusion of elastase from this adsorption-complex to the ^{131}I-elastin is quite slow and can be estimated from these curves (Robert and Robert, unpublished data). This diffusion is in the order of 0.5% of the added enzyme per minute at 37°C. These results confirm the existence of specific fixation sites on the surface of elastic fibers and show that elastase preferentially attacks the fiber to which it is adsorbed. It diffuses only after a certain number of bonds are split, resulting in a conformation of the fiber with distorted fixation sites.

REFERENCES

Kornfeld-Poullain, N. and Robert, L. (1968). Bull. Soc. Chim. Biol. 50, 759.

Mammi, M., Gotte, L. and Pezzin, G. (1968). Nature 220, 371.

Moczar, M. and Robert, L. (1969). J. Atheroscler. Res., submitted for publication.

Partridge, S. M. (1962). Adv. Prot. Chem. 17, 227.

Partridge, S. M. and Davis, H. F. (1955). Biochem. J. 61, 21.

Partridge, S.M., Davis, H. F. and Adair, G.S. (1955) Biochem. J. 61, 11.

Robert, L. and Comte, P. (1968) Life Sciences Part II, 7, 493.

Robert, B., Pignaud, G., Legrand, Y., Caen, J. and Robert, L. (1969). Pathol. Biol. 17, 615.

Robert, L. and Poullain, N. (1963). Bull. Soc. Chim. Biol. 45, 1317.

Robert, L., Robert, B., Moczar,M. and Moczar, E. (1968). In Le Role de la Paroi Artérielle dans l'Athérogénèse (Colloque CNRS, 1967), p. 395.

ELASTICITY AND THERMODYNAMICS OF ELASTIN

Torkel Weis-Fogh and S.O. Andersen

The two best known elastomers in animals are elastin in vertebrate connective tissue and resilin in arthropod cuticle. In the dry state they are both hard and inextensible but become endowed with long-range elasticity when swollen in water and many other polar solvents. However, with respect to chemistry, structure, and elastic behavior they differ considerably (Andersen and Weis-Fogh, 1964). In resilin about 34% of the side chains carry hydrophilic polar groups against 5% in elastin. Swollen resilin behaves as a random network of thermally agitated polypeptide chains in accordance with kinetic theories for swollen rubber, as was found in thermodynamical (Weis-Fogh, 1961a), mechanical, and optical studies (Weis-Fogh, 1961b). The classical investigation by Meyer and Ferri (1936) on elastin and the more recent ones by Hoeve and Flory (1958) have been interpreted as meaning that swollen elastin is also a rubber in the sense that the elastic force is caused by thermal agitation of the kinetically free chains whose configurational entropy decreases with strain, while the changes in internal energy remain zero or are negligible, $(dO/dL)_{T,V} = 0$. The swelling of elastin is very temperature dependent and the experimental difficulty which this gives rise to was overcome by Hoeve and Flory (1958) who used a mixed solvent system (ethylene glycol-water, 30:70 v/v) in which the swelling of elastin is almost independent of temperature. Volpin and Ciferri (these proceedings, p. 691) point out that mixed solvent systems introduce a further complication because the equilibrium distribution of the solvent components between the elastin sample and the surrounding medium is not independent of temperature. However, they found that the swelling of elastin in pure water is almost constant between 50 and 70°C, and within this range their results indicate that about 85% of the isometric force is caused by changes in configurational entropy while the remaining 15% must be attributed to changes in internal energy. This applies to an extension ratio of about $\lambda = 1.25$.

The interpretation put forward by Volpin and Ciferri (these proceedings, p.691) may indeed turn out to be correct as far as the mechanical force is concerned. However, the basic approach is based on an application of the Wiegand and Snyder (1934) equation, whether in its simple or more complicated form (Hoeve and Flory, 1962), and this presupposes not only that the system is reversible but also that it is free of chemical reaction, as discussed by Weis-Fogh (1961a).

The main points which we want to make in this preliminary report are (a) that when elastin is deformed under physiological conditions (in water), the strain introduces a reversible chemical change which involves changes in internal energy ΔU far greater than those corresponding to the change in Helmholtz free energy ΔF, (b) that these changes could contribute significantly to the increase in isometric force with temperature and, therefore that a thermodynamic analysis of elastin will have to take contribtuions from chemical reactions and interfacial forces into consideration. Indeed, as a swollen elastomer, elastin may involve ' the most extraordinary circumstances' for which Hoeve and Flory (1962) had to make exceptions.

I EXPERIMENTAL PROCEDURE

Elastin free of collagen and lipid was prepared from adult bovine <u>ligamentum nuchae</u> according to the purification scheme of Partridge, Davis and Adair (1955). The only modification was that the ligament was purified in the form of thin strips instead of being finely minced. This made it necessary to autoclave the preparation about six times to obtain biuret-negative extracts.

Samples about 35mg dry weight, 15-20 mm long and about 3 mm^2 in cross sectional area, were suspended inside the reaction chamber of a microcalorimeter originally designed by Clarke and Rothschild (1957). The chamber has a capacity of 2.3 ml and was connected to the exterior by means of a long metal chain so that the sample could be stretched, relaxed, the force extension curve measured, and the changes in stored energy ΔF estimated in slow reversible deformations. The calorimter is suitable for detecting rates of heat production, dQ/dt, of the order of 1 mcal/hr. When the amount of change was about 3-5 mcal and when it took place during the first minute after the deformation, the calorimeter could be used as an integrating device where the heat produced or absorbed, $Q = \int_{t=0}^{t=t} dQ/dt$, could be estimated within about 5% in the course of about 15 min (Fig. 1).

It turned out that the amount of heat produced during stretching was always about equal to the heat absorbed when the sample was relaxed (Table I). Since the stress-strain curves were also reversible, this means that the sample plus the surrounding solvent in the container can be considered as a reversible and closed thermodynamic system at constant temperature (T) and pressure, and with very small volume change, if any. We then have that the reversible heat exchange $Q^{(rev)} = T\,\Delta S$, where Q is the heat absorbed by the system and ΔS is the change of entropy. Furthermore, $W^{(rev)} = -\Delta F$, where W is the work done by the system on the surroundings and ΔF is the change in free energy. Since the fundamental equation for a closed system at constant temperature is

$$\Delta F = \Delta U - T\,\Delta S \qquad (1),$$

we can now estimate the change in internal energy ΔU within the accuracy of the calorimeter by inserting the two measured quantities as

$$\Delta U = Q^{(rev)} - W^{(rev)} \qquad (2).$$

TABLE I

Heat Exchange Q and Mechanical Work when Elastin Samples were Extended and Relaxed.

SAMPLE	Mechanical Work (mcal)	Q extend. (mcal)	Q relax (mcal)	Ratio, Q relax./ Q extend.
1	1.33	-5.53	+5.60	1.01
2	1.02	-5.60	+6.10	1.09
		-5.71	+5.32	0.93
		-6.13	+6.00	0.98
3	1.08	-5.73	+5.50	0.96
		-5.92	+5.41	0.91

A positive sign means that heat was absorbed by the system.

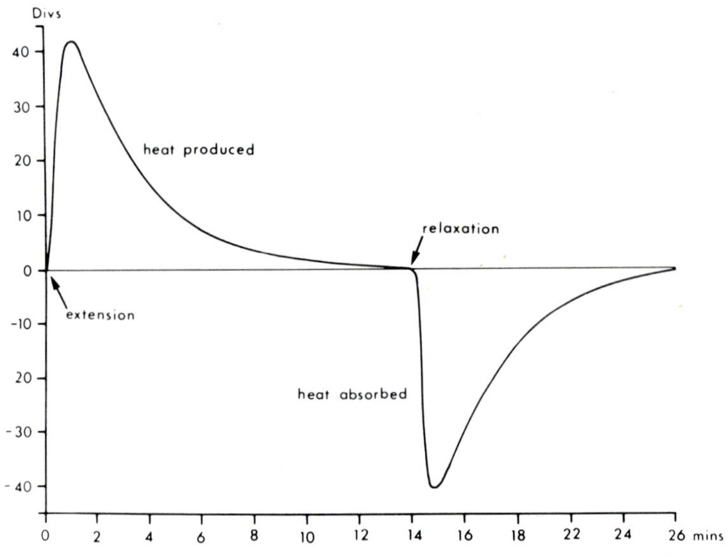

Fig. 1. Heat exchange measured in the calorimeter when a sample of elastin is extended (stretched) or relaxed. One division on the ordinate equals 0.046 mcal/min

II EXPERIMENTAL RESULTS

In an ideal "dry" rubber or in an ideal rubber isotropically swollen in a solvent in which there is no chemical affinity between the chains and the solvent but only a mutual tendency for diffusion, there should be no change in internal energy with deformation ($\Delta U = 0$) and $Q^{(rev)} = W^{(rev)}$. This is far from being the case in elastin placed in pure water or in a dilute phosphate buffer, as can be seen from Table I.

It is seen that the amount of heat given off during extension is about five times larger than the change in free energy so that, typically, $\Delta U = -5 - (-1) = -4$ mcal when the sample is stretched from the swollen length $\lambda = 1.00$ to $\lambda = 1.35$. Conversely, during the succeeding relaxation $\Delta U = +4$ mcal. In other words, the results prove that deformation of elastin in water entails a reversible chemical change which is several times larger in terms of energy than that corresponding to the mechanical change. In this respect elastin differs fundamentally from an ordinary rubber.

When we first found this large heat exchange during stretching of elastin samples we thought that it might be due to some reversible chemical process having a high heat of reaction. In an attempt to characterise this process further we changed the medium surrounding the sample to see whether this would alter the heat exchange. Figure 2 shows that changes in pH have very little effect, indicating that charged groups are not involved to any significant extent.

Figure 3 shows that the entrophy term is strongly influenced by the presence of aliphatic alcohols in the medium and that the effect is larger with alcohols having longer hydrocarbon chains. The concentration of alcohol in the medium is also important as shown in Figure 4. At ethanol concentrations exceeding 30% the entropy term changes sign so that there is a heat uptake instead of a heat output during stretching. In a mixture of ethylene glycol: water (30:70 v/v) the work was numerically about equal to the entropy change, as would be expected in the relatively simple systems discussed by Hoeve and Flory (1958).

The pronounced effect which results from changes in the composition of the medium indicates that the reaction characterised by the large entropy does not only involve

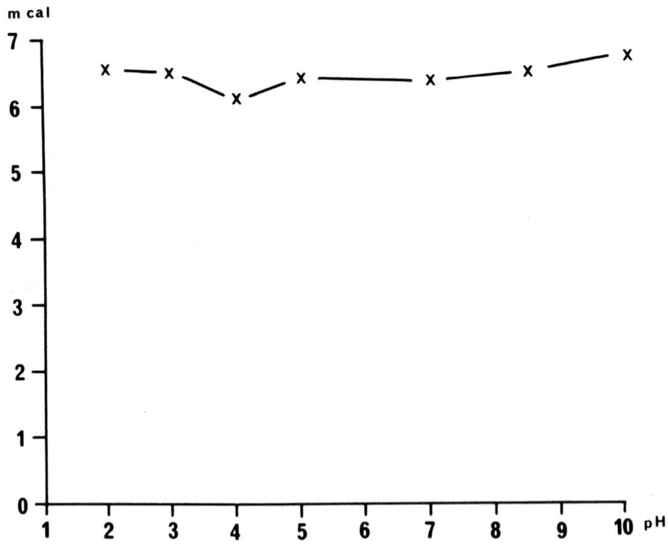

Fig. 2. The effect of pH on the heat production when a sample of elastin is stretched.

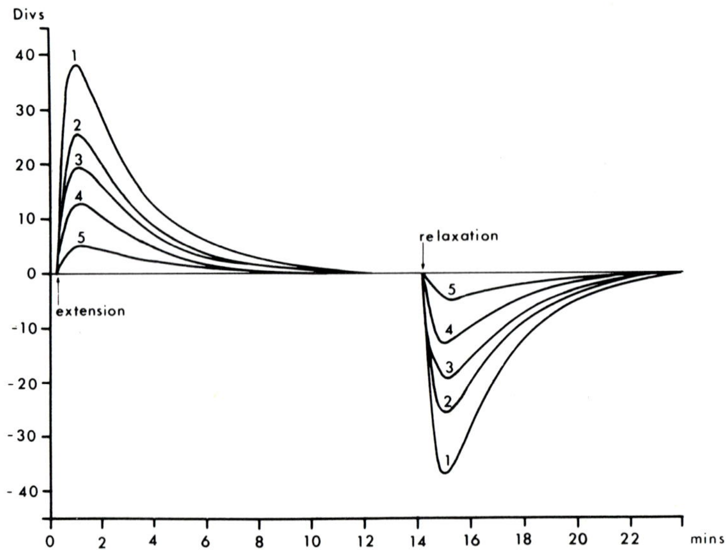

Fig. 3 The effect of organic solvents on the heat exchange of elastin. 1; in water; 2; in 2 M methanol; 3; in 2 M ethanol; 4; in 2 M n-propanol; 5; in formamide. One division on the ordinate equals 0.046 mcal/min.

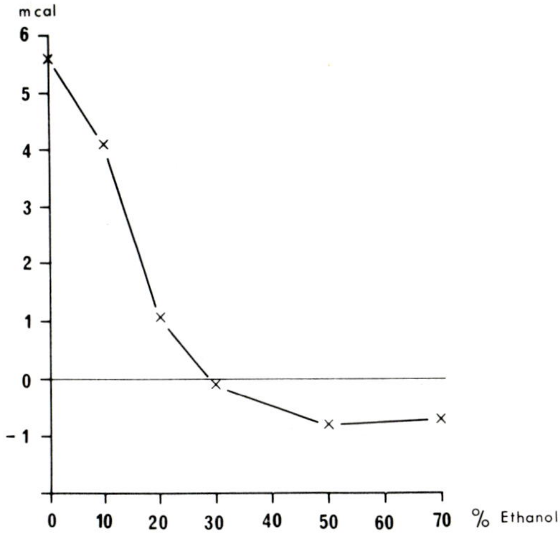

Fig. 4. The effect of the concentration of ethanol on the heat production on stretching a sample of elastin.

the elastin but also the medium. One type of reaction which could be involved is a transfer of hydrophobic groups from a hydrophobic environment into a water phase, as such transfers are characterised by a large decrease in entropy (Nemethy and Scheraga, 1962). The results of Partridge (1967) using columns packed with elastin fibres for gel-filtration indicate that elastin behaves as a two-phase system: the volume in the column accessible for hydrophobic alcohols is considerably greater than the volume accessible for hydrophilic compounds like sugars. Partridge (1966, and these proceedings, p.593) has suggested a molecular structure of elastin which explains his findings. He envisages that elastin is composed of globular molecules which have hydrophobic groups packed in the interior and the hydrophilic groups on the surface where they are exposed to the water phase which also fills the space between the globules. The globules are interlinked by means of the various crosslinks discussed elsewhere in these proceedings.

Such a two-phase model of elastin may be suitable for explaining both our results from the calorimetric measurements in Figs. 1-4 and the elastic properties discussed in the next section.

III POSSIBLE IMPLICATIONS: TWO TYPES OF ELASTOMERS

A. NEW TYPE: "LIQUID DROP" ELASTOMERS.

The classical and, indeed, the traditional elastomers consist of a random network of kinetically free chains linked together at intervals by means of stable crosslinks: in the case of rubber, by sulphur bridges, and in resilin, by di-and tri-tyrosine residues (Andersen, 1966). However, the problems posed by the elastin have led us to believe that another type of elastomer may exist which is fundamentally different from a rubber-like one.

Consider long-chain hydrophobic molecules suspended in a hydrophilic liquid, or hydrophilic molecules in a hydrophobic liquid. This is of course a dispersed two-phase system. Assume, moreover, that a chain is kinetically free when the links are surrounded by its own kind. Such a suspended molecule will tend to behave as a spherical droplet of liquid because the interfacial tension will tend to keep the interfacial area ("surface") at a minimum. Since the "droplet" is in fact a thermally agitated chain, it is possible by means of suitable groups and reactions to crosslink neighbouring molecules at a few points and thereby to form an isotropic material consisting of spatially fixed spherical molecules surrounded by solvent, apart from where the covalent crosslinks bridge the distance between spheres. Such an assembly of interconnected spheres will behave as an elastomer, and we believe that this has not been recognised so far. On uni-directional deformation the spheres will tend to be drawn out into prolate spheroids and the interfacial areas will increase causing both a decrease in configurational entropy of the chains (as in ordinary rubber but with steric restrictions) <u>and</u> an increase in free energy due to the work done against interfacial forces. If it were possible to interconnect liquid droplets suspended in another liquid phase in which they were not soluble, such a system would behave as an ideal "liquid-drop" elastomer in which the changes in configurational entropy would be minimal and the elastic force would be caused mainly by the energy term, in this case due to work done against interfacial forces. Both the ideal random network and the liquid-drop assembly could form stable elastic structures with no flow or faults, but, in other respects, they would be very different and endowed with different potentialities with respect to modification and mode of formation.

B. ELASTIN COMPARED WITH NEW MODEL

With our present knowledge of water-swollen elastin it is reasonable to consider this elastomer as an isotropic assembly of globules with a hydrophobic core and with the relatively few hydrophilic groups scattered at the surfaces (interfaces), as suggested by Partridge. According to recent determinations, the molecular weight of tropoelastin is 67,000 (Sandberg, Hackett and Carnes, according to Partridge, these proceedings, p.593). If the density of the dry protein is 1.33 g/cm^3, the diameter of the spherical molecule will be about 54 Å and the surface area about 9,000 Å^2. Since only about 5% of the amino acid side chains in elastin carry polar groups, calculations show that the available polar groups cannot in any way cover the surface of the globules. This means that an increase of the surface area as a consequence of stretching will bring nonpolar groups to the surface where they will interact with water. Can this (a) explain the large changes in entropy and (b) affect the energy terms and the elastic force?

At present, any calculations must be tentative and of a preliminary nature and we shall only attempt to illustrate the sign, the principles, and the order of magnitude of the effects. Let us first consider the change in surface area as a function of the extension ration λ (Fig. 5, solid line). It is seen that the area changes slowly to begin with and later increases almost linearly with λ. The surface area of an elastin molecule will increase by about 3% corresponding to 270 Å^2 when the sample is stretched from $\lambda = 1.00$ to $\lambda = 1.35$. This corresponds to the area occupied by 22 tightly packed spherical CH_3-groups, each of diameter 3.7 Å and a cross-sectional area of 12 Å^2. In a sample of 35 mg

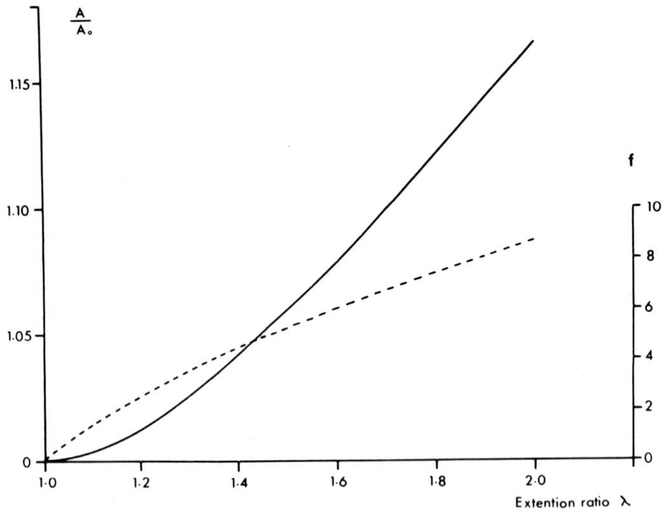

Fig. 5. Fully drawn line: The relative surface area, A/A_o, of a sphere being deformed into a prolate spheroid by a unidirectional force. The area is caluclated according to the formula:

$$A = 1/2A_o\left(\lambda^{-1} + \lambda^{1/2}\frac{\sin^{-1}\sqrt{1-\lambda^{-3}}}{\sqrt{1-\lambda^{-3}}}\right)$$

Broken line: Tensile force, f, as a function of extension ratio, λ, calculated according to the formula for swollen isotropic rubbers: $f = Gxv^{1/3}(\lambda-\lambda^{-2})$, using values for G = 6.4 kg/cm^2 and v = 0.45.

dry elastin this corresponds to a transfer of 1.1 x 10^{-5} mole CH_3-from the core to the surface. According to Nemethy and Scheraga (1962), the transfer of an alanine side chain from water into a nonpolar phase at 25°C is accompanied by the following changes: $\Delta F°_{tr}$ = -1.3 kcal/mole, and $\Delta H°_{tr}$ = +1.5 kcal/mole, and $\Delta S°_{tr}$ = +9.4 entropy units/mole. In the case of the reversible transport in the opposite direction from the core of the molecule to the water-exposed surface, we assume that the side chains do not become completely surrounded by water molecules so that the actual values will be about half those corresponding to transfer from bulk phase to bulk phase. The transport from a hydrophobic core to the surface should then result in the following approximate changes in our calorimeter vessel:

$$\Delta F_{tr} = 0.5 \times 1.3 \times 10^{6} \times 1.1 \times 10^{-5} = 7.2 \text{ mcal}$$

$$T\Delta S_{tr} = 0.5 \times 9.4 \times 1.1 \times 10^{-5} \times 298 = -15.4 \text{ mcal}$$

$$\Delta U = \Delta F + T\Delta S = -8.2 \text{ mcal}$$

In other words, the changes in entropy and internal energy are of the same sign and of the same general order of magnitude at 25°C as in our experiment.

It is also of importance that the work required to transfer a hydrophobic group from a hydrophobic environment to a hydrophilic one increases with temperature (Nemethy and Scheraga, 1962). In other words, interfacial forces will tend to increase their potential contribution to the isometric force of such a system when the temperature is increased. At the same time, the entropy change decreases numerically, and in our latest experiments in a modified calorimeter we have found that $T\Delta S$ decreased continuously with temperature (Fig. 6), as would be expected, while the force increased at constant relative extension (based on length at equilibrium swelling at the temperature in question).

The sign and magnitude of the internal energy changes imply that interfacial forces must be taken into account and could exert a significant influence on the force-extension relationship. The actual curves for elastin swollen in water at different temperatures (Fig. 7) resemble the area-extension relationship in Figure 5 more than does the stress-strain curve for an ordinary rubber (broken curve in Fig. 5). This may be fortuitous, as suggested by Hoeve and Flory (1958), but it deserves further study in the light of the new evidence.

It is even possible that the shape of the curve in Fig. 5 (solid line) which illustrates the relationship between area increase and extension ratio might represent the relationship between axial elastic tension f (ordinate) and relative extension $\varepsilon = \lambda - 1$ (abscissa). The stored elastic energy is $W = \int_0^{\varepsilon} f(\varepsilon)\, d\varepsilon$, which at medium and large extensions approaches proportionality with ε^2 due to the almost linear force-extension curve. This differs from the case of simple surface tension where the inter-

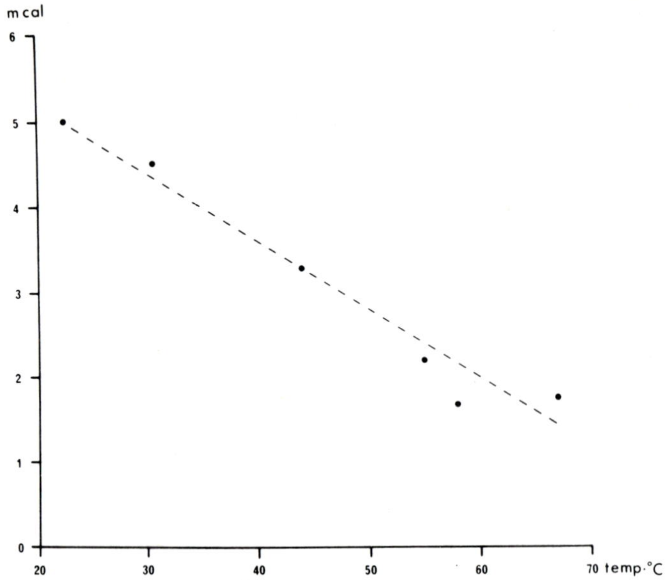

Fig. 6. The effect of temperature on the heat produced when stretching a sample of elastin at constant temperature.

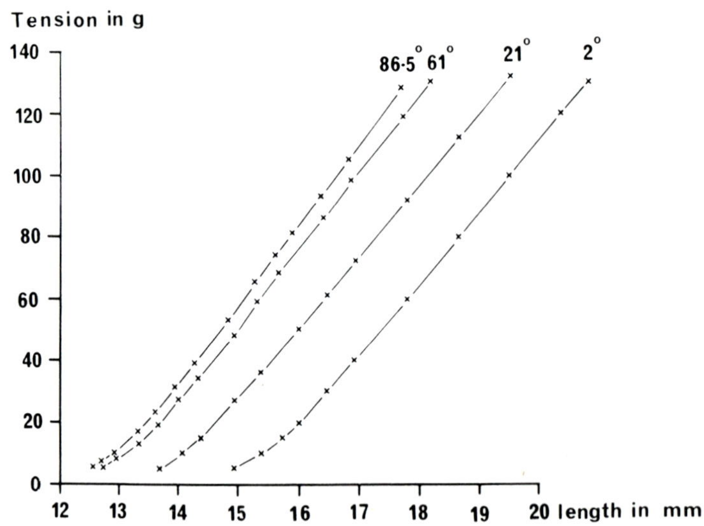

Fig. 7. Length-tension curves for a sample of elastin stretched at different temperatures.

facial tension γ is constant and $W = \gamma \Delta A$ so that W is proportional to ε. In the case of elastin one must namely envisage that the interfacial tension increases with increasing area due to the increased surface concentration of hydrophobic groups. The system is therefore different from the simple two-phase case but is analogous to a system in which a third, surface active substance is present in limited amounts and where, within a wide range, the interfacial tension is dependent on the ratio between the groups which constitute the surface.

It is obvious that the mechanical behaviour of elastin must be studies in considerably greater detail than hitherto.

IV CONCLUSIONS

It is too early to decide to what extent elastin behaves as an ideal liquid-drop elastomer. However, in biology as well as in technology this new type of elastomer is a possibility to be reckoned with. In particular, single molecules with liquid-drop properties could assemble linearly and form single-chain stable springs with ideal elastomeric properties and of molecular width, which would not be feasible in the stable, random network of crosslinked rubber-like material. It should be mentioned that the pronounced elastic properties of insect flight muscle has neither been localized nor understood at the molecular level (Pringle, 1967), and there are probably many other tissues and cells in which elastomeric structures are of functional importance.

ACKNOWLEDGEMENTS

We wish to thank Mr. M.J. Hubbard and Mr. M.J. Pearson, B.A., for their able assistance.

This research has been sponsored in part by the American Air Force through the European Office of Aerospace Research, OAR, United States Air Force under Contract no. F6 1052-67-C-0012.

REFERENCES

Andersen, S.O. (1966). Acta Physiol. Scand. 66, suppl. 263, 1.

Andersen, S.O. and Weis-Fogh, T. (1964). Advanc. Insect Physiol. 2,1.

Clarke, E.W. and Rothschild, Lord. (1957). Proc. Roy. Soc. B, 147, 316.

Hoeve, C.A.J. and Flory, P.J. (1958). J. Amer. Chem. Soc. 80, 6523.

Hoeve, C.A.J. and Flory, P.J. (1962). J. Polymer Sci. 60, 155.

Meyer, K.H. and Ferri, L. (1936). Pflug. Arch. ges. Physiol. 238, 78.

Nemethy, G. and Scheraga, H.A. (1962). J. Phys. Chem. 66, 1773.

Partridge, S.M. (1966). In The Physiology and Biochemistry of Muscle as a Food. pp. 327-339, Ed. by Briskey, Cassens and Trautman. The University of Wisconsin Press, Madison, Wisconsin.

Partridge, S.M. (1967). Nature, 213, 1123.

Partridge, S.M., Davis, H.F. and Adair, G.S. (1955). Biochem. J. 61, 11.

Pringle, J.W.S. (1967). Progr. Biophys. Mol. Biol, 17, 1.

Weis-Fogh, T. (1961a). J. Mol. Biol. 3, 520.

Weis-Fogh, T. (1961b). J. Mol. Biol. 3, 648.

Wiegand, W.B. and Snyder, J.W. (1934). I.R.I. Trans. 10, 234.

INVESTIGATIONS ON THE PHYSICOCHEMICAL AND CONFORMATIONAL PROPERTIES OF ELASTIN

L. Gotte, M. Mammi and G. Pezzin

I SOLUBLE ELASTIN

α-Elastin, the soluble protein which is obtained from the native elastin by treatment with oxalic acid (Partridge and Davis, 1955), was prepared from ox ligamentum nuchae elastin free from collagen, muco- and glycoproteins (Gotte and Serafini-Fracassini, 1963). The amino acid composition of the recovered α-elastin, which accounted for 75% of the starting material, was found not to differ much from that of the parent protein (Mammi, Gotte and Pezzin, 1968), in agreement with Partridge and Davis (1955) and, more recently, Bentley and Hanson (1969). The characterization of this soluble protein was carried out by several chemical and physicochemical methods.

The viscosity of solutions of α-elastin in water was rather low and the intrinsic viscosity, [η] was found to be only about 3 ml/g, close to that reported for most globular proteins (Tanford, 1961). The refractive index increments dn/dc at 546 mμ were 0.16 ml/g in water and 0.19 in trifluoroethanol (TFE). Using these values, which are near to those usually found for proteins, the weight-average molecular weight, M_w, was obtained by light scattering measurements on solutions in water and in TFE, by means of a Sofica photometer.

The values found were of the order of 10^6, suggesting that the α-elastin molecules may be associated in solution. Evidence for association was also given by the curvature and by the negative slope of the Zimm plots (Fig. 1). This

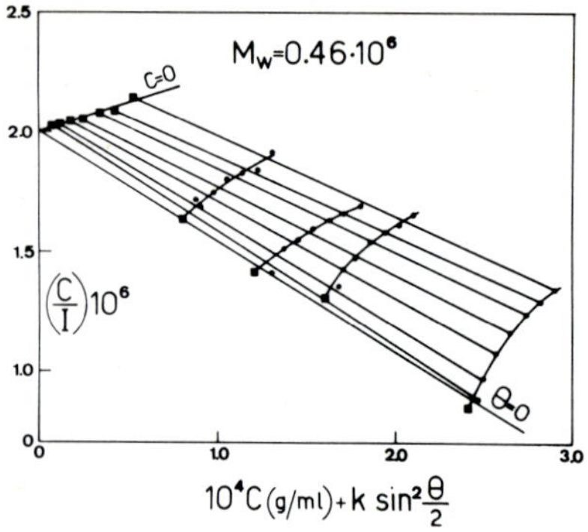

Fig. 1. Light scattering results for water solutions of soluble elastin, plotted according to the Zimm method. C is the concentration and I is the light intensity scattered at the angle Θ.

hypothesis seems to be further supported by the large number of N-terminal residues (about 20 moles per 10^5g of α-elastin). This value was determined by the 3,5-dinitropyridylderivative procedure (Signor, Previero and Terbojevich, 1965) and is very close to that found by Partridge and Davis (1955) by the conventional DNP method.

The conformational properties of α-elastin have been investigated by measuring the far ultraviolet circular dichroism of solutions in water, sulphuric acid, methanesulphonic acid, ethylene glycol, ethanol and trifluoroethanol and in mixtures of these solvents with water.

Some typical results are shown in Fig. 2. The spectra of TFE solutions, as well as those in 97% ethanol (Mammi et. al., 1968) and in ethylene glycol, which are known to favour helical conformations, showthe typical features of the right-handed α-helix, whereas those of sulphuric acid and methanesulphonic acid solutions strictly resemble that of a random coil. The spectrum of solutions in water, which shows a negative band at about 200 mμ and a smaller band at about 222 mμ, exhibits intermediate features and indicates that the α-helix content is of the order of 10% (Mammi et al., 1968), as estimated from the ellipticity value of the negative band at 222 mμ.

The ellipticity of this band changed smoothly and gradually when the amount of sulphuric acid, ethylene glycol and ethanol in the water was increased, while a sharper variation in the range from 0 to 20% was found with TFE, suggesting the occurance of a random coil to helix transition.

On raising the temperature from 5 to 60°C the α-helix content increased in water and decreased in TFE, although the variations were rather small. No conformational changes seemed to occur in solutions of pure ethylene glycol. These temperature effects were also confirmed by optical rotatory power measurements at 436 mμ.

Quite similar CD patterns were shown by α-elastin obtained from human aorta.

II NATIVE ELASTIN

The analysis of several physicochemical properties of native elastin suggested the presence of some ordered structure also in the undegraded protein (Gotte, Mammi and Pezzin, 1968). As a matter of fact, while amorphous polymers usually show no more than two diffuse diffraction rings, the patterns of elastin fibres exhibited four rings at 9, 4.4, 2.2 and 1.12 Å, the first two appearing strengthened in the equatorial region upon stretching. Moreover a fibril structure was supported by electron microscope investigations on appropriately prepared samples, in agreement with the reports of other authors (Kawase, 1962; Fahrenbach, Sandberg and Cleary, 1966; Serafini-Fracassini and Tristam, 1966; Bartman, 1968). An anisotropic behaviour of native elastin samples was also found by measurements of their equilibrium swelling and tensile modulus (Gotte, et. al., 1968). However, no definite conclusions could be drawn on the actual conformation of native elastin from these results and from analysis of the thermal and dynamical-mechanical properties. More recently some indication was obtained by studying the thermoelastic behaviour of this protein (Volpin and Ciferri, 1969). Further, it was also found that the native and soluble elastin show quite similar IR and X-ray patterns. Unfortunately, oriented films or fibers of α-elastin, which would allow a

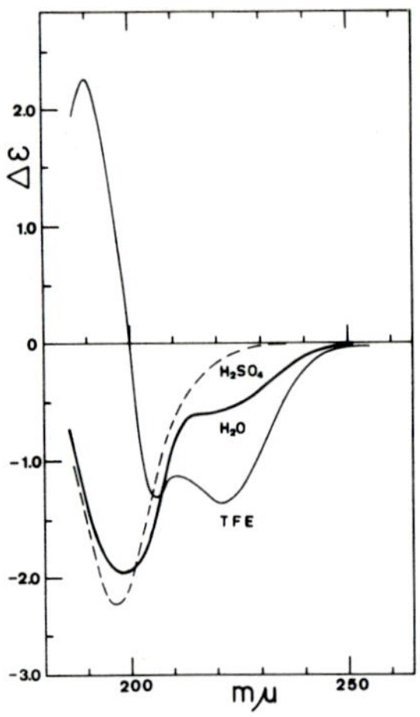

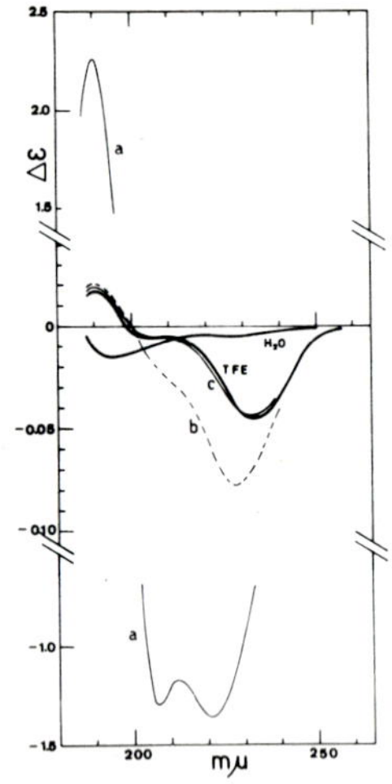

Fig. 2. Far ultraviolet CD spectra of α-elastin, obtained with a Roussel Jouan 185 Medel II Dichrograph. The Δε values were calculated using the mean molecular weight of 80.7.

Fig. 3. Far ultraviolet CD spectra of suspensions of elastin particles in H_2O and in TFE and of solution of α-elastin in TFE (curve a). (b) is curve a after correction for flattening absorption and (c) after correction for flattening absorption and dispersion distortion.

more detailed X-ray analysis, have not been prepared so far, possibly on account of the crosslinked structure of the macromolecules.

More striking evidence of the conformation of native elastin was obtained by measuring its circular dichroism spectra and comparing them with those of α-elastin. The CD patterns of fine particles, about 30 μ in diameter, suspended in water and in TFE (Fig. 3) are characterized by their very low ellipticity values. In the same figure, the spectrum of TFE solutions of α-elastin is also shown for a comparison (curve a).

Recently Urry and Ji (1968) demonstrated that the CD patterns of suspensions of spherical particles are related to those of true solutions by an equation which takes into account two factors, namely the flattening of the UV absorption spectrum (Duysens, 1956) and the dispersion distortion due to light scattering of the particles, both arising from the particulate nature of the systems. By applying these corrections to the spectra of soluble elastin, a satisfactory comparison is obtained with those of the native protein. The agreement is exceptionally good, as shown in Fig. 3 where in the case of the TFE solutions, a mean particle diameter of 28 μ and a K_D value of 20.10^{-20} cm^{-4} are used. Curve a is first reduced to curve b by the flattening-absorption correction and then to curve c by further correcting for the dispersion distortion.

The above results clearly indicate that a right-handed α-helical conformation is present also in the native elastin, although, on account of uncertainties in the physical parameters used for the corrections, it cannot be stated that the helical content is the same as in soluble elastin.

REFERENCES

Bartman, J. (1968). J. Microscopie 7, 355.

Bentley, J.P. and Hanson, A.N. (1969). Biochim.Biophys. Acta 175, 339.

Duysens, L.N.M. (1956). Biochim.Biophys. Acta 19, 1.

Fahrenbach, W.H., Sandberg, L.B. and Cleary, E.G. (1966). Anat. Rec. 155, 563.

Gotte, L., Mammi, M. and Pezzin, G. (1968). In Symposium on Fibrous Proteins, Australia 1967, p. 236. Ed. Crewther, W.G., Butterworths, London.

Gotte, L. and Serafini-Fracassini, A. (1963). J. Atheroscler. Res. 3, 247.

Kawase, O. (1962). In Medical and Clinical Aspects of Aging, Proc. Fifth Congr. Int. Assn. Gerontology, p. 523.

Mammi, M., Gotte, L. and Pezzin, G.(1968). Nature 220, 371.

Partridge, S.M. and Davis, H.F. (1955). Biochem J. 61, 21.

Serfini-Fracassini, A. and Tristram, G.R. (1966). Proc. Roy. Soc. Edinburgh. B69, 334.

Signor, A., Previero, A. and Terbojevich, M. (1965). Nature 205, 597.

Tanford, C. (1961). In Physical Chemistry of Macromolecules, p 394. Wiley, New York.

Urry, D.W. and Ji, T.H. (1968). Arch. Biochem. Biophys. 128, 802.

Volpin, D. and Ciferri, A. (1969). This book, p. 691.

THE ELASTIC BEHAVIOUR OF ELASTIN

D. Volpin and A. Ciferri

Investigations of elastic and thermoelastic behaviour of elastin include the early studies of Meyer and Ferri (1936), Wöhlisch, Weitnauer, Gruning and Rohrbach (1943) and the more recent ones by Hoeve and Flory (1958). Interest in this kind of study arises from the opportunity to combine the thermodynamic behaviour of elastin subjected to a tensile force with the theory of rubber elasticity.

A central problem in elastic and thermoelastic studies is to define experimental conditions which permit a relatively unambiguous molecular interpretation of the measured thermodynamic components of the stress.

The energy and entropy components of the stress required to characterize the molecular chain deformation, for a network in equilibrium swelling with a diluent, are those measured at constant volume and at fixed composition, i.e.

$$f = f_e + f_s = \left(\frac{\partial E}{\partial L}\right)_{VTN} - T\left(\frac{\partial S}{\partial L}\right)_{VTN} = \left(\frac{\partial E}{\partial L}\right)_{VTN} + T\left(\frac{\partial f}{\partial T}\right)_{VTN} \quad (1)$$

where f is the tensile force; E,L,V,T is the internal energy, the length, the volume and the temperature of the network respectively, and N indicates constancy of the mole number of the individual components. In fact, only in this case, is it possible to ignore the contributions to the stress due to dilational and compositional changes.

In practice, it is convenient to measure stress-temperature coefficients under equilibrium swelling at constant pressure and length, i.e. $(\partial f/\partial T)_{pLeq}$ and a method for converting the latter to $(\partial f/\partial T)_{VLN}$ should then be used if a proper interpretation of the fundamental elastic mechanism is to be made (Bashaw and Smith, 1968).

In fact, for elastin Meyer and Ferri (1936) and Wöhlisch et. al. (1943) found a large negative value for the energy component of the stress measured at constant length, constant pressure and under equilibrium swelling in water, which they attributed to stress-induced crystallization. Hoeve and Flory (1958), however, rejected the latter conclusion and attributed the internal energy changes to a reduction of the degree of swelling of elastin in water on increasing temperature. They attempted to circumvent this effect by performing a thermoelastic analysis in a water-glycol mixture where the total volume of the (unstressed) swollen polymer was independent of temperature, i.e., $(\partial V/\partial T)_{peq} = 0$. Under these conditions Hoeve and Flory (1958, 1962) and Bashaw and Smith (1968) have shown that

$$\left(\frac{\partial f}{\partial T}\right)_{pLeq} = \left(\frac{\partial f}{\partial T}\right)_{VLN} \qquad (2)$$

Hoeve and Flory (1958, 1962) concluded that elastin behaved essentially as an ideal rubber, i.e., $f_e = 0$, the elastic mechanism being a purely entropic one.

While the above approach appears a reasonable one in the case of a one-component diluent, the above authors and Oplatka, Michaeli and Katchalsky (1960) have pointed out that its application to a multicomponent diluents must be considered with caution on account of a possible effect due to solvent disproportion during the measurements. In fact, in the case of an elastin sample equilibrated with the 70/30 water-glycol mixture used by Hoeve and Flory (1958), we have determined (by gas chromatography analysis of the composition of the mixture outside the network) the composition of the mixture inside the gel. The latter was found to be 76/24 at 5°C and 65/35 at 48°C.

Occurance of this compositional change of the diluent should be of particular concern in the case of a protein network where strong selective interactions may drastically alter chain conformation and crystallization (Orofino, Ciferri and Hermans, 1967). In particular, the results of

Mammi, Gotte and Pezzin (1968, see page 685) indicate a noticable difference in the temperature coefficient of the α-helix for soluble elastin dissolved in water or glycol.

Because of the above complicating possibilities, the determination of $(\partial f/\partial T)_{pLeq}$ in a single-component diluent should constitute a more satisfactory approach. However, it is not generally easy to find a single-component diluent which satisfies the condition $(\partial V/\partial T)_{peq} = 0$. Recourse to when $(\partial V/\partial T)_{peq} \neq 0$. A method for correcting $(\partial f/\partial T)_{pLeq}$ into $(\partial f/\partial T)_{VLN}$ was recently proposed by Bashaw and Smith and it is based both on the molecular theory of rubber elasticity and on the Flory-Huggins theory of polymer solutions. In terms of the energy component f_e, defined in equation (1), the method of Bashaw and Smith (1968) results in the following relationship:

$$\frac{f_e}{f} = 1 - \frac{T}{f}\left(\frac{\partial f}{\partial T}\right)_{pLeq} - \frac{5}{6}\,\frac{\beta T}{(\alpha^{5/2} - 1)} \qquad (3)$$

where $\beta = \frac{1}{V}\left(\frac{\partial V}{\partial T}\right)_{peq}$, and α is the extension ratio. When $\left(\frac{\partial V}{\partial T}\right)_{peq} = 0$, the last term in equation (3) drops out and equation (3) becomes an alternative expression of equations (1) and (2).

In the course of thermoelastic experiments with elastin in several solvents, we noticed that in water the dimensions of unstressed samples decreased with increasing temperature up to about 50°C and remained constant from ∿50°C up to ∿70°C. The effect is represented in Fig. 1. Thus, this system affords an opportunity to determine f_e/f when $(\partial V/\partial T)_{peq} = 0$ (corresponding to Hoeve and Flory's method when any complications due to disproportion is avoided) and when $(\partial V/\partial T)_{peq} \neq 0$ (corresponding to Bashaw and Smith's method and based on equation 3.)

We have used elastin samples obtained from frozen ox ligamentum nuchae by cutting the samples in the direction parallel to the fiber axis of the ligament. In the case of stress-temperature measurements, the samples used were about 2 cm long and about 0.03 cm^2 in cross-sectional area.

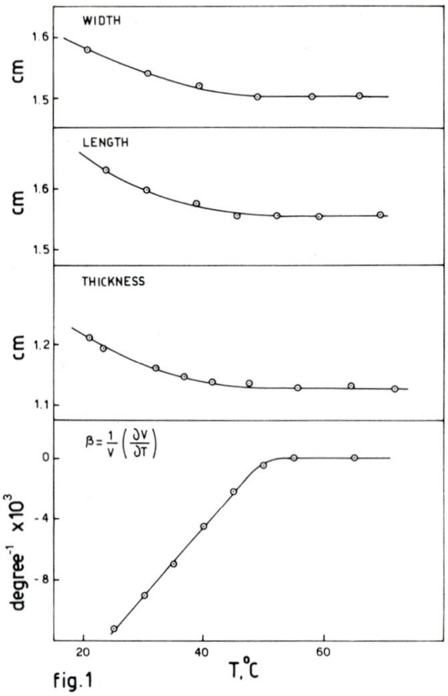

Fig. 1. Variation with temperature of the length, width, thickness and volume expansion coefficient β of an elastin sample immersed in water.

For the determination of expansion coefficients, samples having cross-sectional areas about 1 cm^2 were used. The samples were freed from collagen by autoclaving them at 120°C for 12 hrs. This is different from the material used by Hoeve and Flory (1958) which contained collagen. Samples were stored in vacuo in a refrigerator for periods never exceeding 2 months. Before use, they were placed in a large excess of water until equilibrium swelling was reached. After equilibration in water at 22°C, the length, width and thickness of a dry sample had increased by 10.6%, 11.4% and 11.4%, respectively.

Stress-temperature measurements were performed as described by Puett, Ciferri and Rajagh (1965). The relaxed sample, maintained in swelling equilibrium with water, was extended at the highest temperature used and allowed to relax again. Thereafter, the temperature was lowered and the stress recorded as soon as it appeared constant (i.e. after about 30 min). The stress measured during increasing temperature always corresponded to that seen during de-

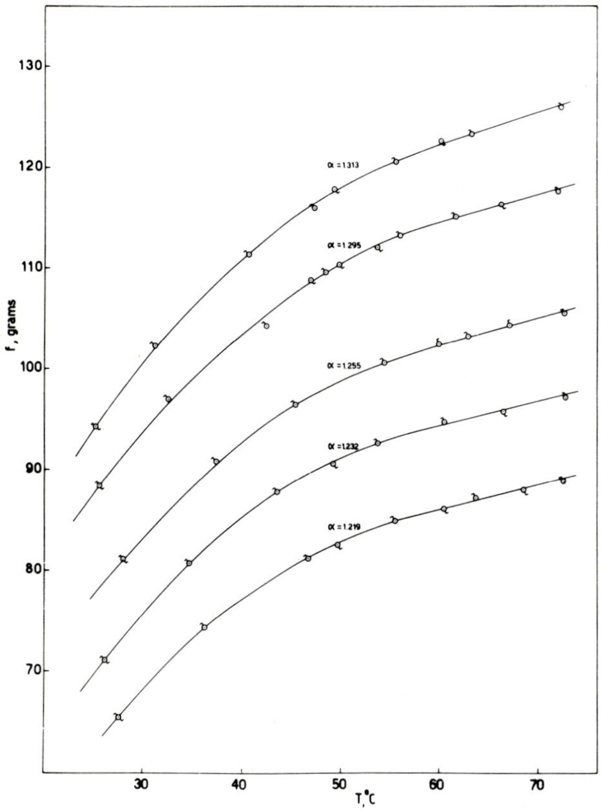

Fig. 2. Variation of the tensile force with temperature for an elastin sample in water. The elongation ratios α were measured at 50°C: ⌐o decreasing temperature; ǫ: increasing temperature.

creasing temperature. The set at the rest length was found to be negligible.

Typical stress-temperature data in water are reported in Fig. 2. The elongation ratios are based on the unstrained, swollen length measured at 50°C. The stress-temperature coefficient is strongly positive and a large curvature is exhibited, particularly at low temperatures. This is not surprising since the expansion coefficient β (cf. Fig. 1) is strongly negative at low temperatures, and this accentuates the decrease of stress with decreasing temperature due to rubber-like behaviour. The values of the stress-temperature coefficient measured between 50°C and 74°C (corresponding to the region where $\beta=0$, cf. Fig. 1) are reported in Table I together with the ratio f_e/f obtained using equation (3) for $\beta=0$. Data for different samples are included. The results indicate the occurrence of a

TABLE I

Thermoelastic data for elastin in equilibrium swelling with water in the temperature range 50°C-74°C.

$\alpha_{50°C}$	T = 62°C f,g	β = 0 $(\frac{\partial f}{\partial T})_{pLeq}$	f_e/f
Sample 1 (dry cross-section 0.0327 cm^2)			
1.219	86.8	0.233	0.10
1.232	95	0.241	0.15
1.254	103	0.255	0.17
1.295	115.2	0.282	0.18
1.313	123	0.319	0.13
Sample 2 (dry cross-section 0.02638 cm^2)			
1.222	75.1	0.200	0.11
1.255	86.4	0.227	0.12
1.288	97.4	0.253	0.13
Sample 3 (dry cross-section 0.04 cm^2)			
1.266	129.4	0.348	0.11
		Average =	$\overline{0.14}$

positive energy contribution which amounts to about 15% of the total retractive force.

The stress-temperature analysis at T<50°C is reported in Table II. Since β is not constant with termperature, f_e/f was calculated (using equation 3) at different temperatures, the β values being determined at the corresponding temperatures. The results indicate that $f_e/f=0.10$, a value consistent with that reported in Table I.

The agreement obtained by using Hoeve and Flory's method (applied to a one-component diluent) and the Bashaw and Smith equation (applied to small temperature intervals along with the corresponding value of volume expansion coefficients) is a gratifying one. In contrast to the reports of Meyer and Ferri (1936) there is no evidence of a stress-induced crystallization for elastin samples. Moreover the fundamental elastic mechanism for elastin in water is not a purely entropic one, as was suggested by Hoeve and Flory (1958). In terms of the current rubber

TABLE II

Thermoelastic data for elastin in equilibrium swelling with water in the temperature range 20-50°C.

	T = 30°C	$\beta = -9.2 \cdot 10^{-3}$		T = 40°C	$\beta = -4.6 \cdot 10^{-3}$	
$\alpha_{50°}$	f,g	$(\frac{\partial f}{\partial T})_{pLeq}$	f_e/f	f,g	$(\frac{\partial f}{\partial T})_{pLeq}$	f_e/f
Sample 1						
1.219	68.1	1.02	0.10	77.1	0.67	0.15
1.234	75.6	1.06	0.16	85.2	0.71	0.15
1.254	83.3	1.07	0.14	92.7	0.73	0.11
1.295	93.9	1.08	0.08	103.3	0.75	0.08
1.313	100.5	1.10	0.07	110.9	0.78	0.03
Sample 2						
1.222	59.6	0.88	0.10	67.6	0.59	0.11
1.255	69.7	0.91	0.10	77.3	0.61	0.10
1.288	80	0.93	0.12	89	0.65	0.08
Sample 3						
1.266	105.2	1.32	0.10	116.3	0.89	0.10
		Av.	0.10		Av.	0.10

elasticity theory (Flory, Ciferri and Hoeve, 1960), the occurrence of a non-vanishing energy component of the stress under constant volume conditions can be related to the temperature-coefficient of the unperturbed mean-square end-to-end distance of a polymer molecule, i.e.

$$\frac{f_e}{f} = T \left(\frac{d \ln \langle r^2 \rangle_o}{d T}\right)$$

Thus, the results obtained indicate a temperature coefficient of $\langle r^2 \rangle_o$ of $\sim 0.3 \times 10^{-3}$. This could be associated with the occurrence of minima favoring coiled conformations in the potentials of internal rotation of the polypeptide chain. However, the possibility of inter- and intramolecular hydrogen bonding, hydrophobic bonding and strong selective solvent interactions render the interpretation of f_e/f considerably more difficult than in the case of ordinary synthetic polymers.

REFERENCES

Bashaw, J. and Smith, K.J. (1968). J. Polymer Sci. 6, 1041

Flory, P.J., Ciferri, A. and Hoeve, C.A.J. (1960). J. Polymer Sci. 45, 235.

Hoeve, C.A.J. and Flory, P.J. (1958). J. Am. Chem. Soc. 80, 6523.

Hoeve, C.A.J. and Flory, P.J. (1962). J. Polymer Sci. 60, 155.

Mammi, M., Gotte, L. and Pezzin, G. (1968). Nature 220, 371.

Meyer, K.H. and Ferri, C. (1936). Pflüg. Arch. ges. Physiol. 238, 78.

Oplatka, A., Michaeli, I. and Katchalsky, A. (1960). J. Polymer Sci. 46, 365.

Orofino, T.A., Ciferri, A. and Hermans, J.J. (1967). Biopolymers 5, 773.

Puett, D., Ciferri, A. and Rajagh, L.V. (1965). Biopolymers 3, 461.

Wöhlisch, E., Weitnauer, H., Gruning, W. and Rohrbach, R. (1943). Kolloidzschr. 104, 14.